Fundamentals of Nursing

made Incredibly Easy!

Second Edition

Clinical Editor

Tracy A. Taylor, MSN, RN
Associate Professor, Division of Nursing
Kettering College
Kettering, Ohio

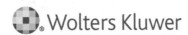

. Wolters Kluwer

Philadelphia • Baltimore • New York • London
Buenos Aires • Hong Kong • Sydney • Tokyo

Staff

Acquisitions Editor
Shannon W. Magee

Product Development Editor
Maria M. McAvey

Senior Marketing Manager
Mark Wiragh

Editorial Assistant
Zachary Shapiro

Production Project Manager
Marian Bellus

Design Coordinator
Elaine Kasmer

Manufacturing Coordinator
Kathleen Brown

Prepress Vendor
Absolute Service, Inc.

2nd edition

Copyright © 2015 Wolters Kluwer Health.

Copyright © 2007 Lippincott Williams & Wilkins.

9 8 7 6 5 4 3 2 1

Printed in China

LWW.com

Library of Congress Cataloging-in-Publication Data

Fundamentals of nursing made incredibly easy! / clinical editor, Tracy A. Taylor. — 2nd edition.
    p. ; cm.
Includes bibliographical references.
ISBN 978-1-4511-9424-1
I. Taylor, Tracy A., editor.
[DNLM: 1. Nursing Care—United States. WY 100 AA1] RT41
610.73—dc23

                                    2014038944

RRS1409

Contributors

Angel Boling, MSN, RN
Assistant Professor
Baptist College of Health Sciences
Memphis, Tennessee

Mary Ann Edelman, MS, RN
Professor
Kingsborough Community College
Brooklyn, New York

Rosemary Macy, PhD, RN, CNE
Associate Professor
Boise State University
Boise, Idaho

Beverly McLean, MSN, RN
Assistant Professor
Kettering College
Kettering, Ohio

Donna Moore, MSN, RN, COI
Associate Professor/Skills Lab Coordinator
Kettering College
Kettering, Ohio

Rhonda Sansone, MSN, RN, CRNP
Assistant Professor of Nursing
Wheeling Jesuit University
Wheeling, West Virginia

Patricia A. Slachta, PhD, RN, APRN, ACNS-BC, CWOCN
The Queen's Medical Center
Honolulu, Hawaii

Previous edition contributors

Elizabeth A. Archer, RN, EdD

Rita Bates, RN, MSN

Mary Ann Edelman, RN, MS, CNS

Erica Fooshee, RN, MSN

Sally Gaines, RN, MSN

Rebecca Crews Gruener, RN, MS

Mari S. Hunter, RN, APN-C, MSN

Rosemary Macy, RN, PhD(c)

Susan O'Dell, RN, APRN-BC, MSN, FNP

Rhonda M. Sansone, RN, MSN, CRNP

Sandra Waguespack, RN, MSN

Preface

I have taught many areas of nursing in my years of educating students and enjoy the excitement of new students as they begin their journey to the study of nursing. My favorite part of teaching fundamentals is watching the mastery of basic skills and the urge to learn more and grow as a student. I admire students' curiosity and tenacity as they try to master the content of this respected profession. As an educator, it's important to explain the content in an interesting and easy-to-understand manner, especially when discussing the foundation of nursing. As such, *Fundamentals of Nursing Made Incredibly Easy*, second edition is a quick resource for the nursing student *and* the instructor. In addition, practicing nurses can review the foundation of nursing and skills.

The content is logically organized into three sections. The first, "Foundational concepts," provides an overview of nursing and information on health care, ethical and legal considerations, and the nursing process. The second section, "General nursing skills," covers communication, health assessment, vital signs, infection, and key medication information. Finally, "Physiologic needs" contains information on oxygenation, patient self-care, mobility, skin integrity, pain management, nutrition, and urinary and bowel elimination.

Each chapter in *Fundamentals of Nursing Made Incredibly Easy* starts with a brief outline of the content of the chapter, allowing readers to quickly determine where they should focus. Practice National Council Licensure Examination (NCLEX) questions at the end of each chapter serve to challenge readers on how much information they absorbed. *Memory joggers* offer simple tricks to help readers remember key information. Fun illustrations and cartoons make learning fun—the surest way to keep readers interested!

In addition, icons draw your attention to important issues:

Teacher's lounge—provides patient-teaching tips on such topics as procedures, equipment, and home care

Ages and stages—identifies areas and procedures in which age could impact the nurse's care

Stay on the ball—focuses on critical areas involving possible dangers, risks, complications, contraindications, or ways to ensure safety

Take note!—offers tips on documentation.

Important topics added to this new edition include:

- Healthy People 2020
- Nutrition has been updated to include MyPlate.gov
- Includes social media relating to the profession of nursing
- Wound care current practice
- Medication and bar code scanning

Fundamentals of Nursing Made Incredibly Easy is a helpful addition to the *Incredibly Easy* series, serving as an invaluable guide for nursing students as they prepare for their nursing career and as a handy reference for newly graduated and experienced nurses.

Tracy A. Taylor, MSN, RN
Associate Professor, Division of Nursing
Kettering College
Kettering, Ohio

Contents

Part I   Foundational concepts

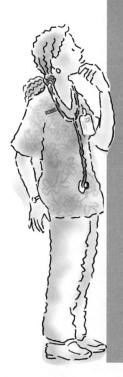

1

Overview of nursing

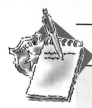

Just the facts

In this chapter, you'll learn:

♦ the historical roots of nursing and its emergence as a profession

♦ practice guidelines and the educational background required for nursing

♦ functions and roles of nurses in various care settings

♦ the guiding principles behind nursing theories and patient care.

Historical evolution of nursing

As we progress through the 21st century, the role of the nurse continues to expand. The increasing reliance on technology in nursing education and practice, the pressures of health care reform, and the continuing crisis of noninsured or underinsured persons have combined to make nursing practice more complex than ever.

The nursing profession has developed a reputation for successfully delivering high-quality, cost-effective care. In fact, a survey of public attitudes toward health care and nurses conducted in the United States revealed that the public admires nurses and that most people are willing to have an increasing portion of their care delivered by registered nurses.

The birth of nursing

Nursing's origins lie in religious and military traditions that demanded unquestioning obedience to authority. Florence Nightingale challenged these traditions by emphasizing

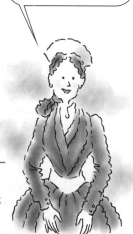

Florence Nightingale challenged traditional views of nursing by emphasizing critical thinking, patients' needs, and respect. Way to go, Flo!

critical thinking, attention to patients' individual needs, and respect for patients' rights.

Go with Flo

Nightingale proposed that schools of nursing be independent of hospitals and that they provide nursing education but not patient care. She demanded that her schools accept only qualified candidates and that the students learn to teach as well as provide care.

Money, money, money

The first schools of nursing based on Nightingale's model opened in the United States in 1873 and in Canada in 1874. Her ideas were soon discarded, however, when nursing schools realized that they couldn't survive without the hospitals' financial support. At the same time, hospitals recognized that nursing students were a major source of cheap, disciplined labor. They began to hire student nurses instead of more experienced—and more expensive—graduate nurses.

A specialist emerges

This situation changed after World War II, when major scientific discoveries and technological advancements altered the nature of hospital care. Increasingly, the care of hospitalized patients required experienced, skilled nurses. The development of intensive and coronary care units gave rise to the concept of the advanced clinician: a nurse qualified to give specialized care and the forerunner of today's clinical nurse specialist.

Advanced knowledge and skills

After the war, nursing responded to greater public interest in health promotion and disease prevention by creating another new role: the nurse practitioner. Using advanced knowledge and skills, the nurse practitioner helps promote health and helps prevent illness while caring for the minor health concerns of patients.

Question, analyze, and argue

Another crucial change in nursing stemmed from a midcentury shift in attitudes about education for women. The practice of extending full educational opportunities to women has significantly altered the role that nurses play in today's health care system. Armed with a strong educational base, nurses have the confidence necessary to question, analyze, and argue for family-centered health care—and to secure a major role for nursing in delivering that care.

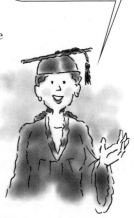

A strong educational base gives me the confidence to question, analyze, argue for, and deliver quality patient care.

Nursing as a profession

Florence Nightingale believed that a nurse's goal should be "to put the patient in the best condition for nature to act upon him." Definitions of nursing have changed over time, but nursing has retained a common focus: providing humanistic and holistic care to each patient.

Focus, focus

The American Nurses Association's (ANA) definition of nursing shares this focus: "The practice of nursing by a registered nurse is defined as the process of diagnosing human responses to actual or potential health problems; providing supportive and restorative care, health counseling and teaching, case finding and referral; collaborating the implementation of the total health care regimen; and executing the medical regimen under the direction of a licensed physician or dentist."

Not just a job

Most people use the term "nursing professionals" to describe a group of people who practice nursing. However, not everyone agrees that nursing has the full autonomy that it needs to distinguish itself as a profession rather than an occupation.

We've got the power

Nursing already has achieved some degree of autonomy. It exercises control over its education and practice. It has achieved legal recognition through licensure. Every state and Canadian province now has a nurse practice act, which requires nurses to pass state board examinations in order to practice and regulates the scope of their practice. Nursing also has a code of ethics, which is regularly updated to reflect current ethical issues.

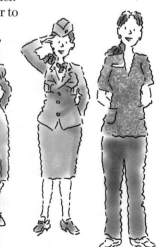

The face of nursing continues to change with the times, growing more autonomous and more professional.

Independence is key

The key to professional nursing autonomy, however, is to function independently of any other profession or external force. For many nurses, this remains a goal to be achieved. As employees of large, sometimes inflexible organizations, nurses seldom enjoy full latitude in deciding on patient care within the defined scope of nursing practice. However, by striving for individual excellence, each nurse can help this emerging profession become a full-fledged profession.

Educational preparation

The ANA has identified two categories of nursing practice—professional and associate—and established educational requirements for each. According to the ANA's guidelines, the minimum requirement for beginning professional nurses is a baccalaureate degree in nursing (BSN), whereas the minimum requirement for beginning associate nurses is an associate's degree in nursing (ADN).

Options abound

Besides pursuing a BSN at a 4-year college or university or an ADN at a junior or community college, today's undergraduate student nurses have a third option: hospital-operated diploma programs. However, regardless of which option she chooses, a graduate of any of these three programs is eligible to sit for the same registered nurse (RN) licensing examination.

Graduate level

After the nurse receives her baccalaureate degree, she may choose to advance her education at the graduate level. She can choose from a number of graduate fields, including nursing. She can choose a Master of Arts (MA) in nursing, Master in Nursing (MN), or Master of Science in Nursing (MSN). A master's degree qualifies a nurse to serve as a nurse educator, clinical nurse specialist, nursing administrator, or nurse practitioner.

Is there a doctor in the house?

Doctoral education in nursing is expanding. Most doctoral programs in nursing lead to a Doctor of Philosophy (PhD) degree or a doctorate in nursing practice (DNP).

A nurse with a doctorate might assume a leadership position in a practice setting or as an educator of beginning nurses and those seeking advanced clinical and educational preparation, including research in nursing.

Practice guidelines

The way you practice your profession of nursing should be guided by two sets of care documents: standards of nursing care and nurse practice acts. The standards of nursing care are administered by the ANA, and the nurse practice acts are administered by individual states or provinces.

Standards of nursing care

Standards of care set minimum criteria for your proficiency on the job, enabling you and others to judge the quality of care you and your nursing colleagues provide. They help to ensure high-quality care and, in the legal arena, they serve as criteria to help determine whether adequate care was provided to a patient. States may refer to standards in their nurse practice acts. Unless included in a nurse practice act, professional standards aren't laws; they're guidelines for sound nursing practice.

Pie in the sky?

Some nurses regard standards of nursing care as pie-in-the-sky ideals that have little bearing on the reality of working life. This opinion is a dangerous misconception. You're expected to meet standards of nursing care for every nursing task you perform.

The ANA standards include two lists:
• standards of professional performance, which include guidelines for quality of care, performance appraisal, education, collegiality, ethics, collaboration, research, resource utilization, and leadership
• standards of practice, which outline professional responsibilities in assessment, diagnosis, outcome identification, planning, implementation, and evaluation. (See *ANA standards of nursing practice*, pages 8 to 12.)

> No part of standards of nursing care is pie in the sky. Professional standards help us all deliver the best care. Care for a slice?

Nurse practice acts

The nurse practice act of each state defines the practice of nursing for that state. Nurse practice acts are broadly worded, and the wording varies from state to state. Understanding your nurse practice act's general provisions will help you stay within the legal limits of nursing practice. With the emergence of more autonomous and expanded roles for nurses, many states have started to revise their nurse practice acts to reflect the greater responsibilities associated with current nursing practice.

Not an easy task

Interpreting your nurse practice act isn't always easy. One problem stems from the fact that nurse practice acts are statutory laws. So, any amendment to a nurse practice act must be accomplished by means of the inevitably slow legislative process. Because of the time involved in pondering, drafting, and enacting laws, amendments to the nurse practice acts lag well behind the changes in nursing.

(Text continues on page 12.)

ANA standards of nursing practice

The standards below are adapted from standards of nursing practice published by the American Nurses Association (ANA). The ANA developed the standards (last revised in 2010) to provide registered nurses with guidelines for determining quality nursing care. The courts as well as hospitals, nurses, and patients may refer to these standards. The standards of nursing practice are divided into the *standards of practice*, which define care provided to patients, and the *standards of professional performance*, which explain the level of behavior expected of the nurse in a professional role.

Each standard below is followed by measurement criteria that give key indicators of competent practice for that standard. This adaptation of the standards doesn't present the standards that are specific only to advanced practice nurses.

STANDARDS OF PRACTICE

Standard 1: Assessment
The nurse collects patient health data.
Measurement criteria
1. Data collection is systematic and ongoing.
2. Data collection involves the patient, partners, and health care providers when appropriate.
3. Priority of data collection activities is determined by the patient's immediate condition or needs.
4. Pertinent data are collected using appropriate evidence-based assessment techniques and instruments.
5. Analytical models and problem solving tools are used.
6. Patterns and variances are identified by synthesizing relevant data and knowledge.
7. Relevant data are documented in a retrievable form.

Standard 2: Diagnosis
The nurse analyzes the assessment data in determining the diagnosis.
Measurement criteria
1. Diagnoses are derived from the assessment data.
2. Diagnoses are validated with the patient, partners, and health care providers when possible.
3. Diagnoses are documented in a manner that facilitates the determination of the expected outcomes and care plan.

Standard 3: Outcomes identification
The nurse identifies expected outcomes individualized to the patient.
Measurement criteria
1. Identification of outcomes involves the patient, family, and health care providers when possible and appropriate.
2. Outcomes are culturally appropriate and are derived from the diagnoses.
3. Outcomes are formulated taking into account any associated risks, benefits, costs, current scientific evidence, and clinical expertise.
4. Outcomes are defined in terms of the patient, the patient's values, ethical considerations, environment, or situation along with any associated risks, benefits, costs, and current scientific evidence.
5. Outcomes include a time estimate for attainment.
6. Outcomes provide direction for continuity of care.
7. Outcomes are modified based on the patient's status.
8. Outcomes are documented as measurable goals.

Standard 4: Planning
The nurse develops a care plan that prescribes interventions to attain expected outcomes.
Measurement criteria
1. The plan is individualized to the patient's condition or needs.
2. The plan is developed with the patient, partners, and health care providers.
3. The plan includes strategies that address each of the diagnoses.
4. The plan provides for continuity of care.
5. The plan includes a pathway or timeline.
6. Priorities for care are established with the patient, family, and others when appropriate.
7. The plan provides directions to other health care providers.
8. The plan reflects current statutes, rules and regulations, and standards.
9. The plan integrates current trends and research.
10. The economic impact of the plan is considered.
11. The plan is documented using standardized language and terminology.

ANA standards of nursing practice *(continued)*

Standard 5: Implementation
The nurse implements the plan.
Measurement criteria
 1. Interventions are implemented in a safe and timely manner.
 2. Interventions and any modifications to the plan are documented.
 3. Interventions are evidence-based and specific to the diagnosis.
 4. Interventions include community resources and systems.
 5. Implementation includes collaboration with other health care providers.

Standard 5a: Coordination of care
The nurse coordinates care delivery.
Measurement criteria
 1. The nurse coordinates implementation of the plan.
 2. The nurse manages consumer care to maximize independence and quality of care.
 3. The nurse assists with identification of options with alternative care.
 4. The nurse communicates with the consumer, family, and health care system during transitions of care.
 5. The nurse advocates for dignified and humane care by the interprofessional team.
 6. The coordination of care is document.

Standard 5b: Health teaching and health promotion
The nurse promotes health and a safe environment.
Measurement criteria
 1. Health teaching includes healthy lifestyles, risk-reducing behaviors, developmental needs, activities of daily living, and preventive self-care.

 2. Health promotion and teaching are appropriate to the patient's needs.
 3. Feedback is received on the effectiveness of health promotion and teachings.
 4. Information technology is used to communicate health promotion and disease prevention information.
 5. Information is provided to consumers concerning intended effects, as well as potential adverse effects of proposed therapies.

Standard 6: Evaluation
The nurse evaluates the patient's progress toward attaining outcomes.
Measurement criteria
 1. Evaluation is systematic, ongoing, and criteria-based.
 2. The patient, partners, and health care providers are involved in the evaluation process.
 3. The effectiveness of the plan is evaluated in relation to the patient's responses and outcomes.
 4. The results of the evaluation are documented.
 5. Ongoing assessment data are used to revise diagnoses, outcomes, and the care plan as needed.
 6. Results of the evaluation are disseminated to the patient and other health care providers involved with the patient's care in accordance with all laws and regulations.

STANDARDS OF PROFESSIONAL PERFORMANCE
Standard 7: Ethics
The nurse integrates ethics in all areas of practice.

Measurement criteria
 1. The nurse's practice is guided by the *Code for Ethics for Nurses with Interpretive Statements* (ANA, 2001).
 2. The nurse preserves and protects patient autonomy, dignity, and rights.
 3. The nurse maintains patient confidentiality.
 4. The nurse acts as a patient advocate and assists patients in developing skills so they can advocate for themselves.
 5. The nurse maintains a therapeutic and professional patient-nurse relationship within professional role boundaries.
 6. The nurse is committed to practicing self-care, managing stress, and connecting with self and others.
 7. The nurse helps resolve ethical issues, including participating in ethics committees.
 8. The nurse reports illegal, incompetent, or impaired practices.

Standard 8: Education
The nurse acquires current knowledge and competency in nursing practice.
Measurement criteria
 1. The nurse participates in ongoing educational activities related to knowledge bases and professional issues.
 2. The nurse is committed to lifelong learning through self-reflection and inquiry to identify learning needs.
 3. The nurse seeks experiences that reflect current practice to maintain current clinical practice and competency.
(continued)

ANA standards of nursing practice *(continued)*

4. The nurse seeks knowledge and skills appropriate to the practice setting.

5. The nurse seeks experiences and formal and independent learning activities to maintain and develop clinical and professional skills and knowledge.

6. The nurse identifies learning needs based on nursing knowledge, roles assumed, and changing needs of the population.

7. The nurse participates in formal/informal consultation to address issues in nursing practice.

8. The nurse shares educational findings, experiences, and ideas with peers.

9. The nurse contributes to the work environment conducive to the education health care professionals.

10. The nurse maintains professional records that evidence competency and lifelong learning.

Standard 9: Evidence-Based Practice and Research

The nurse uses research findings in practice.

Measurement criteria

1. The nurse uses the best available evidence, including research findings, to guide practice decisions.

2. The nurse participates in research activities as appropriate to her position and education. Such activities may include:
- identifying clinical problems suitable for nursing research
- participating in data collection
- participating in a formal committee or program

- sharing research findings with others
- conducting research
- critiquing research for application to practice
- using research findings in the development of policies, procedures, and standards for patient care
- incorporating research as a basis for learning.

Standard 10: Quality of practice

The nurse systematically enhances the quality and effectiveness of nursing practice.

Measurement criteria

1. Quality is demonstrated by documenting the application of nursing process in a responsible, accountable, and ethical manner.

2. The nurse uses the results of quality-of-care activities to initiate changes in nursing practice and throughout the health care delivery system.

3. The nurse uses creativity and innovation to improve care delivery.

4. The nurse participates in quality improvement activities. Such activities may include:
- identifying aspects of care important for quality monitoring
- identifying indicators used to monitor quality and effectiveness of nursing care
- collecting data to monitor quality and effectiveness of nursing care
- analyzing quality data to identify opportunities for improving care
- formulating recommendations to improve nursing practice or patient outcomes

- implementing activities to enhance the quality of nursing practice
- developing policies, procedures, and practice guidelines to improve quality of care
- participating on interdisciplinary teams that evaluate clinical practice or health services
- participating in efforts to minimize cost and unnecessary duplication
- analyzing factors related to safety, satisfaction, effectiveness, and cost-benefit options
- analyzing organizational barriers
- implementing processes to remove or decrease organizational barriers
- incorporating new knowledge to initiate change in nursing practice if outcomes aren't achieved.

Standard 11: Communication

The nurse communicates effectively in all areas of practice.

Measurement criteria

1. The nurse assesses communication preferences of health care consumers, families, and colleagues.

2. The nurse assesses his/her own communication skills with health care consumers, families, and colleagues.

3. The nurse seeks continuous improvement of communication and conflict resolution skills.

4. The nurse conveys information to health care consumers, families, the interprofessional team, and others to promote effective communication.

5. The nurse questions rationales and decisions of patient care processes and decisions, discloses

ANA standards of nursing practice (continued)

observations or concerns related to hazards or errors in care, maintains communication with other providers to optimize safe patient care.

6. The nurse contributes his/her professional perspective with discussions with the interprofessional team.

Standard 12: Leadership
The nurse shows leadership in the practice setting and in the profession.
Measurement criteria

1. The nurse is a team player and a team builder.

2. The nurse creates and maintains healthy work environments.

3. The nurse is able to define clear visions, associated goals, and plans to implement and measure progress.

4. The nurse is committed to continual, lifelong learning for self and others.

5. The nurse teaches others to succeed by mentoring and other strategies.

6. The nurse is creative and flexible through changing times.

7. The nurse exhibits energy, excitement, and passion for quality work.

8. The nurse takes accountability of self and others.

9. The nurse inspires loyalty through valuing people as the most precious asset in an organization.

10. The nurse directs the coordination of care across settings and among caregivers, including licensed and unlicensed personnel.

11. The nurse serves on committees, councils, and administrative teams.

12. The nurse promotes the advancement of the profession by participating in professional organizations.

Standard 13: Collaboration
The nurse collaborates with the patient, family, and others in providing patient care.
Measurement criteria

1. The nurse communicates with the patient, family, and health care providers regarding patient care and the nurse's role in providing that care.

2. The nurse involves the patient, family, and others in creating a documented plan focused on outcomes and decisions related to care and the delivery of services.

3. The nurse collaborates with others to effect change and get positive outcomes for patient care.

4. The nurse makes and documents referrals, including provisions for continuity of care.

5. The nurse documents plans, communications or collaborative discussions, and rationales for plan changes.

Standard 14: Professional practice evaluation
The nurse evaluates her own nursing practice in relation to professional practice standards and relevant statutes and regulations.
Measurement criteria

1. The nurse provides culturally and ethnically sensitive and age-appropriate care.

2. The nurse engages in self-evaluation of practice on a regular basis, identifying areas of strength

as well as areas where professional development would be beneficial.

3. The nurse seeks constructive feedback regarding his or her own practice.

4. The nurse participates in systematic peer review as appropriate.

5. The nurse takes action to achieve goals identified during the evaluation process.

6. The nurse provides rationales for practice beliefs, decisions, and actions as part of the evaluation process.

7. The nurse interacts with peers and colleagues to enhance his/her professional nursing practice or role performance.

8. The nurse provides peers with formal/informal constructive feedback regarding roles and practice.

Standard 15: Resource utilization
The nurse considers factors related to safety, effectiveness, cost, and impact in planning and delivering patient care.
Measurement criteria

1. The nurse evaluates factors related to safety, effectiveness, availability, cost and benefits, efficiencies, and impact when choosing practice options that would result in the same expected patient outcome.

2. The nurse assists the patient and family in securing appropriate health-related services.

3. The nurse delegates tasks as appropriate.

4. The nurse assists the patient and family in becoming informed consumers about health care treatment.

(continued)

ANA standards of nursing practice *(continued)*

Standard 16: Environmental Health
The nurse practices in an environmentally safe and healthy manner.
Measurement criteria
1. The nurse maintains knowledge of environmental health concepts.
2. The nurse assesses and promotes a practice environment that reduces associated health risks.

3. The nurse uses scientific evidence to determine safety of products, communicates potential environmental hazards, and advocates for appropriate use of products in health care.
4. The nurse participates in strategies to promote healthy communities.

Reprinted with permission from American Nurses Association. (2010). *Nursing: Scope and standards of practice* (2nd ed.). Silver Spring, MD: Nursesbook.org.

> It's not enough to know just your state nurse practice act ... today's nurses need to keep up-to-date with policies, procedures, and nursing trends.

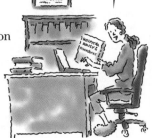

A nursing dilemma

You may be asked to perform tasks that seem to be within the accepted scope of nursing but in fact violate your state's nurse practice act. Your state's nurse practice act isn't a word-for-word checklist on how you should do your work. You must rely on your own education and knowledge of your facility's policies and procedures.

Limits of practice

Make sure you're familiar with the legally permissible scope of your nurse practice act, as defined in your state's nurse practice act and board of nursing rules and regulations. Otherwise, you're inviting legal trouble.

It's all in the certification

This list includes some of the nursing specialty certifications and their appropriate credentials.

Addictions nursing
Certified Addictions Registered Nurse (CARN)

Advanced practice nursing
Acute Care Nurse Practitioner (APRN, BC)
Adult Nurse Practitioner (ANP)
Family Nurse Practitioner (FNP)
Gerontological Nurse Practitioner (GNP)
Pediatric Nurse Practitioner (PNP)

Psychiatric and Mental Health Nurse Practitioner (PMHNP)

Childbirth educators
Lamaze Certified Childbirth Educator (LCCE)

Critical care nursing
Adult Critical-Care Registered Nurse (CCRN)
Cardiac Medicine Certification (CCRN-CMC)

Cardiac Surgery Certification (CCRN-CMS)
Clinical Nurse Specialist in Acute and Critical Care; Adult, Neonatal, or Pediatric (CCNS)
Neonatal Critical-Care Registered Nurse (CCRN)
Pediatric Critical-Care Registered Nurse (CCRN)
Progressive Care Certified Nurse (PCCN)

It's all in the certification *(continued)*

Diabetes educators
Certified Diabetic Educator (CDE)

Emergency nursing
Certified Emergency Nurse (CEN)

Flight nursing
Certified Flight Registered Nurse
(CFRN)

Gastroenterology nursing
Certified Gastroenterological Registered Nurse (CGRN)

Genetic nursing
Advanced Practice Nurse in Genetics
(APNG)
Genetics Clinical Nurse (GCN)

Health care quality nursing
Certified Professional in Healthcare
Quality (CPHQ)

HIV-AIDS nursing
AIDS Certified Registered Nurse
(ACRN)

Holistic nursing
Holistic Nursing Certification (HNC)

Hospice and palliative nursing
Certified Hospice and Palliative Nurse
(CHPN)

Infection control nursing
Certified in Infection Control (CIC)

Infusion nursing
Certified Registered Nurse of Infusion
(CRNI)

Lactation consultant
International Board Certified Lactation Consultant (IBCLC)

Legal nurse consulting
Legal Nurse Consulting Certification
(LNCC)

Managed care nursing
Certified Managed Care Nurse
(CMCN)

Maternal-neonatal nursing
Inpatient Obstetric Nurse (RNC, INPT)
Low Risk Neonatal Nurse (RNC, LRN)
Maternal Newborn Nurse (RNC, MN)
Neonatal Intensive Care Nurse (RNC,
NIC)

Medical-surgical nursing
Certified Medical Surgical Registered
Nurse (CMSRN)

Nephrology nursing
Certified Nephrology Nurse (CNN)

Neuroscience nursing
Certified Neuroscience Registered
Nurse (CNRN)

Nurse administration: Long-term care
Certified Director of Nursing,
Administration in Long-Term Care
(CDONA/LTC)

Nurse anesthetist
Certified Registered Nurse Anesthetist (CRNA)

Nurse midwifery and midwifery
Certified Nurse Midwife (CNM)

Nutrition support nursing
Certified Nutrition Support Nurse
(CNSN)

Occupational health nursing
Certified Occupational Health Nurse
(COHN)
Certified Occupational Health Nurse/
Case Manager (COHN/CM)

Oncology nursing
Certified Oncology Nurse (OCN)

Ophthalmic nursing
Certified Registered Nurse Ophthal-
mology (CRNO)

Orthopedic nursing
Orthopedic Nurse Certified (ONC)

Pediatric nursing
Certified Pediatric Nurse (CPN)
Certified Pediatric Nurse Practitioner
(CPNP)

Pediatric oncology nursing
Certified Pediatric Oncology Nurse
(CPON)

Perianesthesia nursing
Certified Post Anesthesia Nurse
(CPAN)
Certified Ambulatory Perianesthesia
Nurse (CAPA)

Perioperative nursing
Certified Nurse Operating Room
(CNOR)
RN, First assistant (CRNFA)

Rehabilitation nursing
Certified Rehabilitation Registered
Nurse (CRRN, CRRN-A)

School nursing
National Certified School Nurse
(NCSN)

Urology nursing
Certified Urologic Registered Nurse
(CURN)
Certified Urologic Nurse Practitioner
(CUNP)

Licensure and certification

All nurses must be licensed in the state in which they practice. The National Council Licensure Examination (NCLEX) must be taken and passed by all RN candidates. The test is exactly the same in all states.

The practicing nurse may choose to be certified in a specialty area in which she works. Each certification has minimum requirements, such as education and current work experience. After the nurse has met these requirements and passed an examination, she maintains the certification by continuing education and clinical or administrative practice. (See *It's all in the certification*, pages 12 and 13.)

Professional organizations

Professional organizations are an important part of your nursing profession. They provide current information and resource material and allow you a voice in your profession. (See *Individual state nurses associations*.)

Nursing organizations include the ANA, the National League for Nursing, the International Council of Nurses, and the National Student Nurses Association. Nurse specialty groups include the Association of Critical Care Nurses, Sigma Theta Tau, the American Association of Nurse Anesthetists, and the Academy of Medical Surgical Nursing, to name just a few.

Individual state nurses associations

Contacting your state nurses association is only a click away. Can you find the Web site for your state's association in this list?

Alabama State Nurses' Association (ASNA)
www.alabamanurses.org

Alaska Nurses Association (AaNA)
www.aknurse.org

Arizona Nurses Association (AzNA)
www.aznurse.org

Arkansas Nurses Association (ArNA)
www.arna.org

ANA/California (ANA/C)
www.anacalifornia.org

Colorado Nurses Association (CNA)
www.nurses-co.org

Connecticut Nurses Association (CNA)
www.ctnurses.org

Delaware Nurses Association (DNA)
www.denurses.org

District of Columbia Nurses Association (DCNA)
www.dcna.org

Florida Nurses Association (FNA)
www.floridanurse.org

Georgia Nurses Association (GNA)
www.georgianurses.org

Hawaii Nurses Association (HNA)
www.hawaiinurses.org

Individual state nurses associations (continued)

Idaho Nurses Association (INA)
www.nursingworld.org/snas/id

Illinois Nurses Association (INA)
www.illinoisnurses.com

Indiana State Nurses Association
(ISNA)
www.indiananurses.org

Iowa Nurses Association (INA)
www.iowanurses.org

Kansas State Nurses Association
(KSNA)
www.nursingworld.org/snas/ks

Kentucky Nurses Association (KNA)
www.kentucky-nurses.org

Louisiana State Nurses Association
(LSNA)
www.lsna.org

ANA-Maine (ANA-ME)
www.anamaine.org

Maryland Nurses Association (MNA)
www.marylandrn.org

Massachusetts Association of
Registered Nurses (MARN)
www.marnonline.org

Michigan Nurses Association (MNA)
www.minurses.org

Minnesota Nurses Association
(MNA)
www.mnnurses.org

Mississippi Nurses Association
(MNA)
www.msnurses.org

Missouri Nurses Association (MONA)
www.missourinurses.org

Montana Nurses Association (MNA)
www.mtnurses.org

Nebraska Nurses Association (NNA)
www.nursingworld.org/snas/ne/

Nevada Nurses Association (NNA)
www.nvnurses.org

New Hampshire Nurses Association
(NHNA)
www.nhnurses.org

New Jersey State Nurses Association (NJSNA)
www.njsna.org

New Mexico Nurses Association
(NMNA)
www.nmna.org

New York State Nurses Association
(NYSNA)
www.nysna.org

North Carolina Nurses Association
(NCNA)
www.ncnurses.org

North Dakota Nurses Association
(NDNA)
www.ndna.org

Ohio Nurses Association (ONA)
www.ohnurses.org

Oklahoma Nurses Association (ONA)
www.oknurses.com

Oregon Nurses Association (ONA)
www.oregonrn.org

Pennsylvania State Nurses Association (PSNA)
www.panurses.org

Rhode Island State Nurses Association (RISNA)
www.risnarn.org

South Carolina Nurses Association
(SCNA)
www.scnurses.org

South Dakota Nurses Association
(SDNA)
www.nursingworld.org/snas/sd/

Tennessee Nurses Association (TNA)
www.tnaonline.org

Texas Nurses Association (TNA)
www.texasnurses.org

Utah Nurses Association (UNA)
www.utahnurses.org

Vermont State Nurses Association,
Inc. (VSNA)
www.vsna-inc.org/

Virginia Nurses Association (VNA)
www.virginianurses.com

Washington State Nurses Association (WSNA)
www.wsna.org

West Virginia Nurses Association
(WVNA)
www.wvnurses.org

Wisconsin Nurses Association
(WNA)
www.wisconsinnurses.org

Wyoming Nurses Association (WNA)
www.wyonurse.org

In addition, each state has its own nursing association that's a division of the ANA.

Functions of nurses

Recent changes in health care reflect changes in the population that require nursing care and a philosophical shift toward health promotion rather than treatment of illness. The role of the nurse has broadened in response to these changes. Nurses are caregivers, as always, but now they're also educators, advocates, leaders and managers, charge agents, and researchers.

> Today's nurse is a model of independence and an inspiration to caring people everywhere!

Caregiver

Nurses have always been caregivers, but the activities this role encompasses changed dramatically in the 20th century. Increased education of nurses expanded nursing research, and the consequent recognition that nurses are autonomous and informed professionals have caused a shift from a dependent role for the nurse to one of independence and collaboration.

A model of independence

Unlike earlier models, medical-surgical nurses now conduct independent assessments and implement patient care based on their knowledge and skills. They also collaborate with other members of the health care team to implement and evaluate that care.

Educator

With greater emphasis on health promotion and illness prevention, the nurse's role as educator has become increasingly important. The nurse assesses learning needs, plans and implements teaching strategies to meet those needs, and evaluates the effectiveness of the teaching. To be an effective educator, the nurse must have effective interpersonal skills and be familiar with principles of adult learning.

Before you go

Patient teaching is also a major part of discharge planning. Along with teaching come responsibilities for making referrals, identifying community and personal resources, and arranging for necessary equipment and supplies for home care.

Advocate

As an advocate, the nurse helps the patient and his family members interpret information from other health care providers and make decisions about his health-related needs. The nurse must accept and respect a patient's decision, even if it differs from the decision the nurse would make.

Coordinator

All nurses practice leadership and manage time, people, resources, and the environment in which they provide care. They carry out these tasks by directing, delegating, and coordinating activities.

Call a huddle

All health care team members, including the nurse, provide patient care. Although the doctor is usually considered the head of the team, the nurse plays an important role in coordinating the efforts of all team members to meet the patient's goals and may conduct team conferences to facilitate communication among team members.

> Sometimes it's necessary to huddle up, especially when the game plan—the patient's care plan—needs adjusting.

Change agent

As a change agent, the nurse works with the patient to address his health concerns and with staff members to address organizational and community concerns. This role demands knowledge of change theory, which provides a framework for understanding the dynamics of change, human responses to change, and strategies for effecting change.

Doing what's right

In the community, nurses serve as role models and assist people in bringing about changes to improve the environment, work conditions, or other factors that affect health. Nurses also work together to bring about change through legislation by helping to shape and support the laws that mandate the use of car safety seats and motorcycle helmets.

Discharge planner

As a discharge planner, the nurse assesses the patient's needs at discharge, including the patient's support systems and living situation. The nurse also links the patient with available community resources.

Researcher

The primary tasks of nursing research are to promote growth in the science of nursing and to develop a scientific basis for nursing practice. Every nurse should be involved in nursing research and apply research findings to her nursing practice.

> Every nurse should be involved in nursing research and apply research findings to her nursing practice.

Identify and incorporate

Although not all nurses are trained in research methods, each nurse can participate by remaining alert for nursing problems and asking questions about care practices. Many nurses who give direct care identify such problems, which then serve as a basis for research. Nurses can improve nursing care by incorporating research findings into their practice and communicating the research to others.

Roles of nurses

In today's nursing profession, nurses have a broad area of opportunity. They may be staff nurses, nurse educators, nurse managers, case managers, clinical nurse specialists, nurse practitioners, and nurse researchers.

Staff nurse

The staff nurse functions as a primary caregiver by independently making assessments, planning and implementing patient care, and providing direct nursing care. For example, a staff nurse may make clinical observations and execute interventions, such as administering medications and treatments and promoting such activities of daily living as bathing and toileting.

Nurse educator

As the emphasis on health promotion and illness prevention has increased, the nurse's role as educator has become increasingly important. The nurse educator's students include patients and family members as well as other health professionals.

Many hats, one nurse

The nurse assesses patients' and family members' learning needs, plans and implements teaching strategies to meet those needs, and evaluates the effectiveness of the teaching.

    To be an effective educator, the nurse must have excellent interpersonal skills and be familiar with the appropriate developmental stages of children, adolescents, and adults as well as the principles of learning for each age-group.

Nurse manager

The nurse manager acts as a staff nurse and an administrative representative of the unit, ensuring that effective and quality nursing care is being provided in a timely and fiscally managed environment.

Being a case manager means coordinating every aspect of my patient's care and staying on top of all the details—from start to finish!

Case manager

To counter the trend toward fragmented, depersonalized nursing care, hospitals have developed the role of case manager. This role enables the nurse to manage comprehensive care of an individual patient.

TLC for TPC (that's total patient care!)

Case management is a systematic approach to delivering total patient care within specified time frames and economic resources. Case management encompasses the patient's entire illness episode, crosses all care settings, and involves the collaboration of all personnel who care for the patient.

The case manager is also involved in planning for discharge, making referrals, identifying community and personal resources, and arranging for equipment and supplies needed by the patient on discharge.

Clinical nurse specialist

The clinical nurse specialist has obtained an MSN and acquired expertise in a clinical specialty, such as critical care, emergency care, or maternal-neonatal care. The clinical nurse specialist provides evidence-based nursing care by participating in education and direct patient care, consulting the patient and family members, and collaborating with other nurses and health care team members to deliver high-quality patient care.

As your nurse practitioner, I thought we should take a few minutes to go over your medical history.

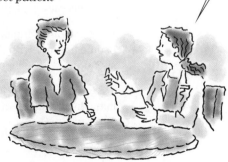

Nurse practitioner

A nurse practitioner has also obtained an MSN and specializes in a clinical area such as critical care. The nurse practitioner provides primary health care to patients and families and can function independently. The nurse practitioner may obtain histories and conduct physical examinations, order laboratory and diagnostic tests and interpret results, diagnose disorders, treat patients, counsel and educate patients and family members, and provide continual follow-up care after patients are discharged from the critical care unit.

Nurse researcher

The nurse researcher promotes the science of nursing by investigating problems related to nursing. The goal is to develop and refine nursing knowledge and practice. Staff nurses participate in nursing research by reading current nursing literature, applying the information in practice, and then collecting data. Advanced practice nurses (clinical nurse specialists and nurse practitioners) can assist staff nurses by conducting the research study and serving as a consultant to the nurses during implementation of a research study.

Nursing theories

Many nursing leaders believe that the profession must establish itself as a scientific discipline to enhance its reputation. To do that, nursing needs a theoretical base that simultaneously shapes and reflects its practice.

Concepts common to nursing theories

Four themes guide the development of nursing theory:

principles and laws that govern life processes, well-being, and the optimal functioning of people—sick or well

patterns of human behavior that describe how people interact with the environment in critical life situations

processes for bringing about positive changes in the health status of individuals

nursing's key role as the central focus of all nursing theories.

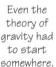

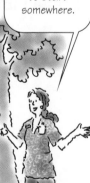

I think I'm on to something here!

Even the theory of gravity had to start somewhere.

Functional health patterns

A holistic way of organizing nursing information is by using functional health patterns—patterns that outline human needs. These patterns, described by Marjory Gordon, focus on behaviors that occur over time and present a total picture of the patient. The patterns represent the patient's basic health needs and are unique and interrelated. (See *Gordon's functional health patterns*.)

Nursing theorists

Theorists and researchers are now collaborating with practicing nurses in the development, testing, and refining of nursing theory. (See *Comparing nursing theories*, pages 22 and 23.)

Gordon's functional health patterns

These health patterns represent broad categories within the wellness–illness continuum. The categories focus on a person's functional abilities.

1. Health perception–health management pattern
   - Perceived pattern of health and well-being
   - How health is managed
2. Nutritional-metabolic pattern
   - Food and fluid consumption relative to metabolic need
   - Pattern indicators of local nutrient supply
3. Elimination pattern
   - Patterns of excretory function
4. Activity-exercise pattern
   - Exercise, activity, leisure, and recreation
5. Sleep-rest pattern
   - Pattern of sleep, rest, and relaxation
6. Cognitive-perceptual pattern
   - Sensory-perceptual pattern
   - Cognitive pattern

7. Self-perception–self-concept pattern
   - Perceptions of self
   - Self-concept pattern
8. Role-relationship pattern
   - Role engagement—family, work, social
   - Relationships
9. Sexuality-reproductive pattern
   - Patterns of satisfaction
   - Dissatisfaction with sexuality pattern
   - Reproductive pattern
10. Coping–stress tolerance pattern
    - General coping pattern and effectiveness
    - Effectiveness of the pattern in terms of stress tolerance
11. Value-belief pattern
    - Values, beliefs (including spiritual), and goals

Adapted with permission from Gordon, M. (1994). *Nursing diagnosis: Process and application* (3rd ed.). St. Louis, MO: Mosby–Year Book.

Comparing nursing theories

Nursing theories differ in their assumptions about patients and health, the goals of nursing, and the methods for research and practice. Together, the theories help define nursing's domain. A nursing theory is expressed as a conceptual model, which usually includes a definition of nursing; a statement of nursing's purpose; and definitions of person, health, and environment. This chart describes seven models.

Model	Definition of nursing	Purpose of nursing	Definition of person	Definition of health	Definition of environment
Nightingale	• A profession for women that seeks to discover and use nature's laws governing health to serve humanity	• To put the person in the best condition for nature to restore or preserve health • To prevent or cure disease and injury	• A being composed of physical, intellectual, and metaphysical attributes and potentials	• To be free from disease and able to use one's own powers to the fullest	• External elements that affect the healthy or sick person
Levine	• A human interaction incorporating scientific principles into the nursing process	• To provide individualized holistic care • To support each person's adaptations	• A complex individual who interacts with internal and external environments and adapts to change	• To possess a pattern of adaptive change • To be whole	• Internally, the person's physiology • Externally, perceptual, operational, and conceptual components
Orem	• A human service designed to overcome limitations in health-related self-care	• To make judgments responding to a person's need for self-care in order to sustain life and health	• A person who functions biologically, symbolically, and socially	• A state of wholeness or integrity of the individual, his or her parts, and modes of functioning	• A subcomponent of the person (Together, they compose an integrated system related to self-care.)
Roy	• An analysis and action related to the care of an ill or potentially ill person	• To manipulate stimuli within a prescribed process of nursing assessment and intervention	• A biopsychosocial being in constant interaction with a changing environment • An open, adaptive system	• Part of the health-illness continuum, a continuous line representing states or degrees of health or illness that a person might experience at a given time	• All conditions, circumstances, and influences surrounding and affecting the development of an organism or group of organisms

Comparing nursing theories (continued)

Model	Definition of nursing	Purpose of nursing	Definition of person	Definition of health	Definition of environment
Neuman	• A profession concerned with the variables that affect the person's response to stressors	• To reduce a person's encounter with stressors • To mitigate the effect of stressors	• A physiologic, psychological, sociocultural, and developmental being • A person who must be viewed as a whole	• A state of wellness or illness determined by physiologic, psychological, sociocultural, and developmental variables that are relative and in a state of flux	• Internally, the state of the person in terms of physiologic, psychological, sociocultural, and developmental variables • Externally, all that exists outside the person
King	• A human interaction between nurse and client	• To exchange information with the patient and take action together to attain mutually set goals	• A being with an open system with permeable boundaries that permit the exchange of matter, energy, and information with the environment	• Dynamic adjustment to stressors in the internal and external environment • To make optimal use of resources to achieve maximum potential for daily living	• An open system with permeable boundaries that permit the exchange of matter, energy, and information with human beings
Rogers	• A learned profession that promotes and maintains health and that includes professionals who care for and rehabilitate the sick and disabled	• To promote harmonious interaction between the environment and person	• A being with a four-dimensional energy field identified by pattern and organization and manifesting characteristics and behaviors that differ from those of its parts and that can't be predicted from knowledge of the parts	• A value word broadly defined by cultures and individuals to describe behaviors considered to be of high or low value	• A four-dimensional energy field identified by pattern and organization and encompassing all that exists outside any given human field

Non-nursing theories

Many theories not specifically developed for nursing have been adopted by the nursing profession to provide guidelines for practicing excellent patient care.

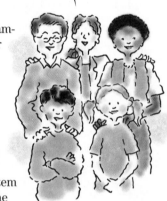

A system can be an individual, a family, or a community.

Systems theories

In systems theory, a system can be an individual, a family, or a community. System theories are the basis for holistic nursing when the patient is viewed not as a whole but as many parts that are interrelated.

The sum of its parts

In general, system theories include a purpose (or goal), content (the information obtained from the system), and a process used to achieve the goal. The whole (be it an individual, family, or community) is broken down, and all of the parts are examined. System theories integrate each part of the whole and examine how each part affects the whole.

Human need theories

Human needs are the physiologic or psychological factors that must be met for an individual to have a healthy existence. These are basic needs that were categorized by Maslow according to importance. Lower level physiologic needs, such as the need for oxygen, food, elimination, temperature control, sex, rest, and comfort, must be met before higher level needs, such as a sense of self-worth and self-respect, can be met. These theories are useful when applying nursing diagnoses. (See *Maslow's hierarchy of needs*.)

According to one developmental theory, I'm working on developing my sense of autonomy by banging this bottle on the table right now.

Developmental theories

Developmental theories classify an individual's behavior or tasks according to their age or development. These theories use categories to describe characteristics associated with the majority of individuals at periods when distinctive developmental changes occur. However, they don't take into account individual differences. These types of theories focus on only one type of development, such as cognitive, psychosocial, psychosexual, and moral or faith

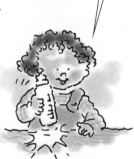

Maslow's hierarchy of needs

To formulate nursing diagnoses, you must know your patient's needs and values. Of course, physiologic needs—represented by the base of the pyramid in the diagram below—must be met first.

Self-actualization
Recognition and realization of one's potential, growth, health, and autonomy

Self-esteem
Sense of self-worth, self-respect, independence, dignity, privacy, and self-reliance

Love and belonging
Affiliation, affection, intimacy, support, and reassurance

Safety and security
Safety from physiologic and psychological threat, protection, continuity, stability, and lack of danger

Physiologic needs
Oxygen, food, elimination, temperature control, sex, movement, rest, and comfort

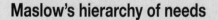

development. Even so, developmental theories do allow the nurse to describe typical behavior within a certain age-group, which can be helpful during patient teaching and counseling.

Nursing research

Research is the foundation on which all sciences are based. Its reliance on observations made in a controlled setting limits confusion over which factors actually produce the results. Health care professionals have long recognized the importance of research in the laboratory setting but recently have begun to develop ways to make research information more useful in the clinical setting.

Supported by evidence

The goal of research is to improve the delivery of care and, thereby, improve patient outcomes. Nursing care is commonly based on evidence that's derived from research. Evidence can be used to support current practices or to change practices. (See *Research and nursing*.)

The best way to get involved in research is to be a good consumer of nursing research. You can do so by reading nursing journals and being aware of the quality of research and reported results.

Share and share alike

Don't be afraid to share research findings with colleagues. Sharing promotes sound clinical care, and all involved may learn about easier and more efficient ways to care for patients.

Good evening, ladies and germs. I'd like to share with you my latest research findings on the importance of humor in the clinical setting . . .

Evidence-based care

One of the newest ways to make research results more useful in clinical practice is by delivering evidence-based care.

Research and nursing

All scientific research is based on the same basic process.

Research steps
The research process consists of these steps:

1. **Identify a problem.** Identifying problems in the critical care environment isn't difficult. An example of such a problem is skin breakdown.
2. **Conduct a literature review.** The goal of this step is to see what has been published about the identified problem.
3. **Formulate a research question or hypothesis.** In the case of skin breakdown, one question is, "Which type of adhesive is most irritating to the skin of a patient on bed rest?"
4. **Design a study.** The study may be experimental or nonexperimental. The nurse must decide what data are to be collected and how to collect that data.
5. **Obtain consent.** The nurse must obtain consent to conduct research from the study participants. Most facilities have an internal review board that must approve such permission for studies.
6. **Collect data.** After the study is approved, the nurse can begin conducting the study and collecting the data.
7. **Analyze the data.** The nurse analyzes the data and states the conclusions derived from the analysis.
8. **Share the information.** Lastly, the researcher shares the collected information with other nurses through publications and presentations.

Evidence-based care isn't based on traditions, customs, or intuition. It's derived from various concrete sources, including:

- formal nursing research
- clinical knowledge
- scientific knowledge.

An evidence-based example

Research results may provide insight into the treatment of a patient who, for example, doesn't respond to a medication or treatment that seems effective for other patients.

In this example, you may believe that a certain drug should be effective for pain relief based on previous experience with that drug. The trouble with such an approach is that other factors can contribute to pain relief, such as the route of administration, the dosage, and concurrent treatments.

> Always remember to use sound clinical judgment when providing patient care.

First, last, and always

Regardless of the value of evidence-based care, you should always use professional clinical judgment when dealing with critically ill patients and their families. Remember that each patient's condition ultimately dictates treatment.

References

American Association of Colleges of Nursing. (n.d.). *Your guide to graduate nursing programs.* Retrieved from http://www.aacn.nche.edu/publications/GradStudentsBrochure.pdf

American Nurses Association. (2010). *Nursing: Scope and standards of practice* (2nd ed.). Silver Springs, MD: Nursesbook.org.

Quick quiz

1. The way you practice your profession of nursing should be guided by standards of nursing care and which of the following?
    A. Nurse practice acts
    B. Joint Commission on Accreditation of Healthcare Organizations
    C. Facility policy
    D. American Medical Association

Answer: A. The way you practice your profession of nursing should be guided by two sets of care documents: standards of nursing care and nurse practice acts.

2. The standards of nursing care are administered by the:
  A.   National Council of State Boards of Nursing.
  B.   American Medical Association.
  C.   American Nurses Association (ANA).
  D.   National Institutes of Health.

Answer: C. The standards of nursing care are administered by the ANA.

3. Nurse practice acts are administered by your:
  A.   health care facility.
  B.   school of nursing.
  C.   licensing bureau.
  D.   individual state.

Answer: D. The nurse practice acts are administered by your individual state.

4. A nurse who can obtain histories, conduct physical examinations, order laboratory and diagnostic tests, interpret results, diagnose disorders, and treat patients has what nursing credentials?
  A.   Clinical nurse specialist
  B.   Case manager
  C.   Nurse practitioner
  D.   Nurse manager

Answer: C. The nurse practitioner may obtain histories, conduct physical examinations, order laboratory and diagnostic tests, interpret results, diagnose disorders, and treat patients.

5. The easiest way to participate in research is to:
  A.   be a good consumer of research.
  B.   do a meta-analysis of related studies.
  C.   conduct a research study.
  D.   participate on your institution's internal review board.

Answer: A. Nurses should start by reading research articles and judging whether or not they're applicable to their practice. Research findings aren't useful if they aren't incorporated into actual practice.

6. The purpose of evidence-based practice is to:
  A.   validate traditional nursing practices.
  B.   improve patient outcomes.
  C.   dispute traditional nursing practices.
  D.   establish a body of knowledge unique to nursing.

Answer: B. Although evidence-based practices may validate or dispute traditional practice, the purpose is to improve patient outcomes.

Scoring

☆☆☆ If you answered all six questions correctly, fantastic! You're building a good nursing foundation.

☆☆ If you answered four or five questions correctly, super! Your foundation is getting strong.

☆ If you answered fewer than four questions correctly, don't worry! With a little review, your foundation will be strong before you know it.

2

Basics of health and illness

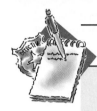

Just the facts

In this chapter, you'll learn:
- ♦ how different people define health and illness
- ♦ common factors affecting health and illness
- ♦ the effects of illness on the family and aging
- ♦ the national goals established in *Healthy People 2020*.

The health-illness continuum

How people view themselves—as individuals and as part of the environment—affect the way health is defined. Many people view health as a continuum, with wellness—the highest level of function—at one end and illness and death at the other. All people are somewhere on this continuum and, as their health status changes, their location on the continuum also changes.

> Although *health* is a commonly used term, definitions abound!

Health defined

Throughout history, the definition of health has changed depending on the knowledge and beliefs of the time. Some cultures have regarded health and disease as reward or punishment for their actions. Others have viewed health as soundness or wholeness of the body.

What is it?

Although *health* is a commonly used term, definitions abound. No single definition is universally accepted. A common one describes health as a disease-free state, but this definition describes an either-or situation—a person as healthy or ill.

WHO says . . . ?

The World Health Organization (WHO) calls health "a state of complete physical, mental, and social well-being and not merely the absence of disease or infirmity." This definition doesn't allow for degrees of health or illness. It also fails to reflect the concept of health as dynamic and constantly changing.

It's about culture

Sociologists view health as a condition that allows the pursuit and enjoyment of desired cultural values. These values include the ability to carry out activities of daily living, such as working and performing household chores.

It's about levels

Many people view health as a level of wellness. According to this definition, a person is striving to attain his full potential. This definition allows a more holistic, subjective view of health.

Factors affecting health

One of the nurse's primary functions is to assist patients in reaching an optimal level of wellness. When assessing patients, the nurse must be aware of factors that affect their health status and plan to tailor interventions accordingly. Such factors include:
• genetics (biological and genetic makeup that causes illness and chronic conditions)
• cognitive abilities (which affect a person's view of health and ability to seek out resources)
• demographic factors, such as age and gender (because certain diseases are more prevalent in a certain age-group or gender)
• geographic locale (which predisposes a person to certain conditions)
• culture (which determines a person's perception of health, the motivation to seek care, and the types of health practices performed)
• lifestyle and environment (such as diet, level of activity, and exposure to toxins)
• health beliefs and practices (which can affect health positively or negatively)
• previous health experiences (which influence reactions to illness and the decision to seek care)
• spirituality (which affects a person's view of illness and health care)
• support systems (which affect the degree to which a person adapts and copes with a situation).

Because so many factors have a bearing on your health, we'll need to consider each one carefully and tailor interventions accordingly.

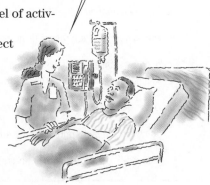

Illness defined

Nurses must understand the concept of illness, particularly how illness may affect the patient. Illness may be defined as a sickness or deviation from a healthy state. It's considered a broader concept than disease. Disease commonly refers to a specific biological or psychological problem that's supported by clinical manifestations and results in a body system or organ malfunction. (See *Disease development.*) Illness, on the other hand, occurs when a person is no longer in a state of perceived "normal" health. A person may have a disease but not be ill all the time because his body has adapted to the disease.

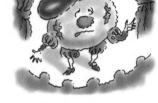

To be ill or not to be ill . . . That is the question!

What does it mean to you?

The meaning of illness also depends on how the patient interprets the disease's source and importance, how the disease affects his behavior and relationships with others, and how he tries to remedy the problem. Another significant component is the meaning that a person attaches to the experience of being ill.

Disease development

A disease is usually detected when it causes a change in metabolism or cell division, which, in turn, causes signs and symptoms. How the cells respond to disease depends on the causative agent and the affected cells, tissues, and organs. In the absence of intervention, resolution of the disease depends on many factors functioning over a period of time, such as the extent of disease and the presence of other diseases. Manifestations of disease may include hypofunction, hyperfunction, or increased or decreased mechanical function.

Disease stages

Typically, diseases progress through these stages:

exposure or injury—target tissue exposed to a causative agent or injury

latency or incubation period—no evident signs or symptoms

prodromal period—generally mild, nonspecific signs and symptoms

acute phase—disease at its full intensity, possibly with complications; called the *subclinical acute phase* if the patient still functions as though the disease wasn't present

remission—second latency phase that occurs in some diseases and is commonly followed by another acute phase

convalescence—progression toward recovery

recovery—return to health or normal functioning; no remaining signs or symptoms of disease.

Types of illness

Illness may be acute or chronic. *Acute illness* usually refers to a disease or condition that has a relatively abrupt onset, high intensity, and short duration. If no complications occur, most acute illnesses end in a full recovery, and the person returns to the previous or a similar level of functioning.

Regain and maintain

Chronic illness refers to a condition that typically has a slower onset, less intensity, and a longer duration than acute illness. The goal is to help the patient regain and maintain the highest possible level of health, although some patients fail to return to their previous level of functioning.

Effects of illness

When a person experiences an illness, one or more changes occur that signal its presence. These may include:
- changes in body appearance or function
- unusual body emissions
- sensory changes
- uncomfortable physical manifestations
- changes in emotional status
- changes in relationships.

Ch-ch-ch-ch-changes . . .

Most people experience a mild form of some of these changes in their daily lives. However, when the changes are severe enough to interfere with usual daily activities, the person is usually considered ill.

Perception and reaction

People's reactions to feeling ill vary. Some people seek action immediately, and others take no action. Some may exaggerate their symptoms, and others may deny that their symptoms exist. A patient's perception of and reaction to illness are unique and are usually based on his culture, knowledge, view of health, and previous experiences with illness and the health care system.

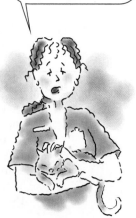

I can't quite put my finger on it, but something's not right. I think I'll need to use a sick day and stay home and cuddle with Fluffy here.

Effects of illness on family

The presence of illness in a family can have a dramatic effect on the functioning of the family as a unit. The type of effect depends on these factors:
- which member is ill
- the seriousness and duration of the illness

• the family's social and cultural customs (each member's role in the family and the tasks specific to that role).

Which member?

The types of role change that occur also vary, depending on the family member affected. For example, if the affected member is the primary breadwinner, other members may need to seek employment to supplement the family income. As the primary breadwinner assumes a dependent role, the rest of the family must adjust to new roles. If the affected family member is a working single parent, serious economic and child care problems may result. That person must depend on support systems for help or face additional stress.

Health promotion

Research shows that poor health practices contribute to a wide range of illnesses, a shortened life span, and increased health care costs. Good health practices have the opposite effect: fewer illnesses, a longer life span, and lower health care costs.

> The earlier in life good practices are started, the fewer poor habits have to be overcome.

Better late than never

Good health practices can benefit most people no matter when they're started. Of course, the earlier in life good practices are started, the fewer poor habits have to be overcome. Even so, later is better than never. For example, stopping cigarette smoking has immediate and long-term benefits. Immediately, the patient will experience improved circulation, pulse rate, and blood pressure. After 10 years without smoking, he'll cut his risk of dying from lung cancer in half.

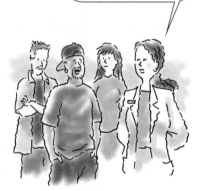

What is health promotion?

Quite simply, health promotion is teaching good health practices and finding ways to help people correct their poor health practices.

But what specifically should you teach? The project *Healthy People 2020* sets forth comprehensive health goals for the nation with the aim of reducing mortality and morbidity in all ages. These objectives make a useful teaching plan (U.S. Department of Health and Human Services, n.d.-b).

Healthy People 2020: Selected objectives

Healthy People 2020 sets forth four major goals for U.S. citizens:
- increase the quality and years of life
- eliminate health disparities among segments of the population (e.g., those that occur by gender, race, education, disability, geographic location, or sexual orientation), achieve health equity, and improve the health of all groups
- create social and physical environments that promote good health for all
- promote quality of life, healthy development, and healthy behaviors across all life stages.

The following target objectives will help measure the nation's progress toward achieving these goals.

Increase
- To at least 100% of the proportion of people younger than 65 years of age to have insurance coverage and to at least 84% of proportion of people to have a usual primary care provider
- To at least 80% of the proportion of children ages 19 months to 35 months to be fully immunized
- To at least 60% the proportion of adults age 18 and older with hypertension to have controlled blood pressure with treatment.

Decrease
- To no more than 30% of the incidence of obese adults age 20 and older
- To no more than 15% of the incidence of obese children between the ages of 2 and 19
- To no more than 12% the incidence of cigarette smoking among adults age 18 and older
- To no more than 10% of suicides per 100,000
- To no more than 16% of the proportion of adults 18 years and older with diagnosed diabetes with poor glycemic control.

Adult health care

Adults between ages 25 and 64 may fall victim to several health problems, including heart disease and cancer. Although some of these problems stem from genetic predisposition, many are linked to unhealthy habits, such as overeating, smoking, lack of exercise, and alcohol and drug abuse. Your teaching can help an adult recognize and correct these habits to ensure a longer, healthier life.

Geriatric health care

Today, people live longer than ever before. In the past century, life expectancy in the United States has increased from 47 years to about 76 years. Fortunately, most elderly people maintain their independence, with few needing to be institutionalized.

Wait up, Grandmom and Granddad! How much further is it to the yogurt stand?

Cope and avoid

Even so, most elderly people suffer from at least one chronic health problem. With the nurse's help, they can cope with existing health problems and learn to avoid new ones. Doing so will improve their quality of life and allow them to continue contributing to society.

References

U.S. Department of Health and Human Services. (n.d.-a). *Healthy people 2020*. Retrieved from http://healthypeople.gov/2020/LHI/infographicGallery.aspx

U.S. Department of Health and Human Services. (n.d.-b). *LHI infographic gallery*. Retrieved from http://www.healthypeople.gov/2020/LHI/inforgraphicGallery.aspx

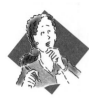

Quick quiz

1. Which of the following is an example of health promotion?
   A. Administering antibiotics to a patient
   B. Splinting a patient's fractured bone
   C. Assisting a patient in stopping smoking
   D. Inserting an I.V. catheter

Answer: C. Health promotion involves teaching good health practices as well as helping people correct their poor health practices. Helping a patient stop smoking helps him to correct a poor health practice.

2. The effect of illness on a family unit depends on several factors, including:
   A. when the illness occurs.
   B. which family member is affected.
   C. whether the illness is due to poor health habits.
   D. at what point the patient sought care.

Answer: B. The effect of illness on a family unit depends on which family member is affected, the seriousness and duration of the illness, and the family's social and cultural customs.

3. One of the goals of *Healthy People 2020* is to decrease the incidence of obese adults age 20 and older to no more than:
- A. 5%.
- B. 10%.
- C. 30%.
- D. 20%.

Answer: C. One of the goals of *Healthy People 2020* is to decrease to no more than 30% the incidence of obese adults age 20 and older.

4. When describing disease development, which disease stage is described as producing generally mild, nonspecific signs and symptoms?
- A. Latent
- B. Acute
- C. Second latency
- D. Prodromal

Answer: D. The prodromal period is described as producing generally mild, nonspecific signs and symptoms.

Scoring

☆☆☆ If you answered all four questions correctly, super! Your understanding of the spectrum of health and illness is spectacular.

☆☆ If you answered three questions correctly, great! You sure have been practicing your nursing practice.

☆ If you answered fewer than three questions correctly, don't despair! Keep "continuum" to review, and you'll soon have a healthy understanding of the chapter.

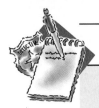

3

Ethical and legal considerations

Just the facts

In this chapter, you'll learn:

♦ the significance of values and ethics in providing nursing care

♦ how to approach ethical dilemmas in patient care

♦ the nurse's role and responsibilities in ensuring patients' rights

♦ the difference between intentional and unintentional torts.

Values

Values are strongly held personal and professional beliefs about worth and importance. The word *values* derives from the Latin *valere* (to be strong). Values are key to developing ethical consciousness and guide us in making important life decisions. Because values are highly individualized yet subject to influence from outside sources, it isn't surprising that value conflicts are common among nurses, doctors, patients, families, and health care facility administrators.

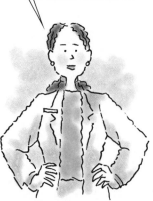

Clarifying your values is an important part of developing a professional ethic.

Personal values

Clarifying your own values is an important part of developing a professional ethic. A person may become more aware of their values by consciously examining their statements and behavior. (See *Developing values awareness*.)

Developing values awareness

Nurses, like all people, sometimes rely on hearsay, opinions, or prejudice instead of developing a strong sense of their own values. Sometimes, they don't stop to reflect on the values that are mirrored in their conversation and behavior.

Consider the following dialogue in which three nurses express various value judgments. As you read, ask yourself: What values does each nurse express? Do the values of the three conflict? Are individual nurses expressing consistent values? Do they show a high regard for patient autonomy?

Shop talk

Kate: I can't believe it. I have to float to the ICU—and it's only my second week on the job. I hate floating, especially to intensive care.

Dean: So do I. The last time I floated to ICU, I was assigned to a 300-lb patient who had been driving drunk and wasn't wearing a seat belt. The guy was badly hurt, and I had to do all the positioning myself because the unit was so short-staffed. I just about killed my back. It isn't fair that they always assign male nurses to obese patients.

Pat: Floating is really a tough issue. I try to see it from the patient's side, though. I mean maybe you were assigned to care for this patient because you're a good nurse and could give him the best care.

Kate: What bugs me is having to care for patients like that drunk driver, who obviously don't care how they live. They don't watch their weight, they drive drunk, they don't use seat belts, and we get pulled from the work we're comfortable with to care for them. I can't even find time for a cigarette break.

Pat: Don't forget, Kate, we're supposed to take care of patients regardless of their health habits or lifestyle. No one's perfect, after all.

Kate: Yeah, I guess you're right, but floating makes me nervous anyway. I'm scared I'll really mess up because everything's so unfamiliar.

Dean: Let me give you some advice. No matter what you think about floating, don't say anything. If you're pegged as a complainer around here, your career is over.

Pat: You sound like you think nurses shouldn't ever speak out if something is wrong with the system. I think nurses do have the power to change things for the better, but that won't happen if we aren't willing to take some risks.

Dean: You're an idealist. I'm a realist. I ask, what's worth risking your job?

Pat: I think being a nurse means not being willing to compromise your standards of care just to keep a job.

Kate: What happened to the 300-lb patient? Is he still in ICU? Do you think I might get assigned to him?

Dean: Well, no. It's the craziest thing. He was a quadriplegic after the accident. So we put all this time and effort into stabilizing his condition and keeping him infection-free, and one day, the doctor decides it isn't worth it, so they just turned everything off. Now I ask you, is that right?

Examining values

The nurses in this scenario make various moral judgments. By analyzing their attitudes, you can come to a better understanding of your own values:

• Kate criticizes the health habits of an obese trauma patient but insists on her own right to have time for a cigarette break. What values are guiding her opinions? Do you think her outlook is consistent?

• Dean thinks that Kate should take an assignment for which she isn't prepared rather than risk losing favor with the administration. Do you think this attitude is irresponsible or merely realistic?

• Pat is accused of being an idealist. Is that a fair judgment?

• What values are mirrored in each nurse's attitude about the practice of floating?

• At the end of the conversation, Dean mentions that the doctor decided to withdraw treatment from the quadriplegic patient. If the three nurses were to discuss the ethical questions raised by the doctor's decision, how do you think each nurse would respond?

• Would these three nurses have similar or conflicting views about what it means to be a patient advocate?

Values clarification

Each nurse and patient brings values to the health care system. These values include beliefs about such concepts as life, death, a higher power, and who should and shouldn't receive health care as well as such complex issues as organ transplantation and the right to die. The patient's values may change when they are faced with illness, injury, and possible death.

Values clarification refers to the process of raising consciousness so that value conflicts can be resolved. You're likely to encounter many conflicting sets of values in the course of your professional career. To provide optimal support to the patient, you must undergo your own values clarification process.

First reflect . . .

Exercises, such as analyzing conversations between coworkers, offer one way to clarify values. Reflecting on one's own statements and actions is another way.

. . . then choose . . .

You must choose among competing values to establish your own. Then you need to incorporate chosen values into your everyday thoughts and actions. You'll then be better prepared to act on chosen values when you're confronted with difficult choices.

. . . and, finally, clarify

Making values decisions need not be haphazard. By clarifying your own values and checking to see if they're consistent with the established standards of the nursing profession, you can enhance your ability to make responsible judgments.

Ethics

Ethics is defined as conduct appropriate for all members of a group. Health care workers today deal with many ethics issues. These issues have risen as a result of technology and increased knowledge about disease and the body's reaction to disease.

OK, boys, how would you handle a hypothetical situation like this . . . ?

ETHICS DISCUSSION

PLATO   DESCARTES   HIPPOCRATES   ROUSSEAU

Code of ethics

A code of ethics is a group of fundamental beliefs about what's morally right or wrong, along with reasons for maintaining those beliefs. (See *Ethical codes for nurses.*)

Ethical codes for nurses

Two of the most important ethical codes for registered nurses are the American Nurses Association (ANA) code and the Canadian Nurses Association (CNA) code. Licensed practical nurses (LPNs) also have an ethical code. The International Council of Nurses (ICN), an organization based in Geneva, Switzerland, that seeks to improve the standards and status of nursing worldwide has also published a code of ethics.

ANA code of ethics
The ANA views nurses and patients as individuals who possess basic rights and responsibilities and whose values and circumstances should command respect at all times. The ANA code provides guidance for carrying out nursing responsibilities consistent with the ethical obligations of the profession.

According to the ANA code, the nurse:
• provides services with respect for human dignity and the uniqueness of the patient, unrestricted by considerations of social or economic status, personal attributes, or the nature of health problems
• safeguards the patient's right to privacy by judiciously protecting information of a confidential nature
• acts to safeguard the patient and the public when health and safety are affected by the incompetent, unethical, or illegal practice of any person
• assumes responsibility and accountability for individual nursing judgments and actions
• maintains competence in nursing
• exercises informed judgment and uses individual competence and qualifications as criteria in seeking consultation, accepting responsibilities, and delegating nursing activities to others
• participates in activities that contribute to the ongoing development of the profession's body of knowledge
• participates in the profession's efforts to implement and improve standards of nursing
• participates in the profession's efforts to establish and maintain conditions of employment conducive to high-quality nursing care
• collaborates with members of the health professions and other citizens in promoting community and national efforts to meet the health care needs of the public.

CNA code of ethics
The CNA code consists of eight primary values that form the basis of nursing obligations:
• *Safe, competent, and ethical care*—nurses value the ability to provide safe, competent, and ethical care that allows them to fulfill their ethical and professional obligations to the people they serve.
• *Health and well-being*—nurses value health promotion and well-being and assisting persons to achieve their optimal level of health in situations of normal health, illness, injury, or disability, or at the end of life.
• *Choice*—nurses respect and promote the autonomy of persons and help them to express their health needs and values and also to obtain desired information and services so they can make informed decisions.
• *Dignity*—nurses recognize and respect the inherent worth of each person and advocate the respectful treatment of all persons.
• *Confidentiality*—nurses safeguard information learned in the context of a professional relationship and ensure that it's shared outside the health care team only with the person's informed consent, as may be legally required, or where the failure to disclose would cause significant harm.
• *Justice*—nurses uphold principles of equity and fairness to assist persons in receiving a share of health services and resources proportionate to their needs and in promoting social justice.

(continued)

Ethical codes for nurses *(continued)*

• *Accountability*—nurses are answerable for their practice, and they act in a manner consistent with their professional responsibilities and standards of practice.

• *Quality practice environments*— nurses value and advocate for practice environments that have the organizational structures and resources necessary to ensure safety, support, and respect for all persons in the work setting.

Code for LPNs

The code for LPNs seeks to provide a motivation for establishing, maintaining, and elevating professional standards. This code requires these nurses to:

• regard conservation of life and disease prevention as a basic obligation
• promote and protect the physical, mental, emotional, and spiritual well-being of the patient and his family
• fulfill all duties faithfully and efficiently
• function within established legal guidelines
• take personal responsibility for actions and seek to earn the respect and confidence of all members of the health care team
• keep confidential all information about the patient obtained from any source
• give conscientious service and charge reasonable fees
• learn about and respect the religious and cultural beliefs of all patients

• meet obligations to patients by staying abreast of health care trends through reading and continuing education
• uphold the laws of the land and promote legislation to meet the health needs of its people.

ICN code of ethics

According to the ICN, the fundamental responsibility of the nurse is fourfold:

1. promote health
2. prevent illness
3. restore health
4. alleviate suffering.

The ICN further states that the need for nursing is universal. Inherent in nursing is respect for life, dignity, and the rights of humanity. It's unrestricted by considerations of nationality, race, color, age, gender, politics, or social status.

Nurses and people

• The nurse's primary responsibility is to people who require nursing care.
• The nurse, in providing care, respects the beliefs, values, and customs of the individual.
• The nurse holds in confidence personal information and uses judgment in sharing this information.

Nurses and practice

• The nurse carries personal responsibility for nursing practice and maintaining competence by continual learning.
• The nurse maintains the highest standards of nursing possible within the reality of a specific situation.

• The nurse uses good judgment in relation to individual competence when accepting and delegating responsibilities.
• The nurse, when acting in a professional capacity, should at all times maintain standards of personal conduct that would reflect credit upon the profession.

Nurses and society

• The nurse shares with other citizens the responsibility for initiating and supporting actions to meet the health and social needs of the public.

Nurses and coworkers

• The nurse sustains a cooperative relationship with coworkers in nursing and other fields.
• The nurse takes appropriate actions to safeguard the patient when his care is endangered by a coworker or another person.

Nurses and the profession

• The nurse plays the major role in determining and implementing desirable standards of nursing practice and nursing education.
• The nurse is active in developing a core of professional knowledge.
• The nurse, acting through the professional organization, participates in establishing and maintaining equitable social and economic working conditions in nursing.

An unbreakable code

The American Nurses Association (ANA) has established a code of ethics. The *ANA Code of Ethics for Nurses* guides the practicing nurse in how to use their professional skills to provide the most effective holistic care possible, such as serving as a patient advocate and striving to protect the health, safety, and rights of each patient.

Confidentiality

The Health Insurance Portability and Accountability Act (HIPAA) of 1996 went into effect in the spring of 2003 to strengthen and protect patient privacy. Health care providers (such as doctors, nurses, pharmacies, hospitals, clinics, and nursing homes), health insurance plans, and government programs (such as Medicare and Medicaid) must notify patients about their rights to privacy and how their health information will be used and shared. This health information includes information in the patient's medical record, conversations about the patient's care between health care providers, billing information, and the health insurer's computerized records.

I've got rights!

Under HIPAA, the patient has the right to access their medical information, know when health information is shared, and make changes or corrections to their medical record. Patients also have the right to decide if they want to allow their information to be used for certain purposes, such as for marketing or research.

For your eyes only

Patient records with identifiable health information must be secured so that they aren't accessible to those who don't have a need for them. Identifiable health information may include the patient's name, Social Security number, medical record number, birth date, admission and discharge dates, and health history.

Social Media

Social media is defined as "a form of electronic communication through which users create online communities to share information, ideas, personal messages, and other content (as videos)." It is the nurse's responsibility to know their employer's policies regarding the use of social media in the workplace. Nurses also need to be cognizant that unauthorized disclosure of a patient's personal information via social media outside of the work place may result in a violation of patient privacy and confidentiality.

Sign here, please

When a patient receives health care, they must sign an authorization form before protected health information can be used for purposes other than routine treatment or billing. The form should be placed in the patient's medical record.

Ethical decisions

Every day, nurses make ethical decisions in their nursing practice. These decisions may involve patient care, actions related to coworkers, or nurse–doctor relationships. At times, you may find yourself trapped in the middle of an ethical dilemma, pulled in every direction by your duties and responsibilities to your patient, your employer, and yourself. Even after you make a decision, you may ask yourself, "Did I make the right decision?"

It isn't automatic

There are no automatic solutions to all ethical conflicts. Although such conflicts may be painful and confusing, particularly in nursing, you don't have to be a philosopher to act ethically or to make decisions that fall within nursing's ethical codes. Nonetheless, you need to understand the principles of ethics that guide your nursing practice. Legally, nurses are responsible for using their knowledge and skills to protect the comfort and safety of their patients. Ethically, nurses, in their role as patient advocates, are responsible for safeguarding their patients' rights.

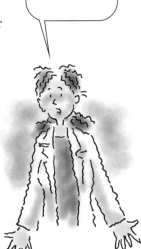

Did I make the right decision?

Being an advocate

Although a nurse isn't legally responsible for obtaining a patient's informed consent, for example, the nurse is ethically responsible as the patient's advocate for reporting to the doctor a patient's misunderstanding about treatment or withdrawal of consent. To be an effective advocate, a nurse must understand the ethical and legal principles of informed consent, including that the patient's consent isn't valid unless they understand their condition, the proposed treatment, treatment alternatives, potential risks and benefits, and relative chances of success or failure.

Ethical conflicts

Rapid advances in medical research have outpaced society's ability to solve the ethical problems associated with new health care technology. For nurses, ethical decision making in clinical practice is complicated by sociocultural factors, legal controversies, growing professional autonomy, and consumer involvement in health care.

Decisions, decisions

Major areas of ethical conflict may include end-of-life decisions, determining medical futility, withholding or withdrawing treatment, advance directives, and organ donation. No matter what your nursing specialty, you'll probably encounter at least one of these conflicts during your nursing career.

End-of-life decisions

End-of-life decisions are almost always difficult for patients, families, and health care professionals to make. Nurses are in a unique position as patient advocates assisting patients and their families through the process of death.

Unsolvable mysteries

Your primary role as a patient advocate is to promote the patient's wishes. In many instances, however, the patient's wishes aren't known. That's when ethical decision making takes priority. Decisions aren't always easy to make, and the answers aren't usually clear-cut. At times, such ethical dilemmas may seem unsolvable.

Question of quality

It's sometimes difficult to determine what can be done to achieve a good quality of life and what can simply be achieved technologically speaking.

Years ago, death was considered a natural part of life and most people died at home, surrounded by their families. Today, most people die in hospitals, and death is commonly regarded as a medical failure rather than a natural event. Sometimes, it's hard to know whether you're assisting in extending the patient's life or merely delaying the patient's death.

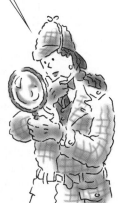

Deducing the patient's wishes isn't always easy. In fact, at times, it may seem unsolvable.

Consulting the committee

Most hospitals have ethics committees that review ethical dilemmas. (See *The ethics committee*, page 46.) The nurse may consider consulting the ethics committee if:
• the doctor disagrees with the patient or their family regarding treatment

The ethics committee

The ethics committee addresses ethical issues regarding the clinical aspects of patient care. It provides a forum for the patient, his family, and health care providers to resolve conflicts.

The functions of an ethics committee include:
• policy development (such as developing policies to guide deliberations over individual cases)
• education (such as inviting guest speakers to visit your health care facility and discuss ethical concerns)
• case consultation (such as debating the prognosis of a patient who's in a persistent vegetative state)
• addressing a single issue (such as reviewing all cases that involve a no-code or do-not-resuscitate [DNR] order)
• addressing problems of a specific population group (e.g., the American Academy of Pediatrics recommending that hospitals have a standing committee called the "infant bioethical review committee")
• addressing issues of organization ethics (such as business practice, marketing, admission, and reimbursement).

Pros and cons

Properly run, an ethics committee provides a safe outlet for venting opposing views on emotionally charged ethical conflicts. The committee process can help lessen the bias that interferes with rational decision making. It enables members of disparate disciplines, including doctors, nurses, clergy, social workers, hospital administrators, and ethicists, to express their views on treatment decisions.

Critics of the ethics committee think that committee decision making is too bureaucratic and slow to be useful in clinical crises. They also point out that one dominating committee member may intimidate others with opposing views. Furthermore, they contend that doctors may view the committee as a threat to their autonomy in patient-care decisions. For these reasons, many ethics committees use a "rapid response team" of committee members who are on call to respond quickly in emergent ethical

dilemmas. The rapid response team usually consists of three or four committee members, including a doctor, who have had special training in negotiation and mediation. The entire committee will then review each case.

Selection of committee members

Committee members should be selected for their ability to work cooperatively in a group. The American Hospital Association recommends the following ratio of committee members: one-third doctors, one-third nurses, and one-third others, including laypersons, clergy, and other health professionals. Regulations of the Joint Commission on Accreditation of Healthcare Organizations require that nursing staff members participate in the hospital ethics committee.

The nurse's role on a hospital ethics committee

Because of the nurse's close contact with the patient, their family, and other members of the health care team, the nurse is commonly in a position to identify ethical dilemmas, such as when a family is considering a DNR order for a relative. In many cases, the nurse is the first to recognize conflicts among family members or between the doctor and the patient or his family.

Before ethics committees were widely used, nurses had no official outlet for voicing their opinions in ethical debates. In many situations, doctors made ethical decisions about patient care behind closed doors. Nursing supervisors would commonly call meetings to alert nursing staff about treatment decisions and discourage protest. Now, ethics committees provide nurses with an avenue to express their views, hear the opinions of others, and understand more deeply the rationale behind ethical decisions.

- health care providers disagree among themselves about treatment options
- family members disagree about what should be done.

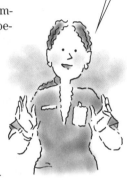

Be advised . . . ethical dilemmas are chock-full of controversies.

Determining medical futility

Medical futility refers to treatment that isn't likely to benefit the patient even though it may appear to be effective. For example, a patient with a terminal illness who's expected to die experiences cardiac arrest. Cardiopulmonary resuscitation (CPR) may be effective in restoring a heartbeat but may be deemed futile because it doesn't change the patient's outcome. CPR must be initiated unless written otherwise by the patient or doctor's order.

Withholding or withdrawing treatment

The issue of withholding or withdrawing treatment can certainly present some ethical dilemmas. When withdrawing treatment from a patient—even at the patient's request—controversy over the principle of *nonmaleficence* (to prevent harm) exists.

Harm alarm

Such controversy revolves around the definition of *harm*. Some feel that removing a patient from a ventilator and allowing death is an intentional infliction of harm. Others argue that keeping a person on a ventilator against the patient's will—thus prolonging death—is an intentional infliction of harm. (See *Approaching ethical decisions*.)

Approaching ethical decisions

When faced with an ethical dilemma, consider these questions:
- What health issues are involved?
- What ethical issues are involved?
- What further information is necessary before a judgment can be made?
- Who will be affected by this decision? (Include the decision maker and other caregivers if they'll be affected emotionally or professionally.)
- What are the values and opinions of the people involved?

- What conflicts exist between the values and ethical standards of the people involved?
- Must a decision be made and, if so, who should make it?
- What alternatives are available?
- For each alternative, what are the ethical justifications?
- For each alternative, what are the possible outcomes?

Dealing with cardiac arrest

In cases of cardiac arrest (sudden stoppage of the heart), a critically ill patient may be described by a code status. This code status relates the orders written by the doctor describing what resuscitation measures should be carried out by the nurse and should be based on the patient's wishes regarding resuscitation measures. When cardiac arrest occurs, you must ensure that resuscitation efforts are initiated or that unwanted resuscitation doesn't occur.

Who decides?

The wishes of a competent, informed patient should always be honored. However, when a patient can't make decisions, the health care team—consisting of the patient's family, nursing staff, and doctors—may have to make end-of-life decisions for the patient.

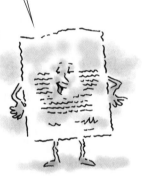

Remember, you're required by law to ask whether your patient has an advance directive or a durable power of attorney.

Advance directives

Most people prefer to make their own decisions regarding end-of-life care. It's important that patients discuss their wishes with their loved ones; however, many don't. Instead, total strangers may be asked to make important health care decisions when a patient can't do so. That's why it's important for people to make choices ahead of time and to make these choices known by developing advance directives.

The Patient Self-Determination Act of 1990 requires hospitals and other institutions to make information available to patients on advance directives. However, it isn't mandatory for patients to have advance directives.

Where there's a will, there's a law

There are two types of advance directive:
• treatment directive, sometimes known as a *living will*
• appointment directive, sometimes known as a *durable power of attorney for health care.*

A living will states what treatments a patient will accept and refuse in case terminal illness renders the patient unable to make those decisions at the time. For example, a patient may be willing to accept artificial nutrition but not hemodialysis.

Durable power of attorney is the appointment of a person chosen by the patient to make decisions on the patient's behalf if the patient can no longer do so. Durable power of attorney for health care doesn't give the chosen individual authority to access business accounts; the power is strictly related to health care decisions.

It takes two

After an advance directive is written, two witnesses must sign it. This document can be altered or canceled at any time. For more information, check the laws regarding advance directives for your state in which you practice.

Organ donation

When asked, most people say that they support organ donation. However, only a small percentage of qualified organs are ever donated. Tens of thousands of names are on waiting lists for organs in the United States alone. Organ transplantation is successful for many patients, giving them additional, high-quality years of life.

The Uniform Anatomical Gift Act governs the donation of organs and tissues. In addition, most states have legislation governing the procurement of organs and tissues. Some require medical staff to ask about organ donation on every death. Other states require the staff to notify a regional organ procurement agency that then approaches the family. Become familiar with the state laws and the policies of the facility in which you practice.

With so many people needing transplants, it's a shame to let a healthy guy like me go to waste. Learn all you can about organ donation in your state.

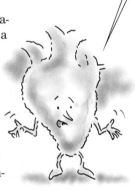

Who died?

Medical criteria for organ donation vary from state to state. Many organ procurement agencies want to be notified of all deaths and imminent deaths so that they, not the medical staff, can determine whether the patient is a potential candidate for organ donation.

No, thank you

These conditions usually preclude any organ or tissue donation:
• advanced age
• metastatic cancer
• history of hepatitis, HIV, or AIDS
• sepsis.

Discuss among yourselves

When ethical problems arise, discuss them candidly with other members of the health care team, especially the patient's doctor. Also, consider calling on social workers, psychologists, the clergy, and ethics committee members to help you resolve difficult ethical problems. By learning as much as possible, you can facilitate the decision-making process for the patient, his family, his doctor, and yourself.

Laws

Laws are binding rules of conduct enforced by authority. Ideally, laws are based on what's right and good. Realistically, though, the relation between laws and ethics is complex. When a law is challenged as unjust or unfair, the challenge usually reflects some underlying clinical principle. Even so, there's a strong connection between ethics and laws regarding the nurse's role as a patient advocate. Most nurses realize that many malpractice suits result from a patient's dissatisfaction with care. When a patient believes he hasn't been treated with respect or dignity or that his needs and rights have been ignored or violated, he's more likely to initiate legal action.

Torts

Torts are personal civil injuries that reside outside a contractual relationship. Torts result in a civil trial to assess compensation for the plaintiff. Torts can be *intentional* or *unintentional*.

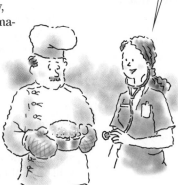

No, that's a lovely tart, but I said "tort!" You know, an injury that resides outside a contractual relationship.

Intentional torts

Intentional torts include fraud, assault and battery, invasion of privacy, false imprisonment, and defamation of character.

Unintentional torts

Unintentional torts include negligence and malpractice. *Negligence* is a mistake or the failure to be careful. *Malpractice* is defined as a professional person's wrongful conduct, improper discharge of professional duties, or failure to meet standards of care that results in harm to another person.

Better get CSI

Patients typically file malpractice lawsuits against nurses when they perceive their nursing care to be substandard or the cause of unforeseeable injuries. Keep in mind, however, that malpractice is more than an undesired outcome; in order for a patient to successfully file a malpractice lawsuit against a nurse, there must be evidence that some action or inaction that the nurse was obligated to perform resulted in harm to the patient. If the patient doesn't have compelling evidence, they may still file the suit, but the court may find the suit to be frivolous and the suit will generally be unsuccessful.

Regulation of nursing practice

The practice of nursing requires rules and regulations to ensure patient safety and a competent level of behavior in the professional role as a nurse. Nursing licensure allows you to practice as a professional nurse. Standards of nursing practice help ensure high-quality care and serve as criteria in legal questions of whether adequate care was rendered.

Licensure

Your nursing license entitles you to practice as a professionally qualified nurse. However, like most privileges, your nursing license imposes certain responsibilities. As a licensed registered nurse (RN), or licensed practical nurse (LPN), you're responsible for providing quality care to your patients. To meet this responsibility and protect your right to practice, you must understand the professional and legal significance of your nursing license.

Get the scoop on the scope of practice

Each nurse practice act contains licensing laws. They establish qualifications for obtaining and maintaining a nursing license. They also broadly define the legally permissible scope of nursing practice. Although they vary from state to state, most licensing laws specify:
• qualifications a nurse must have to be granted a license
• license application procedures for new licenses and reciprocal (state-to-state) licensing arrangements
• application fees
• authorization to use the title of Registered Nurse, Licensed Practical Nurse, or Vocational Nurse to applicants who receive their license
• grounds for license denial, revocation, or suspension
• license renewal procedures.

> Having a license to practice nursing makes you part of an elite health care team—and that's an awesome responsibility!

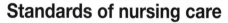

Standards of nursing care

Standards of nursing care set minimum criteria for your proficiency on the job, enabling you and others to judge the quality of care you and your nursing colleagues provide. States may refer to standards in their nurse practice act. Unless included in a nurse practice act, professional standards aren't laws but guidelines for sound nursing practice. You're expected to meet standards of nursing care for every nursing task you perform.

Legal issues affecting nursing

Nurses are faced with legal issues that may affect their nursing care. Patient rights and documentation are two of the most common issues nurses face.

Patient rights

At one time, nurses were forbidden to give patients even the most basic information about their care or health but, in the 1960s, attitudes changed. Patients began demanding more information about their care and turned to nurses to assist them in getting the information.

A patients' bill of rights that's endorsed by major health care providers and consumer groups has helped to reinforce the public's expectation of quality care. This document defines a person's rights while receiving health care. (See *NLN's Patients' Bill of Rights*.)

> Whether using a quill or a computer, drafting a "Bill of Rights" is all about protecting the basic rights of individuals.

Not a new idea

For years, hospitals and extended care facilities have had their own published patients' bills of rights and those of the American Hospital Association to inform consumers of some of their rights in the health care setting. These privately drafted bills of rights are designed to protect such basic rights as human dignity, privacy, confidentiality, and refusal of treatment.

Tell me all about it

They also ensure the patient's right to receive a full explanation of the cost of medical care, be fully informed, and be required to give consent before participating in experimental treatments because the patient exercises control over his own health care. These bills emphasize the patient's right to acquire information about all aspects of his care.

Informed consent

Being adequately informed about proposed treatment, procedures, surgery, or research in order to properly consent is a patient's legal right. So, it isn't surprising that the topic of informed consent appears in all current medical and nursing texts and that a signed informed consent form must be in the patient's records when invasive or experimental procedures, treatment, or surgery is contemplated.

NLN's Patients' Bill of Rights

In 1977, the National League for Nursing (NLN) published its Patients' Bill of Rights. It states that the NLN believes nurses are responsible for upholding these rights of patients:

• People have the right to health care that's accessible and that meets professional standards, regardless of the setting.

• Patients have the right to courteous and individualized health care that is equitable, humane, and given without discrimination as to race, color, creed, sex, national origin, source of payment, or ethical or political beliefs.

• Patients have the right to information about their diagnosis, prognosis, and treatment—including alternatives to care and risks involved—in terms they and their families can readily understand, so that they can give their informed consent.

• Patients have the legal right to informed participation in all decisions concerning their health care.

• Patients have the right to information about the qualifications, names, and titles of personnel responsible for providing their health care.

• Patients have the right to refuse observation by those not directly involved in their care.

• Patients have the right to privacy during interview, examination, and treatment.

• Patients have the right to privacy in communicating and visiting with persons of their choice.

• Patients have the right to refuse treatments, medications, or participation in research and experimentation, without punitive action being taken against them.

• Patients have the right to coordination and continuity of health care.

• Patients have the right to appropriate instruction or education from health care personnel so that they can achieve an optimal level of wellness and an understanding of their basic health needs.

• Patients have the right to confidentiality of all records (except as otherwise provided for by law or third-party payer contracts) and all communications, written or oral, between patients and health care providers.

• Patients have the right of access to all health records pertaining to them, the right to challenge and to have their records corrected for accuracy, and the right to transfer of all such records in the case of continuing care.

• Patients have the right to information on the charges for services, including the right to challenge these.

• Above all, patients have the right to be fully informed as to all their rights in all health care settings.

Reprinted with permission from the National League for Nursing.

In the know

Informed consent basically means that the patient—or someone acting on his behalf—has enough information to know what's at risk in undergoing the proposed treatment and the possible consequences should consent to the treatment be refused or withdrawn. Nurses may provide patients and their families with information that's within a nurse's scope of practice and knowledge base. However, a nurse shouldn't substitute her knowledge for a doctor's input.

Capacity to consent

Under certain circumstances, people with mental disorders may be held incompetent to consent. When there's a question about an individual's capacity to give consent, a legal determination may be sought from the appropriate court or an ethics committee. The bottom line in determining capacity must be whether the person giving consent is impaired in their capacity or judgment to the extent that they do not know what they are getting into before the treatment begins.

How good are your instincts?

To assess capacity to consent, a nurse may need to rely on their instincts as well as professional judgment. If the nurse believes the patient doesn't understand, they should reassess and discuss the consent issue with the patient, the guardian (if applicable), and the doctor before the treatment begins.

HIPAA

The Health Insurance Portability and Accountability Act (HIPAA) protects the privacy, confidentiality, and security of all medical information. Only those who have a need to know patient information in order to provide care for the patient and those authorized by the patient to have access to information can lawfully receive oral, written, or electronic information. Failure to comply with HIPAA, intentionally or unintentionally, could result in criminal or civil penalties. (See *Patient rights under HIPAA*.)

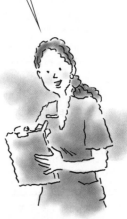

By all means, provide your patient with the information he needs to give an informed consent—only, make sure it's within your scope of practice and nursing knowledge base.

Patient rights under HIPAA

The goal of the HIPAA is to provide safeguards against the inappropriate use and release of personal medical information, including all medical records and identifiable health information in any form (electronic, paper, and verbal). Patients are the beneficiaries of this privacy rule, which includes these six rights:

- right to give consent before information is released for treatment, payment, or health care operations

- right to be educated about the provider's policy on privacy protection

- right to access their medical records

- right to request that their medical records be amended for accuracy

- right to access the history of nonroutine disclosures (disclosures that didn't occur in the course of treatment, payment, or health care operations, or those not specifically authorized by the patient)

- right to request that the provider restrict the use and routine disclosure of information he has. (Providers aren't required to grant this request, especially if they think the information is important to the quality of patient care.)

Documentation

Accurate documentation shows that the care you provide meets the patient's needs and expressed wishes. It also proves that you're following the accepted standards of nursing care mandated by the law, your profession, and your health care facility. Always document your nursing care and your patient's response to that care.

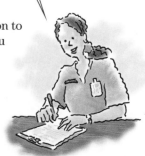

Proper documentation communicates crucial information to caregivers and just might save your license in a legal dispute.

The evidence speaks for itself

Proper documentation communicates crucial information to caregivers so they make fewer errors. How and what you document can determine whether you or your employer wins or loses a legal dispute. Medical records are used as evidence in cases involving disability, personal injury, and mental competency. Poor documentation is the pivotal issue in many malpractice cases.

References

National Council of State Boards of Nursing (NCSBN). (2011). *White paper: A nurse's guide to the use of social media*. Retrieved from https://www.ncsbn.org/Social_media_guidelines.pdf

Social media. (2011). In *Merriam-Webster's online dictionary* (11th ed.). Retrieved from http://www.merriam-webster.com/dictionary/social%20media

Spector, N., & Kappel, D. (2012). Guidelines for using electronic and social media: The regulatory perspective. *Online Journal of Issues in Nursing, 17*(3), 1.

Quick quiz

1. The Code of Ethics for Nurses provides information that's necessary for the practicing nurse to:
   A. document her nursing care appropriately.
   B. make ethical decisions about patient care.
   C. use her professional skills in providing the most effective holistic care possible.
   D. strengthen and protect patient privacy.

Answer: C. The Code of Ethics for Nurses provides information that's necessary for the practicing nurse to use her professional skills in providing the most effective holistic care possible.

2. Which of the following is a type of unintentional tort?
    A.   Invasion of privacy
    B.   Malpractice
    C.   Assault and battery
    D.   Defamation of character

Answer: B. Unintentional torts include negligence and malpractice. Intentional torts include invasion of privacy, fraud, assault and battery, false imprisonment, and defamation of character.

3. The Patient Self-Determination Act of 1990 states that:
    A.   all hospitalized patients must have an advance directive.
    B.   hospitals must make information about advance directives available to all patients.
    C.   it's the responsibility of the doctor to obtain information about advance directives.
    D.   patients may have only a living will or a durable power of attorney for health care, not both.

Answer: B. This act requires hospitals and many other institutions to make information about advance directives available to patients. However, patients aren't required to have an advance directive.

4. Which part of the medical record can be used as evidence in court?
    A.   Entire record
    B.   Medical orders
    C.   Care plan
    D.   Nursing notes

Answer: A. The entire medical record is a legal document that's admissible in court.

Scoring

☆☆☆ If you answered all four questions correctly, bravo! Your understanding of ethics is beyond reproach.

☆☆ If you answered three questions correctly, way to go! You've judged correctly on most legal issues in this chapter.

☆ If you answered fewer than three questions correctly, don't fret! It isn't grounds for malpractice. Review the chapter, and try again.

4

Nursing process

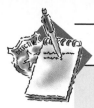

Just the facts

In this chapter, you'll learn:

♦ guidelines for performing an assessment based on the nursing process

♦ methods for formulating a nursing diagnosis

♦ ways to write nursing care plans with expected outcomes and appropriate interventions

♦ how to evaluate and document nursing interventions and outcomes.

A look at the nursing process

The nursing process is a problem-solving approach to nursing care. It's a systematic method for determining the patient's health problems, devising a plan to address them, implementing the plan, and evaluating the effectiveness of the care provided.

The nursing process emerged in the 1960s as team health care came into wider practice and nurses were increasingly called upon to define their specific roles. The roots of the nursing process can be traced to World War II, however, when technology, medical advances, and a growing need for nurses began to change the nursing profession.

Going through the phases

The nursing process consists of six distinct phases:

 assessment

 nursing diagnosis

 outcome identification

planning care

    implementation

evaluation.

These six phases are dynamic, and they commonly overlap. Together, they resemble similar steps that many other professionals take to identify and correct problems.

Assessment

The first step in the nursing process—assessment—begins when you first see the patient. According to the American Nurses Association guidelines, data should accurately reflect the patient's life experiences and his patterns of living. Assessment continues through the patient's care as you obtain more information about his changing condition.

Getting the whole picture

During assessment, you collect relevant information from various sources and analyze it to form a complete picture of your patient. As you collect this information, you need to document it accurately for two reasons:

It guides you through the rest of the nursing process, helping you formulate nursing diagnoses, expected outcomes, and nursing interventions.

It serves as a vital communication tool for other team members—as a baseline for evaluating a patient's progress and for use as legal documentation.

First impressions

In your initial assessment, consider the patient's immediate and emerging needs, including not only their physical needs but also the psychological, spiritual, and social concerns. Historical assessment is the most important part of the assessment. The physical assessment comes second. The questions you ask the patient about medications, health history, presentation, and reason for seeking health care are extremely important in the assessment. The initial assessment helps you determine what care the patient needs and sets the stage for further assessments. The inferences you make from your assessments help to guide the patient care you provide. Remember that a patient's family, culture, and religion are important factors in the patient's response to illness and treatment.

Assessment types

There are four types of assessments. When you use them depends on the clinical situation, the time available, the purpose of the data you need to collect, and the status of the patient.

Initial assessment

An initial, or admission, assessment occurs when the patient first comes to the health care facility. The initial assessment helps you determine what care the patient needs and sets the stage for further assessments. The most important item to find out at this stage is why the patient is seeking health care today. Get the story. Is the patient at the hospital for planned surgery or did the patient come through the emergency room (ER)? Gathering the background data is crucial.

Focus assessment

A focus assessment is used to collect data about a specific problem that has been identified. You must determine if the problem still exists and whether the status of the problem has changed by improving, worsening, or resolving.

Time-lapsed reassessment

Time-lapsed reassessment takes place after the initial assessment to evaluate changes in the client's functional health. Like the focus assessment, it's used to determine the status of already identified problems. It may involve periodic outpatient clinic visits, health developmental screenings, or home care visits.

Emergency assessment

An emergency assessment occurs during a life-threatening situation. Rapid identification of and interventions for the patient's health problem is foremost. These difficulties usually center around the patient's ABCs (airway, breathing, and circulation). An emergency assessment isn't a comprehensive assessment.

An emergency assessment usually focuses only on the basics. Remember your ABCs!

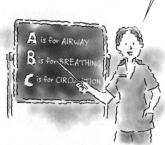

A is for AIRWAY
B is for BREATHING
C is for CIRCULATION

Health history

A health history includes physical, psychological, cultural, spiritual, and psychosocial data. It's the main source of information about the patient's health status and guides the physical examination that follows.

The history you collect helps you:
• plan health care by anticipating needs
• assess the impact of illness on the patient and members of their family
• evaluate the patient's health education needs
• initiate discharge planning.

Effective techniques

To obtain the most benefit from a health history interview, try to ensure that the patient feels comfortable and respected and believes they can trust you. Use effective interview techniques to help the patient identify resources and improve problem-solving abilities. Remember, however, that successful techniques in one situation may not be effective in another. Your attitude and the patient's interpretation of your questions can vary. In general, you should:
• allow the patient time to think and reflect
• encourage the patient to talk
• encourage the patient to describe a particular experience
• indicate that you've listened to the patient such by paraphrasing the patient's response.

Ask specific questions related to the patient's conditions and events. Ask specific questions about history of present illness and chief complaint. The patient should answer the question, "What brought you to seek health care today?"

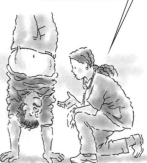

I think you might be a little more comfortable completing your health history in one of the chairs behind me.

Know right from wrong

Although there are many right ways to communicate with a patient, there are also some wrong ways that can hamper your interview. (See *Interview techniques to avoid.*)

Interview techniques to avoid

Some interview techniques cause problems between the nurse and patient. Avoid:
• asking "why" or "how" questions
• asking probing or persistent questions
• using inappropriate language
• giving advice

• giving false reassurance
• changing the subject or interrupting
• using clichés or stereotypical responses
• giving excessive approval or agreement
• jumping to conclusions
• using defensive responses.

Conducting the interview

The physical surroundings, psychological atmosphere, interview structure, and questioning style can all affect the interview flow and outcome. So can your ability to adopt a communication style that fits your patient's needs and the situation at hand. To enhance the interviewing process, close the door to help prevent interruptions and try to arrange yourself so that you're facing the patient, slightly offset from them, to create a friendly feeling.

Start at the very beginning

Begin by introducing yourself. Establish an interview time frame, and ask whether the patient has questions about the interview procedure. Spend a few minutes chatting informally before beginning the interview.

A note on notes

Lengthy note taking may distract the patient, who may wonder whether you're listening. If you must take notes, tell the patient before the interview starts. Finish the interview by summarizing salient interview points, telling the patient the interview results, explaining how the physical assessment will be conducted, and discussing follow-up plans.

Short and sweet

A patient who's ill, experiencing pain, or sedated may have difficulty completing the health history. In such instances, obtain only the information pertaining to the immediate problem. To avoid tiring a seriously ill patient, obtain the history in several sessions or ask a close family relative or friend to supply essential information. However, because of Health Insurance Portability and Accountability Act (HIPAA) policies, personal information cannot be disclosed to family members or friends without the express consent of the patient.

> Lengthy note taking may distract the patient or make them wonder whether you're listening.

Two types

Typically, the health history includes two types of questions: open-ended, which permit more subtle and flexible responses, and closed-ended, which require only a yes-or-no response. Open-ended questions usually result in the most useful information and give patients the feeling that they're actively participating in and have some control over the interview. Closed-ended questions help eliminate rambling conversations. They're also useful when the interview requires brevity—for example, when a patient reports extreme pain or digresses frequently.

Logical and patient

Whatever question type you use, move logically from one history section to the next. Allow the patient to concentrate and give complete information on a subject before moving on.

Obtaining health history data

There are two sources of data: primary and secondary. The patient is the source of primary data. These data are considered the most reliable unless circumstances prevent you from obtaining information directly from the patient, as when the patient has an altered level of consciousness, impending surgery, or severe pain. The patient would also be an unreliable source if he's confused or suffers from a mental condition that alters thinking, judgment, and memory.

Secondary sources provide information that supports, validates, clarifies, and supplements the information gathered from the patient. These sources include family members or significant others, laboratory results, the health care record, diagnostic procedures, and health team members.

Biographic data

Begin obtaining the patient's health history by collecting personal information. This data section identifies the patient and provides important demographic information. By filling out a form, you usually gather such facts as the patient's address, telephone number, age, sex, birth date, Social Security number, place of birth, race, nationality, marital status, occupation, education, religion, cultural background, and emergency contact person.

Health and illness patterns

Health and illness patterns include the patient's chief complaint; current, past, and family health history; status of physiologic systems; and developmental considerations.

Mind his P's and Q's

Determine why the patient is seeking health care by asking, "What brings you here today?" If the patient has specific symptoms, record that information in the patient's own words. Ask the patient with a specific symptom or health concern to describe the problem in detail, including the suspected cause. To ensure that you don't omit pertinent data, use the PQRSTU mnemonic device,

Memory jogger

PQRSTU: What's the story?

Use the **PQRSTU** mnemonic device to fully explore your patient's chief complaint. When you ask the questions below, you'll encourage him to describe his symptoms in greater detail.

Provocative or Palliative	Quality or Quantity	Region or Radiation	Severity	Timing	Understanding
Ask the patient: • What provokes or relieves the symptom? • Do stress, anger, certain physical positions, or other things trigger the symptom? • What makes the symptom worsen or subside?	Ask the patient: • What does the symptom feel like, look like, or sound like? • Are you having the symptom right now? If so, is it more or less severe than usual? • To what degree does the symptom affect your normal activities?	Ask the patient: • Where in the body does the symptom occur? • Does the symptom appear in other regions? If so, where?	Ask the patient: • How severe is the symptom? How would you rate it on a scale of 1 to 10, with 10 being the most severe? • Does the symptom seem to be diminishing, intensifying, or staying the same?	Ask the patient: • When did the symptom begin? • Was the onset sudden or gradual? • How often does the symptom occur? • How long does the symptom last?	Ask the patient: • What do you think caused the symptom? • How do you feel about the symptom? Do you have fears associated with it? • How is the symptom affecting your life? • What are your expectations from the health care team?

which provides a systematic approach to obtaining information. (See *PQRSTU: What's the story?*)

Think back

Document from the history, childhood and other illnesses, injuries, previous hospitalizations, surgical procedures, immunizations, allergies, and medications taken regularly.

Tell me about your mother

Information about the patient's relatives can also unmask potential health problems. Some diseases, such as cardiovascular disease, alcoholism, depression, and cancer, may be genetically linked. Others, such as hemophilia, cystic fibrosis, sickle cell anemia, and Tay-Sachs disease, are genetically transmitted.

Genogram . . . and grandpa, too

Determine the general health status of the patient's immediate family members, including maternal and paternal grandparents, siblings, aunts, uncles, and children. If they're deceased, record the year and cause of death. Use a genogram to organize family history data. Information about the patient's past and current physiologic status (also called *review of systems*) is another health history component. A careful assessment helps identify potential or undetected physiologic disorders. (See *Developing a genogram*.)

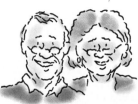

Don't forget about us! Remember, it's all in the family.

Developing a genogram

A genogram provides a visual family health summary. It includes the patients and their spouse, children, and parents. To develop a genogram, first draw the relationships of family members to the patient, as shown, and then fill in the ages of living members and note deceased members and the ages at which they died. Also record diseases that have a familial tendency (such as Huntington's chorea) or an environmental cause (such as lung cancer from exposure to coal tar).

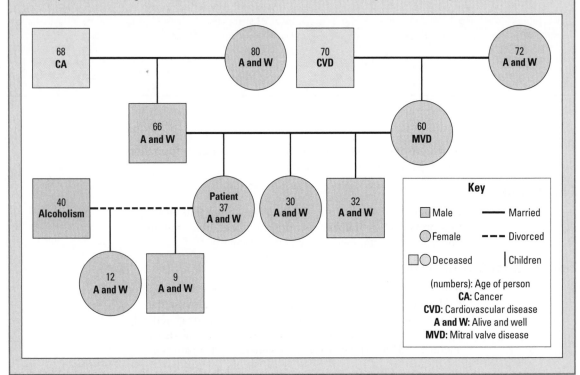

There are times when there is not enough time for a genogram such as in an emergent situation. If this is the case, the nurse must focus on family questioning based on the patient's reason for hospitalization. For example, if a patient presents in the ER with cardiac chest pain as a 40-year-old man, it would be pertinent for the nurse to ask about any family member who may have suffered heart attacks.

Physical examination

The second half of the assessment process involves performing a physical examination. Use the following techniques to conduct the examination:
- inspection
- palpation
- percussion
- auscultation.

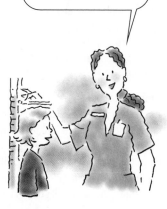

Don't forget . . . besides measuring height and weight and taking vital signs, you'll need to review major body systems.

There is one exception to this rule—abdominal assessment. With this assessment, auscultation comes before palpation and percussion. Think . . . look . . . listen . . . and feel.

The objective data that you gather during the physical examination may be used to confirm or rule out health problems that were suggested or suspected during the health history. You rely on these findings when you develop a care plan and when you conduct patient teaching. For example, if the patient's blood pressure is high, they may need a sodium-restricted diet and instruction on how to control hypertension.

It's in the details

How detailed should your examination be? That depends on the patient's condition, the clinical setting, and the policies and procedures established by your health care facility. The main components of the physical examination include:
- height
- weight
- vital signs
- review of the major body systems. (See *Rapid review of the physical assessment*.)

Rapid review of the physical assessment

During a physical examination, your main task is to record the patient's height, weight, and vital signs and review the major body systems. Here's a typical body system review for an adult patient.

Respiratory system

Note the rate and rhythm of respirations, and auscultate the lung fields. Watch for flaring or retractions as the patient breathes. Inspect the lips, mucous membranes, and nail beds. Also inspect the sputum, noting color, consistency, and other characteristics. If the patient has a cough, always distinguish whether the cough is productive. If not, make a notation that it is a dry cough. Some medications have dry cough as a side effect so this information may be of importance.

Cardiovascular system

Note the color and temperature of the extremities, and assess the peripheral pulses. Check for edema and hair loss on the extremities. Inspect the neck veins, and auscultate for heart sounds. Assess for regularity of apical pulse.

Neurologic system

Assess the patient's level of consciousness, noting his orientation to time, place, and person and his ability to follow commands. Assess pupillary reaction and accommodation (pupils equal, round, reactive to light, and accommodation [PERRLA]). Check the extremities for movement and sensation. Check strength of grip bilaterally.

Eyes, ears, nose, and throat

Assess the patient's ability to see objects with and without corrective lenses. Assess his ability to hear spoken words clearly. Inspect the eyes and ears for discharge and the nasal mucous membranes for dryness, irritation, and blood. Inspect the teeth, gums, and condition of the oral mucous membranes, and palpate the lymph nodes in the neck.

GI system

Auscultate for bowel sounds in all quadrants. Note abdominal distention or ascites. Gently palpate the abdomen for tenderness. Note whether the abdomen is soft, hard, or distended. Assess the condition of the mucous membranes around the anus. Practice tip: It is important to ask if the patient has pain prior to starting abdominal assessment. Assess that area last to avoid guarding through the entire assessment. Ask patient to empty the bladder prior to abdominal assessment.

Musculoskeletal system

Assess the range of motion of major joints. Look for swelling at the joints, contractures, muscle atrophy, or obvious deformity. Assess muscle strength of the trunk and extremities. Assess posture and gait.

Genitourinary and reproductive systems

Note any bladder distention or incontinence. If indicated, inspect the genitalia for rashes, edema, or deformity. (Inspection of the genitalia may be waived at the patient's request or if no dysfunction was reported during the interview.) If indicated, inspect the genitalia for sexual maturity. Also examine the breasts, noting any abnormalities. With history, it is important to ask about patient's current sexual activity. Any adult patient, regardless of age or marital status should be asked especially if the answer would affect treatment. In some instances, patients younger than the age of 18 may be asked about sexual issues.

Integumentary system

Note any sores, lesions, scars, pressure ulcers, rashes, bruises, discoloration, or petechiae. Also note the patient's skin turgor.

Nursing diagnosis

The North American Nursing Diagnosis Association (NANDA) defines nursing diagnosis as a "clinical judgment about individual, family, or community responses to actual or potential health problems of life processes. Nursing diagnoses provide the basis for the selection of nursing interventions to achieve outcomes for which the nurse is accountable." The nursing diagnoses need to be individualized for each patient, based on the patient's medical condition and the medications he's receiving.

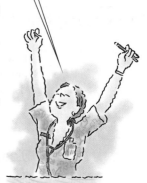

Thank you, NANDA! You make my job that much easier!

Identifying the problem

After clustering significant assessment data and analyzing the pattern, your next step is to label the patient's actual and potential health problems. NANDA has developed a taxonomic scheme to help you do this.

Identify, diagnose, and validate

In forming a nursing diagnosis, you'll identify the patient's problem, write a diagnostic statement, and validate the diagnosis. You'll establish several nursing diagnoses for each patient. Arrange the diagnoses according to priority so that you address the patient's most crucial problems first.

Writing the diagnostic statement

The diagnostic statement consists of a nursing diagnosis and the etiology (cause) related to it. For example, a diagnostic statement for a patient who's too weak to bathe himself properly might be *Bathing or hygiene self-care deficit related to weakness*. A diagnostic statement related to the actual problem might be *Impaired gas exchange related to pulmonary edema*. A statement related to a potential problem might be *Risk for injury related to unsteady gait*.

Stress present, balance absent

The etiology is a stressor or something that brings about a response, effect, or change. A stressor results from the pressure of a stress agent or the absence of an equilibrium factor. Causative agents may include birth defects, inherited factors, diseases, injuries, signs or symptoms, psychosocial factors, iatrogenic factors, developmental phases, lifestyle, or situational or environmental factors.

Validating each diagnosis

Next, validate the diagnosis. Review clustered data. Are they consistent? Does the patient verify the diagnosis? When using a risk for diagnosis, there is no physical data for the diagnosis but it still can be verified—for example, Risk for falls related to weakness. The person cannot have a history of falls because then that would be an actual problem. The risk for indicates that we are watching for the issue and want to avoid it.

Prioritizing the diagnosis

After you've established several nursing diagnoses, categorize them in order of priority. Obviously, life-threatening problems must be addressed first followed by health-threatening concerns. Also, consider how the patient perceives their health problems; their priority problem may differ from yours. In addition, as the patient condition changes, his or her priorities will change.

Maslow's hierarchy

One system of categorizing diagnoses uses Maslow's hierarchy of needs, which classifies human needs based on the idea that lower level, physiologic needs must be met before higher level, abstract needs. For example, if a patient has shortness of breath, they probably aren't interested in discussing relationships. However, as the person improves, the day before discharge, the person may have no issues breathing and their main concern at that point may be the relationship with their daughter.

Planning

After you establish the nursing diagnosis, you'll develop a written care plan. A written care plan serves as a communication tool among health care team members that helps ensure continuity of care. The plan consists of two parts:

patient outcomes or expected outcomes, which describe behaviors or results to be achieved within a specified time frame nursing interventions needed to achieve those outcomes.

Measure and observe

Be sure to state both parts of the care plan in measurable, observable terms and dates. The statement, "The patient will perceive themselves with greater self-worth" is too vague, lacks a time frame, and offers no means to observe the patient's self-perception. A patient outcome such as, "The patient will describe themselves in a positive way within 1 week" provides an observable means to evaluate the patient's behavior and a time frame for the behavioral change. (See *Ensuring a successful care plan*.)

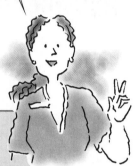

Remember, a nursing care plan contains two important parts: measurable, achievable outcomes and specific interventions for effecting change and achieving the stated outcomes.

Ensuring a successful care plan

Your care plan must rest on a solid foundation of carefully chosen nursing diagnoses. It also must fit your patient's needs, age, developmental level, culture, strengths and weaknesses, and willingness and ability to take part in his care. Your plan should help the patient attain the highest functional level possible while posing minimal risk and not creating new problems. If complete recovery isn't possible, your plan should help the patient cope physically and emotionally with his impaired or declining health.

Using the following guidelines will help ensure that your care plan is effective.

Be realistic

Avoid setting a goal that's too difficult for the patient to achieve. The patient may become discouraged, depressed, and apathetic if they can't achieve expected outcomes. The goal needs to be something the patient can accomplish. An independent nursing goal should be avoided.

Tailor your approach

Individualize your outcome statements and nursing interventions. Keep in mind that each patient is unique; no two patient problems are exactly alike.

Avoid vague terms

Use precise, quantitative terms rather than vague ones. For example, if your patient is restless, describe their specific behavior, such as "pulls at restraints" rather than "patient uncooperative." To indicate that the patient's vital signs are stable, document specific measurements, such as "heart rate less than 100 beats/minute" rather than "heart rate stable."

Intervention options

Before you implement a care plan, review your intervention options and then weigh their potential to succeed. Determine whether you can obtain the necessary equipment and resources. If not, take steps to get what you need or change the intervention accordingly. Observe the patient's willingness to participate in the various interventions and be prepared to postpone or modify interventions, if necessary.

Implementation

The implementation phase is when you put your care plan into action. Implementation encompasses all nursing interventions (including drug therapy) directed at solving the patient's problems and meeting health care needs. While you coordinate implementation, you also seek help from the patient, the patient's family, and other caregivers.

Monitor and gauge

After implementing the care plan, continue to monitor the patient to gauge the effectiveness of interventions and adjust them as the patient's condition changes. Documentation of outcomes achieved should be reflected in the care plan. Expect to review, revise, and update the entire care plan regularly, according to facility policy. Keep in mind that the care plan is usually a permanent part of the patient's medical record. (See *Components of an outcome statement*, and *Writing excellent outcome statements*.)

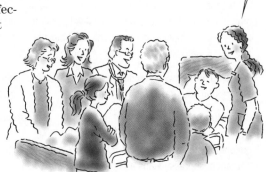

Now, I've got a job for you . . . and you . . . and you . . . and you. . . .

Take note!

Components of an outcome statement

An outcome statement consists of four elements: behavior, measurement, condition, and time.

 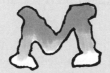

Behavior	**Measurement**	**Condition**	**Time**
A desired behavior for the patient; must be observable	Criteria for measuring the behavior; should specify how much, how long, how far, and so on	The conditions under which the behavior should occur	When the behavior should occur

The two outcome statements below include these four key components:

Ambulate	one flight of stairs	unassisted	by 02/12/06
Demonstrate	measuring radial pulse	before exercising	by 02/12/06

It is important to note that outcomes must represent behavior of the patient, not data about the patient. An outcome statement of "The patient's blood pressure will be 120/80 by the time of discharge" would be incorrect. The patient cannot do anything specific to directly control blood pressure. Instead, think about what behavior may help to regulate blood pressure over time.

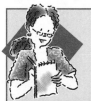

Take note!

Writing excellent outcome statements

These tips will help you write clear, precise outcome statements:
• When writing expected outcomes in your care plan, always start with a specific action verb that focuses on your patient's behavior. By telling your reader how your patient should *look, walk, eat, drink, turn, cough, speak,* or *stand,* for example, you give a clear picture of how to evaluate progress.
• Avoid starting expected outcome statements with *allow, let, enable,* or similar verbs. Such words focus attention on your own and other health care team members' behavior—not the patient's.
• With many documentation formats, you won't need to include the phrase *The patient will* with each expected outcome statement. However, you'll have to specify to which person the goals refer when family, friends, or others are directly involved.

Evaluation

After enough time has elapsed for the care plan to effect the desired changes, you're ready for evaluation, the final step in the nursing process. During evaluation, you must decide whether the interventions carried out have enabled the patient to achieve the desired outcomes. (See *Effective evaluation statements.*)

Start with the finish

Begin by reviewing the patient outcomes stated for each nursing diagnosis. Then observe your patient's behavioral changes, and judge how well they meet the outcomes related to them. Does the patient's behavior match the outcomes or fall short of them?

Consider the evaluation to be positive if the patient's behavior has changed as expected, if the outcomes have been accomplished, or if progress has occurred. Failure to meet these criteria constitutes a negative evaluation and requires new interventions.

A successful resolution

The evaluation phase also allows you to judge the effectiveness of the nursing process as a whole. If the process has been applied successfully, the patient's health status will improve. Their health

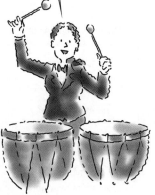

Ending with a big finish is my idea of a job well done!

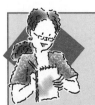

Take note!

Effective evaluation statements

These evaluation statements clearly describe common outcomes. Note that they include specific details of the care provided and objective evidence of the patient's response to care:

• Described the signs and symptoms of hyperglycemia (response to patient education)
• Stated leg pain decreased from 9 to 6 (on a scale of 1 to 10) 30 minutes after receiving I.V. hydromorphone (response to pain medication within 1 hour of administration)
• Ambulated to chair with a steady gait, approximately 10′ unassisted (tolerance of change or increase in activity)
• Unable to tolerate removal of O_2, became dyspneic on room air, even at rest (tolerance of treatments) goal not met

problems will have been solved, or progress will have been made toward achieving their resolution. They will also be able to perform self-care measures with a sense of independence and confidence, and you'll feel reassured that you've fulfilled your professional responsibility.

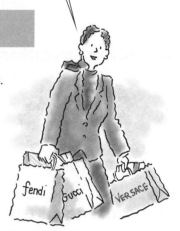

Did someone just mention shopping? Now that's a task I'm well-suited for!

Nursing care plans

The nursing care plan is a vital source of information about the patient's problems, needs, and goals. It contains detailed instructions for achieving the goals established for the patient and is used to direct care. (See *Tips for top-notch care plans*.)

Your patient's nursing care plan may be in one of two styles: *traditional* or *standardized*.

Tips for top-notch care plans

Use a traditional or standardized method for recording your care plan. A *traditional care plan* is written from scratch for each patient. A *standardized care plan* saves time because it's predetermined based on the patient's diagnosis.

No matter which method you use, follow these tips to write an accurate and useful plan:
• Write in ink, and sign your name.
• Use clear, concise language, not vague terms or generalities.
• Use standard abbreviations to avoid confusion.
• Review all your assessment data *before* selecting an approach for each problem; if you can't complete the initial assessment, immediately write *insufficient information* on your records.
• Write an expected outcome and a target date for each problem you identify.
• Set realistic initial goals.
• When writing nursing interventions, consider what to watch for and how often, what nursing

measures to take and how to perform them, and what to teach the patient and their family before discharge.
• Make each nursing intervention specific.
• Make sure your interventions match the staff's resources and capabilities.
• Be creative; include a drawing or an innovative procedure if doing so makes your directions more specific.
• Record all of the patient's problems and concerns so they won't be forgotten.
• Make sure your care plan is implemented correctly.
• Evaluate the results of your plan, and discontinue nursing diagnoses that have been resolved; select new approaches, if necessary, for problems that haven't been resolved.

Traditional care plan

The traditional care plan is written from scratch for each patient. Most have three main columns:

 nursing diagnoses

 expected outcomes

 interventions.

Documenting marathon

When using the traditional care plan, there may be other columns for the date when the care plan was initiated; target dates for expected outcomes; and the dates for review, revisions, and resolutions. Most forms also have a place for you to sign or initial whenever you make an entry or revision. Although this type of care plan allows you to individualize the care of each patient, it requires lengthy documentation.

Standardized care plan

More commonly, your patient will have a *standardized care plan* that's preprinted to save documentation time. Some standardized plans are classified by medical diagnosis; others, by nursing diagnosis.

Individualizing care plans

Even though these care plans are standardized, they allow you to individualize the plan for each of your patients by adding:

• *"related to" (R/T) statements and signs and symptoms for a nursing diagnosis.* If the form provides a root diagnosis, such as "Pain R/T _____," you might fill in "inflammation, as exhibited by grimacing and expressions of pain."

• *time limits for the outcomes to a root statement of the goal.* For example, to the statement "Perform postural drainage without assistance," you might add "for 15 minutes immediately upon awakening on the morning of 11/12."

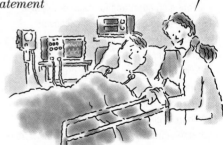

Using standardized care plans frees you up to spend more time caring for your patients—after all, isn't that why you chose to become a nurse in the first place?

Why stand on tradition? Use a standardized plan of care

The standardized care plan below is for a patient with a nursing diagnosis of *Impaired tissue integrity*. To customize it to your patient, complete the diagnosis—including signs and symptoms—and fill in the expected outcomes.

Date _2/15/06_   **Nursing diagnosis**
Impaired tissue integrity related to arterial insufficiency

Target date _2/17/06_   **Expected outcomes**
Attains relief from immediate symptoms: _pain, ulcers, edema_
Voices intent to change aggravating behavior: _will stop smoking immediately_
Maintains collateral circulation: _palpable peripheral pulses, extremities warm and pink with good capillary refill_
Voices intent to follow specific management routines after discharge: _foot care guidelines, exercise regimen as specified by physical therapy department_

> There's a lot less writing with standardized plans.

Date _2/15/06_   **Interventions**
• Provide foot care. Administer and monitor treatments according to facility protocols.
• Encourage adherence to an exercise regimen as tolerated.
• Educate the patient about risk factors and prevention of injury. Refer the patient to a stop-smoking program.
• Maintain adequate hydration. Monitor I/O _q8h._
• To increase arterial blood supply to the extremities, elevate head of bed _6" to 8"_
• Additional interventions: _inspect skin integrity q8h._

Date _____   **Outcomes evaluation**
Attained relief of immediate symptoms: _____
Voiced intent to change aggravating behavior: _____
Maintained collateral circulation: _____
Voiced intent to follow specific management routines after discharge: _____

• *frequency of interventions.* To an intervention, such as "Perform passive range-of-motion exercises," you might add "twice daily: 1× each morning and evening."
• *specific instructions for interventions.* For the standard intervention "Elevate patient's head," you might specify "before sleep, on three pillows." (See *Why stand on tradition? Use a standardized plan of care.*)

Concept mapping

Concept mapping is a way to show the flow of your critical thinking during patient care. Concept mapping allows your clinical instructor to see whether you understand the relationship between important concepts required to provide skillful care to your patient.

A big advantage of concept mapping over nursing care plans is that it requires much less writing time— something all nursing students need! Concept mapping also allows you to be creative and to individualize patient care.

> Instructors use concept mapping as one creative way to test their students' critical thinking skills. Do you think this is what they had in mind?

Developing a concept map

When developing a concept map, don't be too concerned about putting ideas in the "wrong" places. It's more important to write the idea down. The beauty of a concept map is that it allows the student to tell the entire story of the patient rather than focus on 1 to 3 nursing diagnoses. Concept maps allow students to see the big picture when caring for patients.

A fresh start

To develop a concept map, start with a clean sheet of paper. Some students prefer unlined paper and colored pencils or pens to promote creative thinking. Then follow these steps:

After you've assessed your patient, place a box representing the patient in the middle of your paper. In this box, write the patient's medical diagnosis or chief complaint. Be brief! By placing the patient in the center of the page, your focus is clearly patient-centered.

Write the major problems or nursing diagnoses in boxes surrounding the patient with the pertinent supporting data.

Use lines to connect the patient to the nursing diagnoses. Think along the lines of concepts. Perfusion, oxygenation, mobility, nutrition, and pain are some examples. Lines may also be drawn between related nursing diagnoses. For example, for a postoperative patient experiencing constipation caused by use of opioid analgesics, you would draw a line between the nursing diagnoses of *Acute pain* and *Constipation* to show that you understand that they're related.

👋   Prioritize each nursing diagnosis by numbering the boxes.

👋   Write expected outcomes for each nursing diagnosis; place each outcome in its own box because corresponding interventions will be different for each outcome. Connect these boxes by lines to the appropriate nursing diagnoses.

👋✍️   In the same manner, write interventions in a box for each outcome, followed by evaluations. Draw lines between each part of the nursing process to show concepts that are related.

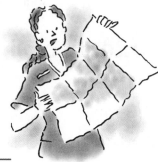

Try to keep your concept map to one page to make it easier to use. Yikes!

A job well done!

Your concept map is complete—for now. You'll need to continually update it throughout the clinical day.

Using a concept map

Use the concept map during your clinical day to guide your patient care. Carry it in your pocket or on your clipboard so you can refer to it often. Keeping it to one page will make it easier to

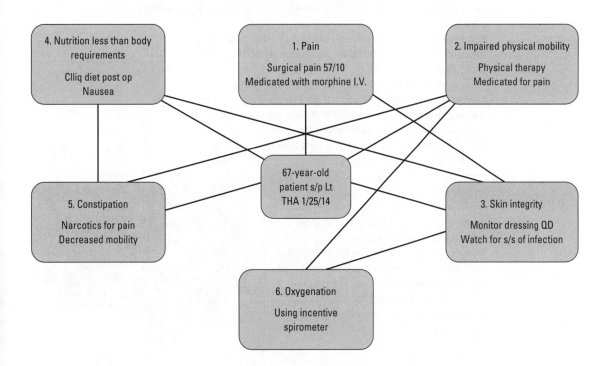

4. Nutrition less than body requirements

Clliq diet post op
Nausea

1. Pain

Surgical pain 57/10
Medicated with morphine I.V.

2. Impaired physical mobility

Physical therapy
Medicated for pain

67-year-old patient s/p Lt THA 1/25/14

5. Constipation

Narcotics for pain
Decreased mobility

3. Skin integrity

Monitor dressing QD
Watch for s/s of infection

6. Oxygenation

Using incentive spirometer

use. Make notes directly on the concept map to update and revise it as necessary.

Your instructor may have you take out the concept map to discuss patient care concepts. For example, you can use the concept map to explain the relationships between incentive spirometers and respiratory assessment findings in your postoperative patient. The concept map allows you to see relationships more clearly at a glance. These also allow you to correlate the patient presentation with the pathophysiology, laboratory data, and medications.

Interdisciplinary team

Nurses aren't the only health care professionals involved in patient care. You'll need to collaborate with an interdisciplinary team to meet the diverse needs of your patients.

Share and share alike

The focus of an interdisciplinary team is on the patient and patient outcomes. Each team member shares responsibility for achieving these outcomes. To provide more effective and comprehensive care, you need to understand each team member's role.

Members of the health care team include the:
• *registered dietitian*, who assesses and monitors nutritional needs, makes nutritional recommendations, and provides patient education
• *social worker*, who provides support and counseling to patients and their families and helps with financial difficulties
• *occupational therapist*, who assists the patient in performing activities of daily living, participating in recreation, and working to their highest functional level
• *physical therapist*, who provides therapy to improve or restore physical functioning and prevent deconditioning
• *respiratory therapist*, who monitors and provides airway management
• *pastoral care specialist*, who provides spiritual and religious support to patients and their families
• *pharmacist*, who reviews, prepares, and dispenses the patient's medications; provides information and guidance in the preparation and administration of medications; and provides patient education.

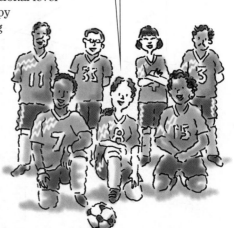

Interdisciplinary teamwork gets the job done!

Passing notes is permitted!

When you're reviewing the patient's chart, be sure to read the progress notes written by other members of the health care team. These notes will provide you with important information about your patient.

If you have questions about the patient's condition or treatment, contact the appropriate team members for more information. For example, the pharmacist can provide information about how to space medications to eliminate drug or food interactions, whereas the physical therapist can provide guidelines on how to transfer a patient with fractures safely from the bed to a chair.

Play well with others

You'll also need to coordinate care with other team members. For example, medicating your postoperative patient before respiratory exercises helps the patient cough and deep-breathe more effectively with the respiratory therapist. When working with the other team members, remember to use good communication skills. Above all, treat all team members with respect, and they'll respect you in turn!

> Thanks for reviewing the patient's meds and breathing exercises with me. It's so busy today. I appreciate your taking the time!

Reference

Cook, L. K., Dover, C., Dickson, M., & Colton, D. L. (2012). From care plan to concept map: A paradigm shift. *Teaching & Learning in Nursing*, 7(3), 88–92.

Quick quiz

1. When obtaining a health history from a patient, ask first about:
   A.   his chief complaint.
   B.   biographic data.
   C.   family history.
   D.   health insurance coverage.

Answer: B. Take care of the biographic data first; otherwise, you might get involved in the patient history and forget to ask basic questions.

2. Expected outcomes are defined as:
 A.   goals the patient should reach as a result of planned nursing interventions.
 B.   goals set by the medical team for each patient.
 C.   goals a little higher than what the patient can realistically reach to help motivate them.
 D.   what a patient and family ask you to accomplish.

Answer: A. Expected outcomes are realistic, measurable goals and their target dates.

3. The primary source of assessment information is:
 A.   the patient's friends.
 B.   the patient's family members.
 C.   the patient.
 D.   medical records.

Answer: C. The patient should be your primary source of assessment information. However, if the patient is sedated, confused, hostile, angry, dyspneic, or in pain, you may have to rely initially on family members or close friends to supply information.

4. What are the three components to a proper patient outcome?
 A.   Realistic, nurse centered, optimistic
 B.   Realistic, time oriented, measurable
 C.   Patient centered, realistic, vague
 D.   Patient centered, realistic, optimistic

Answer: B. A patient outcome should always be patient centered, realistic, measurable, and time oriented.

Scoring

✩✩✩ If you answered all four questions correctly, super! You're a nursing process pro.

✩✩   If you answered three questions correctly, great! You've got the nursing process pretty down pat.

✩   If you answered fewer than three questions correctly, chin up! Process this chapter one more time and try again.

Part II   General nursing skills

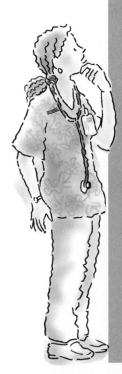

5

Communication

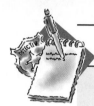

Just the facts

In this chapter, you'll learn:

♦ verbal and nonverbal methods of communication

♦ the phases of a therapeutic relationship

♦ how to incorporate therapeutic use of self

♦ how to identify and handle communication barriers

♦ the importance of communication in documenting patient care.

A look at communication

What is communication? Communication is a way to fulfill a person's basic need to relate to others. Communication is dynamic and ongoing and is a way to interact and develop relationships. It's also a way to effect change.

Nurses encounter many people during the course of their education and nursing career. They communicate with educators, patients, family members, and other members of the health care team. Learning to communicate effectively is a skill that sometimes takes time and effort.

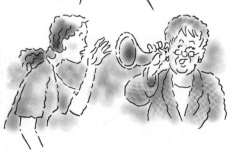

I said, "Learning to communicate effectively is a skill."

Jeez. You don't have to shout. Where'd you learn your skills? A barnyard?

Verbal communication

Verbal communication is the transmission of messages through spoken or written language. For effective verbal communication, six criteria must be met:

 simplicity

 clarity

 timing and relevance

 adaptability

 credibility

 hostile-free patterns of communication.

Simplicity

In verbal communication, you must state complex information in commonly understood terms. This is especially important when communicating with patients. For instance, when explaining a procedure to the patient, you must be careful to use the most appropriate terminology that the patient will understand. Use short sentences that express the idea completely. Long explanations are sometimes difficult for people to understand because the context of the explanation gets lost.

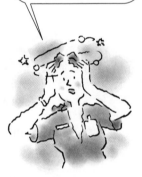

I'm sorry. Your explanation was so long and convoluted, you lost me at "Listen up!"

Avoiding the void

Avoid using medical terminology. For instance, when asking a patient whether they needs to use the bathroom facilities, the patient won't understand, "Do you have to void?" They will better understand what you mean if you ask them if they have to urinate or go to the bathroom.

Clarity

Verbal communication must be clear. You should state exactly what you mean. Communicate in a respectful manner to maintain a hostile-free environment. Don't make the listener guess what you mean or make assumptions.

Say what you mean

For instance, if you're explaining a medication regimen to a patient who has never taken medicine before, don't tell them they must take the medication four times per day. You must be clear and tell them exactly how many hours should elapse before taking the medication.

Timing and relevance

Make sure that the message is communicated at a time when the receiver is ready to receive it. If your patient is in pain, don't try to explain a procedure or do patient teaching. They will be more receptive when the pain subsides.

Score one for format!

Ensure that the message is communicated in an appropriate format. If your patient has trouble visualizing what you're saying, try using written materials or diagrams to complement your verbal explanation to help them to understand better.

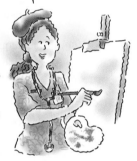

Maybe I can paint a better picture of the procedure this way. Do you prefer watercolors or pastels?

Adaptability

Communication that's effective is adaptable and states the message that reflects the situation. For instance, as you prepare your teaching plan, you may need to adapt the way you communicate if the patient is hearing or visually impaired or speaks another language.

That suits me just fine

Verbal communication also shows appropriateness to the receiver. If the patient is a young child or an infant, it may be necessary to communicate with the parents or guardian instead of the child.

Credibility

In order for communication to be credible, it must be stated in a trustworthy and believable manner.

Honestly now!

It must also be accurate, consistent, and honest. Before you communicate with someone, make sure that you know the content area. Communication commonly spurs continued conversation, so be prepared and well versed in your subject in order to be able to answer any question that arises. If you're asked to explain information that's beyond your scope of practice or your ability, you must be honest with the patient and tell them that you can't answer their question. Explain, however, that you'll convey their concerns to someone who'll be able to answer them.

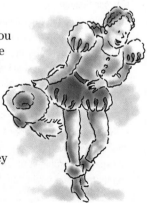

"...and it must follow, as the night the day, thou canest not then be false to any man"...
Actually, I honestly don't know the answer!

Verbal communication strategies

Verbal communication strategies range from alternating between open-ended and closed questions to employing such techniques as silence, facilitation, confirmation, reflection, clarification, summary, and conclusion.

An open . . .

Asking open-ended questions such as "How did you fall?" lets the patient respond more freely. The response may provide answers to many other questions. For instance, from the patient's answer, you might learn that they have fallen previously, that they were unsteady on their feet before they fell, and that they fell just before eating dinner. Armed with this information, you might deduce that the patient had a syncopal episode caused by hypoglycemia.

. . . and shut case

You may also choose to ask closed questions. Although these questions are unlikely to provide extra information, they may encourage the patient to give clear, concise feedback. (See *Two ways to ask.*)

Silence is golden

Another technique is to allow moments of silence during the interview. In addition to encouraging the patient to continue talking,

---

Two ways to ask

Questions can be characterized as *open-ended* or *closed*.

Open-ended questions

Open-ended questions require the patient to express feelings, opinions, and ideas. They also help you gather more information than can otherwise be gathered with closed questions. Open-ended questions encourage a good nurse–patient relationship because they show that you're interested in what the patient has to say. Examples of such questions include:
• "Why did you come to the hospital tonight?"
• "How would you describe the problems you're having with your breathing?"
• "What lung problems, if any, do other members of your family have?"

Closed questions

Closed questions elicit "yes" or "no" answers or one- or two-word responses. They limit the development of the nurse–patient relationship. Although closed questions can help you "zoom in" on specific points, they don't provide the patient with an opportunity to elaborate. Examples of closed questions include:
• "Do you ever get short of breath?"
• "Are you the only one in your family with lung problems?"

this technique also gives you a chance to assess his ability to organize thoughts. You may find this technique difficult (as most people are uncomfortable with silence), but the more often you use it, the more comfortable you'll become.

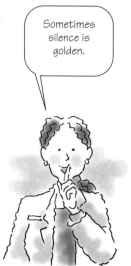

Sometimes silence is golden.

Give 'em a boost

Using such phrases as "please continue," "go on," and even "uh-huh" encourages the patient to continue with their story. Known as *facilitation*, this feedback shows them that you're interested in what they are saying.

Confirmation conversation

Employing the technique of confirmation helps ensure that you and the patient are on the same track. You might say, "If I understand you correctly, you said," and then repeat the information the patient gave. Doing so helps to clear up misconceptions that you or the patient might have.

Check and reflect

Try using reflection—repeating something the patient has just said—to help you obtain more specific information. For example, a patient with a stomachache might say, "I know I have an ulcer." If so, you can repeat, "You know you have an ulcer?" Then the patient might say, "Yes. I had one before, and the pain is the same."

Squawk! I know I have an ulcer!

You know you have an ulcer?

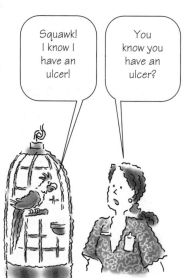

Clear skies

When information is vague or confusing, use the technique of clarification. For example, if your patient says, "I can't stand this," your response might be, "What can't you stand?" or "What do you mean by 'I can't stand this'?" Doing so gives the patient an opportunity to explain their statement.

Put the landing gear down . . .

Get in the habit of restating the information the patient gave you. Known as *summarization*, this technique ensures that the data you've collected are accurate and complete. Summarization also signals that the interview is about to end.

. . . and come in for a safe landing

Signal the patient when you're ready to conclude the interview. This signal gives them the opportunity to gather thoughts and make any pertinent final statements. You can do this by saying, "I think I have all the information I need now. Is there anything you would like to add?"

Nonverbal communication

Nonverbal communication transmits messages without using words. It's commonly referred to as *body language*. Nonverbal communication includes facial expressions, posture, gait, hand gestures, tone of voice, positioning and space, touch, appearance, and level of alertness. Nonverbal communication can convey feelings of sadness, joy, and anxiety. It reflects self-concept, current mood, and health.

> Nonverbal communication transmits messages without using words.

Mixed messages

Nonverbal communication not only aids interpretation of verbal communication but also requires acute observation by the receiver for accurate interpretation of the message. For instance, your patient may state that the pain has subsided, but you notice that they are guarded and clenching the side rails on the bed. Verbal communication tells you one thing, but nonverbal actions reveal something else.

Nonverbal communication strategies

To make the most of nonverbal communication, do the following:
• Listen attentively and make eye contact frequently. (See *Overcoming cultural barriers*.)
• Use reassuring gestures, such as nodding your head, to encourage the patient to keep talking.
• Watch for nonverbal clues that indicate the patient is uncomfortable or unsure about how to answer a question. For example, they might lower their voice or glance around uneasily.
• Be aware of your own nonverbal behaviors that might cause the patient to stop talking or become defensive. For example, if you cross your arms, you might appear closed off from them. If you stand while they are sitting, you might appear superior.

Overcoming cultural barriers

To maintain a good relationship with your patient, remember that their cultural behaviors and beliefs may differ from your own. For example, most people in the United States make eye contact when talking with others. However, people in several other cultures, including Native Americans, Asians, and people from Arabic-speaking countries, may find eye contact disrespectful or aggressive.

If you glance at your watch, you might appear to be bored or rushed, which could keep the patient from answering questions completely.

• Observe the patient closely to see whether he understands each question. If they do not appear to understand, repeat the question using different words or familiar examples. For instance, instead of asking, "Did you have respiratory difficulty after exercising?" ask, "Did you have to sit down after walking around the block?"

Therapeutic relationships

A therapeutic relationship occurs when you interact with a patient in a clinical setting. This interaction is the beginning of the nurse–patient relationship.

The building process

The nurse–patient relationship doesn't just happen; it's created with care and skill and built on the patient's trust of the nurse and on the nurses' respect of the patient. The building process follows a natural progression of four distinct phases:

 pre-interaction

 orientation

 working

 termination.

Pre-interaction phase

During the pre-interaction phase, you can review the patient data that you might already have, such as the medical or surgical history and information gained from family members. If at all possible, after reviewing this information, try to anticipate any concerns or issues that might arise.

> Do your best to make a good first impression by remaining warm, open, and attentive to the patient's needs.

Orientation phase

Orientation is the stage when you first meet the patient. More than likely, it will occur at the bedside when the patient is admitted. This time is the best time for you to talk to the patient and get to know them. However, the meeting commonly isn't leisurely or controlled—especially if the patient is in the emergency department, in pain, or apprehensive. Even in difficult situations, though, you must use your verbal and nonverbal communication skills to ease the patient's fears and begin the relationship.

First impressions

During the orientation phase, the patient will be forming a first impression of your meeting. They will be watching you closely and forming an opinion about your interest in their health care. By presenting a warm, caring manner, you'll make this first impression, one that helps build a good nurse–patient relationship.

Trust building

Trust building is a very important part of the therapeutic relationship you develop with the patient. If the patient doesn't trust you, they won't be open and answer your questions. Take time to sit down with them. Close the curtain so that they feel they have your undivided attention. Sit down in a chair so they do not feel that you're in a hurry to leave. Also, act with integrity so that the patient can develop confidence in you and your abilities.

Role clarification

Patients are becoming increasingly knowledgeable about their bodies. They have access to a wealth of information today via the Internet, newspapers, and magazines. As patients learn more about how to stay healthy, they're taking a more active role in their health care. You must recognize this role and respect it. Patients' growing involvement in their own health care is helping to change the approach of many health care professionals from the authoritarian "Do as I say" attitude to the more cooperative "Here's why I recommend this" approach.

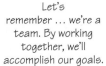

Let's remember ... we're a team. By working together, we'll accomplish our goals.

Sign here

As you begin to develop the therapeutic relationship with your patient, you develop a contract with them that's built on trust and your mutual desire to see that he receives the treatment they need.

Working phase

The working phase is a team-building phase that includes you, the patient, and the entire health care team. During this phase, you encourage the patient and help them to understand their condition and how to set goals. Using therapeutic communication, you encourage the patient to accomplish his goals.

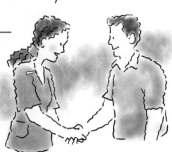

Give and take

This phase is a give-and-take phase because you and the patient have specific roles to play and certain expectations of what will happen during the relationship. You, as the nurse, expect the patient to be willing to participate in their health care by providing accurate information, asking questions about treatments, and participating in treatment procedures as appropriate. The patient, on the other hand, expects that their health care needs will be met by you and the other members of the health care team. They expect you, as the health care advocate, to keep them informed and provide them with the correct treatments and procedures.

Termination phase

As you near the termination phase, you must remind the patient that the termination of the relationship is near. You can do so simply by saying good-bye at the end of your shift. However, termination can be more complex and include discharge planning. At the same time, you may also be paving the way for more relationships to develop with the patient's health care team as you make necessary referrals for home care nurse visits and rehabilitation.

Smooth sailing

By making the termination phase an easy one, you achieve a smooth transition for the patient to other health care team members.

Therapeutic use of self

Using interpersonal skills in a healing way to help the patient is called *therapeutic use of self*. Three important techniques enhance therapeutic use of self:

 exhibiting empathy

 demonstrating acceptance

 giving recognition.

Path to empathy

To show empathy, use phrases that address the patient's feelings, such as "That must have upset you."

Acceptance acts

To show acceptance, use neutral statements, such as "I hear what you're saying" and "I see." Nonverbal

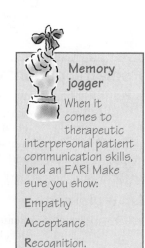

Memory jogger

When it comes to therapeutic interpersonal patient communication skills, lend an EAR! Make sure you show:

Empathy

Acceptance

Recognition.

behaviors, such as nodding or making momentary eye contact, also provide encouragement without indicating agreement or disagreement.

I recognize that

To give recognition, listen actively to what the patient says, occasionally providing verbal or nonverbal acknowledgment to encourage him to continue speaking.

Blocks to communication

Various factors contribute to the communication process and directly affect a person's ability to send and receive messages. In some cases, a patient's special needs can be a deterrent to effective communication. However, these needs shouldn't be an excuse for failing to find alternative ways to promote communication. As a nurse, you need to understand which factors influence communication so that you can clear away any barriers. (See *Considering communication barriers*.)

Don't let communication barriers get in your way. There's always another route around a difficult situation.

Not so obvious

Communication barriers such as speaking another language and being hearing or speaking impaired are obvious communication barriers but aren't insurmountable. What about the not-so-obvious barriers, such as dealing with a young child, an elderly patient, or an unconscious patient?

Pediatric patients

When dealing with a young patient, it's essential to keep in mind the child's developmental level. And in the case of a very young child, such as an infant, you need to communicate with the infant's parents. Always use a caring and compassionate tone with the parents because, more than likely, they're anxious about having their infant hospitalized.

Let's pretend

Remember that children commonly regress to an earlier stage of development when they're ill. Role playing is one way to communicate with children to find out how they're feeling.

Considering communication barriers

This diagram shows the components of nurse–patient communication. Note the factors that affect communication, such as orientation, preconceptions, and language. Your sensitivity to these factors makes the difference between effective and ineffective communication.

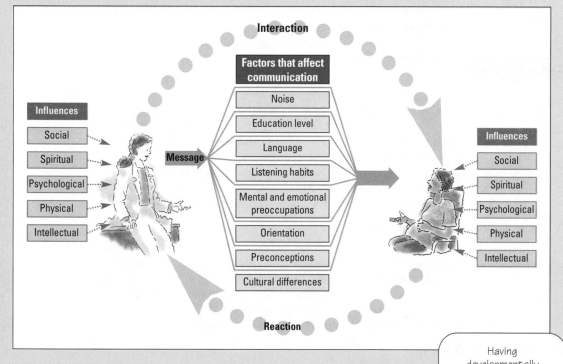

Interaction

Factors that affect communication

Noise

Education level

Language

Listening habits

Mental and emotional preoccupations

Orientation

Preconceptions

Cultural differences

Message

Influences

Social

Spiritual

Psychological

Physical

Intellectual

Influences

Social

Spiritual

Psychological

Physical

Intellectual

Reaction

Always be prepared

When possible, it's ideal to prepare the child for admission to the hospital. The timing of the preparation and the amount of teaching given depend on the child's age, developmental level, and personality, and the length of the procedure or treatment.

Young children may only need a few hours of preparation, whereas older children may benefit from several days of preparation. The use of developmentally appropriate activities will also help the child cope with the stress of hospitalization.

Having developmentally appropriate activities on hand can help a child cope with the stress of hospitalization.

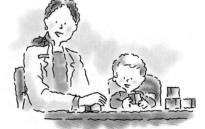

Keep it in the family

To reduce the fear that accompanies hospitalization, you can help the child and family cope by:
• explaining procedures
• answering questions openly and honestly
• minimizing separation from the parents
• structuring the environment to allow the child to maintain as much control as possible.

Elderly patients

Always address an older patient as *Miss, Mrs.,* or *Mr.,* followed by the surname. Experts also recommend the use of touch. For example, shake the patient's hand when you first meet them and say hello; then hold it briefly to convey concern. Use body language, touch, and eye contact to encourage participation. Be patient, relaxed, and unhurried. Suggest mentioning something here about sensory deficits in the elderly (e.g., visual and hearing deficits) and on incorporating devices such as eyeglasses and/or hearing aids.

A little talk goes a long way

Talk to the patient, not at them. Tell the patient how long the process will take. If language poses a problem, enlist the aid of an interpreter, family members, or a friend, as appropriate. Early in the interview, try to evaluate the patient's ability to communicate and their reliability as a historian. If you have doubts, before the interview proceeds further, ask whether a family member or friend can be present.

The more the merrier

Don't be surprised if an older patient requests that someone assist them; they, too, may have concerns about getting through the interview on their own. Having another person present gives you a chance to observe the patient's interaction with this person and provides more data for the history. However, the presence of another person may prevent the patient from speaking freely, so plan a talk privately at some time during your assessment.

Mrs. Dawson, I'll need to ask you some questions.

Oh, my daughter can help you out better than I can.

Be concise and rephrase

Provide carefully structured questions to elicit significant information. Keep your questions concise, rephrase those the patient doesn't understand, and use such nonverbal techniques as facial expressions, pointing, and touching to enhance your meaning.

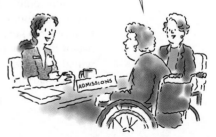

Nix the jargon

Use terms appropriate to the patient's level of understanding; avoid using jargon and complex medical terms. Offer explanations in lay terms, and then use the related medical terms, if appropriate, so the patient can become familiar with them.

To foster your older patient's cooperation, take a little extra time to help them see the relevance of your questions. You may need to repeat an explanation several times during the interview, but don't repeat unnecessarily. Give the patient plenty of time to respond to your questions and directions.

Sound of silence

Remain silent and allow the patient time to collect their thoughts and ideas before responding. Patience is the key to communicating with an older adult who responds slowly to your questions. Even so, don't confuse patience with patronizing behavior. The patient will easily perceive patronization and may interpret it as your lack of genuine concern.

Unconscious patient

When caring for an unconscious patient, don't assume that you don't need to try to communicate with them. Never assume that they can't hear you. Introduce yourself as you would to a conscious patient. Always explain every procedure you're doing. Don't talk about the patient with other people in the room as if the patient weren't present. Always treat the unconscious patient with kindness, consideration, and respect as you would a patient who's conscious.

Communicating by documentation

Patients are cared for by many people who work different shifts, and these various caregivers may speak with one another infrequently. The medical record is the main source of information and communication among nurses, doctors, physical therapists, social workers, and other caregivers. Today, nurses are commonly considered managers of care as well as practitioners, and nurses usually document the most information. Everyone's notes are important, however, because together they represent a complete picture of the patient's care.

Everyone's notes are important because together they represent a complete picture of patient care.

Growing team

As health care facilities continue to streamline and redesign care delivery systems, tasks that were historically performed by nurses are now being assigned to multiskilled workers such as nursing assistants. To deliver highly specialized care, each caregiver must provide accurate, thorough information and be able to interpret what others have written about a patient. Then each can use this information to plan future patient care. Commonly, decisions, actions, and revisions related to the patient's care are based on documentation from various team members. A well-prepared medical record shows the high degree of collaboration among the entire health care team.

References

Berman, A., & Snyder, S. (2012). *Kozier & Erb's fundamental of nursing: Concepts, process, and practice* (9th ed.). Upper Saddle River, NJ: Pearson.

Institute for Safe Medication Practice. (2013). *Unresolved disrespectful behavior in health-care practitioners speak up (again)—Part 1.* Retrieved from http://www.ismp.org/Newsletters/acutecare/showarticle.asp?id=60

Quick quiz

1. When developing a therapeutic nurse–patient relationship, during what phase do you review the patient's surgical history?
    A. Orientation
    B. Working
    C. Pre-interaction
    D. Termination

Answer: C. During the pre-interaction phase, you can review the patient data that you might already have, such as the medical or surgical history.

2. What's a good way to communicate with a very young child?
    A. Role playing
    B. Explaining procedures
    C. Showing him pictures
    D. Showing him a movie

Answer: A. Role playing is an excellent way to communicate with a very young child.

3. What type of behavior provides encouragement during communication without indicating agreement or disagreement?

    A.   Clapping
    B.   Sighing
    C.   Looking away
    D.   Nodding

Answer: D. Nonverbal behaviors, such as nodding and making momentary eye contact, provide encouragement without indicating agreement or disagreement.

4. What's the main source of information and communication among nurses, doctors, physical therapists, social workers, and other caregivers?

    A.   Computer
    B.   Medical record
    C.   Telephone
    D.   Word of mouth

Answer: B. The medical record is the main source of information and communication among nurses, doctors, physical therapists, social workers, and other caregivers.

Scoring

☆☆☆ If you answered all four questions correctly, fantastic! You're a communication connoisseur.

☆☆ If you answered three questions correctly, super! You've got a handle on handling communication strategies.

☆ If you answered fewer than three questions correctly, no worries! Reflect on the chapter and try again.

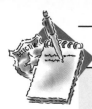

6

Health assessment

Just the facts

In this chapter, you'll learn:

♦ reasons for performing a health history

♦ techniques for effective communication during a health history assessment

♦ essential steps in a complete health history

♦ questions specific to each step of a health history.

A look at health assessment

Knowing how to complete an accurate assessment—from taking the health history to performing the physical examination—will help you uncover significant problems and make an appropriate care plan.

Any assessment involves collecting two kinds of data: objective and subjective. *Objective data* are obtained through observation and are verifiable. For example, a red, swollen arm in a patient who's complaining of arm pain is an example of data that can be seen and verified by someone other than the patient. *Subjective data* can't be verified by anyone other than the patient and are gathered solely from the patient's own account—for example, "My head hurts" or "I have trouble sleeping at night."

Exploring past and present

You'll use a health history to gather subjective data about the patient and explore past and present problems. To begin, ask the patient about their general physical and emotional health. Then ask about specific body systems and structures.

> The health history is an exploration of your patient's health—past and present. Land ho!

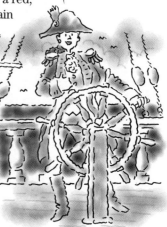

Beginning the interview

Keep in mind that the accuracy and completeness of your patient's answers largely depend on your skill as an interviewer. Therefore, before you start asking questions, review the following communication guidelines.

Create the proper environment

To make the most of your patient interview, you'll first need to create an environment in which the patient feels comfortable. Before asking your first question, try to establish a rapport with the patient and explain what you'll cover during the interview. Consider the following when selecting a location for the interview:

• Choose a quiet, private, well-lit interview setting. Such a setting will make it easier for you and your patient to interact and will help the patient feel more at ease.

• Make sure that the patient is comfortable. Sit facing them, 3′ to 4′ (1 to 1.5 m) away.

• Introduce yourself and explain that the purpose of the health history and assessment is to identify key problems and gather information to aid in planning their care.

• Reassure the patient that everything they say will be kept confidential.

• Tell the patient how long the interview will last, and ask them what they expect from the interview.

• Use touch sparingly. Many people aren't comfortable with strangers hugging, patting, or touching them.

• Assess the patient to see if language barriers exist. For example, do they speak and understand English? Can they hear you? (See *Overcoming interviewing obstacles*, page 100.)

• Speak slowly and clearly using easy-to-understand language. Avoid using medical terms and jargon.

• Address the patient by a formal name, such as Mr. Jones. Don't call him by his first name unless he asks you to. Avoid using terms of endearment, such as "honey" or "sweetie." Treating the patient with respect encourages them to trust you and to provide more accurate and complete information.

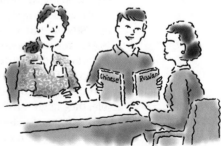

If your patient has difficulty understanding or speaking English, ask your facility's interpreter to sit in on the interview.

Ages and stages

Overcoming interviewing obstacles

With a little creativity, you can overcome barriers to interviewing. For example, if a patient doesn't speak English, your facility may have a bank of interpreters you can call on for help.

A trained medical interpreter—one who's familiar with medical terminology, knows interpreting techniques, and understands the patient's rights—would be ideal. Be sure to tell the interpreter to translate the patient's speech verbatim.

Avoid using one of the patient's family members or friends as an interpreter. Doing so violates the patient's right to confidentiality.

Breaking the sound barrier

Is your patient hearing impaired? You can overcome this barrier, too. First, make sure the light is bright enough for them to see your lips move. Then face them and speak slowly and clearly. If necessary, have the patient use an assistive device, such as a hearing aid or an amplifier. If the patient uses sign language, see if your facility has a sign language interpreter.

Communicate effectively

After you've created a proper environment, you'll want to use various communication strategies to make sure you communicate effectively. Realize that you and the patient communicate nonverbally as well as verbally. Being aware of these forms of communication will aid you in the interview process.

Nonverbal communication strategies

To make the most of nonverbal communication, follow these guidelines:
• Listen attentively, and make eye contact frequently.
• Use reassuring gestures, such as nodding your head, to encourage the patient to keep talking.
• Watch for nonverbal clues that indicate the patient is uncomfortable or unsure about how to answer a question. For example, they might lower their voice or glance around uneasily.
• Be aware of your own nonverbal behaviors that might cause the patient to stop talking or become defensive. For example, if you cross your arms, you might appear closed off from them. If you stand while they are sitting, you might appear superior. If you glance at your watch, you might appear to be bored or rushed, which could keep the patient from answering questions completely.

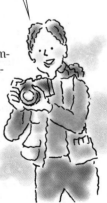

When interviewing a patient, remain focused on the task at hand.

• Observe the patient closely to see if they understand each question. If they don't appear to understand, repeat the question using different words or familiar examples. For example, instead of asking, "Did you have respiratory difficulty after exercising?" ask, "Did you have to sit down after walking around the block?"

Reviewing general health

I'll take "Psychosocial" for $1,000, please.

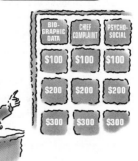

You've learned how to ask questions. Now it's time to learn the right questions to ask when reviewing the patient's general physical and emotional health. Also, remember to maintain a professional attitude throughout this process.

Asking the right questions

A complete health history requires information from each of these categories obtained in this order:

 biographic data

 chief complaint

 medical history

 family history

 psychosocial history

activities of daily living.

Biographic data

Start the health history by obtaining biographic information from the patient. Do this first so you don't forget about this information after you become involved in details of the patient's health. Ask the patient for name, address, telephone number, birth date, age, marital status, religion, and nationality. Find out with whom they live and get the name and telephone number of a person to contact in case of an emergency.

Also, ask the patient about health care, including who is the primary doctor and how they get to the doctor's office. Ask if they have ever been treated for the present problem. Finally, ask if they have advance directive in place. (See *Advance directives*, page 102.)

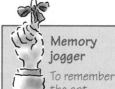

Memory jogger

To remember the categories you should cover in your health history, think "Being Complete Makes For Proper Assessment":

Biographic data

Chief complaint

Medical history

Family history

Psychosocial history

Activities of daily living.

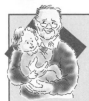

Ages and stages

Advance directives

The Patient Self-Determination Act allows patients to prepare advance directives—written documents that state their wishes regarding health care in the event they become incapacitated or unable to make decisions. Elderly patients in particular may have interest in advance directives because they tend to be concerned with end-of-life issues.

Direction for directives

If a patient doesn't have an advance directive in place, the health care facility must provide them with information about it, including how to establish one.

An advance directive may include:

• name of the person authorized by the patient to make medical decisions if the patient can no longer do so

• specific medical treatment the patient wants or doesn't want

• instructions regarding pain medication and comfort—specifically, whether the patient wishes to receive certain treatment even if the treatment may hasten their death

• information the patient wants to relay to their loved ones

• name of the patient's primary health care provider

• any other wishes.

Take a hint

Your patient's answers to basic questions can provide important clues about their personality, medical problems, and reliability. If they can't furnish accurate information, ask them for the name of a friend or relative who can. Document the source of the information as well as whether an interpreter was necessary.

> Pinpoint your patient's chief complaint. Remember, accuracy is key to a correct diagnosis.

Chief complaint

Try to pinpoint why the patient is seeking health care or his *chief complaint*. Document this information in the patient's exact words to avoid misinterpretation. Ask how and when the symptoms developed, what led the patient to seek medical attention, and how the problem has affected their life and ability to function.

Alphabet soup

To ensure that you don't omit pertinent data, use the PQRSTU mnemonic device (see *PQRSTU: What's the story?* page 63), which provides a systematic approach to obtaining information.

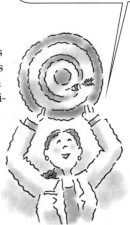

Medical history

Ask the patient about past and current medical problems, such as hypertension, diabetes, and back pain. Typical questions include:
• Have you ever been hospitalized? If so, when and why?
• What childhood illnesses did you have?
• Are you being treated for any problem? If so, for what reason and who's your doctor?
• Have you ever had surgery? If so, when and why?
• Are you allergic to anything in the environment or any drugs or foods or latex? If so, what kind of allergic reaction do you have?
• Are you taking medications, including over-the-counter preparations, such as aspirin, vitamins, and cough syrup? If so, how much do you take and how often do you take it? Do you use home remedies such as homemade ointments? Do you use herbal preparations or take dietary supplements? Do you use other alternative or complementary therapies, such as acupuncture, therapeutic massage, or chiropractic?

Family history

Questioning the patient about family's health is a good way to uncover risks of having certain illnesses. Typical questions include:
• Are your mother, father, and siblings living? If not, how old were they when they died? What were the causes of their deaths?
• If they're alive, do they have diabetes, high blood pressure, heart disease, asthma, cancer, sickle cell anemia, hemophilia, cataracts, glaucoma, or other illnesses?

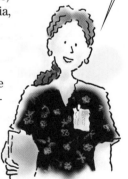

Information about the health of a patient's family can give you clues to risk of developing illnesses.

Psychosocial history

Find out how the patient feels about themselves, their place in society, and relationships with others. Ask about occupation (past and present), education, economic status, and responsibilities. Typical questions include:
• How have you coped with medical or emotional crises in the past? (See *Asking about abuse*, page 104.)
• Has your life changed recently? What changes in your personality or behavior have you noticed?
• How adequate is the emotional support you receive from family and friends?
• How close do you live to health care facilities? Can you get to them easily?
• Do you have health insurance?
• Are you on a fixed income with no extra money for health care?

Asking about abuse

Abuse is a tricky subject. Anyone can be a victim of abuse: a boyfriend or girlfriend, a spouse, an elderly patient, a child, or a parent. Also, abuse can come in many forms: physical, psychological, emotional, and sexual. So, when taking a health history, ask two open-ended questions to explore abuse: When do you feel safe at home? When don't you feel safe?

Watch the reaction

Even when you don't immediately suspect an abusive situation, be aware of how your patient reacts to open-ended questions. Is the patient defensive, hostile, confused, or frightened? Assess how they interact with you and others. Do they seem withdrawn or frightened or show other inappropriate behavior? Keep reac-tions in mind when you perform your physical assessment.

Must report

Remember, if the patient tells you about any type of abuse, you're obligated to report it. Inform the patient that you must report the incident to local authorities.

Activities of daily living

Find out what's normal for the patient by asking them to describe a typical day. Make sure you include the following areas in your assessment.

Diet and elimination

Ask the patient about his appetite, special diets, and food allergies. Can he afford to buy enough food? Who cooks and shops at home? Ask about the frequency of bowel movements and laxative use.

Exercise and sleep

Ask the patient if they have a special exercise program and, if so, why. Ask them to describe it. Ask how many hours they sleep at night, what their sleep patterns are like, and whether they feel rested after sleep. Ask them if they have any difficulties with sleep.

Work and leisure

Ask the patient what they do for a living and what they do during leisure time. Do they have hobbies?

Use of tobacco, alcohol, and other drugs

Ask the patient if they smoke cigarettes. If so, how many packs per day? Do they consume alcohol? If so, how much each day? Ask if there is illicit drug use, such as marijuana or cocaine. If so, how often? Ask if the patient ever smoked cigarettes, drank alcohol, and so forth in the past, and if yes, how much and when did they stop?

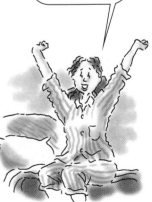

I know I always feel rested after a short catnap in the nurses' lounge.

Fudging the facts

Patients may understate the amount they drink because of embarrassment. If you're having trouble getting what you believe are honest answers to such questions, you might try overestimating the amount. For example, you might say, "You told me you drink beer. Do you drink about a six-pack per day?" The patient's response might be, "No, I drink about half that."

Religious observances

Ask the patient if they have religious beliefs that affect diet, dress, or health practices. Patients will feel reassured when you make it clear that you understand these points.

Maintaining a professional attitude

Don't let your personal opinions interfere with this part of the assessment. Maintain a professional, neutral approach, and don't offer advice. For example, don't suggest that the patient enter a drug rehabilitation program. That type of response puts patients on the defensive, and they might not answer subsequent questions honestly.

Also, avoid saying things like, "The doctor knows what's best for you." Such statements make the patient feel inferior and break down communication. Lastly, don't use leading questions such as "You don't do drugs, do you?" to get the answer you're hoping for. This type of question, based on your own value system, will make the patient feel guilty and might prevent them from responding honestly.

Reviewing structures and systems

The last part of the health history is a systematic assessment of the patient's body structures and systems. A thorough assessment requires that you follow a process while asking specific questions.

Follow a process

Always start at the top of the head and work your way down the body. This helps you avoid skipping an area accidentally. When questioning an elderly patient, remember that they may have difficulty hearing or communicating. (See *Overcoming communication problems in elderly patients.*)

Ages and stages

Overcoming communication problems in elderly patients

An elderly patient may have sensory or memory impairment or a decreased attention span. If your patient is confused or has trouble communicating, you may need to rely on a family member for some or all of the health history.

Ask specific questions

Information gained from a health history forms the basis for your care plan and enables you to distinguish physical changes and devise a holistic approach to treatment. As with other nursing skills, the only way you can improve your interviewing technique is with practice, practice, and more practice. (See *Evaluating a symptom*.)

Here are some key questions to ask your patient about each body structure and system.

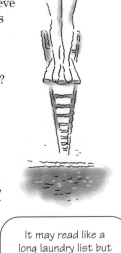

Remember, head first—that's the key to correct assessment!

Head first

Do you get headaches? If so, where are they and how painful are they? How often do they occur, and how long do they last? Does anything trigger them, and how do you relieve them? Have you ever had a head injury? Do you have lumps or bumps on your head?

Vision quest

When was your last eye examination? Do you wear glasses? Do you have glaucoma, cataracts, or color blindness? Does light bother your eyes? Do you have excessive tearing; blurred vision; double vision; or dry, itchy, burning, inflamed, or swollen eyes?

An earful

Do you have loss of balance, ringing in your ears, deafness, or poor hearing? Have you ever had ear surgery? If so, why and when? Do you wear a hearing aid? Are you having pain, swelling, or discharge from your ears? If so, has this problem occurred before and how frequently?

Nose knows

Have you ever had nasal surgery? If so, why and when? Have you ever had sinusitis or nosebleeds? Do you have nasal problems that impair your ability to smell or that cause breathing difficulties, snoring at night, frequent sneezing, or discharge?

Mouth and throat run-through

Do you have mouth sores, a dry mouth, and loss of taste, a toothache, or bleeding gums? Do you wear dentures and, if so, do they fit? Do you have a sore throat, fever, or chills? How often do you get a sore throat, and have you seen a doctor for this?

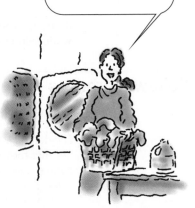

It may read like a long laundry list but all these questions are crucial to a thorough assessment.

Evaluating a symptom

Your patient is vague in describing the chief complaint. Using your interviewing skills, you discover the problem is related to abdominal distention. Now what? This flowchart will help you decide what to do next, using abdominal distention as the patient's chief complaint.

Question the patient to identify the symptom that's bothering them. They tell you, "My stomach gets bloated."

Form a first impression.
Does the patient's condition alert you to an emergency? For example, does he say the bloating developed suddenly?
Do they mention that other signs or symptoms occur with it, such as sweating and light-headedness?
(Both are indicators of hypovolemia.)

 YES

 NO

Take a brief history to gather more clues.
For example, ask the patient if they have severe abdominal pain or difficulty breathing or if they ever had an abdominal injury.

Now, take a thorough history to get an overview of the patient's condition.
Ask about associated signs or symptoms. Especially note GI disorders that can lead to abdominal distention.

Perform a focused physical examination to determine the severity of the patient's condition quickly.
Check for bruising, lacerations, changes in bowel sounds, or abdominal rigidity.

Now, thoroughly examine the patient to evaluate the chief sign or symptom and to detect additional signs and symptoms. Place the patient in a recumbent position and observe for abdominal asymmetry. Inspect the skin, auscultate for bowel sounds, percuss and palpate the abdomen, and measure abdominal girth.

Evaluate your findings. Are emergency signs or symptoms present, such as abdominal rigidity and abnormal bowel sounds?

Based on your findings, intervene appropriately to stabilize the patient. Notify the doctor immediately, place the patient in a supine position, administer oxygen, and start an I.V. line. GI or nasogastric tube insertion and emergency surgery may be needed.

Review your findings to consider possible causes, such as cancer, bladder distention, cirrhosis, heart failure, and gastric dilation.

After the patient's condition is stabilized, review your findings to consider possible causes, such as trauma, large-bowel obstruction, mesenteric artery occlusion, or peritonitis.

Evaluate your findings and devise an appropriate care plan. Position the patient comfortably, administer analgesics, and prepare the patient for diagnostic tests.

Do you have difficulty swallowing? If so, is the problem with solids or liquids? Is it a constant problem or does it accompany a sore throat or another problem? What, if anything, makes it go away?

Neck check

Do you have swelling, soreness, lack of movement, stiffness, or pain in your neck? If so, did something specific cause it to happen such as too much exercise? How long have you had this symptom? Does anything relieve it or aggravate it?

Respiratory research

Do you have shortness of breath on exertion or while lying in bed? How many pillows do you use at night? Does breathing cause pain or wheezing? Do you have a productive cough? If so, do you cough up blood-tinged sputum? Do you have night sweats?

Have you ever been treated for pneumonia, asthma, emphysema, or frequent respiratory tract infections? Have you ever had a chest X-ray or tuberculin skin test? If so, when and what were the results?

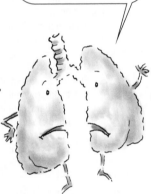

Hey, slow down . . . you're reading too fast! Remember, breathe between sentences—or at least between paragraphs!

Heart health hunt

Do you have chest pain, palpitations, irregular heartbeat, fast heartbeat, shortness of breath, or a persistent cough? Have you ever had an electrocardiogram? If so, when?

Do you have high blood pressure, peripheral vascular disease, swelling of the ankles and hands, varicose veins, cold extremities, or intermittent pain in your legs?

Breast test

Ask women these questions: Do you perform monthly breast self-examinations? Have you noticed a lump, a change in breast contour, breast pain, or discharge from your nipples? Have you ever had breast cancer? If not, has anyone else in your family had it? Have you ever had a mammogram? When and what were the results?

Ask men these questions: Do you have pain in your breast tissue? Have you noticed lumps or a change in contour?

Stomach symptom search

Have you had nausea, vomiting, loss of appetite, heartburn, abdominal pain, frequent belching, or passing of gas? Have you lost or gained weight recently? How often do you have a bowel movement, and what color, odor, and consistency are your stools? Have you noticed a change in your regular elimination pattern? Do you use laxatives frequently?

Have you had hemorrhoids, rectal bleeding, hernias, gallbladder disease, or liver disease?

GU interview

Do you have urinary problems, such as burning during urination, incontinence, urgency, retention, reduced urinary flow, and dribbling? Do you get up during the night to urinate? If so, how many times? What color is your urine? Have you ever noticed blood in it? Have you ever been treated for kidney stones?

Reproduction review

Ask women these questions: How old were you when you started menstruating? How often do you get your period, and how long does it usually last? Do you have pain or pass clots? If you're postmenopausal, at what age did you stop menstruating? If you're in the transitional stage, what perimenopausal symptoms are you experiencing? Have you ever been pregnant? If so, how many times? What was the method of delivery? How many pregnancies resulted in live births? How many resulted in miscarriages? Have you had an abortion?

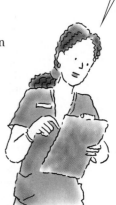

Yep, here we are . . . 67 questions down and only 44 more to go. And this is the short assessment form!

What's your method of birth control? Are you involved in a long-term, monogamous relationship? Have you had frequent vaginal infections or a sexually transmitted disease (STD)? When was your last gynecologic examination and Papanicolaou test? What were the results?

Ask men these questions: Do you perform monthly testicular self-examinations? Have you ever had a prostate examination and, if so, when? Have you noticed penile pain, discharge, lesions, or testicular lumps? Which form of birth control do you use? Have you had a vasectomy? Are you involved in a long-term, monogamous relationship? Have you ever had an STD?

Monitoring muscle

Do you have difficulty walking, sitting, or standing? Are you steady on your feet or do you lose your balance easily? Do you have arthritis, gout, a back injury, muscle weakness, or paralysis?

Central nervous system scrutiny

Have you ever had seizures? Do you ever experience tremors, twitching, numbness, tingling, or loss of sensation in a part of your body? Are you less able to get around than you think you should be? (See *Tips for assessing a severely ill patient,* page 110.)

Tips for assessing a severely ill patient

When the patient's condition doesn't allow a full assessment—for example, if the patient is in severe pain—get as much information as possible from other sources. With a severely ill patient, keep these key points in mind:

• Identify yourself to the patient and the family.

• Stay calm to gain the patient's confidence and allay anxiety.

• Stay on the lookout for important information. For example, if a patient seeks help for a ringing in their ears, don't overlook his casual mention of a periodic "racing heartbeat."

• Avoid jumping to conclusions. Don't assume that the patient's complaint is related to the admitting diagnosis. Use a systematic approach and collect the appropriate information; then draw conclusions.

Endocrine inquiry

Have you been unusually tired lately? Do you feel hungry or thirsty more often than usual? Have you lost weight for unexplained reasons? How well can you tolerate heat or cold? Have you noticed changes in your hair texture or color? Have you been losing hair? Do you take hormone medications?

Circulatory study

Have you ever been diagnosed with anemia or blood abnormalities? Do you bruise easily or become fatigued quickly? Have you ever had a blood transfusion? If so, did you have any type of adverse reaction?

Psychological survey

Do you ever experience mood swings or memory loss? Do you ever feel anxious, depressed, or unable to concentrate? Are you feeling unusually stressed? Do you ever feel unable to cope?

References

Berman, A., & Snyder S. (2012). *Kozier & Erb's fundamentals of nursing: Concepts, process, and practice* (9th ed.). Upper Saddle River, NJ: Pearson.

Sussman, G., & Gold, M. (n.d.). *Guidelines for the management of latex allergies and safe latex use in health care facilities.* Retrieved from http://www.acaai.org/allergist/allergies/Types/latex-allergy/Pages/latex-allergies-safe-use.aspx

Quick quiz

1. Leading questions may initiate untrue or inaccurate responses because such questions:
  A. encourage short or vague answers.
  B. require an educational level the patient may not possess.
  C. prompt the patient to try to give the answer you're looking for.
  D. confuse the patient.

Answer: C. Because of how they're phrased, leading questions may prompt the patient to give the answer you're looking for.

2. When obtaining a health history from a patient, ask first about:
  A. biographic data.
  B. the chief complaint.
  C. health insurance coverage.
  D. family history.

Answer: A. Take care of the biographic data first; otherwise, you might get involved in the patient history and forget to ask basic questions.

3. Silence is a communication technique used during an interview to:
  A. show respect.
  B. change the topic.
  C. encourage the patient to continue talking.
  D. clarify information.

Answer: C. Silence allows the patient to collect his thoughts and continue to answer your questions.

4. Data are considered subjective if you obtain them from:
  A. the patient's verbal account.
  B. your observations of the patient's actions.
  C. the patient's records.
  D. X-ray reports.

Answer: A. Data from the patient's own words are subjective.

5. What allows patients to state their wishes regarding health care if they become incapacitated?

    A.   Patient's Bill of Rights
    B.   The Patient Self-Determination Act
    C.   Health Insurance Portability and Accountability Act
    D.   First Amendment

Answer: B. The Patient Self-Determination Act allows patients to make decisions about their health care when they become incapacitated.

Scoring

☆☆☆ If you answered all five questions correctly, bravo! You're our intrepid interviewer.

☆☆ If you answered four questions correctly, that's cool! You're our hip historian.

☆ If you answered fewer than four questions correctly, that's OK! Review the chapter and you'll know all the questions—and answers.

7

Taking vital signs

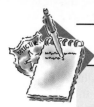

Just the facts

In this chapter, you'll learn:

♦ types of equipment used in vital signs assessment

♦ skills for performing vital signs assessment

♦ tips to interpret vital signs

♦ abnormalities in vital signs.

A look at vital signs assessment

Accurate measurements of your patient's height, weight, and vital signs provide critical information about body functions.

The first time you assess a patient, record the baseline vital signs and statistics. Afterward, take measurements at regular intervals, depending on the patient's condition, doctors' orders, and your facility's policy. A series of readings usually provides more valuable information than a single set.

Vital tips

Always analyze vital signs at the same time because two or more abnormal values provide important clues about your patient's problem. For example, a rapid, thready pulse along with low blood pressure may signal shock.

If you obtain an abnormal value, take the vital sign again after waiting 1 to 2 minutes after the initial readings to make sure it's accurate. Remember that normal readings vary with the patient's age. For example, temperature decreases with age and respiratory rate may increase with age or with an underlying disease.

Also remember that an abnormal value for one patient may be a normal value for another. Each patient has his own baseline values, which is what makes recording vital signs during the initial assessment so important.

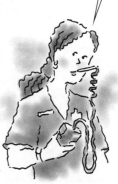

Taking vital signs is a vital part of nursing.

Body temperature

Body temperature represents the balance between heat that's produced by metabolism, muscular activity, and other factors and heat that's lost through the skin, lungs, and body wastes. A stable temperature pattern promotes proper function of cells, tissues, and organs; a change in this pattern usually signals the onset of illness.

Choose one

Oral temperature in adults normally ranges from 97° to 99.5° F (36.1° to 37.5° C). Rectal temperature, the most accurate reading, is usually 1° F (0.6° C) higher. Axillary (armpit) temperature, the least accurate reading, is usually 1° to 2° F (0.6° to 1.1° C) lower. Tympanic (in the ear) temperature reads 0.5° to 1° F (0.3° to 0.6° C) higher. (See *Types of thermometers*.)

Types of thermometers

You can take a patient's oral, rectal, or axillary temperature with an electronic digital thermometer. You can take tympanic temperature with a tympanic thermometer.

For adults who are awake, alert, oriented, and cooperative, use the oral or tympanic route. For infants, young children, and confused or unconscious patients, you may need to use the axillary or rectal route.

Tympanic thermometer

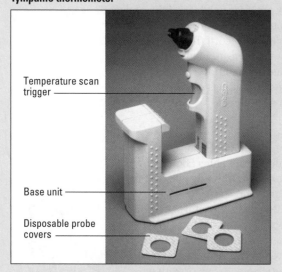

Temperature scan trigger

Base unit

Disposable probe covers

Individual electronic digital thermometer

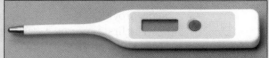

Institutional electronic digital thermometer

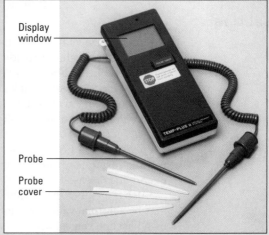

Display window

Probe

Probe cover

Normal ups and downs

Temperature normally fluctuates with rest and activity. Lowest readings typically occur between 4 and 5 a.m.; the highest readings, between 4 and 8 p.m. Other factors also influence temperature. (See *Differences in temperature.*)

From F to C and back again

To convert a Celsius measurement to a Fahrenheit measurement, multiply the Celsius temperature by 1.8 and add 32. To convert Fahrenheit to Celsius, subtract 32 from the Fahrenheit temperature and divide by 1.8. (See *How temperature readings compare*, page 116.)

What you need

Electronic or tympanic thermometer, facial tissue, disposable thermometer sheath or probe cover, gloves and lubricant (for rectal temperature)

How you do it

• Introduce yourself to your patient, explain the procedure, and wash your hands. If you're taking an oral temperature and the patient has had hot or cold liquids, chewed gum, or smoked, wait 20 to 30 minutes before getting started.

Taking an oral temperature

• Put on gloves.
• Insert the probe into a disposable probe cover.
• Position the tip of the probe under the patient's tongue on either side of the frenulum as far back as possible. *Placing the tip in this area promotes contact with superficial blood vessels and ensures a more accurate reading.*
• Instruct the patient to close their lips but to not bite down with his teeth *to avoid breaking the thermometer in his mouth.*
• Leave the probe in place until the maximum temperature appears on the digital display. Then remove the probe and note the temperature and document in the patient's record.

Taking a rectal temperature

• Put on gloves.
• Insert the probe into a disposable probe cover.
• Position the patient on their side with the top leg flexed and drape to *provide privacy.* Then fold back the bed linens *to expose the anus.*
• Lift the patient's upper buttock and insert the thermometer about ½″ (1 cm) for an infant and 1½″ (3.8 cm) for an adult.

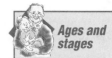

Ages and stages

Differences in temperature

Besides activity level, other factors that influence temperature include gender, age, emotional conditions, and environment. Keep these principles in mind:
• Women normally have higher temperatures than men do, especially during ovulation.
• Normal temperature is highest in neonates and lowest in elderly people.
• A hot external environment can raise temperature; a cold environment lowers it.

How temperature readings compare

You can take your patient's temperature in four ways. This chart describes each method.

Method	Normal temperature	Used with
Oral	97.7° to 99.5° F (36.5° to 37.5° C)	Adults and older children who are awake, alert, oriented, and cooperative
Axillary (armpit)	96.7° to 98.5° F (35.9° to 3.6.9° C)	Infants, young children, and patients with impaired immune systems when infection is a concern
Rectal	98.7° to 100.5° F (37.1° to 38.1° C)	Infants, young children, and confused or unconscious patients
Temporal artery	97.4° to 100.1° F (36.3° to 37.8° C)	Adults, children, infants, conscious and cooperative patients
Tympanic (ear)	98.2° to 100° F (36.8° to 37.8° C)	Adults and children, conscious and cooperative patients, and confused or unconscious patients

• Gently direct the thermometer along the rectal wall toward the umbilicus *to avoid perforating the anus or rectum and to help ensure an accurate reading.* (The thermometer will register hemorrhoidal artery temperature instead of fecal temperature.)
• Hold the thermometer in place for the appropriate length of time *to prevent damage to rectal tissues caused by displacement.*
• Carefully remove the thermometer, wiping it if necessary. Then wipe the anal area *to remove any feces.*
• Remove your gloves, and wash your hands.

Remember, an armpit isn't an enclosed body cavity, so you'll need to keep me in place a little longer for an accurate reading.

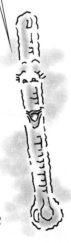

Taking an axillary temperature

• Position the patient with the axilla exposed.
• Put on gloves, and gently pat the axilla dry with a facial tissue *because moisture conducts heat.* Avoid harsh rubbing, *which generates heat.*
• Ask the patient to reach across their chest and grasp the opposite shoulder, lifting the elbow.
• Position the thermometer in the center of the axilla, with the tip pointing toward the patient's head.
• Tell the patient to keep grasping their shoulder and to lower the elbow and hold it against their chest *to promote skin contact with the thermometer.*

• Leave the thermometer in place for the appropriate length of time. Axillary temperatures take longer to register than oral or rectal temperature *because the thermometer isn't enclosed in a body cavity.*
• Grasp the end of the thermometer, and remove it from the axilla. Remove your gloves, and wash your hands and document the results.

With a tympanic thermometer

• Make sure the lens under the probe is clean and shiny. Attach a disposable probe cover.
• Stabilize the patient's head; then gently pull his ear straight back (for children up to age 1) or up and back (for adults and children older than age 1). (See *Taking an infant's temperature.*)
• Insert the thermometer until the entire ear canal is sealed. The thermometer should be inserted toward the tympanic membrane in the same way an otoscope is inserted.
• Press the activation button, and hold for 1 second. The temperature will appear on the display. (See *Tips about temperature*, page 118.)

With a temporal artery thermometer

• Attach a disposable probe cover.
• Place the probe in the middle of the forehead; while keeping the red button depressed, slide the probe across the forehead to the hairline.

> ### Ages and stages
>
> ## Taking an infant's temperature
>
> For infants younger than age 3 months, take three readings and use the highest one.

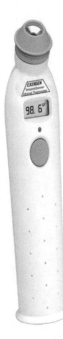

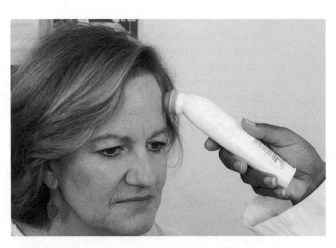

Source: Temporal Artery Thermometer Information
TemporalScanner 2000C
Developed, designed, and manufactured
by Exergen Corporation in the USA
EXERGEN CORPORATION, 400 PLEASANT STREET.

WATERTOWN, MA 02472
PHONE: 617.923.9900 FAX: 617.923.9911
www.exergen.com
P/N 818541 Rev 6
Exergen Corporation. All rights reserved.

Tips about temperature

Keep these tips in mind when taking a patient's temperature:
• Oral measurement is contraindicated in young children and infants and in patients who are unconscious, disoriented, or prone to seizures or those who must breathe through their mouth.
• Rectal measurement is contraindicated in patients with diarrhea, recent rectal or prostatic surgery or injury (because it may injure inflamed tissue), or recent myocardial infarction (because anal manipulation may stimulate the vagus nerve, causing bradycardia or another rhythm disturbance).
• Use the same thermometer for repeat temperature taking to ensure consistent results.
• If your patient is receiving nasal oxygen, know that you can still measure his temperature orally because oxygen administration raises oral temperature by only about 0.37° F (0.21° C).

• Lift the probe from the forehead and touch the client's neck just behind the earlobe and release the button and record temperature.
• Remove the plastic disposable cover and dispose.

Pulse

The patient's pulse reflects the amount of blood ejected with each heartbeat. The recurring wave—called a *pulse*—can be palpated at locations on the body where an artery crosses over bone or firm tissue. To assess the pulse, palpate one of the patient's arterial pulse points and note the rate, rhythm, and amplitude of the pulse. A normal pulse for an adult is between 60 and 100 beats/minute.

The radial pulse

The radial pulse is the most accessible. However, in cardiovascular emergencies, you may palpate for the femoral or carotid pulses. These vessels are larger and more accurately reflect the heart's activity. (See *Pinpointing pulse sites.*)

Rate, rhythm, and volume

Taking a patient's pulse involves determining the number of beats per minute (the pulse rate), the pattern or

Pinpointing pulse sites

You can assess your patient's pulse rate at several sites, including those shown in this illustration.

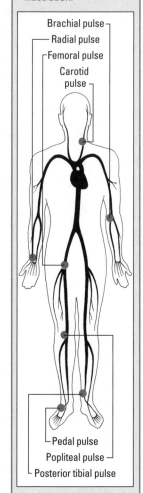

Brachial pulse
Radial pulse
Femoral pulse
Carotid pulse

Pedal pulse
Popliteal pulse
Posterior tibial pulse

irregularity of the beats (the rhythm), and the volume of blood pumped with each beat. (See *Alternate site for taking a pulse.*) If the pulse is faint or weak, consider using a Doppler ultrasound blood flow detector. (See *Using a Doppler device*, page 120.)

What you need

Watch with a second hand, stethoscope (for auscultating apical pulse), Doppler ultrasound blood flow detector, if necessary

How you do it

• Introduce yourself to your patient, wash your hands, and tell the patient that you're going to check their pulse.
• Make sure the patient is comfortable and relaxed *because an awkward, uncomfortable position may affect his heart rate.*

Taking a radial pulse

• Place the patient in a sitting or supine position, with their arms at the side or across the chest.

Keep the thumb out of it

• Gently press your index, middle, and ring fingers on the radial artery inside the patient's wrist. You should feel a pulse with only moderate pressure; *excessive pressure may obstruct blood flow distal to the pulse site.* Don't use your thumb to take the patient's pulse; *the thumb has a strong pulse of its own and may be easily confused with the patient's pulse.*

One, two, three . . . sixty

• After locating the pulse, count the beats for 60 seconds to get the number of beats per minute. *Counting for a full minute provides a more accurate picture of irregularities.*
• While counting the rate, assess pulse rhythm and volume by noting the pattern and strength of the beats. If you detect an irregularity, repeat the count and note whether the irregularity occurs in a pattern or randomly. If you're still in doubt, take an apical pulse. (See *Identifying pulse patterns*, page 121.)

Taking an apical pulse

• Help the patient to a supine position, and drape him if necessary.

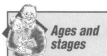

Ages and stages

Alternate site for taking a pulse

The most common site for taking a pulse is the radial artery in the wrist. This holds true for adults and children older than age 3.

For infants and children younger than age 3, however, it's better to listen to the heart with a stethoscope rather than palpate a pulse. Because auscultation is done at the apex of the heart, the pulse measured is the *apical pulse.*

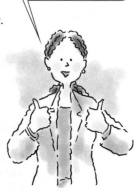

When taking a radial pulse, count for a full minute and keep these guys out of the picture.

Using a Doppler device

More sensitive than palpation for determining pulse rate, the Doppler ultrasound blood flow detector is especially useful when a pulse is faint or weak. Unlike palpation, which detects arterial wall expansion and retraction, this instrument detects the movement of red blood cells. Here's how you use it:
• Apply a small amount of transmission gel to the ultrasound probe.
• Position the probe on the skin directly over the selected artery. In the illustration below, the probe is over the posterior tibial artery.
• When using a Doppler probe with an amplifier (as shown below), turn the instrument on, and moving counterclockwise, set the volume control to the lowest setting.

If your model doesn't have a speaker, plug in the earphones and slowly raise the volume.
• To obtain the best signals, put gel between the skin and the probe and tilt the probe 45 degrees from the artery. Slowly move the probe in a circular motion to locate the center of the artery and the Doppler signal—a hissing noise at the heartbeat. Avoid moving the probe rapidly because this distorts the signal.
• Count the signals for 60 seconds to determine the pulse rate.
• After you've measured the pulse rate, clean the probe with a soft cloth soaked in antiseptic solution or soapy water. Don't immerse the probe.

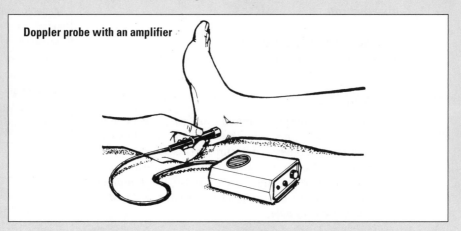

Doppler probe with an amplifier

Warm the scope first, please

• Keeping in mind that the bell of the stethoscope transmits low-pitched sounds more effectively than the diaphragm, warm the bell or diaphragm in your hand. *Placing a cold stethoscope against the patient's skin may startle him and momentarily increase his heart rate.*
• Place the warmed bell or diaphragm over the apex of the heart (normally located at the fifth intercostal space, left of the midclavicular line), and insert the earpieces in your ear.
• Count the beats for 60 seconds, and note their rhythm, volume, and intensity.
• Remove the stethoscope and make the patient comfortable.

Identifying pulse patterns

This chart lists different types of pulse patterns along with their rates, rhythms, and causes and incidence.

Type	Rate	Rhythm	Causes and incidence
Normal	60 to 80 beats/minute; in neonates, 120 to 140 beats/minute		• Varies with such factors as age, physical activity, and gender (Infants and children have higher pulse rates than adults; older adults have lower pulse rates.)
Tachycardia	More than 100 beats/minute		• Accompanies stimulation of the sympathetic nervous system resulting from emotional stress (such as anger, fear, or anxiety) or the use of certain drugs (such as caffeine) • May result from exercise or such health conditions as heart failure, anemia, and fever, which increase oxygen requirements, and thus, pulse rate
Bradycardia	Less than 60 beats/minute		• Accompanies stimulation of the parasympathetic nervous system resulting from drug use, especially cardiac glycosides, and such conditions as cerebral hemorrhage and heart block • May also be present in fit athletes and persons with hypothyroidism
Irregular	Uneven time intervals between beats (e.g., periods of regular rhythm interrupted by pauses or premature beats)		• May indicate cardiac irritability, hypoxia, digoxin toxicity, potassium imbalance, or a more serious arrhythmia if premature beats occur frequently (Occasional premature beats are normal.)

Taking an apical-radial pulse

• Find another nurse to work with you when taking an apical-radial pulse so that she can palpate the radial pulse while you auscultate the apical pulse with a stethoscope or vice versa.

• Help the patient to the supine position, and drape him if necessary.

• Locate the apical and radial pulses, and then determine a time to begin counting. You should both count beats for 60 seconds.

Sometimes, you'll need to fly solo when taking an apical-radial pulse. If that's the case, be sure to keep both hands on the wheel . . . errr . . . patient and watch your timing.

If you need to work alone

- First auscultate the apex of the heart, holding the stethoscope in place with the hand that holds the watch, and then palpate at the radial artery with the other hand. You can feel any discrepancies between the apical and radial pulses.
- Some heartbeats detected at the apex can't be detected at peripheral sites. When this occurs, the apical pulse rate is higher than the radial pulse rate; the difference is the pulse deficit.

Leaps and bounds

You also need to assess the pulse amplitude. To do so, use a numerical scale or descriptive term to rate or characterize the strength. Numerical scales differ slightly among facilities, but the following scale is commonly used:

- *absent pulse*—not palpable; measured as 0
- *weak or thready pulse*—hard to feel, easily obliterated by slight finger pressure; measured as +1
- *normal pulse*—easily palpable, obliterated by strong finger pressure; measured as +2
- *bounding pulse*—readily palpable, forceful, not easily obliterated by pressure from the fingers; measured as +3. (See *Documenting pulse*.)

Take note!

Documenting pulse

When documenting a pulse, be sure to record pulse rate, rhythm, and volume as well as the time of measurement. "Full" or "bounding" describes a pulse of increased volume; "weak" or "thready," a pulse of decreased volume. When recording apical pulse, include the intensity of heart sounds. When recording apical-radial pulse, chart the rate according to the pulse site—for example, A/R pulse = 80/76.

Respiration

Respiration is the exchange of oxygen and carbon dioxide between the atmosphere and the body. External respiration, or breathing, occurs through the work of the diaphragm and chest muscles and delivers oxygen to the lower respiratory tract and alveoli.

Rate, rhythm, depth, and sound

Respiration can be measured according to rate, rhythm, depth, and sound. These measurements reflect the body's metabolic state, diaphragm and chest muscle condition, and airway patency.

Respiratory rate is recorded as the number of cycles per minute, with inspiration and expiration making up one cycle; rhythm, as the regularity of these cycles. Depth is recorded as the volume of air inhaled and exhaled with each respiration; sound is recorded as the audible digression from normal, effortless breathing.

What you need

A watch with a second hand

How you do it

• The best time to assess your patient's respirations is immediately after taking his pulse rate. Keep your fingertips over his radial artery, and don't tell him that you're counting respirations; *otherwise, he'll become conscious of them and the rate may change.*

Watch the movement

• Count respirations by observing the rise and fall of the chest as the patient breathes. Alternatively, position the patient's opposite arm across the chest, and count respirations by feeling its rise and fall. Consider one rise and one fall as one respiration.
• Count respirations for 30 seconds and multiply by 2, or count for 60 seconds if respirations are irregular *to account for variations in respiratory rate and pattern.*
• Observe chest movements for depth of respirations. If the patient inhales a small volume of air, record the depth as shallow; if inhales a large volume, deep.
• Observe the patient for use of such accessory muscles as the scalene, sternocleidomastoid, trapezius, and latissimus dorsi. Such use indicates weakness of the diaphragm and the external intercostal muscles—the major muscles of respiration.

Listen to the sounds

• As you count respirations, watch for and record such breath sounds as stertor, stridor, wheezing, and expiratory grunting.
• *Stertor* is a snoring sound resulting from secretions in the trachea and large bronchi. Listen for it in comatose patients and in patients with a neurologic disorder.
• *Stridor* is an inspiratory crowing sound that occurs in patients with laryngitis, croup, or upper respiratory tract obstruction with a foreign body. (See *How age affects respiration,* page 124.)
• *Wheezing* is caused by partial obstruction in the smaller bronchi and bronchioles. This high-pitched, musical sound is common in patients with emphysema or asthma.
• To detect other breath sounds—such as crackles and rhonchi—or the lack of them, you'll need a stethoscope.
• Watch the patient's chest movements and listen to breathing to determine the rhythm and sound of respirations. (See *Identifying respiratory patterns,* page 125.)
• Respiratory rates of less than 8 breaths/minute or more than 40 breaths/minute are usually considered abnormal and should be reported promptly.
• Observe the patient for signs of dyspnea, such as an anxious facial expression, flaring nostrils, a heaving chest wall, and cyanosis. To detect cyanosis, look for the characteristic bluish discoloration of the nail beds and lips, under the tongue, in the buccal mucosa, and in the conjunctiva.

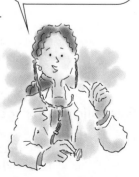

Observing, counting, and listening . . . assessing respirations is an exercise in multi-tasking!

Ages and stages

How age affects respiration

When assessing respirations in pediatric and older patients, keep these points in mind:
• When listening for stridor in infants and children with croup, check for sternal, substernal, and intercostal retractions.
• In infants, an expiratory grunt indicates imminent respiratory distress.
• In older patients, an expiratory grunt indicates partial airway obstruction.

• A child's respiratory rate may double in response to exercise, illness, or emotion.
• Normally, the rate for neonates is 30 to 80 breaths/minute; for toddlers, 20 to 40 breaths/minute; and for children of school age and older, 15 to 25 breaths/minute.
• Children usually reach the adult rate (12 to 20 breaths/minute) at about age 15.

• When assessing a patient's respiratory status, consider personal and family history. Ask if he smokes and, if he does, the number of years and the number of packs per day. (See *Documenting respirations*.)

Accessory to the act . . . of breathing

Use of accessory muscles can enhance lung expansion when oxygenation drops. Patients with chronic obstructive pulmonary disease (COPD) or respiratory distress may use neck muscles, including the sternocleidomastoid muscles, and abdominal muscles for breathing. Patient position during normal breathing may also suggest such problems as COPD. Normal respirations are quiet and easy, so note any abnormal sounds, such as wheezing and stridor.

Blood pressure

Blood pressure, which is the lateral force that blood exerts on arterial walls, is affected by the force of ventricular contractions, arterial wall elasticity, peripheral vascular resistance, and blood volume and viscosity. Blood pressure measurements consist of systolic pressure and diastolic pressure readings.

Systolic (contract) versus diastolic (relax)

Systolic pressure occurs when the left ventricle contracts. It reflects the integrity of the heart, arteries, and arterioles. A normal systolic pressure ranges from

In respiratory disorders, such as COPD, I have to rely on accessory muscles to help me expand.

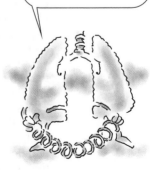

Identifying respiratory patterns

This chart lists types of respirations along with their characteristics, patterns, and possible causes.

Type	Characteristics	Pattern	Possible causes
Apnea	Periodic absence of breathing	———————————	• Mechanical airway obstruction • Conditions affecting the brain's respiratory center in the lateral medulla oblongata
Apneustic	Prolonged, gasping inspiration followed by extremely short, inefficient expiration	∿∿∿∿∿∿∿∿	• Lesions of the respiratory center
Bradypnea	Slow, regular respirations of equal depth	∼∼∼∼∼	• Normal pattern during sleep • Conditions affecting the respiratory center, such as tumors, metabolic disorders, respiratory decompensation, and the use of opiates or alcohol
Cheyne-Stokes	Fast, deep respirations for 30 to 170 seconds punctuated by periods of apnea lasting 20 to 60 seconds	∿∿__∿∿∿__∿∿	• Increased intracranial pressure, severe heart failure, renal failure, meningitis, drug overdose, and cerebral anoxia
Eupnea	Normal rate and rhythm	∿∿∿∿∿	• Normal respiration
Kussmaul	Fast (more than 20 breaths/minute), deep (resembling sighs), labored respirations without pause	∧∧∧∧∧∧∧∧∧∧	• Renal failure and metabolic acidosis, particularly diabetic ketoacidosis
Tachypnea	Rapid respirations, rate rises with body temperature at about 4 breaths/minute for each degree Fahrenheit above normal	∿∿∿∿∿∿∿	• Pneumonia, compensatory respiratory alkalosis, respiratory insufficiency, lesions of the respiratory center, and salicylate poisoning

Take note!

Documenting respirations

Record the rate, depth, rhythm, and sound of the patient's respirations.

100 to 119 mm Hg. *Diastolic pressure* occurs when the left ventricle relaxes. It indicates blood vessel resistance. A normal diastolic pressure ranges from 60 to 79 mm Hg. It's generally more significant as it measures the heart at rest. Both pressures are measured in millimeters of mercury with a sphygmomanometer and a stethoscope, usually at the brachial artery.

Systolic pressure – diastolic pressure = pulse pressure

Pulse pressure or the difference between systolic an diastolic pressures varies inversely with arterial elasticity. Normally, systolic pressure exceeds diastolic pressure by about 40 mm Hg. Narrowed pulse pressure, or a difference of less than 30 mm Hg, occurs when systolic pressure falls and diastolic pressure rises. These changes reflect reduced stroke volume, increased peripheral resistance, or both.

Widened pulse pressure, a difference of more than 50 mm Hg between systolic and diastolic pressures, occurs when systolic pressure rises and diastolic pressure remains constant or when systolic pressure rises and diastolic pressure falls. These changes reflect increased stroke volume, decreased peripheral resistance, or both.

Goin' up

Blood pressure rises with age, weight gain, prolonged stress, and anxiety. (See *Effects of age on blood pressure*.)

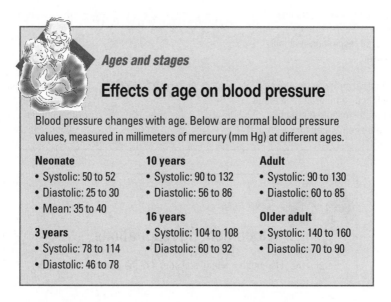

Ages and stages

Effects of age on blood pressure

Blood pressure changes with age. Below are normal blood pressure values, measured in millimeters of mercury (mm Hg) at different ages.

Neonate
- Systolic: 50 to 52
- Diastolic: 25 to 30
- Mean: 35 to 40

3 years
- Systolic: 78 to 114
- Diastolic: 46 to 78

10 years
- Systolic: 90 to 132
- Diastolic: 56 to 86

16 years
- Systolic: 104 to 108
- Diastolic: 60 to 92

Adult
- Systolic: 90 to 130
- Diastolic: 60 to 85

Older adult
- Systolic: 140 to 160
- Diastolic: 70 to 90

What you need

Sphygmomanometer, stethoscope, automated vital signs monitor (if available)

Cuffs come in six standard sizes, ranging from neonate to extra-large adult. Disposable cuffs are available.

The automated vital signs monitor is a noninvasive device that measures pulse rate, systolic and diastolic pressures, and mean arterial pressure at preset intervals. (See *Using an electronic vital signs monitor*, page 128.)

Getting ready

• Carefully choose a cuff of appropriate size for the patient. An excessively narrow cuff may cause a false-high reading; an excessively wide one, a false-low reading.
• To use an automated vital signs monitor, collect the monitor, dual air hose, and pressure cuff. Then make sure the monitor unit is firmly positioned near the patient's bed.

How you do it

• Introduce yourself to your patient, wash your hands, and tell the patient that you're going to take their blood pressure.
• The patient can lie in a supine position or sit erect while you measure their blood pressure. The arm should be extended at heart level and be well supported. *If the artery is below heart level, you may get a false-high reading.* Make sure the patient is relaxed and comfortable when you measure the blood pressure *so it stays at its normal level.*

Don't compromise

• Don't take a blood pressure measurement on the same arm of an arteriovenous fistula or hemodialysis shunt *because blood flow through the device may be compromised.* Don't take a blood pressure measurement on the affected side of a mastectomy *because it may compromise lymphatic circulation, worsen edema, and damage the arm.* Also, don't take blood pressure on the same arm as a peripherally inserted central catheter *because it may damage the device.*
• Be careful, some blood pressure cuffs contain latex. Assess the patient for a latex allergy and use latex-free blood pressure cuff if indicated.
• Wrap the deflated cuff snugly around the patient's upper arm.
• If necessary, connect the appropriate tube to the rubber bulb of the air pump and the other tube to the manometer. Then insert the stethoscope earpieces into your ears.

Using an electronic vital signs monitor

An electronic vital signs monitor allows you to continually track a patient's vital signs without having to reapply a blood pressure cuff each time. What's more, the patient won't need an invasive arterial line to gather similar data. The steps below can be followed with most monitors.

Some automated vital signs monitors are lightweight and battery-operated and can be attached to an I.V. pole for continual monitoring, even during patient transfers. Make sure you know the capacity of the monitor's battery, and plug the machine in whenever possible to keep it charged.

Before using any monitor, check its accuracy. Determine the patient's pulse rate and blood pressure manually, using the same arm you'll use for the monitor cuff. Compare your results when you get initial readings from the monitor. If the results differ, call your supply department or the manufacturer's representative.

Preparing the device

• Explain the procedure to the patient. Describe the alarm system so the patient won't be frightened if it's triggered.
• Make sure the power switch is off. Then plug the monitor into a properly grounded wall outlet. Secure the dual air hose to the front of the monitor.
• Connect the pressure cuff's tubing into the other ends of the dual air hose and tighten the connections to prevent air leaks. Keep the air hose away from the patient so that it isn't accidentally dislodged.
• Squeeze all air from the cuff, and wrap the cuff loosely around the patient's arm or leg, allowing two finger-breadths between the cuff and the arm or leg. Never apply the cuff to a limb that has an I.V. line in place or to an individual who has had breast or lymph node excision on that side or has an arteriovenous graft, shunt, or fistula. Position the cuff's "artery" arrow over the palpated brachial artery. Then secure the cuff for a snug fit.

Selecting parameters

• When you turn on the monitor, it will default to a manual mode. (In this mode, you can obtain vital signs yourself before switching to the automatic mode.) Press the AUTO/MANUAL button to select the automatic mode. The monitor will give you baseline data for the pulse rate, systolic and diastolic pressures, and mean arterial pressure.
• Compare your previous manual results with these baseline data. If they match, you're ready to set the alarm parameters. Press the SELECT button to blank out all displays except systolic pressure.
• Use the HIGH and LOW limit buttons to set the specific parameters for systolic pressure. (These limits range from a high of 240 to a low of 0.) You'll also do this three more times for mean arterial pressure, pulse rate, and diastolic pressure. After you've set the parameters for diastolic pressure, press the SELECT button again to display all current data. If you forget to do this last step, the monitor will automatically display current data 10 seconds after you set the last parameters.

Collecting data

• You also need to tell the monitor how often to obtain data. Press the SET button until you reach the desired time interval in minutes. If you've chosen the automatic mode, the monitor will display a default cycle time of 3 minutes. You can override the default cycle time to set the interval you prefer.
• You can obtain a set of vital signs any time by pressing the START button. Also, pressing the CANCEL button will stop the interval and deflate the cuff. You can retrieve stored data by pressing the PRIOR DATA button. The monitor will display the last data obtained along with the time elapsed since then. Scrolling backward, you can retrieve data from the previous 99 minutes.

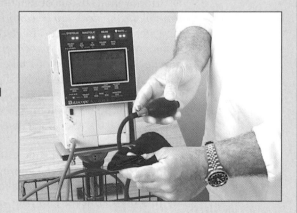

Go with the bell

• Palpate the brachial artery. Center the bell of the stethoscope over the part of the artery where you detect the strongest beats and hold it in place with one hand. *The bell of the stethoscope transmits low-pitched arterial blood sounds more effectively than the diaphragm.* (See *Using a sphygmomanometer.*)

• Using the thumb and index finger of your other hand, turn the thumbscrew on the rubber bulb of the air pump clockwise to close the valve.

• Pump air into the cuff while auscultating for the sound over the brachial artery *to compress and, eventually, occlude arterial blood flow.* Continue pumping air until the mercury column or aneroid gauge registers 160 mm Hg or at least 30 mm Hg above the level of the last audible sound.

• Carefully open the valve of the air pump. Then deflate the cuff no faster than 5 mm Hg/second while

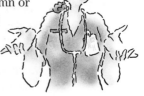

Be aware of preexisting conditions or problems that can compromise the blood pressure reading or your patient's health.

Using a sphygmomanometer

Here's how to use a sphygmomanometer properly:

• For accuracy and consistency, position your patient with his upper arm at heart level and his palm turned up.

• Apply the cuff snugly, 1" (2.5 cm) above the brachial pulse, as shown in the top photo.

• Position the manometer at your eye level.

• Palpate the brachial or radial pulse with your fingertips while inflating the cuff.

• Inflate the cuff to 30 mm Hg above the point where the pulse disappears.

• Place the bell of your stethoscope over the point where you felt the pulse, as shown in the bottom photo. Using the bell helps you better hear Korotkoff sounds, which indicate pulse.

• Release the valve slowly and note the point at which Korotkoff sounds reappear. The start of the pulse sound indicates the systolic pressure.

• The sounds will become muffled and then disappear. The last Korotkoff sound you hear is the diastolic pressure.

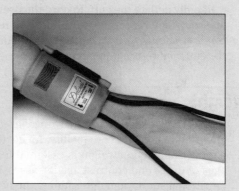

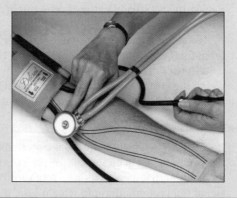

watching the mercury column or aneroid gauge and auscultating for the sound over the artery.

Tune in to the five sounds

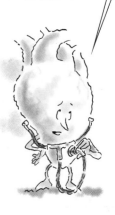

That's one (tap) . . . two (swish) . . . three (tap) . . . four (muffle) . . . five . . .

• When you hear the first beat or clear tapping sound, note the pressure on the column or gauge—that is, the systolic pressure. (The beat or tapping sound is the first of five Korotkoff sounds. The second sound resembles a murmur or swish; the third, crisp tapping; the fourth, a soft, muffled tone; and the fifth, the last sound heard.)
• Continue to release air gradually while auscultating for the sound over the artery.
• Note the diastolic pressure—the fourth Korotkoff sound. If you continue to hear sounds as the column or gauge falls to zero (common in children), record the pressure at the beginning of the fourth sound. *This step is important because, in some patients, a distinct fifth sound is absent.* (For information on situations that can cause false-high or false-low readings, see *Correcting problems of blood pressure measurement.*)

One mo' time

• Rapidly deflate the cuff. Record the pressure, wait 1 to 2 minutes, and then repeat the procedure and record the pressures *to confirm your original findings.* After doing so, remove and fold the cuff, and return it to storage.

Height and weight

Height and weight are routinely measured when a patient is admitted to a health care facility. An accurate record of the patient's height and weight is essential for calculating dosages of drugs and contrast agents, assessing the patient's nutritional status, and determining the height-to-weight ratio. Reassure and steady patients who are at risk for losing their balance on a scale.

Weigh the patient at the same time each day (usually before breakfast), in similar clothing, and using the same scale. If the patient uses crutches, weigh the patient with the crutches. Then weigh the crutches and any heavy clothing and subtract their weight from the total to determine the patient's weight.

What weight tells you

Because body weight is the best overall indicator of fluid status, daily monitoring is important for patients receiving a diuretic or a medication that causes sodium retention. Rapid weight gain may signal fluid retention; rapid weight loss, diuresis.

Correcting problems of blood pressure measurement

This chart lists blood pressure measurement problems along with their causes and appropriate nursing actions.

Causes	Nursing actions
False-high reading	
Cuff too small	Make sure the cuff bladder is 20% wider than the circumference of the arm or leg being used for measurement.
Cuff wrapped too loosely, reducing its effective width	Tighten the cuff.
Cuff deflated too slowly, causing venous congestion in the arm or leg	Never deflate the cuff more slowly than 2 mm Hg per heartbeat.
Mercury column tilted	Read pressures with the mercury column vertical.
Measurement poorly timed (e.g., after the patient has eaten, ambulated, appeared anxious, or flexed their arm muscles)	Postpone the blood pressure measurement or help the patient relax before measuring the blood pressure.
False-low reading	
Arm or leg positioned incorrectly	Make sure the patient's arm or leg is level with the heart.
Mercury column below eye level	Read the mercury column at eye level.
Auscultatory gap (sound fades out for 10 to 15 mm Hg and then returns) unnoticed	Estimate systolic pressure by palpation before measuring it. Then check this pressure against measured pressure.
Low-volume sounds inaudible	Before reinflating the cuff, instruct the patient to raise their arm or leg to decrease venous pressure and amplify low-volume sounds. After inflating the cuff, tell the patient to lower their arm or leg. Then deflate the cuff and listen. If you still fail to detect low volume sounds, chart palpated systolic pressure.

Scales for every position

Weight can be measured with a standing scale, chair scale, or bed scale. Height can be measured with the measuring bar on a standing scale or with a tape measure for a patient confined to a supine position.

What you need

Standing scale with measuring bar or chair or bed scale, wheelchair if needed (to transport patient), tape measure if needed

Getting ready

Select the appropriate scale—usually, a standing scale for an ambulatory patient or a chair or bed scale for an acutely ill or debilitated patient. Then make sure the scale is balanced. Standing scales and, to a lesser extent, bed scales may become unbalanced when transported.

How you do it

• Introduce yourself to the patient. Tell the patient that you're going to measure their height and weight. Explain the procedure to the patient, depending on which type of scale you'll use.

Using a standing scale

• Place a paper towel on the scale's platform.
• Tell the patient to remove their robe and slippers or shoes. If the scale has wheels, lock them before the patient steps on. Assist the patient onto the scale and remain close to them *to prevent falls*.

That's upright balance

• If you're using an upright balance scale, slide the lower rider to the groove representing the largest increment below the patient's estimated weight. Grooves represent 50, 100, 150, and 200 lb.
• Slide the small upper rider until the beam balances. Add the upper and lower rider figures to determine the weight.

That's multiple weight

• If using a multiple-weight scale, move the appropriate ratio weights onto the weight holder to balance the scale; ratio weights are labeled 50, 100, and 200 lb.
• Add ratio weights until the next weight causes the main beam to fall.
• Adjust the main beam poise until the scale balances.
• To obtain the weight, add the sum of the ratio weights to the figure on the main beam.
• Return ratio weights to their rack and the weight holder to its proper place.

That's digital

• If you're using a digital scale, make sure the display reads 0 before use.
• Read the display with the patient standing as still as possible.

Raising the bar

• If you're measuring height, tell the patient to stand erect on the scale's platform. Raise the measuring bar above the patient's head, extend the horizontal arm, and lower the bar until it touches the top of the patient's head. Then read the patient's height.

• Help the patient off the scale and give the patient their robe and slippers or shoes. Then return the measuring bar to its initial position.

Using a chair scale

• Transport the patient to the weighing area or the scale to the patient's bedside.
• Lock the scale in place *to prevent it from moving accidentally*.
• If you're using a scale with a swing-away chair arm, unlock the arm. When unlocked, the arm swings back 180 degrees *to permit easy access*.
• Position the scale beside the patient's bed or wheelchair with the chair arm open. Transfer the patient onto the scale, swing the chair arm to the front of the scale, and lock it in place.
• Weigh the patient by adding ratio weights and adjusting the main beam poise. Then unlock the swing-away chair arm as before, and transfer the patient back to his bed or wheelchair.
• Lock the main beam *to avoid damaging the scale during transport*. Then unlock the wheels and remove the scale from the patient's room.

Using a bed scale

• Cover the bed scale stretcher with a drawsheet. Balance the scale with the drawsheet in place *to ensure an accurate measurement*.
• Provide privacy, and tell the patient that you're going to weigh them on a special bed scale.
• When rolling the patient onto the stretcher, be careful not to dislodge I.V. lines, indwelling catheters, and other supportive equipment.
• Position the scale next to the patient's bed, and lock the scale's wheels. Then turn the patient onto their side, facing away from the scale.
• Release the stretcher frame to the horizontal position, and pump the hand lever until the stretcher is positioned over the mattress. Lower the stretcher onto the mattress, and roll the patient onto the stretcher.
• Raise the stretcher 2″ (5 cm) above the mattress. Then add ratio weights, and adjust the main beam poise as for the standing and chair scales.
• After weighing the patient, lower the stretcher onto the mattress, turn the patient onto their side, and remove the stretcher. Be sure to leave the patient in a comfortable position.

Using a digital bed scale

• Release the stretcher to the horizontal position; then lock it in place. Turn the patient onto their side, facing away from the scale.

- Roll the base of the scale under the patient's bed. Adjust the lever *to widen the base of the scale, providing stability.* Then lock the scale's wheels.
- Center the stretcher above the bed, lower it onto the mattress, and roll the patient onto the stretcher. Then position the circular weighing arms of the scale over the patient, and attach them securely to the stretcher bars.
- Pump the handle with long, slow strokes *to raise the patient a few inches off the bed.* Make sure the patient doesn't lean on or touch the headboard, side rails, or other bed equipment *because doing so will affect weight measurement.*
- Depress the OPERATE button, and read the patient's weight on the digital display panel. Then press in the scale's handle *to lower the patient.*
- Detach the circular weighing arms from the stretcher bars, roll the patient off the stretcher and remove it, and position comfortably in bed.
- Release the wheel lock and withdraw the scale. Return the stretcher to its vertical position.

> When you return the patient to bed after weighing her with a bed scale, be sure to leave the patient in a comfortable position.

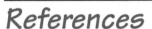

References

Berman, A., & Snyder, S. J. (2012). *Skills in clinical nursing* (7th ed.). Upper Saddle River, NJ: Pearson Education.

Berman, A., Snyder, S. J., & McKinney, D. S. (2011). *Nursing basics for clinical practice.* Upper Saddle River, NJ: Pearson Education.

Treas, L. S., & Wilkinson, J. M. (2014). *Basic nursing concepts, skills, & reasoning.* Philadelphia, PA: F.A. Davis.

Quick quiz

1. Which heart rate in a neonate would be considered normal?
    A. 60 to 80 beats/minute
    B. 100 to 120 beats/minute
    C. 120 to 140 beats/minute
    D. 160 to 200 beats/minute

Answer: C. A heart rate of 120 to 140 beats/minute in a neonate is considered normal.

2. The highest temperature reading would be expected to occur during what time of day?
A.   4 and 5 a.m.
B.   8 and 9 a.m.
C.   4 and 8 p.m.
D.   9 and 11 p.m.

Answer: C. Temperature normally fluctuates with rest and activity. Lowest readings typically occur between 4 and 5 a.m.; the highest readings, between 4 and 8 p.m.

3. Which lung sound is referred to as a snoring sound that results from secretions in the trachea?
A.   Stertor
B.   Stridor
C.   Wheezing
D.   Expiratory grunting

Answer: A. Stertor is a snoring sound that results from secretions in the trachea and large bronchi.

4. Which method for assessing temperature is the least accurate?
A.   Oral
B.   Rectal
C.   Tympanic
D.   Axillary

Answer: D. Axillary temperature, the least accurate reading, is usually 1° to 2° F (0.6° to 1.1° C) lower.

Scoring

✩✩✩ If you answered all four questions correctly, congratulations! You're a vital signs expert.

✩✩ If you answered three questions correctly, great! You've got the pulse on vital signs assessment skills.

✩ If you answered fewer than three questions correctly, don't despair. Take a deep breath, listen to your heart, and know that you still measure up to a good nurse!

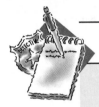

8

Asepsis and infection control

Just the facts

In this chapter, you'll learn:

♦ types of infection

♦ ways infection is spread

♦ proper hand hygiene

♦ ways to put on isolation equipment.

A look at infection

Infection is the invasion and multiplication of microorganisms in or on body tissues that produce signs and symptoms as well as an immune response. Such reproduction injures the host by causing cellular damage from microorganism-produced toxins or intracellular multiplication or competing with host metabolism.

Your own worst enemy

The host's own immune response may compound the tissue damage. The damage may be localized (as in infected pressure ulcers) or systemic. The infection's severity varies with the pathogenicity and number of the invading microorganisms and the strength of host defenses. The very young and the very old are especially susceptible to infections. In addition, individuals who are hospitalized are especially at risk for contracting a hospital-acquired infection.

Factor in . . .

Certain factors contribute to increase the risk of infection. For example, travel can expose people to diseases for which they have little natural immunity. In addition, the expanded use of immunosuppressants, surgery, and other invasive procedures increases the risk of infection.

> Severity of infection depends on invading organisms and the strength of host defenses.

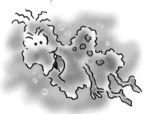

Types of infection

There are three major types of infection:

   Subclinical, also called *silent* or *asymptomatic,* is a laboratory-verified infection that causes no signs and symptoms.

   Colonized is a multiplication of microbes that produces no signs, symptoms, or immune responses.

   Dormant, also called *latent,* occurs after a microorganism has been dormant in the host, sometimes for years. An exogenous infection results from environmental pathogens; an endogenous infection, from the host's normal flora (e.g., *Escherichia coli* displaced from the colon, which may cause urinary tract infection).

   Active infection is when a patient is symptomatic and has an immune response. Because a person with a subclinical infection or colonization may not have symptoms, this person can be a carrier and transmit infection to others.

Types of infecting organisms

The varied forms of microorganisms responsible for infectious diseases include bacteria, spirochetes (a type of bacteria), viruses, rickettsiae, chlamydiae, fungi, and protozoa. Larger organisms such as helminths (worms) may also cause disease.

Bacteria

Bacteria are single-cell microorganisms with well-defined cell walls that can multiply independently on artificial media without the need for other cells. In developing countries, where poor sanitation heightens the risk of infection, bacterial diseases commonly cause death and disability. Even in industrialized countries, they're still the most common fatal infectious diseases. (See *Bacteria: Oh, the damage they can do!,* page 138.)

Shaping up

Bacteria can be classified by shape:
• *spherical*—cocci
• *rod-shaped*—bacilli
• *spiral-shaped*—spirilla.

Bacteria: Oh, the damage they can do!

Bacteria and other infectious organisms constantly infect the human body. Some are beneficial, such as the intestinal bacteria that produce vitamins. Others are harmful, causing illnesses ranging from acute otitis media to life-threatening septic shock.

To infect a host, bacteria must first enter it. They do this by adhering to the mucosal surface and directly invading the host cell or attaching to epithelial cells and producing toxins that invade host cells. To survive and multiply within a host, bacteria or their toxins adversely affect biochemical reactions in cells. The result is a disruption of normal cell functions or cell death (as shown below).

For example, the diphtheria toxin damages heart muscle by inhibiting protein synthesis. In addition, as some organisms multiply, they extend into deeper tissue and eventually enter the bloodstream.

Some toxins cause blood to clot in small blood vessels. The tissues supplied by these vessels may be deprived of blood and damaged (as shown below).

Other toxins can damage the cell walls of small blood vessels, causing leakage. This fluid loss results in decreased blood pressure, which in turn impairs the heart's ability to pump enough blood to vital organs (as shown below).

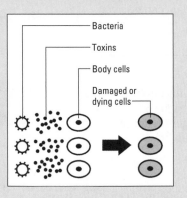

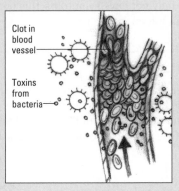

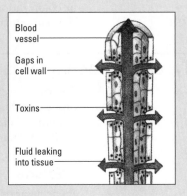

Response, motility, capsulation, spores, and O_2

They also can be classified by:
- response to staining—gram-positive, gram-negative, or acid-fast
- motility—motile or nonmotile
- tendency toward capsulation—encapsulated or nonencapsulated
- capacity to form spores—sporulating or nonsporulating
- oxygen requirements—aerobic (need oxygen to grow) or anaerobic (don't need oxygen).

Spirochetes

A type of bacteria, spirochetes is flexible, slender, undulating spiral rods that have cell walls. Most are anaerobic. The three pathogenic forms in humans include *Treponema*, *Leptospira*, and *Borrelia*.

Viruses

Viruses are subcellular organisms made up of only an RNA or a DNA nucleus covered with proteins. They're the smallest known organisms, so tiny that they're visible only through an electron microscope.

> How can such a tiny little thing cause so much trouble?

An invasion occasion

Viruses can't replicate independent of host cells. Rather, they invade a host cell and stimulate it to participate in the formation of additional virus particles. The estimated 400 viruses that infect humans are classified according to their size, shape (spherical, rod-shaped, or cubic), or means of transmission (respiratory, fecal, oral, or sexual).

Rickettsiae

Relatively uncommon in the United States, rickettsiae are small, gram-negative, bacteria-like organisms that commonly induce life-threatening infections. Like viruses, they require a host cell for replication. Three genera of rickettsiae include *Rickettsia*, *Coxiella*, and *Rochalimaea*.

Chlamydiae

Larger than viruses, chlamydiae have recently been found to be intracellular obligate bacteria. Unlike other bacteria, they depend on host cells for replication. However, unlike viruses, they're susceptible to antibiotics.

> Don't look now, but I think there's a fungus among us.

Fungi

Fungi are single-cell organisms that have nuclei enveloped by nuclear membranes. They have rigid cell walls like plant cells but lack chlorophyll, the green matter necessary for photosynthesis. They also show relatively little cellular specialization. Fungi occur as yeasts (single-cell, oval-shaped organisms) or molds (organisms with hyphae or branching filaments). Depending on the environment, some fungi may occur in both forms. Fungal diseases in humans are called *mycoses*.

Protozoa

Protozoa are the simplest single-cell organisms of the animal kingdom, but they show a high level of cellular specialization. Like other animal cells, they have cell membranes rather than cell walls, and their nuclei are surrounded by nuclear membranes.

Helminths

The three groups of helminths that invade humans include nematodes, cestodes, and trematodes. Nematodes are cylindrical, unsegmented, elongated helminths that taper at each end; this shape has earned them the designation *roundworm*. Cestodes, better known as *tapeworms*, have bodies that are flattened front to back with distinct, regular segments. Tapeworms also have heads with suckers or sucking grooves. Trematodes have flattened, unsegmented bodies. They're called *blood, intestinal, lung, or liver flukes*, depending on their infection site.

Modes of transmission

Infectious diseases are transmitted directly (by contact) or indirectly. Indirect transmission may occur via airborne transmission, vector-borne transmission, or vehicle-borne transmission.

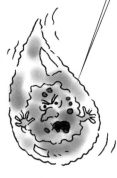

I'll find a way in— one way or another!

Close contact

In contact transmission, the susceptible host comes into direct contact (as in sexually transmitted diseases) or indirect contact (contaminated inanimate objects) with the source. Direct transmission may also occur via droplet spread—the close-range spray of contaminated droplets into the conjunctiva or mucous membranes.

How's the air?

Airborne transmission results from inhalation of contaminated evaporated saliva droplets (as in pulmonary tuberculosis), which sometimes are suspended in airborne dust particles or vapors. These airborne particles are small and light that's why they are airborne. (Think droplet = larger particles that drop to the ground vs. airborne = lighter particles that float in the air.)

Hector vector

Vector-borne transmission occurs when an intermediate carrier (vector), such as a flea or a mosquito, transfers an organism. Vehicle-borne transmission occurs when water, food, or blood products introduce organisms into a susceptible host via ingestion or inoculation.

Health care–associated infections

Formerly known as *nosocomial infections*, health care–associated infections (HAIs) develop while a patient is in a health care

Preventing health care–associated infections

Here's how to help prevent HAIs:
• Follow good hand-washing techniques and encourage other staff members to do the same.
• Follow strict infection control procedures.
• Document hospital infections as they occur.
• Identify outbreaks early and take steps to prevent their spread.
• Eliminate unnecessary procedures that contribute to infection.
• Strictly follow necessary isolation techniques.
• Observe all patients for signs of infection, especially patients who are at high risk for infection.
• Keep staff members and visitors with obvious infection as well as known carriers away from susceptible patients.

facility or another facility. According to the Centers for Disease Control and Prevention (CDC), every day, about 1 in every 20 hospitalized patients has an infection caused by receiving medical care. Annually, at least 2 million people will become infected with bacteria that are resistant to antibiotics in the United States alone. In addition, the number of people who will die each year as a direct result of these infections will topple over 23,000 patients. Most infections of this type result from group A *Streptococcus pyogenes, Staphylococcus, Escherichia coli, Klebsiella, Proteus, Pseudomonas, Haemophilus influenzae, Candida albicans,* and hepatitis viruses.

HAIs are usually transmitted by direct contact. Less commonly, they're transmitted by inhalation of or wound invasion by airborne organisms or contaminated equipment and solutions.

Many risks for many reasons

HAIs continue to pose a problem because most facility patients are older and more debilitated than in the past. The advances in treatment that increase longevity in patients with diseases that alter immune defenses also create a population at high risk for infection. Moreover, the growing use of invasive and surgical procedures, immunosuppressants, and antibiotics predisposes patients to infection and superinfection and helps create new strains of antibiotic-resistant bacteria. The growing number of facility personnel that come in contact with each patient increases the risk of exposure. (See *CDC isolation precautions,* pages 142 and 143.)

CDC isolation precautions

The CDC's *Guidelines for Isolation Precautions in Hospitals*, developed by the CDC and the Hospital Infection Control Practices Advisory Committee, help facilities maintain up-to-date isolation practices.

Standard precautions

The guidelines contain two tiers of precautions. The first—called *standard precautions*—are those designated for the care of all facility patients regardless of their diagnosis or presumed infection. Standard precautions are the primary strategy for preventing HAI. These precautions apply to:
• blood
• all body fluids, secretions, and excretions, except sweat, regardless of whether they contain visible blood
• skin that isn't intact
• mucous membranes.

Transmission-based precautions

The second tier of precautions, *transmission-based precautions*, are instituted for patients who are known to be or suspected of being infected with a highly transmissible infection—one that needs precautions beyond those set forth in the standard precautions. There are three types of transmission-based precautions: airborne precautions, droplet precautions, and contact precautions.

Airborne precautions

Airborne precautions apply to patients known or suspected to be infected with microorganisms transmitted by airborne droplet nuclei. These precautions are designed to reduce the risk of airborne transmission of infectious agents. Microorganisms carried through the air can be dispersed widely by air currents, making them available for inhalation or deposit on a susceptible host in the same room or a longer distance away from the infected patient. Airborne precautions include special air handling and ventilation procedures to prevent the spread of infection. They require the use of respiratory protection such as a mask—in addition to standard precautions—when entering an infected patient's room. This should be either N95 or PAPR. This patient must be placed in a special room known as an *airborne infection isolation room*.

Airborne infection isolation room

At a minimum, airborne infection isolation room (AIIR) rooms must:
  Provide negative pressure room with a minimum of 6 air exchanges per hour
  Exhaust directly to the outside or through HEPA (High Efficiency Particulate Air) filtration

Droplet precautions

These precautions are designed to reduce the risk of transmitting infectious agents through large-particle (exceeding 5 micrometers) droplets. Such transmission involves contact of infectious agents with the conjunctivae or the nasal or oral mucous membranes of a susceptible person. Large-particle droplets don't remain in the air and generally travel short distances of 3' (1 m) or less. They require the use of a mask—in addition to standard precautions—to protect the mucous membranes.

Contact precautions

These precautions are designed to reduce the risk of transmitting infectious agents by direct or indirect contact. Direct-contact transmission can occur through patient care activities that require physical contact. Indirect-contact mission involves a susceptible host coming in contact with a contaminated object, usually inanimate, in the patient's environment. Contact precautions require the use of gloves, a mask, and a gown—in addition to standard precautions—to avoid contact with the infectious agent. Stringent hand washing is also necessary after removal of the protective items.

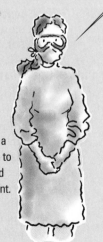

Always take precautions and wear personal protective gear when warranted!

CDC isolation precautions (continued)

Always take the right precautions! This chart shows the different types of precautions and provides examples of infections for which specific precautions would be used.

Precautions	Indications
Standard precautions	Designated for all patients regardless of diagnosis or presumed infection
Airborne precautions (used in addition to standard precautions)	Patients known to have or suspected of having a serious illness transmitted by airborne droplet nuclei, such as: • measles • tuberculosis • varicella • severe acute respiratory syndrome (SARS).
Droplet precautions (used in addition to standard precautions)	Patients known to have or suspected of having a serious illness transmitted by large-particle droplets, such as: • invasive *Haemophilus influenzae* type b disease, including meningitis, pneumonia, epiglottitis, and sepsis • invasive *Neisseria meningitides* disease, including meningitis, pneumonia, and sepsis • other serious bacterial respiratory infections spread by droplets, such as diphtheria; *Mycoplasma* pneumonia; pertussis; pneumonic plague; and streptococcal (Group A) pharyngitis, pneumonia, or scarlet fever in infants and young children • other serious viral infections spread by droplets, including adenovirus, influenza, mumps, parvovirus B19 (with most serious risk to fetuses), and rubella.
Contact precautions (used in addition to standard precautions)	Patients known to have or suspected of having a serious illness that can be transmitted by direct patient contact or by contact with items in the patient's environment. Examples of such illnesses include: • GI, respiratory, skin, or wound infections or colonization with multidrug-resistant bacteria judged by the infection control program (based on current state, regional, or national recommendations) to be of special clinical and epidemiologic significance • enteric infections with a low infectious dose or prolonged environmental survival, including *Clostridium difficile* or, for diapered or incontinent patients, enterohemorrhagic *Escherichia coli* O157:H7, *Shigella*, hepatitis A, or rotavirus • respiratory syncytial virus, parainfluenza virus, or enteroviral infections in infants and young children • skin infections that are highly contagious or that may occur on dry skin, including diphtheria (cutaneous); herpes simplex virus (neonatal or mucocutaneous); impetigo; major (noncontained) abscesses, cellulitis, or decubiti; pediculosis; scabies; staphylococcal furunculosis in infants and young children; zoster (disseminated or in an immunocompromised host) • viral or hemorrhagic conjunctivitis • viral hemorrhagic infections (Ebola, Lassa, or Marburg). Neutrophils are immature WBCs and are the important warrior cells that our body uses to fight infection. In certain patients, especially those receiving chemotherapy, these neutrophils are extremely lowered. In these patients, they can become infected from their environment. Precautions include: • No live flowers, fruits, or vegetables. All food must be well cooked. • Private room • Patient must wear a mask when out of the room. Health care providers should wear a mask if any illness persists. • Strict handwashing.

Need for accurate assessment

Accurate assessment helps identify infectious diseases and prevents avoidable complications. Complete assessment consists of a patient history, a physical examination, and diagnostic tests.

All the details

The history should include the patient's gender, age, address, occupation, and place of work; known exposure to infection; and date of disease onset. It should also detail information about recent hospitalization, blood transfusions, blood donation denial by the Red Cross or other agencies, vaccination, travel or camping trips, and exposure to animals. If a patient has contracted an HAI in the recent past, depending on the policy of the institution, the patient may be put in isolation precautions.

Diseases, drugs, diet . . .

If applicable, ask the patient about possible exposure to sexually transmitted diseases and about drug abuse. Also ask him about his usual dietary patterns, unusual fatigue, and factors that may predispose the patient to infection, such as neoplastic disease and alcoholism. Notice if the patient is listless or uneasy, lacks concentration, or has any obvious abnormality of mood or affect.

Suspicions? See the skin

In suspected infection, a physical examination includes assessment of the skin, mucous membranes, liver, spleen, and lymph nodes. Check for and note the location and type of drainage from skin lesions. Record skin color, temperature, and turgor; ask if the patient has pruritus. Skin with a warm or red appearance is always suspected.

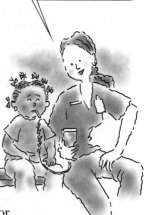

Always remember that a fever is often the best sign of infection.

Follow the fever

Monitor the patient's temperature, using the same route consistently, and watch for a fever, the best indicator of many infections. Note and record the pattern of temperature change and the effect of antipyretics. Many times you will avoid the use of antipyretics. Be aware that certain analgesics may contain antipyretics, which will mask a fever. Watch for seizures in cases of high fever, above 105° F, especially in children.

Mostly up, sometimes down

Check the patient's pulse rate. Infection commonly increases the pulse rate, but some infections such as typhoid fever may decrease it. In severe infection or when complications are possible, monitor the patient for hypotension, hematuria, oliguria, hepatomegaly, jaundice, palpable and painful lymph nodes, bleeding from gums or into joints, and altered level of consciousness. Obtain diagnostic tests and appropriate cultures, as ordered.

Preventing infection

Comprehensive immunization (including immunization of travelers to or emigrants from endemic areas); improved nutrition, living conditions, and sanitation; and correction of other environmental factors are some broad steps the health care community can take to prevent infection.

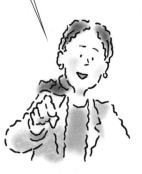

Immunizations and improved living conditions are great, but there's a lot YOU can do to prevent infection, too!

What YOU can do

Individual health care professionals can also prevent infection by:
• employing drug prophylaxis when necessary
• using strict hand-hygiene technique
• following standard precautions
• using correct isolation garb.

Drug prophylaxis

Although prophylactic antibiotic therapy may prevent certain diseases, the risk of superinfection and the emergence of drug-resistant strains may outweigh the benefits. So prophylactic antibiotics are usually reserved for patients at high risk for exposure to dangerous infection.

Hand hygiene

The hands are the conduits for almost every transfer of potential pathogens from one patient to another, from a contaminated object to the patient, or from a staff member to the patient. Hand hygiene is the single most important procedure in preventing infection. To protect patients from HAIs, hand hygiene must be performed routinely and thoroughly.

Keep it real

In effect, clean and healthy hands with intact skin; short, natural fingernails; and no rings minimize the risk of contamination. Artificial nails may serve as a reservoir for microorganisms, and microorganisms are more difficult to remove from rough or chapped hands.

Present arms

Before participating in any sterile procedure or whenever your hands are grossly contaminated, remember to wash your forearms and clean under your fingernails and in and around the cuticles with a fingernail brush, disposable sponge brush, or plastic cuticle stick. Use these softer implements because brushes, metal files, or other hard objects may injure your skin and, if reused, may be a source of contamination.

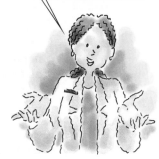

Think of your hands as healing tools. Always keep them clean, healthy, and ready to assist . . . naturally!

Soap for most

Follow your facility's policy concerning when to wash with soap and when to use an antiseptic cleaning agent. Typically, you'll wash with soap before coming on duty; before and after direct or indirect patient contact; before and after performing any bodily functions, such as blowing your nose or using the bathroom; before preparing or serving food; before preparing or administering medications; after direct or indirect contact with a patient's excretions, secretions, or blood; and after completing your shift.

Antiseptic when susceptible

Use an antiseptic cleaning agent before performing invasive procedures, wound care, and dressing changes and after contamination. Antiseptics are also recommended for hand washing in isolation rooms, newborn nurseries, and before caring for any highly susceptible patient.

Hold the alcohol

If your hands aren't visibly soiled, an alcohol-based hand rub is preferred for routine decontamination. Don't use alcohol-based hand sanitizer if you might come in contact with items contaminated with *Clostridium difficile* or *Bacillus anthracis* (Anthrax). These organisms can form spores and alcohol will not kill spores. Wash hands with soap and water or antiseptic soap and water if either of these organisms is known or suspected to be present.

Care and contact

Wash your hands before and after performing patient care or procedures or having contact with contaminated objects, even though you may have worn gloves. Always wash your hands after removing gloves.

Home sweet home

If you're providing care in the patient's home, bring your own supply of soap and disposable paper towels. If there's no running water, disinfect your hands with an alcohol-based hand sanitizer.

What you need
Hand washing
Hand washing soap or detergent ✳ warm running water ✳ paper towels ✳ optional: antiseptic cleaning agent, fingernail brush, disposable sponge or plastic cuticle stick

Hand sanitizing
Hands sanitizing alcohol-based hand rub

How you do it
Hand washing
• Remove rings or artificial fingernails as facility policy dictates *because they harbor dirt and skin microorganisms.*
• Remove your watch or wear it well above the wrist. *Long natural nails may harbor more microorganisms*; keep nails short, no more than ¼″ beyond the end of the finger.

> Hand washing should be such an automatic part of your daily routine that, after a while, you'll feel like your hands are leading you to the sink!

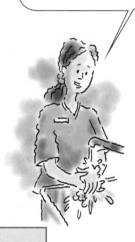

Proper hand-washing technique

To minimize the spread of infection, follow these basic hand-washing instructions. With your hands angled downward under the faucet, adjust the water temperature until it's comfortably warm.

Lather up
Work up a generous lather by scrubbing vigorously for 10 seconds. Make sure you clean beneath your fingernails, around your knuckles, and along the sides of your fingers and hands.

Pat dry
Rinse your hands completely to wash away suds and microorganisms. Pat dry with a paper towel. To prevent recontamination on your hands on the faucet handles, cover each one with a dry paper towel when turning off the water.

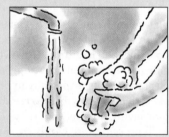

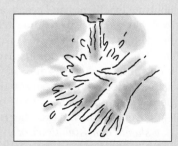

- Wet your hands and wrists with warm water and apply soap from a dispenser. Don't use bar soap *because it allows cross-contamination.*
- Hold your hands below elbow level *to prevent water from running up your arms and back down, thus contaminating clean areas.* (See *Proper hand-washing technique,* page 147.)
- Work up a generous lather by rubbing your hands together vigorously for about 10 seconds. *Soap and warm water reduce surface tension and this reduced tension, aided by friction, loosens surface microorganisms, which wash away in the lather.*
-     Pay special attention to the area under fingernails and around cuticles and to the thumbs, knuckles, and sides of the fingers and hands *because microorganisms thrive in these protected or overlooked areas.* If you don't remove your wedding band, move it up and down your finger to clean beneath it.
- Avoid splashing water on yourself or the floor *because microorganisms spread more easily on wet surfaces and because slippery floors are dangerous.* Avoid touching the sink or faucets *because they're considered contaminated.*
- Rinse hands and wrists well *because running water flushes suds, soil, and microorganisms away.*
- Pat hands and wrists dry with a paper towel. Avoid rubbing, *which can cause abrasion and chapping.*
- If the sink isn't equipped with knee or foot controls, turn off the faucets by gripping them with a dry paper towel *to avoid recontamination of your hands.*
- Because frequent hand washing strips the skin of natural oils, this simple procedure can result in dryness, cracking, and irritation. However, these effects are probably more common after repeated use of antiseptic cleaning agents, especially in people with sensitive skin. *To help minimize irritation,* rinse your hands thoroughly, making sure they're free from residue.
- *To prevent your hands from becoming dry or chapped,* apply an emollient hand cream after each washing or switch to a different cleaning agent. Make sure that the hand cream or lotion you use won't cause the material in your gloves to deteriorate. Avoid creams and lotions with strong perfume as they may irritate a patient with asthma or cause nausea in some patients. If you develop dermatitis, you may need to be evaluated by your employee health care provider *to determine whether you should continue to work until the condition resolves.*

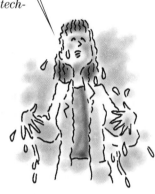

Just being clean isn't enough . . . it's all in the technique!

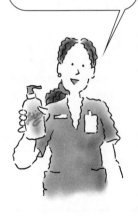

Use hand cream to avoid dry, chapped hands caused by frequent hand washing. But make sure that the lotion you use won't deteriorate your gloves. Use lotion provided by the facility.

Hand sanitizing
• Apply a small amount of the alcohol-based hand rub to all surfaces of the hands.
• Rub hands together until all the product has dried (usually about 30 seconds).

Standard precautions

The CDC recommends that the following standard blood and body fluid precautions be used for *all* patients. These standard precautions are especially important in emergency care settings where the risk of blood exposure is increased and the patient's infection status is usually unknown. Implementing standard precautions doesn't eliminate the need for other transmission-based precautions, such as airborne, droplet, and contact precautions.

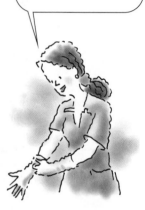

Gloves—the perfect accessory for every nursing occasion . . . no matter which scrubs I wear!

Sources of potential exposure

Standard precautions apply to blood, semen, vaginal secretions, cerebrospinal fluid, synovial fluid, pleural fluid, peritoneal fluid, pericardial fluid, and amniotic fluid. These fluids are most likely to transmit HIV. Standard precautions also apply to other body fluids—including stool, nasal secretions, saliva, sputum, tears, vomitus, and breast milk.

Barrier precautions

• Wear gloves when touching blood and body fluids, mucous membranes, or broken skin of all patients; when handling items or touching surfaces soiled with blood or body fluids; and when performing venipuncture and other vascular access procedures.
• Change gloves when they become soiled and wash hands before and after contact with each patient.
• Wear a mask and protective eyewear or a face shield to protect mucous membranes of the mouth, nose, and eyes during procedures that may generate drops of blood or other body fluids.
• In addition to a mask and protective eyewear or a face shield, wear a gown or an apron during procedures that are likely to generate splashing of blood or other body fluids.
• After removing gloves, thoroughly wash hands and other skin surfaces that may be contaminated with blood or other body fluids.

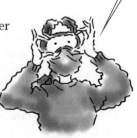

Like I always say . . . when in doubt, goggle up!

Precautions for invasive procedures

• During all invasive procedures, wear gloves. Also wear a surgical mask and goggles or a face shield.
• During procedures that commonly generate droplets or splashes of blood or other body fluids or bone chips, wear protective eyewear and a mask or face shield.
• During invasive procedures that are likely to cause splashing or splattering of blood or other body fluids, wear a gown or an impervious apron.
• If you perform or assist in vaginal or cesarean deliveries, wear gloves and a gown when handling the placenta or the infant and during umbilical cord care.

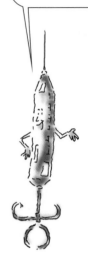

Handling syringes is sticky business. Take all necessary precautions to avoid injury and infection.

Work practice precautions

• Prevent injuries caused by needles, scalpels, and other sharp instruments or devices when cleaning used instruments, disposing of used needles, and handling sharp instruments after procedures.
• To prevent needle-stick injuries, don't recap used needles, bend or break needles, remove them from disposable syringes, or manipulate them. Use safety-protected needles and needleless I.V. systems whenever possible.
• Place disposable syringes and needles, scalpel blades, and other sharp items in puncture-resistant containers for disposal, making sure these containers are located near the area of use.
• Place large-bore reusable needles in a puncture-resistant container for transport to the reprocessing area.
• If the glove tears or a needle-stick or other injury occurs, remove the gloves, wash your hands, and wash the site of the needle stick thoroughly; then put on new gloves as quickly as patient safety permits. Remove the needle or instrument involved in the incident from the sterile field. Promptly report injuries and mucous membrane exposure to the appropriate infection control officer.
• Never reuse a one-time use needle or vial.

Additional precautions

• Make sure mouthpieces, one-way valve masks, resuscitation bags, or other ventilation devices are available in areas where the need for resuscitation is likely.
• If you have exudative lesions or weeping dermatitis, refrain from direct patient care and handling patient-care equipment until the condition resolves.

Using isolation equipment

Isolation procedures may be implemented to prevent the spread of infection from patient to patient, from the patient to health care workers, or from health care workers to the patient. They may also be used to reduce the risk of infection in immunocompromised patients. Central to the success of these procedures is the selection of proper equipment and adequate training of those who use it.

> I wouldn't have guessed in a million years it would be so easy breaking in through all that armor . . .

Once is enough

Use gowns, gloves, goggles, and masks only once, and discard them in the appropriate container before leaving a contaminated area. If your mask is reusable, retain it for further use unless it's damaged or damp. Be aware that isolation garb loses its effectiveness when wet because moisture permits organisms to seep through the material. Change masks and gowns as soon as moisture is noticeable or according to the manufacturer's recommendations or your facility's policy.

What you need

Materials required for isolation typically include barrier clothing, an isolation cart or anteroom for storing equipment, and a door card stating that isolation precautions are in effect.

Barrier clothing: Gowns ✳ gloves ✳ goggles ✳ masks (Each staff member must be trained in their proper use.)

Isolation supplies: Specially marked laundry bags (and water-soluble laundry bags, if used) ✳ plastic trash bags

An isolation cart may be used when the patient's room has no anteroom. It should include a work area (such as a pull-out shelf), drawers or a cabinet area for holding isolation supplies and, possibly, a pole on which to hang coats or jackets.

> Barrier clothing isn't what it used to be, thank goodness! Now you need gowns, gloves, goggles, and masks—a bit more comfortable if you ask me!

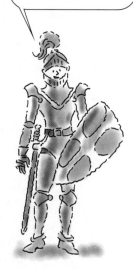

Getting ready

• Remove the cover from the isolation cart, if necessary, and set up the work area. Check the cart or anteroom to ensure that correct and sufficient supplies are in place for the designated isolation category.

Recommended standard precautions

Component	Recommendations
Hand hygiene	After touching blood, body fluids, secretions, excretions, contaminated items; immediately after removing gloves; between patient contacts.
Personal protective equipment (PPE)	
Gloves	For touching blood, body fluids, secretions, excretions, contaminated items; for touching mucous membranes and nonintact skin
Gown	During procedures and patient-care activities when contact of clothing/exposed skin with blood/body fluids, secretions, and excretions is anticipated
Mask, eye protection (goggles), face shield	During procedures and patient-care activities likely to generate splashes or sprays of blood, body fluids, secretions, especially suctioning, endotracheal intubation
Patient placement	Prioritize for single-patient room if patient is at increased risk of transmission, is likely to contaminate the environment, does not maintain appropriate hygiene, or is at increased risk of acquiring infection or developing adverse outcome following infection.

Table adapted from Centers for Disease Control and Prevention (CDC). (2004). *Recommendations for application of standard precautions for the care of all patients in all healthcare settings*. Retrieved from http://www.cdc.gov/sars/guidance/I-infection/app1.html

How you do it

- Remove your watch (or push it well up your arm) and your rings according to facility policy. *These actions help prevent the spread of microorganisms hidden under your watch or rings.*
- Wash your hands with an antiseptic cleaning agent to prevent the growth of microorganisms under gloves.

Putting on isolation garb

- Put the gown on and wrap it around the back of your uniform. Tie the strings or fasten the snaps or pressure-sensitive tabs at the neck. Make sure your uniform is completely covered from the neck to the knees and the arms to the end of your wrists, and secure the gown at the waist.
- Place the mask snugly over your nose and mouth. Secure ear loops around your ears or tie the strings behind your head high enough so the mask won't slip off. Squeeze the adjustable nose

DONNING PERSONAL PROTECTIVE EQUIPMENT

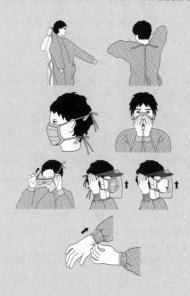

REMOVING PERSONAL PROTECTIVE EQUIPMENT

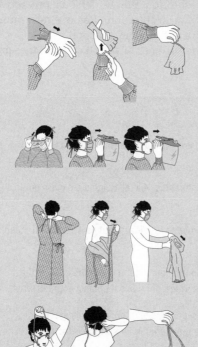

Putting on a face mask

To avoid spreading airborne particles, wear a sterile or nonsterile face mask as indicated. Position the mask to cover your nose and mouth, and secure it high enough to ensure stability.

Get all tied up
Tie the top strings at the back of your head above the ears. Then tie the bottom strings at the base of your neck. Adjust the metal nose strip if the mask has one.

Limit the spread of infection by
- Keeping hands away from your face
- Limiting surfaces touched while in isolation
- Changing gloves while caring for a patient if become visibly soiled or heavily contaminated

bridge to fit your nose firmly but comfortably. If you wear eyeglasses, tuck the mask under their lower edge. Ensure that the mask fits snugly to your face and below your chin.
- Put on the gloves. Pull the gloves over the cuffs to cover the edges of the gown's sleeves.

Removing isolation garb
- Except for N95 mask or respirator, remove personal protective equipment (PPE) at doorway or in anteroom. Remove respirator after leaving the patient room and closing the door.
- Remember that the outside surfaces of your barrier clothes are contaminated.

Removing contaminated gloves

Proper removal techniques are essential for preventing the spread of pathogens from gloves to your skin surface. Follow these steps carefully:

Grasp outside of opposite hand glove with dominant hand. Avoid allowing the glove's outer surface to buckle inward against your wrist.

Peel off glove by pulling downward, allowing the glove to turn inside out as it comes off. Keep the right glove in your left hand after removing it.

Now insert the first two fingers of your ungloved nondominant hand under the edge of the dominant hand glove. Avoid touching the glove's outer surface or folding it against your left wrist.

Pull downward so that the glove turns inside out as it comes off. Continue pulling until the glove completely encloses the other glove and its uncontaminated inner surface is facing out.

Discard the gloves in the trash container that contains a plastic trash bag.

- Wearing gloves, untie the gown's waist strings.
- Untie your mask, holding it only by the strings. The front of the mask is contaminated. Discard the mask in the trash container. If a patient has airborne precautions, the mask must be removed outside the room with the door shut.
- Untie the neck straps of your gown. The gown front and sleeves are contaminated. Grasp the outside of the gown at the back of the shoulders and pull the gown down over your arms, turning it inside out as you remove it to ensure containment of the pathogens.
- Holding the gown well away from your uniform, fold it inside out. Discard it in the specially marked laundry bags or trash container, as necessary.
- If the sink is inside the patient's room, wash your hands and forearms with soap or antiseptic before leaving the room. Turn off the faucet using a paper towel and discard the towel in the room. Grasp the door handle with a clean paper towel to open it, and discard the towel in a trash container inside the room. Close the door from the outside with your bare hand.
- If the sink is in an anteroom, wash your hands and forearms with soap or antiseptic after leaving the room.

References

Centers for Disease Control and Prevention (CDC). (n.d.). *Sequence for donning and removing personal protective equipment PPE poster*. Retrieved from http://www.cdc.gov/HAI/pdfs/ppe/ppeposter1322.pdf

Centers for Disease Control and Prevention (CDC). (2013). *Antibiotic resistance threats in the United States, 2013*. Retrieved from http://www.cdc.gov/drugresistance/threat-report-2013/pdf/ar-threats-2013-508.pdf

Siegel, J. D., Rhinehart, E., Jackson, M., & Chiarello, L. (2007). *Guideline for isolation precautions: Preventing transmission of infectious agents in healthcare settings*. Retrieved from http://www.cdc.gov/hicpac/pdf/isolation/isolation2007.pdf

Quick quiz

1. What's the most effective method of infection control?
    A. Isolation precautions
    B. Hand washing
    C. Neutropenic precautions
    D. Wearing sterile gloves

Answer: B. Hand washing with soap and water or an alcohol-based hand sanitizer is the most effective infection control method.

2. Which type of mask or respirator is used for airborne precautions?

    A.   Standard surgical mask

    B.   Face shield

    C.   N95 mask

    D.   None is needed.

Answer: C. The N95 mask is specially fitted to each individual provider and is used as the particles with airborne precautions are smaller than the surgical mask can filter.

3. What type of transmission occurs when an intermediate carrier, such as a flea or mosquito, transfers an organism?

    A.   Vector-borne transmission

    B.   Vehicle-born transmission

    C.   Contact transmission

    D.   Airborne transmission

Answer: A. Vector-borne transmission occurs when an intermediate carrier (vector), such as a flea or mosquito, transfers an organism.

4. What's the name for a laboratory-verified infection that causes no signs or symptoms?

    A.   Colonized

    B.   Subclinical

    C.   Latent

    D.   Dormant

Answer: B. A laboratory-verified infection that causes no signs and symptoms is called a *subclinical, silent,* or *asymptomatic infection.*

Scoring

☆☆☆ If you answered all four questions correctly, bravo! You're super at preventing superinfection.

☆☆ If you answered three questions correctly, great! There are no spirochetes on you.

☆ If you answered fewer than three questions correctly, chin up! Review the chapter and you'll be discarding this quiz properly in no time.

9

Medication basics

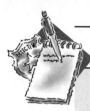

Just the facts

In this chapter, you'll learn:

♦ basics of medication administration

♦ drug administration routes

♦ key concepts of pharmacokinetics and pharmacodynamics

♦ dosage and administration considerations

♦ various drug delivery systems

♦ common medication errors.

A look at medication basics

When you care for a patient in your day-to-day nursing practice, one of the most crucial skills you bring to the bedside is your ability to administer medications. From legal, ethical, and practical standpoints, medication administration is much more than simply a delivery service. It's a highly technical skill that requires you to exercise wide-ranging knowledge, analytical skill, professional judgment, and clinical expertise. Indeed, some would consider the safe, effective administration of medications the foundation of your success as a professional nurse.

To deliver medications accurately, you need a sound working knowledge of:

• drug terminology
• routes by which drugs are delivered
• effects the drugs produce after they're inside the body.

Pharmacology is the scientific study of the origin, nature, chemistry, effects, and uses of drugs. This chapter reviews some concepts basic to pharmacology—and essential to your ability to administer drugs wisely—starting with the most basic of all: drug names.

The name game

The typical drug has three or more names:
- The *chemical name* describes the drug's atomic and molecular structure.
- The *generic name* is a shorter, simpler version of the drug's chemical name.
- The *trade name* (also known as the *brand name* or *propriety name*) is the name selected by the drug company that sells it. Trade names are protected by copyright laws. (See *What's in a name?*)

A class act

Drugs that share similar characteristics are grouped together into pharmacologic classes or families. For example, the class known as *beta-adrenergic blockers* contains several drugs with similar properties.

Drugs can also be grouped according to their therapeutic class, which classifies drugs according to their use. For example, thiazide diuretics and beta-adrenergic blockers are both antihypertensives, but they belong to different pharmacologic classes because they share few characteristics.

Routes of administration

A drug's administration route influences the quantity given and the rate at which the drug is absorbed and distributed. These variables in turn affect the drug's action and the patient's response. Routes of administration that involve the gastrointestinal (GI) tract are known as *enteral routes*, which are from the mouth to the rectum. The enteral routes include oral, sublingual, translingual, buccal, tube feedings and rectal. Those that don't involve the GI tract or respiratory tract and include the use of a needle are known as *parenteral routes*. Parenteral routes can be useful for treating a patient who can't take a drug orally. Compare the advantages and disadvantages of the following routes.

Topical route

The topical route is used to deliver a drug via the skin or a mucous membrane. The advantages of delivering drugs by this route include:
- easy administration
- few allergic reactions

What's in a name?

Most drugs have three names—chemical, generic, and trade/brand—as this example demonstrates. Some drugs may have more than one trade name. The best way to avoid confusion is to use the generic name when speaking or writing about a drug.

Chemical name

> 7-chloro-1,3-dihydro-1-methyl-5-phenyl-2H-1,4-benzodiazepin-2-one

Generic name

> diazepam

Trade name or brand name

> Valium

• fewer adverse reactions than drugs administered by systemic routes.

You can make a real mess of it

Delivering precise doses can be difficult with the topical route. Also, these medications can be messy to apply— and even messier for your patient to wear! They may stain the patient's clothing and bed linens, have a distinctive smell, or get on you as well.

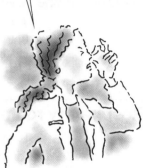

Besides being messy, some topical medications have a very distinctive smell . . . phew!

Ophthalmic administration

Ophthalmic administration involves drugs such as creams, ointments, and liquid drops that are placed in the conjunctival sac or directly onto the surface of the eye. Intraocular inserts and collagen shields can be used to deliver drugs to the eye as well. For all types of ophthalmic administration, take care to avoid contaminating the medication container or transferring organisms to the patient's eye.

Convenience at a price

Ocusert Pilo, one type of intraocular insert, supplies pilocarpine to the ciliary muscles to treat glaucoma. Because this eye medication disk releases the drug for an entire week, it's more convenient than eyedrops. However, intraocular inserts cost much more than eyedrops and they may be uncomfortable. Also, the drug may be absorbed systemically, causing adverse effects.

Wielding the shield

Collagen shields that have been presoaked in a drug solution can be applied to the eye to treat corneal ulcers and severe iridocyclitis (inflammation of the iris and ciliary body). Collagen shields may prove more effective than injections of collagen beneath the conjunctiva, where the substance is poorly absorbed.

Make sure that eardrops are at room temperature before administration. Otherwise, they can cause pain or vertigo.

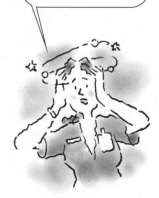

Otic administration

Otic administration involves drugs that are placed directly into the ear. Solutions placed into the ear can be used to treat infection or inflammation of the external ear canal, produce local anesthesia, or soften built-up cerumen (earwax) for removal.

Bring otic solutions to room temperature before administering them because cold solutions can cause pain or vertigo.

Nasal administration

Nasal administration involves drugs that are placed directly into the patient's nostrils. Medicated solutions can be placed into the patient's nostrils from a dropper or as an atomized spray from a squeeze bottle or pump device.

Bypassing the first-pass effect

The highly vascular nasal mucosa allows systemic absorption while avoiding first-pass metabolism by the liver (the liver changes the drug to a more water-soluble form for excretion before it enters circulation).

Respiratory route

Drugs that are lipid-soluble and available as gases can be administered into the respiratory tree. The respiratory tree provides an extensive, highly perfused region for enhanced absorption. Smaller doses of potent drugs can be given by this route to minimize their adverse effects. Because this route is easily accessible, it provides a convenient alternative when other routes are unavailable.

Emergency!

In emergencies, some injectable drugs, such as atropine, lidocaine, and epinephrine, can be given directly into the lungs via an endotracheal tube. A drug administered into the trachea is absorbed into the bloodstream from the alveolar sacs. Surfactant, for example, is administered to premature neonates via the trachea to improve their respiratory function. Also, atropine can be administered to patients with symptomatic bradycardia and no vascular access to increase their heart rate.

Breathing easy? Not so fast!

A major disadvantage of the respiratory route is that few drugs can be given this way. Other disadvantages include:
• difficulty in administering accurate doses—or full doses, if the patient isn't cooperative
• nausea and vomiting when certain drugs are delivered into the lungs
• irritation of the tracheal or bronchial mucosa, causing coughing or bronchospasm
• possible infection from the equipment used to deliver drugs into the lungs.

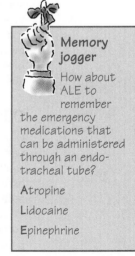

Memory jogger

How about ALE to remember the emergency medications that can be administered through an endotracheal tube?

Atropine

Lidocaine

Epinephrine

Buccal, sublingual, and translingual routes

Certain drugs are given buccally (in the pouch between the cheek and teeth), sublingually (under the tongue), or translingually (on the tongue) to prevent their destruction or transformation in the stomach or small intestine. Drugs given by these routes act quickly because the oral mucosa's thin epithelium and abundant vasculature allow direct absorption into the bloodstream.

Cheeky checklist

These routes can be used if the patient can take nothing by mouth, can't swallow, or is intubated. What's more, the drugs have no first-pass effect in the liver and don't cause GI irritation. However, only drugs that are highly lipid-soluble may be given by these routes, and they may irritate the oral mucosa.

Oral route

Oral administration is usually the safest, most convenient, and least expensive method. For that reason, most drugs are administered by this route to patients who are conscious and able to swallow.

Down in the mouth

The oral route does have some disadvantages:
• It produces variable drug absorption.
• Because it moves drugs through the liver, first-pass metabolism may take place.
• Drugs can't be given orally in most emergencies because of their unpredictable and relatively slow absorption. (See *Enteral administration: Why absorption varies.*)

Enteral administration: Why absorption varies

A drug that's administered enterally—orally or by gastric tube—can undergo variable rates of absorption due to:
• changes in the pH of the GI tract
• changes in intestinal membrane permeability
• fluctuations in GI motility
• fluctuations in GI blood flow
• food in the GI tract
• other drugs in the GI tract.

- Oral drugs may irritate the GI tract, discolor the patient's teeth, or taste unpleasant.
- Oral drugs can be accidentally aspirated if the patient has trouble swallowing or is combative.

Gastric route

The gastric route allows direct instillation of medication into the GI system of patients who can't ingest the drug orally. A variety of tubes can be placed for instillation. Oily medications and enteric-coated or sustained-release tablets or capsules can't be administered by this route.

Rectal and vaginal routes

You may instill suppositories, ointments, creams, or gels into the rectum or vagina to treat local irritation or infection. Some drugs applied to the mucosa of the rectum or vagina can be absorbed systemically. Drugs may also be delivered to the rectum in a medicated enema or to the vagina in a medicated douche.

> Some drugs can be administered by the rectal or vaginal route to treat local irritation or infection.

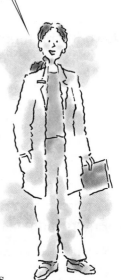

The up side

Drugs administered through the rectal or vaginal routes don't irritate the upper GI tract, as some oral medications do. Also, these drugs avoid destruction by digestive enzymes in the stomach and small intestine.

The down side

However, there are some disadvantages to the rectal and vaginal routes:
- The rectal route is usually contraindicated when the patient has a disorder affecting the lower GI tract, such as rectal bleeding or diarrhea.
- Drug absorption may be irregular or incomplete with these routes.
- The rectal route usually can't be used in an emergency.
- Rectal doses of some drugs may need to be larger than oral doses.
- Because rectal administration typically stimulates the vagus nerve, this route may pose a risk for cardiac patients.
- Drugs given rectally may irritate the rectal mucosa.
- Administering a drug by the rectal or vaginal route may cause discomfort and embarrassment for the patient.

Intradermal route

Intradermal drug administration is used mainly for diagnostic purposes when testing for allergies or tuberculosis. To administer drugs intradermally, inject a small amount of serum or vaccine between the skin layers just below the stratum corneum. Because this route results in little systemic absorption, it produces mainly local effects.

Don't get too deep

You must be sure not to inject the substance too deeply. If you do, you'll have to reinject it, causing added stress, cost, and delay of treatment for the patient.

Subcutaneous route

When using the subcutaneous route, you inject small amounts of a drug beneath the dermis and into the subcutaneous tissue, usually in the patient's upper arm, thigh, or abdomen. Patients with diabetes use this technique to give themselves insulin. The drug is absorbed slowly from the subcutaneous tissue, thus prolonging its effects.

Tissue issues

There are disadvantages to the subcutaneous route:
• Subcutaneous injection may damage tissue.
• The subcutaneous route can't be used when the patient has occlusive vascular disease and poor perfusion because decreased peripheral circulation delays absorption. Exceptions to this are heparin (Lovenox) and insulin.
• The subcutaneous route can't be used when the patient's skin or underlying tissue is grossly adipose, edematous, burned, hardened, swollen at the common injection sites, damaged by previous injections, or diseased.

Implants eliminate noncompliance

Aside from injection, another method of subcutaneous administration is to implant beneath the skin pellets or capsules that contain small amounts of a drug. From the dermis, the medication seeps slowly into the tissues. Goserelin, one such implant, is inserted into the upper abdominal wall to manage advanced prostate cancer.

Because subcutaneous implants require no patient action after they're in place, they eliminate the problem of noncompliance. Their major drawback is the need for minor surgery to insert or remove them.

Intramuscular route

The I.M. route allows you to inject drugs directly into various muscle groups at varying tissue depths. You'll use this route to give aqueous suspensions and solutions in oil and to give medications that aren't available in oral form. The effect of a drug administered by the I.M. route is relatively rapid, and aqueous I.M. medications can be given to adults in doses of up to 5 ml in some sites. The I.M. route also eliminates the need for an I.V. site.

> I.M. injections are helpful in a lot of situations, but they require proper technique to prevent pain, tissue breakdown, nerve injury, and even accidental overdose.

Intramuscular miscues

Despite the advantages, there are many disadvantages to the I.M. route:
• A drug delivered I.M. may precipitate in the muscle, thereby reducing absorption.
• The drug may not absorb properly if the patient is hypotensive or has a poor blood supply to the muscle.
• Improper technique can cause accidental injection of the drug into the patient's bloodstream, possibly causing an overdose or an adverse reaction.
• The I.M. route may cause pain and local tissue irritation, damage bone, puncture blood vessels, injure nerves, or break down muscle tissue, thus interfering with myoglobin—a marker for acute myocardial infarction.

Intravenous route

The I.V. route allows injection of substances directly into the bloodstream through a vein. Appropriate substances include drugs, fluids, diagnostic contrast agents, and blood or blood products. Administration can range from a single dose to an ongoing infusion delivered with great precision.

In the I.V. league

Because the drug or solution is absorbed immediately and completely, the patient's response is rapid. Instant bioavailability (the drug's availability for target tissues) makes the I.V. route the first choice for giving drugs during an emergency to relieve acute pain. This route has no first-pass effect in the liver and avoids damage to muscle tissue caused by irritating drugs. Because absorption into the bloodstream is complete and reliable, large drug doses can be delivered at a continuous rate.

This road can be bumpy

Life-threatening adverse reactions may arise if I.V. drugs are administered too quickly, if the flow rate isn't monitored carefully enough, or if incompatible drugs are mixed together. Also, the I.V. route increases the risk of complications, such as extravasation, vein irritation, systemic infection, and air embolism. Follow the I.V. administration guidelines in chapter 11, Intravenous administration, to help pave your way to success.

Specialized infusions

Under certain circumstances, drug infusion may take place directly at the site of intended activity. Using specialized catheters and devices, drugs and solutions can be delivered to an organ or its blood vessels to manage emergencies, treat disease, infuse tumors, or relieve pain. These infusions may be given by the epidural, intrapleural, intraperitoneal, intra-articular, or intraosseous routes. (See *Reviewing specialized infusions.*)

Reviewing specialized infusions

If drug therapy needs to take a direct route to a specific site in the patient's body, you may use one of the specialized routes of drug administration as shown in this chart.

Route	Characteristics
Epidural infusion	• The drug is injected into the epidural space, outside or above the dura mater. • The drug is absorbed into cerebrospinal fluid and works directly on the central nervous system. • Epidural anesthesia or analgesia is given through a special catheter and is considered safe and versatile. It may be tailored to affect a specific area of the body from the legs up to the upper abdomen. • The drug infused through an epidural catheter must be preservative-free to prevent serious reactions to the preservative. • Epidural catheters should be labeled "for epidural use only" to prevent the accidental injection of other drugs into the epidural space.
Intrapleural infusion	• The drug is injected into the pleural cavity. • The drug crosses the pleural membrane and enters the pleural space, where it works locally at the disease site. • Chemotherapy is an example of a drug given by this type of infusion to minimize systemic effects and increase drug effects on the tumor.
Intraperitoneal infusion	• The drug is injected into the peritoneal cavity. • The drug or solution crosses the peritoneal membrane and enters the peritoneal space where it works locally. • This administration route is used for peritoneal dialysis in which the peritoneum functions as a diffusible semipermeable membrane. • Fluid or electrolyte imbalances can be corrected, toxins removed, and normal renal excretion facilitated using this route.

(continued)

Reviewing specialized infusions *(continued)*

Route	Characteristics
Intra-articular infusion	• The drug is injected into the synovial cavity of a joint to suppress inflammation, prevent contractures, and delay muscle atrophy. • This route is most commonly used to treat rheumatoid arthritis, gout, systemic lupus erythematosus, osteoarthritis, and other joint disorders. • Corticosteroids, anesthetics, and lubricants are most commonly administered into the shoulder, elbow, wrist, finger, knee, ankle, or toe joints. • This route is used sparingly because of the risk of infection.
Intraosseous infusion	• The drug is injected into the rich vascular network of a long bone for rapid absorption. • Drugs and solutions administered through bone marrow are absorbed as rapidly as those administered I.V. • With a special intraosseous access needle, this route has been used successfully in children and adults for emergency infusions when normal vascular access isn't possible.

Pharmacokinetics

A solid understanding of pharmacokinetics—the movement of a drug through the body—can help you predict your patient's response to a prescribed drug regimen and anticipate potential problems. Any time you give a drug, a series of physiochemical events takes place in the patient's body and includes four basic processes:

 absorption

 distribution

 metabolism

 excretion. (See *What happens after drug administration.*)

Absorption

Before a drug can act on the body, it must be absorbed into the bloodstream. How well a patient's body absorbs a drug depends on several factors. These include:
• the drug's physiochemical properties
• the drug's form
• the route of administration

What happens after drug administration

Drug disposition begins as soon as a drug is administered. The drug proceeds through pharmacokinetic, pharmacodynamic, and pharmacotherapeutic phases. This chart shows the various phases, the activities that occur during them, and the factors that influence those activities.

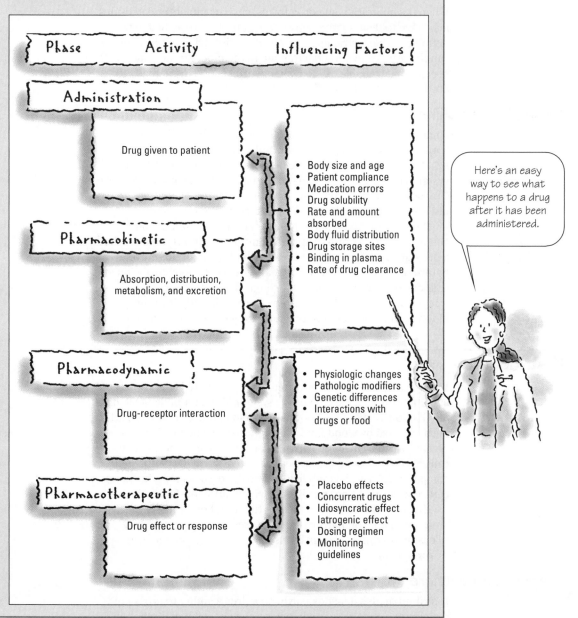

Phase	Activity	Influencing Factors
Administration	Drug given to patient	• Body size and age • Patient compliance • Medication errors • Drug solubility • Rate and amount absorbed • Body fluid distribution • Drug storage sites • Binding in plasma • Rate of drug clearance
Pharmacokinetic	Absorption, distribution, metabolism, and excretion	
Pharmacodynamic	Drug-receptor interaction	• Physiologic changes • Pathologic modifiers • Genetic differences • Interactions with drugs or food
Pharmacotherapeutic	Drug effect or response	• Placebo effects • Concurrent drugs • Idiosyncratic effect • Iatrogenic effect • Dosing regimen • Monitoring guidelines

Here's an easy way to see what happens to a drug after it has been administered.

- the drug's interactions with other substances in the GI tract
- various patient characteristics, especially the site and the condition of the absorbing surface.

These factors can also determine the speed and amount of drug absorption.

Becoming bioavailable

When taken orally, some drug forms, such as tablets and capsules, may have to disintegrate before free particles are available to dissolve in the gastric juices. Only after dissolving in these juices can the drug be absorbed, circulate in the bloodstream, and thus become bioavailable. A bioavailable drug is one that's ready to produce a physiologic effect.

Timing is everything

Some tablets have enteric coatings, which delay disintegration until after the tablets leave the acidic environment of the stomach. Others, such as liposome capsules, have special delivery systems that release the drug only at a specific osmotic pressure. Oral solutions and elixirs, which don't have to disintegrate and dissolve to take effect, are usually absorbed more rapidly.

If the patient has had a bowel resection, anticipate slow absorption of any oral drug you administer. And remember that a drug given I.M. must first be absorbed through the muscle before it can enter the bloodstream. Rectal suppositories must first dissolve to be absorbed through the rectal mucosa. Drugs administered I.V.—thereby placed directly into the bloodstream—are completely and immediately bioavailable.

Distribution

When a drug enters the bloodstream, it's distributed to body tissues and fluids through the circulatory system. To better understand drug distribution, think of the body as a system of physiologic compartments defined by blood flow. The bloodstream and highly perfused organs—such as the brain, heart, liver, and kidneys—make up the central compartment. Lesser perfused areas form the peripheral compartment, which is subdivided into the tissue compartment (viscera, muscle, and skin) and the deep compartment (fat and bone).

Highly perfused tissues receive the drug before lesser perfused areas do. Each compartment then stores portions of the drug, releasing it as plasma drug levels decline. (See *How the body stores a drug.*)

Leaping lipid barriers

Distribution also depends partly on a drug's ability to cross lipid membranes. Some drugs can't cross certain cell membranes and

How the body stores a drug

The body can store a drug in fat, bone, or skin. Knowing the characteristics of each drug storage compartment will help you understand how distribution can affect a drug's duration of action.

Fat storage

A drug that dissolves easily in lipids migrates to adipose tissue (what we commonly think of as fatty tissue). Because this tissue lacks receptors for drug action, the drug remains inactive there. Eventually, it's released by fat cells to exert its pharmacologic effect. With some drugs, this slow, prolonged action is an advantage. For example, slow release of anesthetic barbiturates provides effective anesthesia during surgery. With other drugs, such prolonged action can be dangerous.

Bone storage

Bone acts as a storage compartment for certain drugs. Tetracycline, for example, is distributed throughout bone and may eventually crystallize there. In a growing child, this can cause tooth discoloration. Lead and some chemicals can also accumulate in bone, resulting in prolonged exposure to toxins.

Skin storage

Storage of drugs in the skin typically causes photosensitivity. Tetracycline and amiodarone are examples of drugs that are stored in the skin.

thus have limited distribution. For example, antibiotics have trouble permeating the prostate gland, abscesses, and exudates.

It's got to be free

Distribution can also be affected if the drug binds to plasma proteins, especially albumin. Only a free, unbound drug can produce an effect at the drug receptor site, so such binding greatly influences the drug's effectiveness and duration of action.

Disease disrupts distribution

Certain diseases impede drug distribution by altering the volume of distribution—the total amount of drug in the body in relation to the amount in plasma. Heart failure, dehydration, and burns are examples of such disorders. If the patient has heart failure, expect to increase the dosage because the drug must be distributed to a larger fluid volume. On the other hand, if the patient is dehydrated, expect to decrease the dosage because the drug will be distributed to a much smaller fluid volume. (See *Dosing dilemma*.)

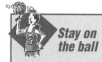

Stay on the ball

Dosing dilemma

Some drugs—such as digoxin, gentamicin, and tobramycin—are poorly distributed to fatty tissue. Therefore, dosing based on actual body weight in a highly obese patient may lead to overdose and serious toxicity.

Go lean

When administering such drugs, calculate the dose based on lean body weight, which you can estimate from actuarial tables that give average weight ranges for various heights.

Metabolism and excretion

Most drugs are metabolized in the liver and excreted by the kidneys. The rate at which a drug is metabolized varies with the individual. Some patients metabolize drugs so quickly that their blood and tissue levels prove therapeutically inadequate. Others metabolize drugs so slowly that even ordinary doses can produce toxic results.

Slow or fast? Here's some help . . .

Drug metabolism may be faster in smokers than in nonsmokers because cigarette smoke contains substances that induce production of hepatic enzymes. Also, a diet high in fat or carbohydrates may slow the metabolism of certain drugs, whereas a diet high in protein may speed metabolism.

Hepatic diseases, or diseases that interfere with hepatic blood flow or transport of drugs to the liver, may affect one or more of the liver's metabolic functions. Thus, in patients with hepatic disease, drug metabolism may be increased or decreased. All patients with hepatic disease must be monitored closely for drug effects and toxic reactions.

The kidneys can be key

Some drugs, such as digoxin and gentamicin, are eliminated almost unchanged by the kidneys. Thus, inadequate renal function causes the drug to accumulate, producing toxic effects. Some drugs can block renal excretion of other drugs, thereby allowing them to accumulate and enhancing their effects. In contrast, some drugs can promote renal excretion of other drugs, thus diminishing their effects.

Different escape routes

Although most drugs are excreted by the kidneys, not all are. Some are excreted hepatically, via the bile and into stool. A few drugs leave the body in sweat, saliva, and breast milk. Certain volatile anesthetics—for example, halothane—are eliminated primarily by exhalation. When natural excretion mechanisms fail, as in drug overdose or renal dysfunction, many drugs can be removed through dialysis.

Underlying disease

Underlying disease can have a marked influence on drug action and effect. For example, acidosis may cause insulin resistance.

Genetic diseases, such as glucose-6-phosphate dehydrogenase (G6PD) deficiency and hepatic porphyria, may turn drugs into toxins. As a result, patients with G6PD deficiency may develop hemolytic anemia when given sulfonamides or certain other drugs.

It's in your genes

A genetically susceptible patient can develop an acute porphyria attack if given a barbiturate.

Toxic conditions

Also, patients with highly active hepatic enzyme systems (rapid acetylators, for example) can develop hepatitis when treated with isoniazid because of the rapid intrahepatic buildup of a toxic metabolite.

Sphere of influence

Other conditions that may influence a patient's response to drug therapy include infection; fever; stress; starvation; hypersensitivity; sunlight; exercise; variations in circadian rhythm; alcohol intake; pregnancy; lactation; immunization; barometric pressure; and GI, renal, hepatic, cardiovascular, and immunologic function. (See *Age-old influence*.)

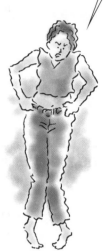

So many conditions and factors can influence a person's response to drug therapy, even genes. There's nothing worse than a pair of tight-fitting genes (or jeans, in my case)!

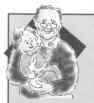

Ages and stages

Age-old influence

The patient's age has an important influence on a drug's overall action and effect. Older adults usually have decreased hepatic function, less muscle mass, and diminished renal function. Consequently, they need lower doses and, sometimes, longer dosage intervals to avoid toxicity.

Neonates have underdeveloped metabolic enzyme systems and inadequate renal function, which can also lead to toxicity. They need highly individualized dosages and careful monitoring.

Types of medication orders

In an outpatient setting, the process of ordering a medication is rather simple. A prescriber typically writes the order on a prescription pad and gives it to the patient. The patient then takes the written prescription and has it filled at a pharmacy.

Where it gets tricky (and where you come in)

In an inpatient setting, however, the process may be somewhat more complex. Several types of medication orders can be used for in patient, including:

- standard orders
- single (or one-time) orders
- stat orders
- p.r.n. orders
- standing orders
- verbal orders
- telephone orders.

Standard orders

A *standard order* is a prescription that remains in effect indefinitely or for a specified period. The prescriber either writes the order—along with instructions, such as for diet, X-rays, and laboratory work—on the order sheet in the patient's chart or enters the order into a computer, and then the order is printed out on a computer-generated patient record.

> Following standard orders is important but complicated. Don't forget to check your facility's policy on certain drugs and dosages.

Following orders

The order must specify the name of the medication, dosage, route of administration, frequency, duration (if time limited), and indication (if p.r.n.). (See *Components of a medication order*.) For example, the order might be written this way: *Amoxil 500 mg P.O. q 8 hr × 10 days*.

It's your job to schedule administration times based on the order, your facility's policies, and pertinent characteristics of the medication itself, such as onset and duration of action and whether it's to be given with or without food.

Wait for further orders

If a standard order doesn't specify a termination time, the order usually remains in effect until the prescriber writes another order to replace or discontinue it. For some types

Components of a medication order

For a hospitalized patient, a prescriber writes a medication order on an order sheet in the patient's chart or enters the order into the computer system. An example of a written order is shown here.

Component list

Whether written or entered into the computer, all drug orders must contain:
- patient's full name
- date and time of the order
- name of the drug being ordered
- dosage form
- dose amount
- administration route
- time schedule for administration
- prescriber's signature or computer code.

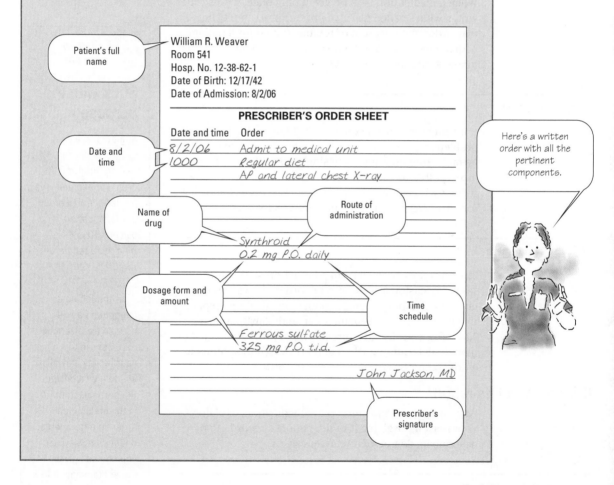

Patient's full name

William R. Weaver
Room 541
Hosp. No. 12-38-62-1
Date of Birth: 12/17/42
Date of Admission: 8/2/06

PRESCRIBER'S ORDER SHEET

Date and time   Order

Date and time

8/2/06   Admit to medical unit
1000   Regular diet
    AP and lateral chest X-ray

Name of drug

Route of administration

Synthroid
0.2 mg P.O. daily

Dosage form and amount

Time schedule

Ferrous sulfate
325 mg P.O. t.i.d.

John Jackson, MD

Prescriber's signature

Here's a written order with all the pertinent components.

of drugs, however, the amount of time covered by the order may be limited by facility policy. For example, opioid orders may have a controlled delivery time of 3 days. Some antibiotics may have a controlled delivery time of 7 days. If the patient still needs the drug after the termination date has passed, the prescriber must write another order. The same is true for postoperative medications; the prescriber must rewrite standard orders for all medications that are to continue after surgery.

Single (one-time) orders

When a medication is to be given only once, a prescriber writes what's called a *single order*. For example, he may order one injection of tetanus toxoid for a patient with a puncture wound who received a primary tetanus toxoid series more than 5 years earlier.

Stat orders

If a patient needs a medication right away for an urgent problem, a prescriber writes a stat order. For example, he may order an immediate single dose of an anti-anxiety drug to calm an acutely agitated patient. For a patient with acute chest pain, he may write a stat order for nitroglycerin (sublingual, spray, or I.V. form).

P.R.N. orders

The term *p.r.n.* comes from a Latin phrase that means "as the occasion arises." A p.r.n. order allows you to give a medication when the patient needs it for a specified problem, such as pain, fever, and constipation. Naturally, you should exercise sound professional judgment in determining when and how often to administer a drug p.r.n. (See *Stick with the purpose.*)

Record it in the record

Any time you administer a p.r.n. medication, explain your reason for giving it in the patient's record. Also, describe its degree of effectiveness.

Standing orders

Also known as *protocols*, standing orders are derived from guidelines created by health care providers for use in specific settings to treat certain diseases or sets of symptoms. Some units of a health care facility

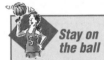
Stay on the ball

Stick with the purpose

Sometimes, a p.r.n. order specifies a reason for giving the drug. For example, the prescriber may order *acetaminophen 650 mg P.O. q 4 hr, p.r.n. for a temperature above 101.3° F (38.5° C).*

Although acetaminophen can be used to treat various problems, in this case, your facility may allow you to give it only for the purpose stated in the medication order. In other words, under such a policy, you couldn't give the acetaminophen ordered above if the patient complained of a headache but had no fever.

(such as the coronary care unit) routinely employ standing orders. For example, the unit may have standing orders for morphine sulfate to treat chest pain and anxiety, for lidocaine to treat ventricular tachycardia, and for furosemide to treat pulmonary congestion.

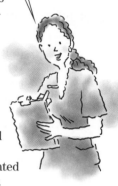

It may sound like double-talk, but make sure your patient's chart includes an order to give a standing order before administering a protocol drug.

Does a standing order need an order? Yes

Standing orders specify which drugs you're permitted to administer and under which circumstances. They must still be individually reviewed and ordered for each patient by his provider. That is, there must be an order to enact the standing orders. Standing orders may also provide guidelines or algorithms for making dosage adjustments. For example, you may need to change the dosage of a heparin infusion based on your patient's anticoagulation studies.

A good test of your skills

Standing orders require considerable judgment and expertise on your part in assessing a patient's need for a drug and detecting any dose-related adverse reactions that could occur. No standing order should be automatically implemented without a careful review regarding its appropriateness for a given patient at a given time.

Verbal and telephone orders

Medication orders given orally rather than in writing are known as *verbal orders*. Whenever possible, avoid them. Why? Because miscommunications can occur and you'll lack a written record of the order. (See *Telephone order accuracy*.)

Stay on the ball

Telephone order accuracy

If you have to take a medication order over the telephone, follow these steps to help ensure its accuracy:
• Have another nurse listen in on the call to confirm that she heard the same order you did.
• Repeat the name of the ordered drug to the prescriber to verify that you heard it correctly. Have the prescriber spell the drug name, if necessary.
• Repeat the individual digits of the dose ordered. For example, you could say, "You ordered fifteen, one-five, milligrams of meperidine; is that right?" The prescriber can then confirm the amount or correct it with something like, "No, I ordered fifty, five-zero, milligrams of meperidine."
• Write out the order, noting that it was a verified telephone order, then sign and date it.
• Administer the medication as ordered.
• The prescriber must cosign your written order within the time allotted by your facility.

You're now entering the danger zone

The danger of miscommunication rises even higher when a prescriber gives a verbal medication order over the telephone. A bad connection, commotion on either end, or the lack of nonverbal communication cues can easily result in medication errors if you fail to clarify exactly what the prescriber wants.

If possible, use a fax machine to obtain a written order, instead of taking a verbal order over the phone.

> Getting a signature after a verbal order is just as important as getting it right!

An emergency? Make it a repeat performance . . .

In urgent situations, you may not be able to avoid verbal orders. Repeat the order aloud so the prescriber can verify that you understood it. For example, your patient goes into hypoglycemic or insulin shock and the doctor tells you to immediately prepare 50 ml of 50% glucose for I.V. administration. To verify the order, show the doctor the label on the empty glucose vial and say the drug's name out loud as you hand him the syringe. That way, he can confirm the accuracy of the drug and its dose.

It may be verbal, but still get a signature

Anytime you accept a verbal order, it's your responsibility to ensure the accuracy of the communication. This holds true even in an emergency. Ask the prescriber to spell the drug's name if you aren't sure what it is. Afterward, write and sign the order that was given to you verbally by the prescriber. Then have the prescriber sign your written copy as soon as possible. Your facility should have a policy that specifies a time frame allotted for a prescriber to sign a verbal order.

> Use your good judgment before administering a medication.

Administration procedures

Making sure you understand a medication order is just the start of your responsibilities when it comes to administering medications correctly. Next, you have to make your own judgment about the correctness of the order based on your knowledge of the medication and your understanding of the patient's condition.

The order looks good, now what?

After you have looked up the drug in the drug guide and you're convinced that a medication order is appropriate for

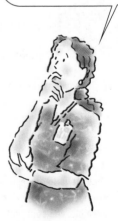

Orders into action

After you receive a written medication order, transcribe it onto a working document approved by your health care facility. For example, your facility may want you to use a medication administration record (MAR), a medication Kardex, medication cards or tickets, or a computer printout.

Stepping away from errors

Each time you copy a medication order, you introduce the possibility of making an error. Make sure you follow these steps:
• Read the order carefully.
• Concentrate on copying it correctly.
• Check it when you're finished.

Don't rely on memory

Next, prepare the medication from the approved copy. Never prepare a medication from memory or from your personal worksheets or notes.

To reduce the risk of overlooking a medication order, your facility may require you to periodically check all MARs against the original order sheets.

the drug and the patient involved, your next step is to prepare the drug correctly for administration. (See *Orders into action*.)

After you transcribe the medication order onto a working document, go to a quiet area to prepare the medication for delivery. Then follow the 6 rights of medication administration.

The 6 rights

Following a tried-and-true set of safeguards known as the *6 rights* can quickly and easily help you avoid the most basic and common sources of medication error. Each time you administer a medication, confirm that you have the:

right drug

right dose

right patient

right time

right route

right documentation.

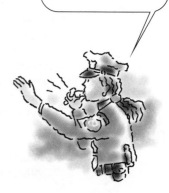

Before giving a drug, make sure you confirm the 6 rights of medication administration. Read the patient their rights!

Right drug

Always compare the name of an ordered drug with the name printed on the container label. Take your time and do it carefully; drugs with similar-sounding and similar-looking names may have very different indications and effects.

Sounds like . . .

For example, Celexa (citalopram hydrobromide) and Celebrex (celecoxib) sound quite similar. But Celexa is a selective serotonin reuptake inhibitor used to treat depression. Celebrex is a nonsteroidal anti-inflammatory drug used to treat osteoarthritis and rheumatoid arthritis. Other similar-sounding drugs may raise a similar risk of mix-ups.

Make sure you aren't unwrapping any surprises

When a medication is individually wrapped in single doses, check the name when removing it from the drawer and again when unwrapping and giving the drug to the patient. Always mention the drug name and the reason you're giving it before actually giving it to the patient.

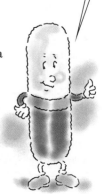

Be a name-dropper . . . before giving me to your patient, mention my name to see what kind of reaction you get.

From the mouth of the patient

Besides carefully checking the ordered drug name against the container label, also check the patient's reaction to the drug as you try to administer it. If he says, "I usually take one pink pill, but you've given me two yellow pills," stop what you're doing and recheck the order. Perhaps you'll simply explain to the patient that the pink pill contains 10 mg of the drug and the yellow ones contain 5 mg each. Or perhaps, you'll discover that you're giving the patient the wrong medication. Either way, you must carefully follow up on any comment a patient makes about changes in a medication before you administer it.

Right dose

The growing use of unit-dose medications (in which a single dose of medication is wrapped and labeled for individual use) has greatly reduced the risk of giving a patient the wrong drug dose. Also, many commercially prepared medications are available in various tablet sizes, decreasing the number of calculations you have to do to determine the dosage.

Even so, you still need to know how and when to perform the appropriate dose calculations. (See *Keeping calculations correct.*)

The buddy system

Whenever possible, double-check all your calculations with another nurse or with a pharmacist. Many hospitals require these

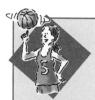

Stay on the ball

Keeping calculations correct

A recent study of 200 equation-based prescribing errors found that more than one half resulted from calculation mistakes. To help keep your medication calculations correct, use these safeguards:

• Think about whether a dosage seems right, given the patient's diagnosis and the drug involved.

• If your calculation indicates that you need more than one or possibly two dosage units to prepare a prescribed dose, double-check the calculation.

• If your calculation indicates that you need a small fraction of a dosage unit to prepare a prescribed dose, double-check the calculation.

• Be especially careful when calculating with decimal points because a mistake can increase or decrease the intended dose many times over.

• Minimize the possibility of confusion anytime you have to write down a dose that contains a decimal point by putting a zero in front of a decimal point that has no other number in front of it. In other words, write *0.25 mg* rather than *.25 mg*, which someone could easily mistake for *25 mg*. Likewise, never write a zero after a dose that includes a decimal point. In other words, don't write *0.250 mg* for a dose of *0.25 mg*.

• Never break an unscored tablet to prepare a calculated dose because you won't get an exact amount. Instead, ask a pharmacist for a form of the drug that you can measure accurately.

double checks when your dosage calculations involve children's medications or drugs with narrow safety margins, such as heparin and insulin.

Know your role on the team

No matter what, never take it upon yourself to alter the drug dosage specified in a prescriber's order. Say, for example, that a doctor orders 75 mg of meperidine for postoperative pain. You give the medication after the patient's surgery, but he says he still has intense pain. Your conclusion may be that 75 mg of meperidine isn't enough and that 100 mg would probably do the trick. But that doesn't give you the authority to change the dose.

Instead, consult with the doctor and obtain a new standard order. However, if the prescriber's original medication order specifies a range of dosages, then you must determine the most appropriate dose for the patient—within that range.

Remember that you're part of a team. Consult with the doctor and pharmacist if you think a drug isn't effective.

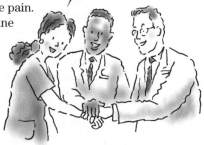

Right patient

To reduce the risk of medication errors, never assume that the patient in a labeled bed is indeed the patient named on the label. Instead, always use two patient identifiers (neither of which should be the patient's room number) before giving any medication. One new identifier used by some hospitals is the bar code medication administration method. The nurse scans their identification badge, the patient's bracelet, and the medication bar code on the drug that is to be administered to the patient. (Follow agency policy for patient identification.)

Roll call

As an additional check, also ask the patient to tell you his name and birthdate. (Don't say something like, "You're John, right?" because the patient could misunderstand you, could be confused, or could be a different John than the one scheduled for a medication.)

Right time

The considerations that make an administration time the "right" time may be therapeutic, practical, or both. For therapeutic purposes, the right time is one that appropriately maintains the level of drug in the patient's bloodstream. For practical purposes, the right time is one that's convenient for the staff and the patient. Naturally, therapeutic goals take precedence over practical ones.

> The right time to give a drug depends on the patient's individual circumstances.

Working around the clock

To meet therapeutic goals, you may need to space the delivery of some medications evenly around the clock. Doing so helps to maintain a consistent level of the drug in the patient's bloodstream. If you don't have a particular need to space the drug delivery over 24 hours, you can space it over the patient's waking hours to avoid disrupting his sleep.

For some drugs, you may need to measure the patient's therapeutic response before determining whether it's the right time to give another dose. For example, you should check the patient's apical pulse rate (determined by cardiac auscultation for 1 minute) before giving digoxin, and you should assess the patient's respiratory rate before giving morphine.

The perfect plan

Besides maximizing the therapeutic effect, giving medications at specified, evenly spaced intervals provides some practical benefits. For one thing, it allows you to plan administration times that don't interfere with meals or especially busy times on the nursing unit. For example, instead of scheduling twice-daily administration times at 8 a.m. and 6 p.m., which are common times for shift changes, schedule them at 9 a.m. and 7 p.m. instead.

Another practical benefit of standardized administration times is that they establish a habit in the patient's mind. This may make it easier for him to keep taking the medication appropriately when he gets home.

If it's on the schedule, you need to be on time

Regardless of the reasons behind the administration times you establish for the patient, you'll need to follow those times carefully. In fact, many facilities consider it a medication error if you fail to give a medication within 30 minutes before or after its scheduled administration time.

Can this possibly be the right route?

Right route

Always pay careful attention to the administration route specified in the medication order, on the product's label, and in the drug guide. Also, make sure the ordered form of the drug is appropriate for the intended route. Only drugs labeled "for injection" should be used for injections of any kind.

Before you give the drug, consider whether the amount ordered is appropriate for the route by which you're preparing

Working with sustained-release drugs

A growing number of drugs are being formulated to exert an effect over many hours. The components of each drug dose dissolve at different rates, thus releasing the drug gradually but continuously into the patient's bloodstream. Convenient for staff and patients, sustained-release drugs require fewer doses per day and provide steadier control over symptoms.

Easy identification
Sustained-release drugs are supplied as plain tablets, coated tablets, and capsules filled with tiny granules. They may be identified by an *SR* (for sustained release) after the drug name, or they may have one of a number of prefixes attached to the name that suggests an extended effect. Some common examples include *Quinaglute Dura-Tabs*, *Dimetapp Extentabs*, *Chlor-Trimeton Repetabs*, and *Desoxyn Gradumets*. You may also see such names as *Spansules* and *Gyrocaps*.

Don't split, crush, or chew
Never split or crush a sustained-release drug. Warn the patient not to chew the drug and to never open a sustained-release capsule to mix the granules into foods or beverages. All of these actions could alter the drug's absorption rate, put too much drug into the patient's bloodstream too quickly, or reduce the drug's overall effect.

to give it. For example, 10 mg is an appropriate amount of morphine sulfate to give by the I.M. route to relieve pain in an adult. If the patient will be receiving it by the I.V. route, however, the equivalent dose would be more like 2 to 4 mg. If they are taking the drug orally, they will need more than 10 mg to achieve the same effect.

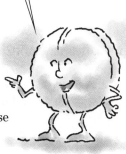

You can increase or decrease the rate of absorption of a drug depending on the application.

Different routes

Remember that the route by which you give a drug affects the rate at which it gets absorbed into the patient's bloodstream. Because certain forms of a drug may be intended for specific routes, be careful not to interfere with a drug's action by changing routes or circumventing the chemical preparation. For example, you wouldn't want to crush an enteric-coated tablet or open a sustained-release capsule. (See *Working with sustained-release drugs*, page 181.)

Different speeds

You can also help increase the speed at which topical nitroglycerin enters a patient's bloodstream by spreading it over a larger skin area and covering it with plastic wrap.

On the other hand, you can decrease the rate of absorption and effectiveness of a drug. For example, if a patient chews or swallows a sublingual drug, such as sublingual nitroglycerin, the rate of absorption and effectiveness will be decreased.

Right documentation

After administration

After administering the medication with the 5 rights completed, your 6th right is to document the administration correctly on the right patient following your facilities policy on documenting medications. There are many ways to document for example: paper charts, computerized charting, finger printing and bar-code scanning.

Procedural safeguards

The 6 rights of medication administration afford you a basic level of protection against medication errors. However, most experts consider them the minimum requirement. Here are some additional measures you should take to help avoid medication errors.

Storage and preparation

Follow these guidelines when storing and preparing drugs:

• Store and handle drugs carefully to maintain their stability and potency. Remember that some drugs can be altered by temperature, air, light, and moisture; make sure you follow all drug-specific precautions. Some drugs may need to be kept in brown bottles. Some I.V. bags may need to be covered with foil to block the light during infusion.

• Always keep drugs in the containers in which the pharmacy dispensed them. Cap all containers tightly. If you see small cylinders in a container, they probably serve to absorb moisture and keep the product fresh; don't remove them.

• Store drugs at room temperature unless you're instructed to refrigerate them. Refrigeration causes moisture to form and could alter some drugs through condensation.

• As required by law, keep opioids and controlled substances under double lock.

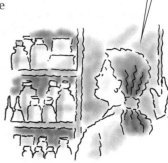

Always follow the manufacturer's recommendations and your facility's guidelines for storing and handling all medications.

Out of date? Out of the question!

• Always note a drug's expiration date—the date after which it loses some amount of potency. Never administer an outdated drug or one that looks or smells unusual.

• If the original package looks like someone may have tampered with it, don't give the drug; instead, return it in its package to the pharmacy for an investigation.

• Check the medication label three times—when you take it from the shelf or drawer, before putting it into the medication cup, and before returning the container to the shelf or drawer—to make sure you're giving the prescribed medication. For a unit-dose medication, check the label just after obtaining the medication and again before discarding the wrapper.

• You may need to reconstitute a drug dispensed as a powder just before you administer it. If medication is left over after you remove your dose, label the container with the date, time, strength, and your initials or signature.

• Never administer a drug that wasn't labeled properly after reconstitution.

• Discard any drug that will reach its expiration date before another dose is scheduled.

• If you find an unlabeled syringe with medication inside, discard it.

• Let a refrigerated drug reach room temperature before administering it, unless you're instructed otherwise.

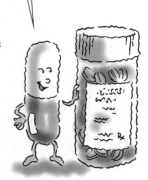

Check all medication labels and packaging carefully. Note the expiration date, too.

Handling orders for bedside medications

If a medication order specifies that you should leave a drug at the patient's bedside for self-administration, label the drug with:
• patient's name
• drug name
• dosage
• instructions the patient needs.

    Drugs commonly left at the patient's bedside include antacids and nitroglycerin tablets.

Supervision requires a super nurse
In most health care facilities, you're responsible for supervising a patient whose drugs are left at the bedside. For example, you must know how many nitroglycerin tablets the patient took, the exact times of self-administration, the degree of relief he obtained, and any unusual reactions he had to the drug. Record this information in the patient's chart, and report it to the prescriber.

Administration

Follow these guidelines when administering drugs:
• Before administering a medication based on new orders, review the patient's medication history for known allergies or other problems. Always ask the patient if they have any allergies to medications including over-the-counter medications.
• If you know a patient has a drug allergy, make sure the chart clearly displays the allergy.
• Never administer a drug to you patient that you haven't given before if you haven't first looked it up in the drug guide.
• When you deliver drugs to a patient's room, stay with the medication cart. Never leave without locking the cart and taking it back to the medication room or its usual storage place.
• Assess the patient's physiologic and psychological condition before administering any medication.
• Stay with the patient until they take the medication to verify that they took it as directed.
• Never leave medication doses at a patient's bedside unless you have a specific order to do so. (See *Handling orders for bedside medications.*)
• Administer only medications you've prepared personally or that the pharmacist prepared.
• Never administer a drug that another nurse asks you to give to their patient.
• Don't open individually prepared doses (unit-dose medications) until you're at the bedside and you've confirmed the patient's identity.
• When administering an oral drug, urge the patient to drink a full glass of water, if appropriate. Doing so helps move the medication out of the esophagus and into the stomach. It also dilutes the drug, thus reducing the chance of gastric irritation.

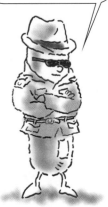

Just following orders ma'am . . . You're under surveillance until we can verify that you took your medication as prescribed.

Write it down!

• Document drugs immediately after you administer them. Delayed charting, especially of p.r.n. medications, can result in repeated doses. Documenting before giving a medication can lead to missed doses.

• Record your observations of the patient's positive and negative responses to the medication. For example, if you give an antibiotic to a patient with pneumonia, chart such positive responses as decreased sputum, reduced fever, and easier breathing to confirm the drug's effectiveness. Also, chart such adverse reactions as skin eruptions or gastric upset. Severe adverse reactions may prompt the prescriber to substitute another drug.

Drug delivery systems

Yet another area of medication administration that you'll need to master is the drug delivery system. Your facility may use one of several systems by which you can obtain ordered drugs from the pharmacy. In each one, you serve a vital coordinating function between the prescriber and the pharmacist.

Room 237-A . . . That's a medium pepperoni with extra cheese and one antacid to go!

Systems analysis

Regardless of the delivery system used by your facility, the doctors, nurses, and pharmacists must collaborate to make it work effectively. Common drug delivery systems include:

• unit-dose system
• automated systems
• individual prescriptions.

Unit-dose system

In a unit-dose system, the pharmacist dispenses a supply of wrapped, labeled individual doses of all forms of drugs: oral, injectable, and I.V. solutions with additives. The pharmacist usually dispenses sufficient drugs and I.V. solutions to last 24 hours; he may also prepare trays of medications for you to administer at specified hours.

Keep it under wraps

The pharmacist may prepare unit doses or purchase them commercially. They usually place each patient's drugs in an individual drawer of a portable medication cart. Keep the drugs in their labeled wrappers until you actually administer them. The unit-dose system reduces the likelihood of drug administration errors.

Automated systems

In essence, an automated drug delivery system is a computerized version of the unit-dose system. A pharmacist fills an electronic drug-dispensing unit and keeps it locked. The unit then delivers individually wrapped and labeled medications when you request them. A computer records all drug transactions on electronic tape and furnishes requested printouts.

To avoid the possibly disastrous effects from computer downtime, facilities that use automated dispensing systems must have a backup plan for dispensing medications and documenting their delivery.

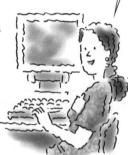

I just love this new automated drug delivery system . . . everything's in the computer and up and running!

Freeing time for patients

An automated system greatly simplifies record keeping because the computer can monitor and track drugs from the original inventory to patient billing. It saves staff time and may allow you to spend more time teaching and consulting with patients. (See *Understanding automated drug delivery*.)

Individual prescriptions

In an individual prescription system, a pharmacist fills a prescription using a container that has been labeled for a particular patient. You then administer the drug to the patient directly from the container. Because the drug is designated for a particular person, this system reduces the risk that you'll give a drug to the wrong patient. However, the system is cumbersome and slow because the medication order must travel from you to the pharmacy and back to you again.

Understanding automated drug delivery

An automated drug delivery system may free you from doing some of what you currently do by hand. For example, you may no longer have to transcribe medication orders or procure and store drugs.

The responsibility stays the same
However, keep in mind that an automated system doesn't relieve you of the responsibility for noting medication orders and administering medications properly. It also can't take your place in unusual patient circumstances in which a computer can't render your professional judgments.

Common medication errors

In addition to following your facility's policies faithfully, you can help prevent medication errors by studying common ones and avoiding the slip-ups that allowed them to happen.

Similar names

As you read earlier, drugs with similar-sounding names can be easy to confuse. Keep in mind, however, that even different-sounding names can look similar when written out rapidly by hand on a medication order: Soriatane and Loxitane, for example, both of which are capsules. Any time a patient's drug order doesn't seem right for the diagnosis, call the doctor to clarify the order. (See *Avoiding med mix-ups.*)

A case of mistaken identity

Drug names aren't the only kinds of words you can confuse. Patient names can cause trouble as well if you fail to verify each person's identity. This problem can be especially troublesome if two patients have the same first name.

> I just need to check your identification . . .

Consider this clinical scenario: Robert Brewer, age 5, was hospitalized for measles. Robert Brinson, also age 5, was admitted after a severe asthma attack. The boys were assigned to adjacent rooms on a small pediatric unit. Each had a nonproductive cough. When Robert Brewer's nurse came to give him an expectorant, the child's mother told the nurse that Robert had already inhaled a medication through a mask.

Stay on the ball

Avoiding med mix-ups

Many nurses have confused an order for morphine with one for hydromorphone (Dilaudid). Both drugs come in 4-mg prefilled syringes. If you give morphine when the doctor really ordered hydromorphone, the patient could develop respiratory depression or even arrest.

Consider posting a prominent notice in your medication room that warns the staff about this common mix-up. Or try attaching a fluorescent sticker printed with "not morphine" to each hydromorphone syringe and a sticker of a different color printed with "not hydromorphone" to each morphine syringe.

Teacher's lounge

Reducing medication errors through patient teaching

You aren't the only one who's at risk for making medication errors. Patients are at an even greater risk because they know so much less about medications than you do.

Clearly, patient teaching is a crucial aspect of your responsibility in minimizing medication errors and their consequences—especially as more patients receive outpatient rather than inpatient care.

Teaching tips
You can help minimize medication errors by:
• teaching the patient about their diagnosis and the purpose of their drug therapy
• providing the patient with their drug information in writing
• asking if they take over-the-counter medications at home in addition to prescribed drugs

• asking about herbal remedies and other nutritional supplements
• telling the patient what kinds of drug-related problems warrant a call to the doctor
• urging the patient to report anything about their drug therapy that concerns or worries them.

The nurse quickly figured out that another nurse, new to the unit, had given Robert Brinson's medication (acetylcysteine, a mucolytic) to Robert Brewer in error. Fortunately, no harmful adverse effects ensued. Had the nurse checked the patient's identity more carefully, however, no error would have occurred in the first place.

Checking ID

Always check each patient's full name and birthdate. Also, teach each patient (or parent) to offer an identification bracelet for inspection and to state a full name and birthdate when anyone enters the room with the intention of giving a medication. In addition, urge patients to tell you if an identification bracelet falls off, is removed, or gets lost. Replace it right away. (See *Reducing medication errors through patient teaching.*)

Allergy alert

After you've verified your patient's full name, take time to check whether he has drug allergies—even if they are in distress. If the patient has an allergy, immediately document the allergy in the appropriate places such as the chart, MAR, wristband, and the pharmacy and report to the doctor.

Stay on the ball

Safe alternative

A patient who's severely allergic to peanuts could have an anaphylactic reaction to Atrovent aerosol given by metered-dose inhaler. Ask the patient or the parents whether they are allergic to peanuts before you administer this drug.

If you find that they have such an allergy, you'll need to use the nasal spray and inhalation solution form of Atrovent. Because it doesn't contain soy lecithin, this form of the drug is safe for patients who are allergic to peanuts.

A re-enaction of an allergic reaction

Consider this real-life example: A doctor issued a stat order for chlorpromazine (Thorazine) for a distressed patient. By the time the nurse arrived with it, the patient had grown more distressed and was demanding relief. Unnerved by the patient's demeanor, the nurse gave the drug without checking the patient's MAR or documenting the order—and the patient had an allergic reaction to it.

Any time you're in a tense situation with a patient who needs or wants medication fast, resist the temptation to act first and document later. Skipping that crucial assessment step could easily lead to a medication error. (See *Safe alternative.*)

An allergic reaction is nothing to sneeze at. Take the time to check for drug allergies before giving any medication.

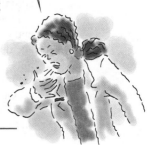

Order errors

Many medication errors stem from compound problems— a mistake that could have been caught at any of several steps along the way. For a medication to be administered correctly, each member of the health care team must fulfill the appropriate role. The doctor must write the order correctly and legibly. The pharmacist must evaluate whether the order is appropriate and then fill it correctly. In addition, the nurse must evaluate whether the order is appropriate and then administer it correctly.

Chain reaction

A breakdown anywhere along this chain of events can lead to a medication error. That's why it's so important for members of the health care team to act as a real team, checking each other and catching any problems that arise before those problems affect the patient's health. Do your best to foster an environment in which professionals can double-check each other.

For example, the pharmacist can help clarify the number of times a drug should be given each day, help you label drugs in the most appropriate way, and remind you to always return unused or discontinued medications to the pharmacy.

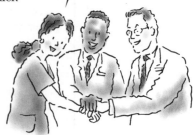

The health care team—always professional and working together!

Clear the confusion

You must clarify any doctor's order that doesn't seem clear or correct. You must also correctly handle and store any multi-dose vials obtained from the pharmacist. Additionally, store drugs in their original containers to avoid errors. (See *Container confusion*.)

Label liability

Only administer drugs that you've prepared personally. Never give a drug that has an ambiguous label or no label at all. Here's an actual example of what could happen if you do: A nurse placed an unlabeled cup of phenol (used in neurolytic procedures) next to a cup of guanethidine (a postganglionic-blocking agent). The doctor accidentally injected the phenol instead of the guanethidine, causing severe tissue damage to a patient's arm. The patient needed emergency surgery and developed neurologic complications.

Obviously, this was a compound problem. The nurse should have labeled each cup clearly, and the doctor shouldn't have given an unlabeled substance to a patient.

Stay on the ball

Container confusion

Even a confusing container can cause a medication error if you aren't careful. For example, it's easy to mistake eyedrops for the developers used for the Hemoccult test. Some patients have sustained permanent eye damage as a result. The best way to avoid this mistake is to keep Hemoccult developers in an appropriate room (such as the utility room). Never keep them in a patient's room.

Route trouble

Many medication errors stem at least in part from problems related to the route of administration. The risk of error increases when a patient has several lines running for different purposes.

Caught in a tangle of lines

Consider this example: A nurse prepared a dose of digoxin elixir for a patient who had a central I.V. line and a jejunostomy tube—and she mistakenly administered the drug into the central I.V. line. Fortunately, the patient had no adverse reaction. To help prevent such mix-ups in administration route, prepare all oral medications in a syringe that has a tip small enough to fit an abdominal tube but too big to fit a central line.

Bubble trouble

Here's another error that could have been avoided: To clear air bubbles from a 9-year-old patient's insulin drip, a nurse disconnected the tubing and raised the pump rate to 200 ml/hour to flush the bubbles through quickly. The nurse then reconnected the tubing and restarted the drip, but she forgot to reset the rate back to 2 units/hour. The child received 50 units of insulin before the error was detected. To prevent this kind of error, never increase a drip rate to clear bubbles from a line. Instead, remove the tubing from the pump, disconnect it from the patient, and use the flow-control clamp to establish gravity flow.

You carry a great deal of responsibility for making sure that patients get the right drugs in the right concentrations at the right times and by the right routes. By diligently applying the guidelines offered here, you can minimize your risk of medication errors and maximize the therapeutic effects of your patients' drug regimens.

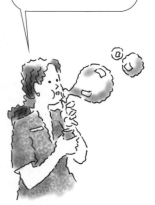

Bubbles can be trouble. Never adjust flow rate to clear bubbles from tubing.

References

Berman, A., & Snyder, S. J. (2012). *Skills in clinical nursing* (7th ed.). Upper Saddle River, NJ: Pearson Education.

Berman, A., Snyder, S. J., & McKinney, D. S. (2011). *Nursing basics for clinical practice.* Upper Saddle River, NJ: Pearson Education.

Hogan, M., Bolten, S., Ricci, M., & Taliaferro, D. (2008). *Nursing fundamentals* (2nd ed.). Upper Saddle River, NJ: Pearson Prentice Hall.

Treas, L. S., & Wilkinson, J. M. (2014). *Basic nursing concepts, skills & reasoning.* Philadelphia, PA: F.A. Davis.

Quick quiz

1. Which branch of pharmacology deals with the study of inter-actions between drugs and living tissues and serves as the basis of drug treatment?
    A.   Pharmacokinetics
    B.   Pharmacodynamics
    C.   Steady-state dosing
    D.   Bioavailability

Answer: B. Pharmacodynamics is the study of the interactions between drugs and living tissues and serves as the basis of drug treatment. It encompasses drug action and drug effect.

2. Which type of order poses the highest risk of error?
    A.   Verbal order in person
    B.   Verbal telephone order
    C.   Standard order
    D.   P.R.N. order

Answer: B. The risk of error is highest when a prescriber gives a verbal order over the telephone.

3. Which type of inpatient medication order remains in effect indefinitely or for a specified period?
    A.   Standard
    B.   Single
    C.   Standing
    D.   Stat

Answer: A. A standard order is a prescription that remains in effect indefinitely or for a specified period.

Scoring

☆☆☆ If you answered all three questions correctly, excellent! You're on the route to greatness.

  ☆☆ If you answered two questions correctly, you're getting the essentials! You used the key concepts to unlock the door to understanding.

    ☆ If you answered fewer than two questions correctly, don't worry! Go back and review this chapter, and soon you'll be pharmaco-dynamite.

10

Medication administration

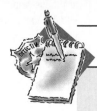

Just the facts

In this chapter, you'll learn:

♦ how to administer drugs by the oral, nasogastric tube, and gastric routes

♦ correct procedures for administering topical, ophthalmic, otic, and nasal drugs

♦ advantages and disadvantages of rectal and vaginal administration methods

♦ how to administer drugs via the respiratory route

♦ principles of injecting drugs

♦ methods for preparing an injection

♦ proper techniques for administering drugs intradermally, subcutaneously, and intramuscularly.

Administering oral drugs

Oral drug administration offers the safest, most convenient, and least costly way to administer a host of drugs. Usually, you'll give tablets, capsules, or liquid drugs (such as an elixir, syrup, or suspension) by the oral route. However, oral drugs are also available as powders, granules, and oils.

Taste test

You may need to mix some drug forms in juice or applesauce before delivery to make them more palatable.

Giving a tablet or capsule

You may give tablets or capsules whole. However, you may need to crush a tablet or split a scored tablet. (See *Crushing a tablet*, and *Splitting a scored tablet*, page 194.)

Splitting a scored tablet

To split a scored tablet, follow these steps:
• Wash your hands.
• If splitting the scored tablet using your fingers, start by placing the tablet in a paper towel.
• Notice the location of the score mark.
• Use both hands to grip the tablet on either side of the score mark, and then push down on the edges to break the tablet along the score line.
• If splitting the tablet using a cutting device, place the tablet into the device so the score mark lines up with the blade.
• Close the lid of the cutting device to force the blade through the tablet.
• Place the correct dose in a medication cup.
• Administer the prescribed dose with sufficient liquid for the patient to swallow it comfortably.

Crushing a tablet

To crush a tablet, follow these steps:
• Check first to see if the medication can be crushed in your drug guide book.
• Never crush an enteric-coated tablet or timed-release capsule.
• Wash your hands.
• Remove the unit-dose tablet from the patient's medication drawer or pour the tablet from its container.
• Make sure the mortar and pestle are clean and contain no remnants of a previously crushed tablet.
• Place the tablet in the mortar and crush it completely with the pestle.
• To save time and keep the mortar and pestle clean, crush a unit-dose tablet in its unopened wrapper. Then make sure you empty the wrapper completely.
• Place the crushed tablet into the fluid or food in which you'll administer it, and mix it thoroughly.

What you need

Prescribed medication in tablet or capsule form ✳ medication cup ✳ glass of water or other liquid to help the patient swallow the drug ✳ mortar and pestle (if crushing a tablet) ✳ paper towel or cutting device (if splitting a scored tablet)

Getting ready

• Verify the order for a tablet or capsule in the patient's chart.
• Wash your hands.

How you do it

• If you're giving a unit-dose tablet or capsule, remove it from the patient's medication drawer. Then place the unwrapped medication into the cup.

Keeping tabs

• If you need to pour the drug from its container, open the container and pour the required number of tablets or capsules into the lid of the container. Then put them in the medication cup.
• Assess your patient's ability to swallow before giving them an oral drug. Impaired swallowing can lead to aspiration.
• Confirm the patient's identity using at least two patient identifiers (not including the patient's room number).
• Help the patient to a sitting position.

One at a time please

- Offer the tablets or capsules one at a time. Have the patient place it in their mouth and take enough liquid to swallow it comfortably.
- If the drug is chewable, make sure the patient chews it thoroughly before swallowing it.

Practice pointers

- Assess the patient's ability to swallow before administering tablets or capsules to prevent choking or aspiration.

Look for the designer label

- Don't give tablets or capsules from a poorly labeled or an unlabeled bottle.
- Never give a tablet or capsule that has been poured by someone else.

No returns, no surprises

- Never return an opened or unwrapped drug to the patient's medication drawer. Instead, properly dispose of it and notify the pharmacy.

Gotta get a witness

- Remember that another nurse must witness and cosign your disposal of an opioid. (See *Documenting oral drug administration.*)
- If the patient questions you about the drug you're giving or the amount you're giving, double-check their medication record.

Take note!

Documenting oral drug administration

After administering a tablet or capsule, be sure to record:
- drug given
- dose given
- date and time of administration
- signing out of the drug on the patient's medication record
- patient's ability to swallow the drug you administered (if the patient has had problems swallowing oral drugs)

- patient's vital signs if you give a drug that could affect them
- adverse reactions that arise
- patient's refusal and notification of a doctor as needed (if a patient refuses a tablet or capsule)
- omission or withholding of a drug for any reason.

If the drug and dose are correct, reassure and inform the patient about the drug and any changes in dosage. (See *Teaching about giving a tablet or capsule.*)

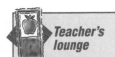

Teacher's lounge

Administering a liquid drug

For an infant, child, or patient who has trouble swallowing pills, you may give a liquid drug. (If the patient has a nasogastric [NG], gastrostomy, or jejunostomy tube, you may give the drug through the tube rather than orally.)

What you need

Measuring cup ✳ damp paper towel ✳ prescribed medication

Getting ready

• Verify the order in the patient's chart.
• Always look up the drug in the drug guide if you have not given the drug before and are not familiar with the purpose, dosage, contraindications, possible side effects, and nursing considerations.
• Wash your hands.
• Take the bottle from the patient's medication drawer or from the shelf.

How you do it

• Shake the bottle well and then uncap it. Place the cap upside down on a clean surface to avoid contaminating the inside surface.

Graduate to the next level

• While holding a graduated medicine cup at eye level, use your thumb to mark the correct level on the cup.
• Hold the bottle so the liquid flows from the side opposite the label so that the liquid won't stain or obscure the label if it runs down the bottle.
• Pour the drug into the cup until the bottom of the meniscus reaches the correct dose mark.
• Set the cup down and read the bottom of the meniscus again—still at eye level—to double-check your accuracy. If you've poured too much, discard the excess rather than pour it back into the bottle.

Teaching about giving a tablet or capsule

• Caution the patient not to chew tablets that aren't supposed to be chewed, especially enteric-coated ones.
• Teach the patient about the drug you're administering, including its name, purpose, and possible adverse effects.
• If the patient will be taking the tablets or capsules independently at home, make sure the patient thoroughly understands and plans to follow the regimen.
• Be sure to tell the patient to report anything that could be an adverse reaction to the drug.

Give lip service

• Remove drips from the lip of the bottle using a damp paper towel. Then clean the sides of the bottle, if necessary.
• Confirm the patient's identity using at least two patient identifiers (not including the patient's room number).
• To administer a liquid drug to an infant, follow the steps outlined in *Administering a liquid drug to an infant*.

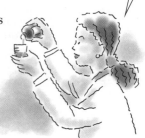

Like everything else in nursing, it's all in the technique.

Practice pointers

• Don't give medication from a poorly labeled or an unlabeled container.
• Never give a medication that has been poured by someone else.

Ages and stages

Administering a liquid drug to an infant

To administer a liquid drug to an infant, be sure to follow these steps:
• Verify the infant's identity using at least two patient identifiers (not including the patient's room number).
• Wash your hands.
• Place a bib or towel under the infant's chin.
• Withdraw the correct amount of liquid drug from the medication bottle by squeezing the bulb on the dropper.
• If the dropper is calibrated, hold it in a vertical position at eye level to check the dose amount.
• If the dropper holds too much of the drug, squeeze some into a sink or trash container. Don't return excess drug to the bottle.
• Hold the infant securely in the crook of your arm and raise his head to about a 45-degree angle.
• Place the dropper at the corner of the infant's mouth so the drug will run into the pocket between the cheek and gum as shown. This action keeps the infant from spitting out the drug and also reduces the risk of aspiration.
• If the dropper isn't calibrated, hold it vertically over the corner of the infant's open mouth and instill the prescribed number of drops.
• You may also place the drug in a nipple and allow the infant to suck the contents. Lift the infant's head and give

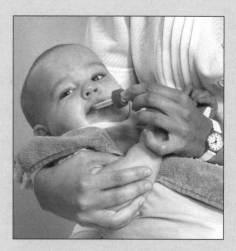

the drug slowly to prevent aspiration. Be sure to never mix a medication in a bottle because if the infant doesn't drink all of the contents of the bottle, they may not receive the full drug dosage.
• If the dropper touches the infant's mouth, wash it thoroughly before returning it to the bottle. Then close the bottle securely.

Swallows of Capistrano

• Assess your patient's ability to swallow before administering a liquid drug.
• If the patient or a parent questions you about the drug you're giving or the amount you're giving, double-check the patient's medication record. If the drug and dose are correct, reassure and inform the patient or parent about the drug and any changes in dosage.

Sip tips

• To avoid damaging or staining the patient's teeth, give acidic drugs or iron preparations through a straw.
• Liquid drugs that have an unpleasant taste are usually more palatable when taken through a straw because the liquid contacts fewer taste buds.
• When administering oral medications to pediatric patients remember the helpful hints listed in *Administering oral medications to pediatric patients*.

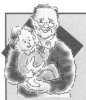

Ages and stages

Administering oral medications to pediatric patients

The oral route of drug administration is the preferred route in children because it's more comfortable and is usually safer and easier to use. When administering oral medications to pediatric patients, use these guidelines:
• An effective liquid medication administration technique for young children involves administering the medication into the corner pocket of the patient's cheek to prevent the medication from running back out.
• If the patient is a toddler, don't mix a drug with food or call it "candy," even if it has a pleasant taste. Have the child drink a liquid drug from a calibrated medication cup, rather than from a spoon, because it's easier and more accurate. Rinsing the device with water before pouring the drug into it keeps the drug from sticking and delivers a more accurate dose. If the drug is available only in tablet form, crush it and mix it with compatible syrup after consulting the pharmacist. Check with the pharmacist first to make sure it's safe to crush the tablet.
• If the patient is an older child who can swallow a tablet or a capsule, have them place the pill on the back of the tongue and swallow it with water or fruit juice. Remember, milk or milk products may interfere with drug absorption.

Gastric administration

If your patient has an NG or a gastrostomy tube, you can deliver drugs directly to the gastric mucosa through the tube. If they have a jejunostomy tube, you can deliver drugs to the intestinal lumen.

Going down the tubes

An NG tube extends from the patient's nose into the stomach. Your patients may have an NG tube in place if they have trouble swallowing or has an altered level of consciousness. In either case, it may be necessary to administer the oral drugs through the tube rather than through the oral route.

Crossing over

Unlike an NG tube, a gastrostomy tube crosses the abdominal wall to enter the stomach. It may be surgically inserted, or it may be placed during an endoscopic, a laparoscopic, or a radiologic procedure.

A gastrostomy tube reduces the risk of aspiration and it's more comfortable for the patient than an NG tube. You'll use the tube to deliver feeding solutions and drugs directly into the patient's stomach.

What you need

Prescribed medication * towel or linen-saver pad * clean gloves * facial tissues * container of water * 50- or 60-ml piston-type, catheter-tipped syringe * pH test strip (to confirm tube placement) * bulb syringe * mortar and pestle for crushing drug * and liquid in which to dissolve the drug just before instilling it (if giving a crushed tablet)

Getting ready

• All drugs delivered through an NG or a gastrostomy tube must be in liquid form so they can pass easily through the tube. If your patient's drug comes in tablet form, you'll need to crush it and dissolve it in water. If the drug comes in capsule form, you'll need to empty the contents of the capsule into water.
• Consult the pharmacist in your facility before crushing a pill or emptying the contents of a capsule to verify that it's an acceptable practice for the drug and its intended action.
• Verify the order in the patient's chart.
• Always look up the drug in the drug guide if you have not given the drug before and are not familiar with the purpose, dosage, contraindications, possible side effects and nursing considerations.
• Check the medication administration record (MAR) and drug allergies.

- Confirm the patient's identity using at least two patient identifiers (not including the patient's room number).
- Check the label on the medication three times before preparing it to make sure you'll be giving the medication correctly.
- If your facility uses a bar code scanning system, be sure to scan your identification badge, the patient's bracelet, and the medication bar code.
- Explain the procedure to the patient.
- Wash your hands and put on clean gloves.

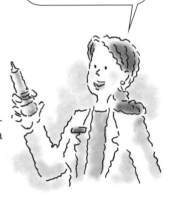

Always aspirate a small amount of stomach contents and check the pH to verify correct tube placement before administering drugs through a gastric tube.

How you do it

- Prepare the drug for delivery by crushing a tablet and mixing it in water or opening a capsule and mixing the contents in water, after consulting the pharmacist.
- Help the patient into semi-Fowler's position.
- Always verify placement of an NG tube before administering any medication. Unclamp the NG tube and attach a bulb syringe to the end of the tubing and aspirate a small amount of stomach contents from the NG tube.

Grassy green

- Examine the aspirate and place a small amount on a pH test strip. Probability of gastric placement is increased if the aspirate has a typical gastric fluid appearance (grassy-green, brown, or clear and colorless with mucus shreds) and the pH is less than or equal to 5.0.
- If no gastric contents appear when you draw back on the syringe, the tube may have risen into the esophagus, and you'll have to advance it before proceeding.
- If you meet resistance when aspirating for gastric contents, stop the procedure. *Resistance may indicate a nonpatent tube or improper tube placement.* (Keep in mind that some smaller tubes may collapse when aspiration is attempted.)
- If examination of the aspirate confirms tube placement in the stomach, resistance probably means that the tube is lying against the stomach wall. *To relieve resistance,* withdraw the tube slightly or turn the patient.
- After you've confirmed that the tube is in the proper position, remove the syringe from the end of the tube.
- Draw water into the piston-type syringe and use it to irrigate the tube with about 30 ml of water. Then remove the syringe from the tube and remove the piston from the syringe.
- Insert the catheter tip into the distal end of the NG tube, making sure it fits snugly.
- With the syringe attached to the opening of the tube, hold the syringe upright and slightly above the level of the patient's nose.
- Slowly pour the drug into the syringe, using it as a funnel.

Slow flow

• Allow the drug to flow slowly through the tube. If it flows too quickly, lower the syringe. If it flows too slowly, raise the syringe slightly.
• As the syringe empties, add more of the drug. *To prevent air from entering the patient's stomach,* don't let the syringe drain completely before you add more of the drug to it.
• After you've given the full dose, pour 30 to 50 ml of water into the syringe.

Getting carried away

• Let the water flow through the tube to rinse it and to carry all of the drug into the patient's stomach.
• Next, clamp the tube and remove the syringe.
• If the tube is attached to suction, clamp it for 30 to 60 minutes after you give a drug, depending on the patient's ability to tolerate it and if the doctor agrees and writes an order.

No backsies

• Have the patient remain in semi-Fowler's position or in a side-lying position for at least 30 minutes after administration *to prevent esophageal reflux* (backward or return flow of stomach contents into the esophagus).
• Clean and store the equipment or dispose of it as appropriate.

Practice pointers

• Remember that all drugs instilled through the tube must be in liquid form. Check with a pharmacist if you aren't sure whether a tablet can be safely crushed or a capsule safely opened.
• Never crush an enteric-coated or a sustained-release drug.

Full follow-through

• *Because capsules tend not to dissolve completely,* always follow them with water to flush the tube and prevent occlusion.
• Dilute liquid drugs with about 30 ml of water to decrease their osmolality.
• If you need to give more than one drug through an NG tube, give each one separately, flushing the tube with 10 to 15 ml of water between doses *to avoid drug interactions.*
• Irrigate the tube with 30 ml of irrigant before and after drug instillation.

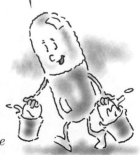

Water flushes between doses are a must to prevent drug interactions.

Free to vent

• If the patient has a Salem sump tube, watch for fluid reflux in the vent lumen. *Reflux means that pressure in the patient's stomach exceeds atmospheric pressure, possibly because the primary lumen is clogged or the suction system was set up incorrectly.* Don't clamp the vent tube in an attempt to stop the reflux.

• Some drugs, such as phenytoin (Dilantin), are altered by the presence of feeding solutions in the patient's stomach. Check with a doctor to see whether you should stop the patient's tube feeding for 1 to 2 hours before or after giving the prescribed drug.

Administering topical drugs

Topical drugs exert their effects after being applied to a patient's skin or the mucous membrane in the patient's mouth or throat.

Most forms are local

Topical drugs may take the form of a lotion, cream, ointment, paste, powder, or spray that you apply to an affected skin area. Other topical drug forms include a spray, mouthwash, gargle, and lozenge to treat a problem in the patient's mouth or throat.

Usually, you'll use these topical administration methods to obtain local, rather than systemic, drug effects. The drug moves through the epidermis and into the dermis, based in part on the vascularity of the region to which it's applied.

Interstate transport

Certain types of topical drugs, known as *transdermal drugs*, are meant to enter the patient's bloodstream and exert a systemic effect after you apply a paste or patch to the patient's skin.

Vive la difference

Keep in mind the differences between lotions, creams, ointments, pastes, and powders:

• A *lotion* contains an insoluble powder suspended in water or an emulsion. When you apply a lotion, it leaves a uniform layer of powder in the film on the patient's skin.
• A *cream* is an oil-in-water emulsion in semisolid form. It lubricates the skin and acts as a barrier.
• An *ointment* is a semisolid substance that, when applied to the skin, helps to retain body heat and provides prolonged contact between the skin and the drug.
• A *paste* is a stiff mixture of powder and ointment. It provides a uniform coat to reduce and repel moisture.
• A *powder* is an inert chemical that may contain medication. It helps dry the skin and reduces maceration and friction. (See *Topical tips for tots.*)

Ages and stages

Topical tips for tots

Remember these tips when giving topical drugs to pediatric patients:

• When applying powder, shake it into your hand, and then apply it; this avoids creating puffs of powder that you or the child could accidentally inhale.
• Use topical corticosteroids cautiously and sparingly on diaper covered body areas. A disposable diaper or rubber pants act like an occlusive dressing, possibly increasing systemic absorption of the drug.

Administering a transdermal drug

Transdermal drugs deliver a constant, controlled amount of medication through the skin and into the bloodstream, thereby achieving a steady, prolonged systemic effect.

Patch him up

To give a transdermal drug, you'll either apply a measured amount of ointment to a selected area of the patient's skin, or you'll apply a transdermal patch that contains medication. (See *Understanding a transdermal patch.*)

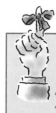

Memory jogger

Trans means "across" or "through"; *dermal* means "related to the skin." A transdermal drug moves through the skin and into the bloodstream.

Understanding a transdermal patch

A transdermal patch is made up of several layers. The outermost layer is an aluminized polyester barrier that holds the drug in the patch. The next layer is the drug reservoir, which contains the main dose of the drug. The next layer—a membrane—controls release of the drug from the reservoir.

Stick with it

The innermost adhesive layer keeps the patch on the patient's skin and holds a small amount of drug as it moves from the patch into the skin. The dots in this illustration show the drug moving through the skin and into the bloodstream.

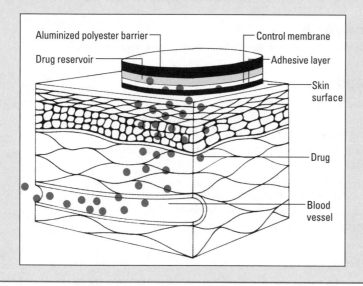

Aluminized polyester barrier — Control membrane
Drug reservoir — Adhesive layer
— Skin surface
— Drug
— Blood vessel

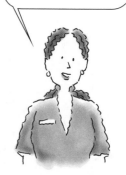

A transdermal patch delivers a constant, controlled amount of medication that achieves a steady, prolonged systemic effect.

The transdermal team

Drugs that are commonly given via the transdermal route include:
- nitroglycerin to control angina
- scopolamine to treat motion sickness
- estradiol to provide hormone replacement after menopause
- clonidine to treat hypertension
- fentanyl to control chronic pain.

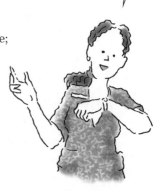

Generally, patches deliver drugs for longer periods of time than ointments do.

A matter of time

The appropriate form—ointment or patch—by which to give the drug depends largely on the desired delivery time; typically, a patch delivers the drug for a longer period. For example, transdermal nitroglycerin ointment dilates coronary vessels for up to 4 hours, whereas a nitroglycerin patch lasts for up to 24 hours. In patch form, scopolamine lasts up to 72 hours, estradiol up to a week, clonidine up to 24 hours, and fentanyl up to 72 hours.

What you need

Transdermal ointment
Prescribed medicated ointment ✳ application strip or measuring paper ✳ semipermeable dressing or plastic wrap ✳ clean gloves ✳ washcloth ✳ soap and warm water ✳ towel ✳ adhesive tape

Transdermal patch
Prescribed medicated patch ✳ washcloth ✳ soap and water ✳ towel

Getting ready

- Verify the order in the patient's chart.
- Always look up the drug in the drug guide if you have not given the drug before and are not familiar with the purpose, dosage, contraindications, possible side effects, and nursing considerations.
- Check the MAR and drug allergies.
- Confirm the patient's identity using at least two patient identifiers (not including the patient's room number).
- Wash your hands and put on clean gloves.

How you do it

Follow these steps for applying a transdermal ointment or a transdermal patch.

Applying a transdermal ointment
- Choose the application site—usually a dry, hairless spot on the patient's chest or arm.
- To promote absorption, wash the site with soap and warm water. Dry it thoroughly.
- If the patient has a previously applied medication strip at another site, remove it and wash this area to clear away drug residue.

Splitting hairs

- If you must use an area that's hairy, clip excess hair rather than shaving it; shaving causes irritation, which may be exacerbated by the drug.
- Squeeze the prescribed amount of ointment on the application strip or measuring paper as shown. Don't let the drug touch your skin.
- Apply the strip, drug side down, directly to the patient's skin.
- Maneuver the strip slightly to spread a thin layer of the ointment over a 3″ (7.5 cm) area, but don't rub the ointment into the skin.
- Secure the application strip to the patient's skin by covering it with a semipermeable dressing.

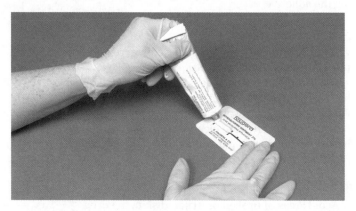

Skin tight

- Press firmly with the palm of one hand to ensure that the dressing adheres well, especially around the edges.
- Label the strip with the date, time, and your initials.
- Remove your gloves and wash your hands.

Applying a transdermal patch
- Remove the old patch. (See *Discarding a patch*, page 206.)
- Choose a dry, hairless application site. Be sure to rotate application sites. Don't attempt to apply the patch to an area with alterations in skin integrity.

Discarding a patch

There's still a substantial amount of drug remaining in a used patch. To avoid possible harm to children or animals, fold the patch in half with the adhesive layer inside and place into a closed container that is not accessible to children or pets.

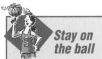

A shocking experience

Don't place a defibrillator paddle on a transdermal patch. The aluminum on the patch can cause electrical arcing during defibrillation, resulting in smoke, thermal burns and, possibly, ineffective electrical cardioversion. If a patient's patch is on a standard paddle site, remove the patch before applying the paddle.

• If necessary, clip any hair from the site, but don't shave the area. The most commonly used sites are the upper arm, the chest, the back, and behind the ear.
• Clean the application site with soap and warm water. Dry it thoroughly.
• Open the drug package and remove the patch.
• Without touching the adhesive surface, remove the clear plastic backing.
• Apply the patch to the application site without touching the adhesive.

Practice pointers
• Apply any transdermal drug at the prescribed intervals to ensure a continuous effect.
• Don't apply the drug if the patient has skin allergies or has experienced skin reactions to the drug.
• Always make sure you have removed the old patch, some patches are clear and are hard to see. Not removing the old patch may cause an adverse reaction.

Saved by his own skin
• Avoid areas of broken or irritated skin; the drug could increase the irritation.
• Don't apply a transdermal drug to scarred or callused skin because either one may impair absorption.
• If you need to defibrillate a patient who has a transdermal patch in place, see *A shocking experience*.
• Teach the patient about taking transdermal drugs. (See *Teaching about transdermal medications*.)

Here are the facts, Jack
• Also be sure to alert the patient to potential adverse reactions to the particular drug being delivered. For example:

> Don't apply transdermal drugs if your patient has skin allergies or has had a previous skin reaction to the drug.

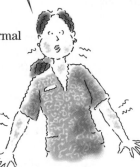

Teacher's lounge

Teaching about transdermal medications

• Review drug-specific precautions the patient must know. For example, make sure the patient knows to thoroughly remove an old application of nitroglycerin ointment before applying a new dose.
• Make sure the patient knows how to choose an appropriate application site, and tell the patient to avoid scarred or callused areas, bony prominences, and hairy surfaces.
• Warn the patient not to get transdermal ointment on their hands and to wash them thoroughly after applying a transdermal drug.

Dry as a bone
• Make the patient aware to keep the area around the application site as dry as possible.
• If the patient will be applying scopolamine, tell the patient not to drive or operate machinery until the patient knows how the drug affects him.
• If the patient will be using clonidine patches, tell the patient to check with their primary health care provider before using nonprescription cough preparations. Over-the-counter preparations may counteract the effects of the drug.
• Warn the patient about the possible adverse reactions that can occur with transdermal drug delivery, such as skin irritation, itching, and rashes.

Take note!

Documenting transdermal drug administration

Be sure to record:
• date and time of a transdermal application
• medication used
• location of the ointment or patch on the patient's body
• effects of the medication
• patient teaching you provided.

– Nitroglycerin may cause headaches and, in elderly patients, postural hypotension.
– Scopolamine most commonly causes a dry mouth and drowsiness.
– Transdermal estradiol may increase the risk of endometrial cancer, thromboembolic disease, and birth defects.
– Clonidine may cause severe rebound hypertension, especially if withdrawn suddenly. (See *Documenting transdermal drug administration.*)

Administering ophthalmic drugs

Typically, you'll give ophthalmic drugs (diagnostic and therapeutic) in the form of drops or ointment. To administer some types of drugs, you'll insert a medicated disk into your patient's eye. Sometimes, you'll need to apply a patch over a patient's eye after you instill an ophthalmic drug.

Instilling eyedrops

Eyedrops can be used for several diagnostic and therapeutic purposes, including:
- dilating the pupil
- staining the cornea to detect abrasions or scars
- anesthetizing the eye
- lubricating the eye
- protecting the vision of a neonate
- treating certain eye disorders, such as infections or glaucoma.

What you need

Prescribed eyedrops ✳ sterile cotton balls ✳ clean gloves ✳ warm water or normal saline solution ✳ sterile gauze pads ✳ facial tissues ✳ eye dressing (if necessary)

Getting ready

- Verify the order in the patient's chart.
- Always look up the drug in the drug guide if you have not given the drug before and are not familiar with the purpose, dosage, contraindications, possible side effects, and nursing considerations.
- Check the MAR and drug allergies.
- Read the label to make sure the drug is intended for ophthalmic use.

Seeing is believing

- Check the expiration date on the eye drop container and inspect the drops for cloudiness, discoloration, and precipitates. If the solution appears abnormal in any way, don't use it.
- Keep in mind that some ophthalmic drugs are in suspension form and normally appear cloudy. When in doubt, check with a pharmacist.

Not the same eye-dea

- Take extra care when verifying an order for eye drops because different drugs or dosages may be ordered for each eye.
- Confirm the patient's identity using at least two patient identifiers (not including the patient's room number).
- Explain the procedure to the patient.
- Wash your hands and put on clean gloves.

How you do it

- If the patient has an eye dressing in place, remove it by gently pulling it down and away from the patient's forehead.

Careful clean up

• If the patient has discharge around the eye, moisten sterile cotton balls or sterile gauze pads with warm water or normal saline solution.
• Wipe the eye gently to clean away debris, moving from the inner canthus to the outer canthus as shown. Use a fresh sterile cotton ball or sterile gauze pad for each stroke.

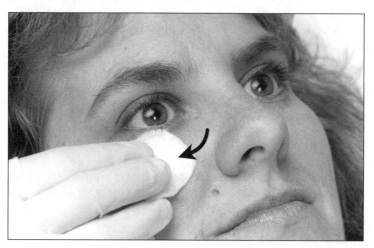

• If the patient has crusted secretions around her eye, moisten a sterile gauze pad with warm water or normal saline solution. Then have the patient close their eye, and place the moist pad over the closed eye for 1 or 2 minutes.
• Remove the pad and reapply new moist sterile gauze pads, as needed, until the secretions become soft enough that you can remove them without injuring the tender ocular tissues.

> When removing discharge from around the eye, remember to wipe from the inner canthus to the outer canthus using a fresh, sterile cotton ball or gauze pad with each swipe.

Full tilt

• To help minimize systemic reactions to eyedrops, see *Minimizing systemic reactions to eyedrops*, page 210.
• Remove the dropper cap from the bottle (unless the bottle has a built-in dropper) and draw the eyedrops into the dropper, taking care not to contaminate the dropper.
• Ask the patient to look up and away *to move the cornea away from the lower lid and minimize the risk of touching the cornea with the dropper if the patient blinks*.

Stay on the ball

Minimizing systemic reactions to eyedrops

Systemic reactions to eyedrops, such as tachycardia, palpitations, flushing, dry skin, ataxia, and confusion, can be minimized by having the patient press a finger over the tear duct at the inner canthus as you instill the drops. This action compresses the nasolacrimal tear ducts, thus preventing the drops from draining out of the eye.

In addition, have your patient tilt their head back and toward the side of the affected eye to ensure that the drops will flow away from the tear duct at the inner canthus. If you'll be placing drops in the left eye, ask your patient to tilt to the left, to the right if you'll be placing drops in the right eye. By tilting her head, the patient will reduce the chance that the drops will drain into the tear duct and cause systemic effects.

• Steady the hand holding the dropper or eye drop bottle by resting it against the patient's forehead. Use your other hand to gently pull down the patient's lower eyelid as shown.

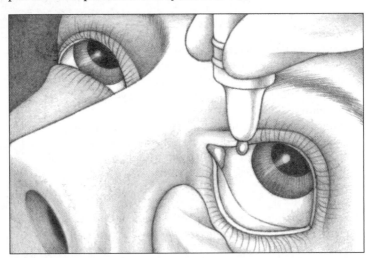

• Instill the prescribed number of drops into the conjunctival sac, not onto the patient's eyeball. Then release the patient's eyelid and have the patient blink to distribute the drops throughout their eye.

Practice pointers

• If you're opening the drug container for the first time, write the date on the label. Once the container has been opened, the drug should be used within 2 weeks or discarded.

• To prevent contamination, never use the same eyedrop container for more than one patient.

Worth the wait

• If the patient needs more than one type of eye medication, wait at least 5 minutes between administering different doses.
• Teach the patient the correct procedure for instilling eyedrops at home, if prescribed. (See *Teaching about eyedrops*.)
• For tips on teaching an older patient, see *Managing eyedrop non-sense*.

Administering ophthalmic ointment

An ointment formulation helps keep an ophthalmic drug in contact with the treatment area for as long as possible—an especially useful tactic for pediatric patients. Usually, you'll use an antibiotic ointment to treat eye infections.

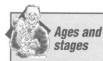

Ages and stages

Managing eyedrop non-sense

If your patient is an older adult, they may have trouble sensing whether a drop has gone into their eye. If so, suggest that the patient chill the eyedrops before using them. Most people find it easier to feel a drop entering the eye when the drop is cold.

Teacher's lounge

Teaching about eyedrops

• Explain why the doctor prescribed the eyedrops.
• Stress the importance of proper hand-washing technique.
• Teach the patient to make sure it is the right medication, the correct number of drops, and the correct eye.
• Tell the patient to warm the drops to room temperature by holding the bottle between their hands for about 2 minutes, unless the patient has troubles getting the drop into the eye, then chilling the eyedrop first helps the patient know if the drop gets into their eye.
• If the patient is using more than one kind of drop, tell the patient to wait 5 minutes between administering them.

• Teach the patient to protect the container from light and heat.
• Teach the patient the potential adverse effects of the medication and when the patient should notify the doctor.
• Stress the importance of never placing any medication in the patient's eyes unless the label reads "For Ophthalmic Use" or "For Use in Eyes."
• If your patient can see through the eyedrop container, teach the patient to hold it up to the light and look at it. If the liquid is discolored or if it contains sediment, tell the patient not to use it but to take the container back to the pharmacy and have it checked.
• Provide written instructions so the patient can review the proper administration steps after the patient gets home.

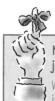

Memory jogger

When instilling eyedrops, remember up, up, and away—have the patient look up and away from you.

What you need

Prescribed eye ointment ✳ sterile cotton balls ✳ clean gloves ✳ warm water or normal saline solution ✳ sterile gauze pads ✳ facial tissues ✳ eye dressing (if necessary)

Getting ready

- Verify the order in the patient's chart.
- Always look up the drug in the drug guide if you have not given the drug before and are not familiar with the purpose, dosage, contraindications, possible side effects, and nursing considerations.
- Check the MAR and drug allergies.
- Read the label to make sure the drug is intended for ophthalmic use.
- Double-check the medication order when administering ophthalmic ointment because different drugs or dosages may be ordered for each eye.
- Confirm the patient's identity using at least two patient identifiers (not including the patient's room number).
- Explain the procedure to the patient.
- Wash your hands and put on clean gloves.

How you do it

- If the patient has an eye dressing in place, remove it by gently pulling it down and away from her forehead.
- If the patient has discharge around the eye, moisten sterile cotton balls or sterile gauze pads with warm water or normal saline solution.
- Gently wipe the eye to clean away debris, moving from the inner canthus to the outer canthus. Use a fresh sterile cotton ball or sterile gauze pad for each stroke.
- If the patient has crusted secretions around their eye, moisten a sterile gauze pad with warm water or normal saline solution. Have the patient close their eye, then place the moist pad over it for 1 or 2 minutes.
- Remove the pad and reapply new moist sterile gauze pads, as needed, until the secretions are soft enough to be removed without injuring the tissue.

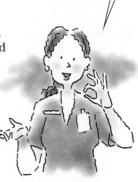

Remember, a little dab'll do ya . . . but avoid touching the tube against the patient's eye.

Conquering crust

- If the tip of the ointment tube has crusted, wipe it with a sterile gauze pad to remove the crust.
- Ask the patient to look up and away *to move the cornea away from the lower lid and minimize the risk of touching the cornea with the tip of the ointment tube if the patient blinks.*

• Steady the hand holding the ointment tube against the patient's forehead. Use your other hand to gently pull down her lower eyelid.

Avoiding eye contact

• Squeeze a small ribbon of ointment along the edge of the conjunctival sac from the inner to the outer canthus as shown. Don't let the tip of the tube touch the patient's eye. (If it does, discard the tube.)

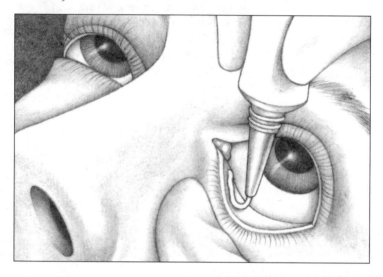

• Cut off the ribbon of ointment by turning the tube. Then release the patient's eyelid and have the patient roll their eyes behind closed lids *to help distribute the drug.*
• Use a clean tissue to remove excess ointment that leaks from the patient's eye. Use a fresh tissue for each eye *to prevent cross-contamination.*
• Lastly, apply a new eye dressing, if indicated.

Practice pointers

• If you're opening the drug container for the first time, write the date on the label. When the container has been opened, the drug should be used within 2 weeks or discarded.

An ounce of prevention

• To prevent contamination, never use the same drug container for more than one patient.
• Systemic reactions are unlikely with ophthalmic ointments because they don't empty quickly into the lacrimal duct, as eyedrops do.

Teaching about ophthalmic ointment

• Explain why the doctor prescribed the ointment, and review the proper steps for using the ointment at home.
• Tell the patient to wash their hands before and after applying eye ointment. Be sure to warn the patient not to contaminate the lid of the ointment tube

or touch the tip of the tube to the eye or to the skin around the eye.
• Tell the patient to apply ointment from the inner to the outer corner of the eye. Let the patient know that their vision may be blurry for several minutes after putting the ointment in their eye.

Documenting ophthalmic drug administration

After administering an ophthalmic drug, be sure to record:
• eye treated
• date and time
• prescribed drug
• dose administered
• patient's response to the instillation procedure (Note the appearance of the patient's eye before and after she receives eyedrops.)
• patient or family teaching you provided.

• Carefully document the procedure. (See *Documenting ophthalmic drug administration*.)
• Teach the patient how to apply ophthalmic ointment for home use, if prescribed. (See *Teaching about ophthalmic ointment*.)

Administering otic drugs

Otic drugs may be instilled to:
• treat infections and inflammation
• soften cerumen for later removal
• produce local anesthesia
• aid removal of a foreign object trapped in the ear.

Instilling eardrops

You probably won't administer otic drugs to a patient with a perforated eardrum (although it may be permitted with certain medications and with sterile technique). Certain otic drugs may be prohibited in other conditions as well—for example, hydrocortisone is contraindicated if the patient has a viral or fungal infection.

What you need

Prescribed eardrops ✳ penlight ✳ facial tissues (or cotton-tipped applicators) ✳ cotton balls ✳ emesis basin for warm water ✳ and clean gloves

Getting ready

- Verify the order in the patient's chart.
- Always look up the drug in the drug guide if you have not given the drug before and are not familiar with the purpose, dosage, contraindications, possible side effects, and nursing considerations.
- Check the MAR and drug allergies.
- To avoid adverse reactions caused by the instillation of cold eardrops (such as vertigo, nausea, and pain), warm the drops to body temperature by placing the container in a basin of warm water.

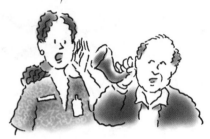

I said, the doctor thinks eardrops might help soften your cerumen a little so that maybe we can loosen the horn that's attached to your ear!

Now hear this

- Don't make the drops too hot; if necessary, test their temperature by placing a drop on your wrist.
- Confirm the patient's identity using at least two patient identifiers (not including the patient's room number).
- Wash your hands.
- Explain the procedure to the patient.

How you do it

- Have the patient lie on his side with his affected ear facing up.
- Straighten the patient's ear canal. (See *Positioning a patient for eardrops*, page 216.)

Light the way

- Using a penlight, examine the ear canal for drainage. If you find any, clean the canal with a tissue or cotton-tipped applicator because drainage can reduce the effectiveness of the drug.
- Straighten the patient's ear canal once again and instill the ordered number of drops. To avoid patient discomfort, aim the dropper so the drops fall against the side of the ear canal, not on the eardrum.

Disappearing act

- Hold the ear canal in position until you see the drug disappear down the canal. Then release the ear.

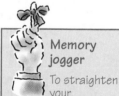

Memory jogger

To straighten your patient's ear canal, remember:

- For an adult or grown-up, gently pull the auricle up and back
- For an infant or young child, get down to his level and gently pull the auricle down and back.

Ages and stages

Positioning a patient for eardrops

Before you instill eardrops, have the patient lie on their side. Then straighten the patient's ear canal to help the drops reach the eardrum. In an adult, gently pull the auricle *up* and *back*; in an infant or young child, gently pull *down* and *back* as shown.

Adult

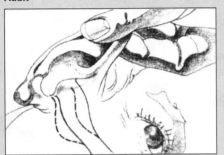

Child

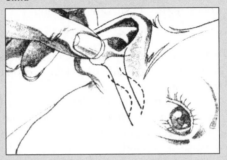

• Tell the patient to remain on their side for 5 to 10 minutes to allow the drug to travel down the ear canal.
• If ordered, tuck a cotton ball loosely into the opening of the ear canal. Don't push it too far into the ear, however, because you'll keep secretions from draining and increase pressure on the eardrum.
• Clean and dry the outer ear.
• Help the patient into a comfortable position.
• Remove your gloves, and wash your hands and document.

Keep in mind that vertigo is possible with eardrop instillation. For safety's sake, keep the bedside rails up.

Practice pointers

• Some conditions make the normally sensitive ear canal quite tender, so be especially gentle when instilling eardrops. (See *Otic tips for tots.*)

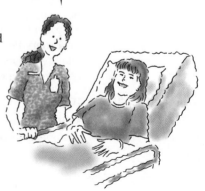

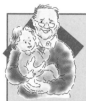

Ages and stages

Otic tips for tots

When teaching parents how to administer eardrops to their child, make sure you include this helpful information:
• Warm the drops for their child's comfort by holding the bottle in their hands for about 2 minutes.
• Gently pull the earlobe down and back to straighten the child's ear canal.

• If necessary to keep the medication from running out of the ear, place a cotton ball moistened with the medication at the very entrance to the ear canal. Remove the cotton after 1 hour. Avoid using dry cotton because it may absorb the medication.

• Take special care not to injure the eardrum. Never insert any object, even a cotton-tipped applicator, so far into the ear canal that you can't see its tip.
• If the patient has vertigo, keep the bedside rails up and assist as necessary. Also, move slowly to avoid aggravating any vertigo.
• Carefully document the procedure. (See *Documenting otic drug administration.*)
• Teach the patient how to instill eardrops if they have been prescribed for home use. (See *Teaching about eardrops.*)

Take note!

Documenting otic drug administration

After administering an otic drug, be sure to record:
• ear treated
• name of the drug instilled
• date and time you instilled it
• dose given, and the patient's response to the instillation procedure
• appearance of the patient's ears before and after instilling eardrops
• teaching aids given to the patient or family.

Teacher's lounge

Teaching about eardrops

• Remind the patient never to insert any object into their ear.
• Review the importance of washing hands thoroughly.
• Make sure the patient knows how many drops to give and into which ear.

• Teach the patient not to use the medication and to call the pharmacist or doctor if the liquid looks discolored or contains sediment.
• Provide written guidelines to parents who will be administering eardrops to a child at home.

Administering nasal drugs

For the most part, nasal drugs produce local effects.

Instilling nose drops

You'll use drops to treat a specific nasal area and sprays and aerosols to diffuse the drug through the nasal passages.

The nose knows

The most commonly administered nasal drugs are:
• vasoconstrictors, which coat and shrink swollen mucous membranes
• local anesthetics, which promote patient comfort during such procedures as bronchoscopy
• corticosteroids, which reduce inflammation caused by allergies or nasal polyps.

What you need

Prescribed nasal medication ✳ clean gloves

Getting ready

• Verify the order on the patient's chart.
• Always look up the drug in the drug guide if you have not given the drug before and are not familiar with the purpose, dosage, contraindications, possible side effects, and nursing considerations.
• Check the MAR and drug allergies.
• Confirm the patient's identity using at least two patient identifiers (not including the patient's room number).
• Explain the procedure to the patient and position them as needed to make sure the drops reach the intended site.

How you do it

• Push up gently on the tip of the patient's nose to open his nostrils completely.
• Place the dropper about ⅓″ (1 cm) inside his nostril. Angle the tip of the dropper slightly toward the inner corner of the patient's eye. Squeeze the dropper bulb to dispense the correct number of drops into each nostril.
• After you've instilled the prescribed number of drops, instruct the patient to keep their head tilted back for about 5 minutes. Encourage the patient to expectorate any medication that runs into the throat.

Practice pointers

• Stay with the patient after administering nose drops. Urge the patient to breathe through their mouth. If the patient coughs, help the patient to sit up. For several minutes, observe the patient closely for possible respiratory problems.

Administering rectal drugs

You may administer a drug rectally to a patient who's unconscious, vomiting, or unable to swallow or take anything by mouth. Rectally administered drugs can produce either local or systemic effects. The most commonly used forms of rectal drugs include:
• suppositories
• medicated enemas.

Dodging digestion and bypassing biotransformation

Because rectal administration bypasses the upper gastrointestinal (GI) tract, drugs given by this method aren't destroyed by digestive enzymes in the stomach or small intestine. Also, these drugs don't irritate the upper GI tract, as some oral drugs can. In addition, rectal drugs bypass the portal system, thus avoiding biotransformation in the liver. Biotransformation or drug metabolism refers to the body's ability to change a drug from its dosage form to a more water-soluble form that can be excreted. Once in the liver, drugs are metabolized by enzymes.

Rectal drug downsides

Rectal drugs do have some disadvantages, however. The administration procedure may cause discomfort or embarrassment to the patient. Also, the drug may be incompletely absorbed, especially if the patient can't retain it or if the rectum contains feces. As a result, the patient may need a higher dose than if taken the same drug in oral form.

Administering rectal suppositories

A suppository is a firm, bullet-shaped object made from a substance that melts at body temperature (such as cocoa butter). As the suppository melts, it releases the drug into the patient's rectum, where it can be absorbed across the rectal mucosa. Most suppositories are about 1½″ (4 cm) long (or smaller for infants and children).

Rectal suppositories commonly contain drugs that reduce fever; induce relaxation; stimulate peristalsis and defecation; or relieve pain, vomiting, and local irritation.

What you need

Prescribed rectal drug ✳ several 4″ × 4″ gauze pads ✳ clean gloves ✳ linen-saver pad ✳ water-soluble lubricant ✳ bedpan (if necessary)

Getting ready

• Verify the order on the patient's chart.
• Always look up the drug in the drug guide if you have not given the drug before and are not familiar with the purpose, dosage, contraindications, possible side effects, and nursing considerations.
• Check the MAR and drug allergies.
• Confirm the patient's identity using at least two patient identifiers (not including the patient's room number).
• Provide privacy.

How you do it

• Place the patient on their left side in Sims' position (semiprone with the right knee and thigh drawn up and the left arm along the patient's back). Cover the patient with the bedcovers, exposing only the buttocks.
• Place a linen-saver pad under the buttocks *to protect the bedding.*
• Wash your hands and put on clean gloves.
• Remove the suppository from its wrapper and apply a water-soluble lubricant to it.
• Using your nondominant hand, lift the patient's upper buttock to expose the anus.

Take a deep breath and relax

• Tell the patient to take several deep breaths through their mouth *to relax the anal sphincter and reduce anxiety and discomfort during insertion.*

Tapered end first

• For information on administering a rectal suppository to a child, see *Using rectal suppositories in pediatric patients.*
• Using your dominant hand, insert the tapered end of the suppository into the patient's rectum. (See *Inserting a rectal suppository in an adult.*)
• Ensure the patient's comfort. Ask the patient to lie quietly and, if applicable, to retain the suppository for an appropriate time. A suppository given to relieve

> Try to have your patient lie quietly after a rectal suppository has been inserted to allow the drug time to take effect.

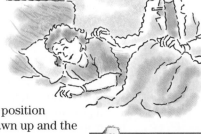

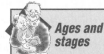

Ages and stages

Using rectal suppositories in pediatric patients

Rectal administration via suppository may be a good alternative when the oral route can't be used, but remember that it's a less reliable method in children than in adults. Remember to insert the suppository only up to the first knuckle joint of your finger. If your patient is an infant, use your little finger to insert the drug.

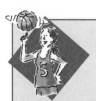

Inserting a rectal suppository in an adult

When inserting a rectal suppository in an adult, use your index finger to direct the suppository along the rectal wall toward the patient's umbilicus, as shown, so the membrane can absorb the drug. Continue to advance it about 3″ (7.5 cm), or about the length of your finger, until it passes the internal anal sphincter.

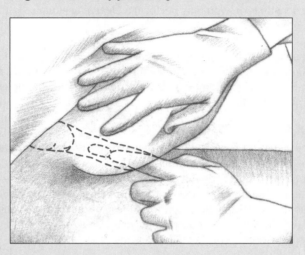

Contraindications for rectal suppositories

You'll want to avoid giving rectal suppositories to a patient who has:

• cardiac arrhythmias or has had a myocardial infarction because inserting a rectal suppository typically stimulates the vagus nerve

• undiagnosed abdominal pain because, if the pain stems from appendicitis, the peristalsis caused by rectal administration could rupture the appendix

• recently undergone colon, rectal, or prostate surgery because rectal suppositories increase the risk of local trauma.

constipation should be retained as long as possible (at least 20 minutes) for it to be effective. If necessary, press on the patient's anus with a gauze pad until the urge to defecate passes.

• If the patient can't retain the suppository and pressing on the anus with a gauze pad doesn't relieve the urge to defecate, place the patient on a bedpan.

Practice pointers

• Store rectal suppositories in the refrigerator, as indicated, to keep them firm and to maintain the drug's effectiveness.

• Before administering rectal medication, inspect the patient's anus. If the tissues are inflamed or if hemorrhoids are present, withhold the suppository and notify a doctor. The drug could aggravate the condition.

• To minimize the risk of local trauma, you may need to avoid this route if the patient has had recent rectal, colon, or prostate surgery.

• Rectal suppositories are contraindicated in certain patients. (See *Contraindications for rectal suppositories.*)

Administering medicated enemas

When you give an enema, you instill fluid into a patient's rectum for a variable amount of time. If you're preparing the patient for a diagnostic or surgical procedure or if you're giving the enema to relieve constipation, you may perform a cleansing enema.

Cleaning crew

A cleansing enema is a procedure that involves instilling unmedicated fluid into a patient's rectum simply to clean the patient's rectum and colon. The patient expels the irrigant almost completely within about 15 minutes.

Pay attention . . . the topic is retention

Enemas can also be used to deliver such drugs as lactulose, which acidifies the colon contents and lowers blood ammonia levels. To deliver a drug, you'll probably give a retention enema. A retention enema is a type of enema that requires the patient to retain the fluid in his rectum and colon for 30 to 60 minutes, if possible, before expelling it. A retention enema can also be used as an emollient to soothe irritated colon tissues.

Enema enemies

Enemas stimulate peristalsis by distending the colon and stimulating nerves in the rectal walls. Consequently, you shouldn't give an enema to a patient who has had:
- recent colon or rectal surgery
- myocardial infarction
- undiagnosed abdominal pain, which could be caused by appendicitis (Giving an enema to a patient with appendicitis can irritate the inflamed area of the appendix and precipitate perforation.)

Most importantly, give an enema cautiously to any patient who has cardiac arrhythmias because inserting anything into the rectum stimulates the vagus nerve and could cause an increase in the cardiac arrhythmias.

What you need

Prescribed solution (usually in a premixed, commercially prepared container) ✳ disposable enema kit ✳ clean gloves, 4″ × 4″ gauze pads ✳ bedpan ✳ toilet paper ✳ emesis basin ✳ linen-saver pad ✳ water-soluble lubricant (see *Choosing enema supplies.*)

Grab bag

If you need to prepare the solution for a patient's enema or you need a large volume of fluid, you'll use an enema bag to perform the procedure instead of commercially prepared solution and a disposable

Choosing enema supplies

When choosing supplies for an enema, you should consider the drug prescribed as well as your patient's age, size, and condition. Remember that physical size is always more important than age. For example, if your patient is a small 9-year-old, you'll want to use the smallest tube possible for their age-group.

Remember to use smaller tubing and a smaller volume of fluid when giving a retention enema, so you'll create less pressure in the patient's rectum and make it easier to retain the fluid.

Retention enema

Follow these general guidelines when selecting supplies for your patient's retention enema:
• *Adult*—#14 to #20 French rectal tube using 150 to 200 ml of fluid
• *Child older than age 6*—#12 to #14 French rectal tube using 75 to 150 ml of fluid.

Nonretention enema

Follow these general guidelines when selecting supplies for your patient's nonretention enema:
• *Adult*—#22 to #30 French rectal tube using 750 to 1,000 ml of fluid
• *Child older than age 6*—#14 to #18 French rectal tube using 300 to 500 ml of fluid
• *Child ages 2 to 6*—#12 to #14 French rectal tube using 250 to 350 ml of fluid
• *Child younger than age 2*—#12 French rectal tube using 150 to 250 ml of fluid.

enema kit. You may need an I.V. pole from which to hang the enema bag and a bath thermometer to test the temperature of the solution.

Getting ready

• Verify the order on the patient's chart.
• Confirm the patient's identity using at least two patient identifiers (not including the patient's room number).
• Explain the procedure to the patient.
• To minimize peristalsis, have the patient empty their bladder and rectum before you begin.

Explain the need to retain

• Explain to the patient, after you instill the enema solution, to retain it in the rectum for a prescribed length of time until the drug is absorbed.
• Have the patient wear a gown, and provide privacy.

How you do it

• Help the patient onto the left side in Sims' position. If the patient is uncomfortable in that position, reposition onto the right side or, if necessary, onto the back. Place a linen-saver pad under the patient *to protect the bedding.*

For disposable enemas

• Put on clean gloves, and remove the cap from the rectal tube.
• Check the amount of lubricant that's already on the tube. If needed, squeeze water-soluble lubricant onto a 4″ × 4″ gauze pad and dip the tip of the rectal tube into the lubricant.
• Gently squeeze the enema container to expel air.
• With your nondominant hand, lift the patient's upper buttock *to expose the anus*.

Waiting to inhale

• Tell the patient to take a deep breath. As the patient inhales, insert the rectal tube into the rectum, pointing the tube toward the umbilicus.
• If the patient is an adult, advance the tube about 4″ (10 cm). Pediatric patients require different guidelines. (See *Administering enemas to children*.)

Squeeze until empty

• Squeeze the solution container until it's empty. Then remove the rectal tube and discard the used enema container, the packaging it came in, and your gloves.

For enema bags

• Prepare the prescribed solution and warm it to 105° F (40.6° C). Test the temperature using a bath thermometer, or pour a small amount of solution over your wrist.
• Put on gloves, close the clamp on the enema tubing, and fill the enema bag with the solution.
• Hang the enema bag on an I.V. pole, and adjust the bag so it's slightly above bed level.

Tip of the day

• Remove the protective cap from the end of the enema tubing. The tip of the tubing should be prelubricated. If it isn't, lubricate it with a small amount of water-soluble lubricant.
• Unclamp the tubing, flush solution through it, then reclamp the tubing.
• With your nondominant hand, lift the patient's upper buttock. While holding the tube in your other hand, touch the patient's anal sphincter with the tip of the tube to stimulate contraction. Then insert the tube into the patient's anus.

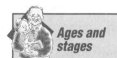

Ages and stages

Administering enemas to children

For a child age 11 or older, advance the rectal tube about 4″ (10 cm). For a child ages 4 to 10, advance the tube about 3″ (7.5 cm). For a child ages 2 to 4, advance the tube about 2″ (5 cm). For an infant, advance the tube about 1″ (2.5 cm).

Flow rate
Regulate the flow rate by lowering or raising the bag according to the patient's retention ability and level of comfort. Don't raise it higher than 12″ (30.5 cm) for a child or 6″ to 8″ (15 to 20 cm) for an infant.

• As the sphincter relaxes, tell the patient to breathe deeply through the mouth as you gently advance the tube.

Hold on

• Release the clamp on the tubing. Make sure you continue holding the tube in the patient's rectum because bowel contractions and pressure from the anal sphincter can expel the tube.
• Regulate the flow rate by lowering or raising the bag according to the patient's retention ability and level of comfort. Don't raise it higher than 18″ (45.7 cm) for an adult.

Blocked!

• If the flow stops, the tubing may be blocked with feces or wedged against the rectal wall. Gently turn the tubing *to free it without stimulating defecation.*
• If the tubing becomes clogged, withdraw it, flush it with solution, and then reinsert it.
• *To avoid inserting air into the patient's rectum,* clamp the tubing to stop the flow just before the enema bag empties.
• Remove the tubing, and dispose of the setup.

A matter of time

• Tell the patient to retain the solution for the prescribed time. If necessary, hold a 4″ × 4″ gauze pad against the anus until the patient's urge to defecate passes.
• If the patient is apprehensive, place him on a bedpan and have the patient hold toilet tissue or a rolled washcloth against the patient's anus.
• Dispose of your gloves, and place the call button within easy reach. Tell the patient to call for help to get out of bed, especially if the patient feels weak or faint.

Practice pointers

• Before giving a retention enema, check the patient's elimination pattern. A constipated patient may need a cleansing enema *to keep feces from interfering with drug absorption.* A patient with a fecal impaction may need to have the drug delivered by another route.
• Keep in mind that a patient with diarrhea may not be able to retain the enema solution for the prescribed time.
• Before administering a rectal medication, inspect the patient's anus for hemorrhoids, *which could make insertion more difficult and painful for the patient.*

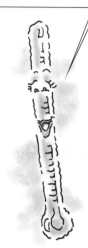

It's important to test the temperature of enema solution before instillation. 105° F is perfectly comfortable!

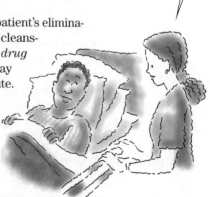

I've instilled the enema solution and removed the tubing. You should remain in bed for a while. I've placed the call bell within reach.

Administering vaginal drugs

Vaginal drugs are available in many forms, including:
- suppositories
- creams
- gels
- ointments
- solutions.

These medicated preparations can be inserted to treat infection (particularly *Trichomonas vaginalis* and candidiasis), treat inflammation, or prevent conception. Vaginal administration is most effective when the patient can remain lying down afterward to retain the drug.

Giving a vaginal drug

Most vaginal drugs come packaged in or with an applicator that you or the patient can use to insert the drug into the anterior and posterior fornices. When in contact with the vaginal mucosa, suppositories melt, diffusing the drug as effectively as creams, gels, and ointments.

What you need

Prescribed vaginal drug (with an applicator, if necessary) ✳ clean gloves ✳ water-soluble lubricant ✳ small sanitary pad ✳ absorbent towel ✳ linen-saver pad, small drape ✳ cotton balls ✳ 4″ × 4″ gauze pad ✳ paper towel ✳ soap and water (if necessary)

Getting ready

- Verify the order on the patient's chart.
- Always look up the drug in the drug guide if you have not given the drug before and are not familiar with the purpose, dosage, contraindications, possible side effects, and nursing considerations.
- Check the MAR and drug allergies.
- If possible, plan to give the drug at bedtime when the patient is recumbent.
- Confirm the patient's identity using at least two patient identifiers (not including the patient's room number).
- Explain the procedure to the patient, and provide privacy.
- Ask the patient to empty their bladder.

Self-administration is an option

- Ask the patient whether they would rather insert the medication herself. If so, provide appropriate instructions.

How you do it

- If the patient decides not to self-administer, help her into the lithotomy position.
- Place a linen-saver pad under her buttocks and a small drape over their legs. Expose only the perineum.
- Wash your hands and put on clean gloves.
- Squeeze a small portion of water-soluble lubricant onto a 4″ × 4″ gauze pad.

Package deal

- Unwrap the suppository, and coat it with the lubricant. If the drug is a small suppository in a prepackaged applicator, lubricate the tip of the suppository with water-soluble lubricant. If the drug is a foam or gel, fill the applicator as prescribed, and lubricate the tip of the applicator with the water-soluble lubricant.
- Separate the patient's labia.

Examination before administration

- Examine the patient's perineum. If you find that it's excoriated, withhold the drug and notify a doctor. The patient may need a different type of drug.
- If you see discharge, wash the area.
- To wash the area, soak several cotton balls in warm, soapy water.
- While holding the labia open with one hand, wipe once down the left side of the patient's perineum with a cotton ball.
- Discard the cotton ball, pick up another one, and use the new cotton ball to wipe once down the right side of the perineum.
- Discard the cotton ball, pick up another one, and use it to wipe once down the middle of the patient's perineum.

You'll need at least three cotton balls to clean your patient's perineum, so you'd better have a supply on hand.

Rounded tip first

- With the patient's labia still separated, insert the rounded tip of a suppository into her vagina, advancing it 3″ to 4″ (7.5 to 10 cm) along the posterior wall of the vagina or as far as it will go.
- If you're using an applicator, insert it into the patient's vagina. (See *How to administer a vaginal drug using an applicator*, page 228.)

Time to lie down

- Tell the patient to lie down for 5 to 10 minutes with her knees flexed *to help promote absorption and allow the medication to flow into the posterior fornix*. If you inserted a suppository, tell her to remain recumbent for at least 30 minutes *to allow time for it to melt*.

How to administer a vaginal drug using an applicator

If you're using an applicator to administer a vaginal drug to your patient, follow these steps:
• Use your dominant hand to insert the applicator about 2″ (5 cm) into the patient's vagina. Direct the applicator down initially, toward the patient's spine, and then back up toward the cervix, as shown.
• Press the plunger until you empty all of the medication from the applicator.
• Remove the applicator, and place it on a paper towel to prevent the spread of microorganisms.
• Discard the applicator, or wash it with soap and warm water before storing it, as appropriate.

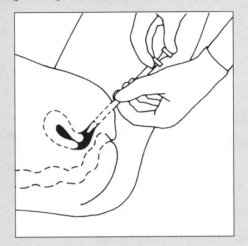

• Place a small sanitary pad in the patient's underwear *to keep her clothes or bedding from becoming soiled.*

Practice pointers

• Refrigerate vaginal gels, foams, and suppositories that melt at room temperature.

Administering respiratory medication

Several devices and procedures can be used to produce a fine, drug-carrying mist that a patient can inhale deep into his lungs.

Quick route to the capillaries

When the drug enters the lungs, it moves almost immediately into the lining of the patient's bronchi or alveoli and then into the adjacent capillaries. Drugs are administered in this way because the inhaled route is the most effective method to get the medicine where it's supposed to go—directly to the airways. In addition, the total dose is low and there's little chance for systemic effect.

A breath of fresh air

To deliver drugs to the respiratory tract, you'll typically use some type of handheld inhaler (sometimes with special attachments that are holding chambers called *spacers*) or a nebulizer.

Using a metered-dose inhaler

Many inhalant drugs, such as bronchodilators (which help to open the bronchial airways of the lungs) and corticosteroids (used as effective anti-inflammatory agents), are available in small canisters that are inserted into a metered-dose inhaler, also known as a *puffer*. A metered-dose inhaler is a device that can be used to trigger the release of measured doses of aerosol drug from a canister. The patient can then inhale the fine mist deep into his lungs.

What you need

Metered-dose inhaler device ✳ prescribed drug ✳ normal saline solution

Getting ready

- Verify the order on the patient's chart.
- Always look up the drug in the drug guide if you have not given the drug before and are not familiar with the purpose, dosage, contraindications, possible side effects, and nursing considerations.
- Check the MAR and drug allergies.
- Confirm the patient's identity using at least two patient identifiers (not including the patient's room number).
- Place the patient in a comfortable sitting position.

How you do it

- Shake the inhaler canister well.
- Remove the cap from the canister, turn the canister upside down, and insert the stem of the canister into the small hole in the flattened portion of the mouthpiece as shown.

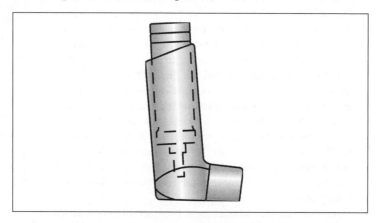

- Ask the patient to exhale, then hold the inhaler about 1″ (2.5 cm) in front of their open mouth (two to three fingerwidths from the mouth).

• Tell the patient to inhale slowly through the mouth and to continue inhaling until the lungs feel full.

Once is enough

• As the patient begins to inhale, compress the drug canister into the plastic housing of the inhaler to release a metered dose of the drug. Do this only once.

Whistle while you work

• Tell the patient to hold their breath for 10 seconds or as long as possible. Then instruct the patient to exhale slowly through pursed lips, as though whistling. Doing so produces back pressure, which helps to keep the bronchioles open, thus increasing absorption and diffusion of the drug.

Practice pointers

• If the patient can't coordinate well enough to inhale the drug as soon as you discharge it, you may need to put a spacer device on the inhaler.
• Some inhaled bronchodilators may cause restlessness, palpitations, nervousness, and hypersensitivity reactions, such as rash, urticaria, and bronchospasm.

Horse sense

• If the patient takes an inhaled corticosteroid, watch for evidence of hoarseness or fungal infection in the mouth or throat.
• To give inhaled drugs to pediatric patients, see *Giving inhaled drugs to pediatric patients*.
• Have the patient rinse their mouth and gargle with normal saline solution or water to remove the drug from the mouth and the back of the throat. This step helps to prevent oral fungal infections. Warn the patient not to swallow after gargling but rather to spit out the liquid.
• Instruct the patient to call the doctor if the patient's shortness of breath worsens, the drug becomes less effective, or the patient develops palpitations, nervousness, or hypersensitivity reactions such as a rash.
• If the patient takes a bronchodilator and a corticosteroid by inhaler, administer the bronchodilator 5 minutes before the corticosteroid. That way, the bronchial tubes will be as open as possible when the patient takes the corticosteroid.
• Have the patient wait at least 1 minute between doses of a single inhaled drug.

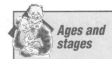

Ages and stages

Giving inhaled drugs to pediatric patients

When giving inhaled drugs to pediatric patients, remember these tips:
• If you need to give an inhaled drug to an infant or young child, have a parent or assistant hold the child to gain their cooperation.
• Give the drug through an aerosol nebulizer or spacer so the child doesn't have to hold their breath to retain the drug.
• For an older child, consider using a metered-dose inhaler, but only after you explain its use and you're satisfied that they understand the device and can use it properly. Don't use this type of inhaler if you doubt the patient's ability to get an appropriate dose into the lungs rather than into the mouth and throat.

Identification, please!

- If the patient takes an inhaled corticosteroid, urge the patient to carry medical identification announcing the possibility of needing supplemental corticosteroids during stress or a severe asthma attack.

Preparing an injection

The ability to inject drugs into a patient's skin, subcutaneous tissue, or muscle is a key nursing skill that you must exercise with great accuracy and care.

Quick and potent

These routes of administration promote a rapid onset of drug action and high drug levels in a patient's blood, in part, because they sidestep the breakdown that can take place in the GI tract and liver.

It calls for preparation

To prepare for an injection, you need to know how to correctly choose a needle and withdraw liquid drug from a vial or ampule. You may need to reconstitute the drug or combine drugs in a single syringe. Then you'll need to administer the injection to the appropriate site using proper techniques.

After administering the injection, don't recap the needle. Dispose of the syringe in the nearest sharps container.

Start at the very beginning

Typically, unless you're using one of the special needleless injection systems described later in this chapter, the first step in preparing for an injection is to choose the proper syringe and needle. Consider the route of administration, the size of the patient, and the most likely injection site when you select a syringe and needle. (See *Selecting syringes and needles*, pages 232 and 233.) Next, you'll need to withdraw the drug from its vial or ampule into a syringe—possibly together with another drug.

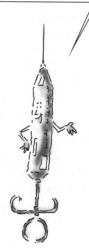

Being able to inject drugs into a patient's skin is a test of your nursing skill. It requires a great deal of accuracy and care—get my point?

Withdrawing a drug from a vial

Withdrawing a drug from a vial may require you to perform two steps:

 reconstitution

 withdrawal.

Selecting syringes and needles

Success at giving injections greatly improves with your ability to choose the proper syringe and needle for the task.

Syringes

Illustrated here are four types of commonly used syringes, shown without the protection devices to prevent needle-stick injuries.

Standard syringe

The standard syringe is available in 3-, 5-, 10-, 20-, 25-, 30-, 35-, and 50-ml sizes. It's used to administer numerous drugs in various settings. It consists of a plunger, barrel, hub, and needle. The dead space is the volume of fluid remaining in the syringe and needle when the plunger is depressed completely.

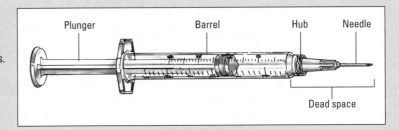

Plunger   Barrel   Hub   Needle

Dead space

Insulin syringe

The insulin syringe has an attached 25G needle and no dead space. It's divided into units rather than milliliters and should be used only for insulin administration.

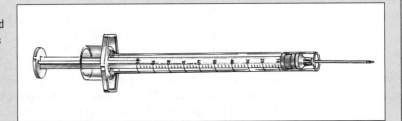

Tuberculin syringe

The tuberculin syringe holds up to 1 ml and is typically used for intradermal (I.D.) injections. It can also be used to give small doses, as may be required in pediatric and intensive care units.

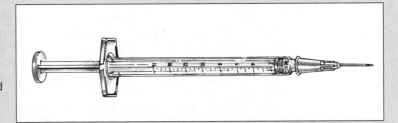

Unit-dose syringe

The unit-dose syringe is prefilled with a measured drug dose in a ready-to-dispense plastic cartridge. You only need to attach a needle.

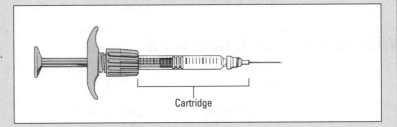

Cartridge

Selecting syringes and needles *(continued)*

Needles

You'll choose different types of needles based on whether you're giving an I.D., subcutaneous (subQ), or I.M. injection. Needles come in various lengths, diameters (or gauges), and bevel designs.

Intradermal needle

For an I.D. injection, select a needle that's ⅜" to ⅝" in length and 25G in diameter, with a short bevel.

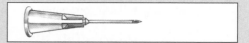

Subcutaneous needle

For a subQ injection, select a needle that's ⅝" to ⅞" in length and 23G to 25G in diameter, with a medium bevel.

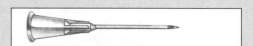

Intramuscular needle

For an I.M. injection, select a needle 1" to 3" in length and 18G to 23G in diameter, with a medium bevel.

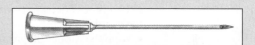

Shielded needle

To reduce the risk of needle-stick injury and the disease transmission that could result, a safety device built onto the syringe can be used to cover the needle when you're finished giving an injection, thus eliminating the temptation to recap a used needle.

After you've completed an injection, simply grasp the syringe flanges with one hand and push the shield forward with the other hand until it clicks, as shown below. The shield is now locked firmly in place over the needle.

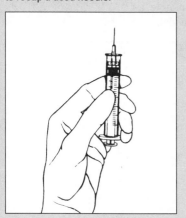 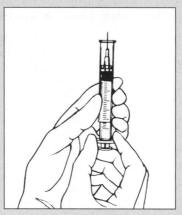 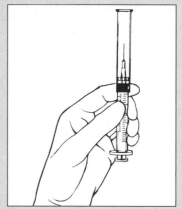

What you need

Medication vial ✻ vial or ampule of an appropriate diluent ✻ alcohol pads ✻ syringe ✻ two needles of appropriate size ✻ filter needle (if indicated, to screen particles that may be created during reconstitution)

Getting ready

- Verify the order on the patient's chart.
- Always look up the drug in the drug guide if you have not given the drug before and are not familiar with the purpose, dosage, contraindications, possible side effects, and nursing considerations.
- Check the MAR and drug allergies.
- Wash your hands.

How you do it

- Place the vial on a countertop.
- Wipe the rubber diaphragm on top of the vial with an alcohol pad.
- Avoid rubbing the diaphragm vigorously *because doing so can move bacteria from the nonsterile rim of the vial onto the diaphragm.*
- Wipe the rubber diaphragm on the top of the diluent vial with a fresh alcohol pad.

Give it some space

- Pick up the appropriate syringe, uncap the needle, and pull back on the plunger until the air-filled space inside the syringe equals the amount of diluent desired.
- While holding the base of the vial to keep it steady, puncture the rubber diaphragm of the diluent vial with the needle, as shown, and inject the air from the syringe into the vial.

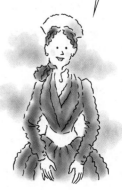

Knowing how to withdraw a drug from a vial is a fundamental procedure that every nurse must learn . . . it's as basic—and old a skill—as rolling bandages. Oh my, I'm dating myself, aren't I?

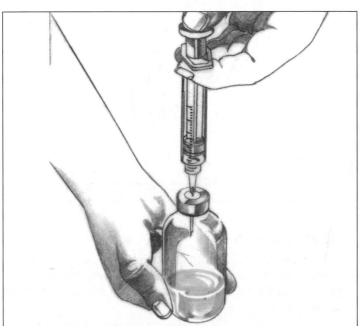

• Draw up the appropriate amount of diluent into the syringe.
• Turn to the drug vial. While holding the base to keep the vial steady, inject the diluent into it and withdraw the needle.

Gently roll

• Do not shake the vial, roll it between your hands to mix the drug and diluent thoroughly. *Shaking the vial traps air in the drug.*
• If the drug vial contains its own diluent compartment, remove the protective cap and use your finger to depress the rubber plunger. *This forces the lower stopper to fall to the bottom of the vial along with the diluent.* Gently roll the vial between your hands to mix the drug and diluent.
• If you need to draw the drug through a filter needle, remove the original needle from the syringe, attach the filter needle, and then uncap it. If you don't need a filter needle, simply leave the original needle on the syringe.

Be sure to replace the needle with a new one after withdrawing a drug from a vial. Puncturing the rubber stopper can dull the tip or get rubber particles in the syringe.

Pump up the volume

• Pull back on the plunger until the volume of air in the syringe equals the volume of drug to be given.
• Puncture the diaphragm of the drug vial, and inject the air.
• Invert the vial, as shown below, and withdraw the amount of drug to be given.

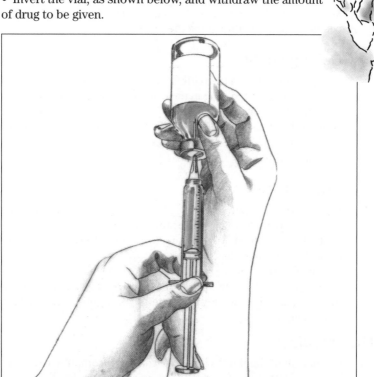

New needle needed

- Remove the needle from the syringe, and replace it with a new sterile needle. *You should do so because puncturing a rubber diaphragm can dull a needle and increase the pain of injection, and also because drug stuck to the outside of the used needle could irritate the patient's tissues.*
- Label the drug-filled syringe to finish preparing it for administration.

Practice pointers

- When inserting a needle through a rubber diaphragm, hold the needle bevel up and exert slight lateral pressure as the needle goes through the diaphragm. By using this technique, you'll avoid cutting a piece of rubber out of the stopper and pushing it into the drug in the vial.

Withdrawing a drug from an ampule

You may be required to withdraw a drug from an ampule.

What you need

Medication ampule ✳ dry 2″ × 2″ gauze pad ✳ syringe ✳ filter needle ✳ needle for injecting the drug

Getting ready

- Verify the order on the patient's chart.
- Always look up the drug in the drug guide if you have not given the drug before and are not familiar with the purpose, dosage, contraindications, possible side effects, and nursing considerations.
- Check the MAR and drug allergies.
- Wash your hands.

How you do it

- Check to make sure that all of the fluid is in the bottom of the ampule. If you see fluid in the stem or the top of the ampule, gently flick the stem *to knock the fluid out of the stem and into the bottom of the ampule.*
- If flicking the stem doesn't force all of the fluid to the bottom of the ampule, try holding the ampule by the stem, raising it to about eye level, and then quickly and carefully swinging it downward at arm's length.

Bottom of the ampule

- When all of the fluid is in the bottom of the ampule, wrap it in a dry 2″ × 2″ gauze pad *so the pad covers the ampule's stem.*

• Hold the body of the ampule with one hand and the top portion of the ampule between the thumb and first two fingers of your other hand.

It's a snap!

• While pointing the ampule away from you and others, snap off the top.
• With a filter needle on the syringe, aspirate the correct amount of drug from the open ampule. The filter needle strains out small pieces of glass that might have fallen into the drug.

New needle needed (again)

• Replace the filter needle with a fresh needle appropriate for injecting the drug. *Changing needles prevents drug on the outside of the filter needle from irritating the patient's tissues.*
• Label the drug-filled syringe *to finish preparing it for administration.*

Practice pointers

• An opened ampule doesn't contain a vacuum, so you don't have to inject air as you do with a vial.

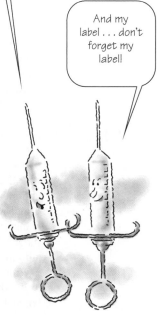

Don't forget to replace my needle.

And my label . . . don't forget my label!

Combining drugs in a syringe

Combining two drugs in one syringe or cartridge avoids the discomfort of two separate injections. Typically, you can combine drugs from:
• two multi-dose vials (as with regular and long-acting insulin, for example)
• one multi-dose vial and one ampule
• two ampules
• a multi-dose vial or an ampule into a partially filled cartridge injection system.

Bad combinations

Don't combine drugs in a syringe if the drugs are incompatible or if the combined doses exceed the amount of solution that can be absorbed from a single injection site.

What you need

Drug vials or ampule ✳ alcohol pads ✳ syringe ✳ one or more needles of appropriate size

Getting ready

- Verify the order on the patient's chart.
- Always look up the drug in the drug guide if you have not given the drug before and are not familiar with the purpose, dosage, contraindications, possible side effects, and nursing considerations.
- Check the MAR and drug allergies.
- Wash your hands.

How you do it

For two multi-dose vials

- Using an alcohol pad, wipe the rubber stopper on the first vial.
- Pull back the plunger of the syringe until the volume of air in the syringe equals the volume of drug to be withdrawn from the first drug vial.

Don't touch!

- Without inverting the first drug vial, insert the needle into the vial. Make sure the needle tip doesn't touch the liquid in the vial.
- Inject the air into the vial, and then withdraw the needle.

Moving to vial #2 . . .

- Using an alcohol pad, wipe the rubber stopper on the second drug vial.
- Pull back the plunger of the syringe until the volume of air in the syringe equals the volume of drug to be withdrawn from the second vial.
- Insert the needle into the second vial, inject the air, invert the vial, and withdraw the correct amount of drug.
- Wipe the rubber stopper of the first vial again, insert the needle, invert the vial, and withdraw the correct amount of drug.

Change needles if possible

- Ideally, to avoid contaminating the second drug drawn into the syringe, you should change the needle on the syringe. In reality, however, this isn't always possible because many disposable syringes don't have removable needles.
- If possible, replace the needle with a fresh needle before you administer the drug.

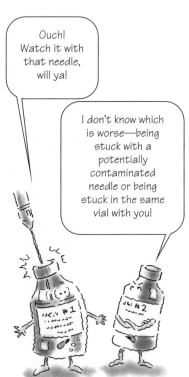

For a multi-dose vial and ampule

• Wipe the vial's rubber stopper with an alcohol pad, inject an amount of air equal to the drug dose to be given, invert the vial, and withdraw the correct dose.
• Place the sterile cover back on the needle, and place the syringe on the counter.

Bottoming out

• Make sure all of the drug is in the bottom of the ampule, wrap the ampule with a dry 2″ × 2″ gauze pad, and snap the neck of the ampule away from you.
• Replace the needle on your syringe with a filter needle, insert the needle into the ampule, and withdraw the correct drug dose into the syringe. Be careful not to touch the outside of the ampule with the needle.
• Change back to a regular needle to give the injection.

For two ampules

• Make sure all of the fluid is in the bottom of the first ampule, wrap the ampule with a dry 2″ × 2″ gauze pad, and snap the neck of the ampule away from you.
• Repeat this process for the second ampule.
• Use a filter needle to draw up the required amount of both drugs, one after the other.
• Change to a regular needle to give the injection.

For a cartridge-injection system

• If the cartridge has a removable needle with a rubber stopper, gently remove the capped needle from the cartridge *to expose the rubber stopper.*
• Wipe the rubber stopper with an alcohol pad, and insert the needle of an empty syringe into the partly filled cartridge. Don't let the needle touch the drug inside the cartridge.

And now for my next nursing feat, I'll change you back into a regular needle before giving the injection. Poof!

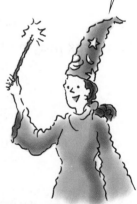

Equal volume

• Aspirate from the cartridge a volume of air equal to the volume of drug you'll be adding to the cartridge, and then withdraw the needle.
• Draw the correct amount of drug from a vial or an ampule into the syringe.

Rewipe

• Wipe the rubber stopper on the cartridge again, and insert the needle of the syringe into the cartridge.
• Inject the correct amount of compatible drug into the partly filled cartridge.
• Replace the needle on the cartridge using aseptic technique.

In addition . . .

- If the cartridge doesn't have a rubber stopper, you can add a compatible drug by holding the cartridge needle up, pulling back the plunger until it reaches a level equal to the combined drug volume, and then inserting the needle into an inverted, single-dose drug vial (after cleaning the diaphragm with an alcohol pad). Advance the needle until the tip is above the liquid in the vial. Inject into the vial an amount of air equal to the volume to be withdrawn from the vial, and then pull the needle into the liquid and withdraw the drug into the cartridge. Remove the needle from the vial, expel excess air, and replace the needle guard.

Always make sure you know the correct amount of air to inject or solution to draw up before taking the plunge with that needle.

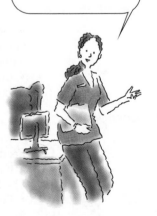

Irreconcilable differences

- After mixing drugs in a syringe or cartridge, check for signs of incompatibility, such as discoloration and precipitation.
- Label the drug-filled syringe to finish preparing it for administration.

Practice pointers

- Never combine drugs unless you're sure they're compatible, and never combine more than two drugs.
- Although drug incompatibility usually causes a visible reaction—such as clouding, bubbling, or precipitation—it may not. Always check a reputable drug reference or ask a pharmacist if you aren't sure about compatibility.

The clock may be ticking

- Some drugs should be given within 15 minutes after they're mixed; ask a pharmacist if you aren't sure about this timing.
- To reduce the risk of drug contamination, most facilities dispense parenteral drugs in single-dose vials. Insulin is the main exception. Check your facility's policy before you mix insulins.

Drug compatibility is a serious issue. Don't make assumptions or leave it to chance. Check with the pharmacist or a reputable drug reference if in doubt!

Administering intradermal drugs

In intradermal (I.D.) drug administration, you inject a small amount of liquid (usually 0.5 ml or less) into the outer layers of a patient's skin. A substance administered in this way undergoes little systemic absorption.

Identifying I.D.

You'll use the I.D. route to deliver substances that test for allergies and tuberculosis (TB). You also may use it to deliver a local anesthetic, such as lidocaine, before the patient undergoes a venipuncture procedure. Although the most common site for I.D. injection is the ventral forearm, other sites can be used. (See *Intradermal injection sites.*)

> One common use for intradermal injections is allergy testing. Now you may feel a bit itchy after this.

Giving an I.D. injection

You may be required to give an I.D. injection, such as:
- TB testing
- allergy testing
- certain vaccines
- local anesthetics.

What you need

Tuberculin syringe with a 26G or 27G ✳ ½″ or ⅝″ needle ✳ prescribed test antigen (or drug) ✳ clean gloves ✳ marking pen ✳ alcohol pads

Getting ready

- Verify the order on the patient's chart.
- Always look up the drug in the drug guide if you have not given the drug before and are not familiar with the purpose, dosage, contraindications, possible side effects, and nursing considerations.

Intradermal injection sites

The most common I.D. injection site is the ventral forearm. Other sites (indicated by dotted areas in these illustrations) include the upper chest, upper arm, and shoulder blades. Skin in these areas is usually lightly pigmented, thinly keratinized, and relatively hairless, facilitating detection of adverse reactions.

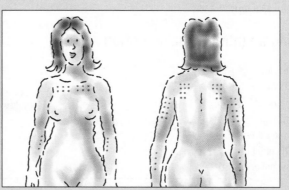

- Check the MAR and drug allergies.
- Check the drug's expiration date.
- Wash your hands.
- Confirm the patient's identity using at least two patient identifiers (not including the patient's room number).

Stand by please

- Explain the procedure to the patient, and tell the patient to stay nearby for about 30 minutes after the time of injection in case the patient has a severe allergic reaction to it.

How you do it

- Select an injection site.
- To use the ventral forearm, have the patient sit up and extend one arm. Make sure the arm is supported.
- Put on clean gloves. Then use an alcohol pad to clean the ventral forearm two or three fingerwidths distal to the antecubital space. Make sure the site is free of hair and blemishes. Let the skin air-dry.
- While holding the patient's forearm in your nondominant hand, stretch the skin taut. (See *Giving an intradermal injection.*)
- Withdraw the needle at the same angle you inserted it.

Missing wheals

- If no wheal or bleb forms, you've probably injected the antigen too deeply. Give another dose at least 2″ (5 cm) from the first site.
- If you're giving more than one I.D. injection, space them about 2″ apart.

Stay on the ball

Giving an intradermal injection

To give an I.D. injection, first secure the forearm. Then insert the needle bevel up at a 10- to 15-degree angle so that it just punctures the skin's surface, as shown. The antigen should raise a small wheal or bleb as it's injected.

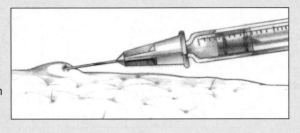

Keeping track

• Circle and label each test site with a marking pen so you can track the response to each substance given.
• Dispose of your gloves, needles, and syringes according to standard precautions.

Practice pointers

• Be prepared to deal with a possible anaphylactic reaction. (See *Don't get caught off guard*.)
• Notify a doctor immediately if an allergic reaction occurs.
• Don't rub the site after you give an I.D. injection. Doing so could irritate the underlying tissue and alter test results.
• Assess the patient's response to the skin testing in 24 to 48 hours.

Check the response

• When interpreting the patient's response, keep in mind that erythema without induration (a hard, raised area) isn't significant. If the test area is indurated, measure the diameter in millimeters.
• Induration of more than 5 mm after a tuberculin test may indicate a positive test result. After allergy tests, induration and erythema of more than 3 mm may indicate a positive result. The larger the affected area, the stronger the allergic reaction.

> ### Don't get caught off guard
>
> A patient who's hypersensitive to the test antigen may have an anaphylactic reaction. Be prepared to inject epinephrine immediately and perform emergency resuscitation procedures.

Administering subcutaneous drugs

In subcutaneous (subQ) administration, you inject a small amount of liquid drug (usually 0.5 to 2 ml) into the subcutaneous tissue beneath the patient's skin. From there, the drug is absorbed slowly into nearby capillaries.

Steady and safe

As a result, a dose of concentrated drug can have a longer duration of action than it would by other injection routes. Plus, subQ injection causes little tissue trauma and offers little risk of striking large blood vessels and nerves.

Subcutaneous contraindications

Typically, heparin and insulin are given by subQ injection. However, a subQ injection is contraindicated in areas that are inflamed, edematous, scarred, or covered by a mole, birthmark, or other lesion. It may also be contraindicated in patients with impaired coagulation.

Giving a subcutaneous injection

You may be required to give a drug subQ, such as:
- heparin
- insulin
- ovulation-stimulating drugs (or fertility drugs).

What you need

Prepared drug (with an appropriate syringe) ✳ needle of appropriate size (usually 25G to 27G and ⅝″ or ½″ long) ✳ clean gloves ✳ two alcohol pads

For insulin administration

Insulin infusion pump or subQ injector is optional. (See *Understanding insulin administration aids*.)

Understanding insulin administration aids

These days, patients have insulin delivery options beyond standard subQ injections, such as subQ infusion, an implanted catheter, or needle-free insulin delivery.

Subcutaneous infusion

In continuous subQ insulin infusion, the patient carries a portable infusion pump that holds insulin and is programmed to deliver precise insulin doses—both baseline and bolus—over a 24-hour period. (The device can be used for pain management as well.) Some insulin pumps allow you to track daily bolus doses, review the last 12 alarms, and download the device's long-term memory.

To deliver the infusion, the patient will need a 25G to 27G subQ needle inserted at a 30- to 45-degree angle into the abdomen, thigh, or arm. The insertion site should be rotated every 2 to 3 days according to standard precautions. After needle insertion, cover the site with a transparent adhesive dressing. Teach the patient how to recognize and when to report possible problems with the device insertion site.

Implanted catheter

Some patients may prefer an indwelling subQ catheter, such as an Insuflon catheter, rather than a needle. After insertion, the catheter remains in the fatty tissue of the abdomen. A small adhesive foam pad protects the insertion site and catheter and allows the patient to bathe, shower, and engage in sports or other activities. After 3 to 7 days, the catheter should be removed and inserted in the opposite side of the abdomen, 1″ to 2″ (2.5 to 5 cm) away from previously used sites.

Needle-free insulin delivery

Needle-free insulin delivery uses a device that looks something like a syringe without a needle. A spring inside the device triggers a plunger that expels a prescribed dose of insulin through a tiny hole at the tip. When the patient holds the device against the skin surface and discharges it, a thin column of insulin penetrates the skin and disperses within the subcutaneous tissue. This device is popular for home use, especially by patients (including children) who are afraid of needles.

Getting ready

- Verify the order on the patient's chart.
- Always look up the drug in the drug guide if you have not given the drug before and are not familiar with the purpose, dosage, contraindications, possible side effects, and nursing considerations.
- Check the MAR and drug allergies.
- Check the drug's color, clarity, and expiration date.
- Confirm the patient's identity using at least two patient identifiers (not including the patient's room number).
- Explain the procedure to the patient.
- Select an appropriate injection site. (See *SubQ injection sites.*)

Give your patient the cold shoulder

- Before giving the injection, you may apply a cold compress to the injection site to minimize pain.
- Wash your hands and put on clean gloves.

How you do it

- Position and drape the patient, if necessary.

Bubble trouble

- If you're giving insulin, gently invert and roll the vial *to mix the drug*. Don't shake the vial *because air bubbles could get into the syringe and reduce the dose given.*

SubQ injection sites

Potential subQ injection sites (as indicated by the dotted areas in these illustrations) include the fat pads on the abdomen, upper hips, upper back, and lateral upper arms and thighs.

Preferred injection sites for insulin are the arms, abdomen, thighs, and buttocks. The preferred injection site for heparin is the lower abdominal fat pad, just below the umbilicus.

When you repeat, rotate

For subQ injections administered repeatedly, such as insulin, rotate the injection sites. Choose one injection site in one area, move to a corresponding injection site in the next area, and so on. When returning to an area, choose a new site in that area.

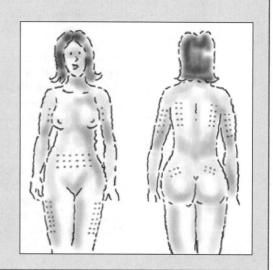

- Clean the injection site with an alcohol pad, starting at the center of the site and moving outward in a circular motion. Let the skin air-dry to avoid stinging.
- If you wish, open a second alcohol pad and place it between the index and middle fingers of your non-dominant hand.
- Remove the protective needle sheath.

Hold the fat

- With your nondominant hand, grasp the skin around the injection site and firmly elevate the subcutaneous tissue to form a 1″ (2.5 cm) fat fold (½″ [1.3 cm] for heparin). If the patient is large, you may be able to spread the skin taut rather than forming a fold. (See *Technique for subQ injections*.)
- Position the needle with the bevel up, and tell the patient that he'll feel a prick as you insert it quickly—in one motion—at a 45-degree angle.
- Pull back the plunger slightly to check for blood return unless you aren't administering heparin or insulin; if none returns, inject the drug slowly. (Check agency policy on aspirating medications).

Try not to be irritating

- After injection, remove the needle gently but quickly at the same angle used for injection. However, when injecting heparin or insulin, leave the needle in place for 5 seconds; then withdraw it.
- Cover the injection site with an alcohol pad, and DO NOT massage if you're administering heparin or insulin.
- Document the medication given.

Just checking

- Check the injection site for bleeding or bruising. If bleeding continues, apply pressure. If a bruise develops, apply ice. Watch for adverse reactions at the injection site for 30 minutes.
- Dispose of the equipment according to standard precautions. To avoid needle-stick injuries, don't recap the needle.

Practice pointers

- If your patient is of average weight, you can reach subcutaneous tissue by using a ½″ needle and inserting it at a 90-degree angle; if your patient is thin, use a ⅝″ needle and insert it at a 45-degree angle. If your patient is a child, you may also give certain drugs by the subQ route. (See *Giving a child a subQ or I.D. injection.*)

Do a double take

- If you're giving insulin, double-check that you have the correct type, unit dose, and syringe. Before mixing insulins in a syringe,

Technique for subQ injections

Before giving a subQ injection, elevate the subcutaneous tissue at the site by grasping it firmly, as shown. Insert the needle at a 45- or 90-degree angle to the skin surface, depending on needle length and the amount of subcutaneous tissue at the site. Some medications, such as heparin, should always be injected at a 90-degree angle.

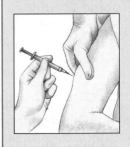

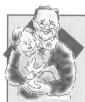

Ages and stages

Giving a child a subQ or I.D. injection

You may give certain drugs to children by the subQ or I.D. route. For example, insulin, hormone replacement, allergy desensitization, and some vaccines are given by subQ injection. Tuberculin testing, local anesthesia, and allergy testing are given by I.D. injection. The procedure for subQ or I.D. injection differs little from that used for an adult patient.

In a child, you can reach subcutaneous tissue by using a ⅝" needle and inserting it at a 45-degree angle.

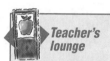

Teacher's lounge

Teaching about subQ injections

• If the patient will be giving their own subQ injections at home, teach them the correct way to perform the procedure. Send home written instructions to support your teaching.
• Inform the patient that different brands of syringes have differing amounts of space between the bottom line and the needle. Suggest that the doctor or pharmacist is notified if they change the brand of syringe used.

make sure they're compatible and that you have a doctor's order to do so. Follow your facility's policy about which insulin to draw up first. Don't mix insulins of different purities or origins.

Remember to rotate

• If you'll be giving repeated subQ injections, as with insulin, rotate the injection sites.
• Don't administer heparin injections within 2" (5.1 cm) of a scar, a bruise, or the umbilicus.
• Don't aspirate for blood when giving insulin or heparin because it's unnecessary to do so with insulin and may cause a hematoma with heparin.
• Don't massage the site if you've given insulin or heparin.
• Teach your patient the correct way to give a subQ injection if on insulin or requires other injections at home. (See *Teaching about subQ injections*.)
• Teach your patients, especially the older adults, how to use compliance aids. (See *Using compliance aids*, page 248.)

Administering intramuscular drugs

An I.M. injection deposits a drug deep into muscle tissue that's richly supplied with blood. As a result, the injected drug moves rapidly into the systemic circulation. Other advantages include:
• bypassing damaging digestive enzymes
• relatively little pain (because muscle tissue contains few sensory nerves)
• delivery of a relatively large volume of drug (the usual dose is 3 ml or less, but you may give up to 5 ml into a large muscle).

Teacher's lounge

Using compliance aids

To help your patient safely comply with injectable drug therapy, you or a family member or other caregiver can pre-measure doses for them using compliance aids, such as the ones shown here. Most pharmacies or community service agencies can supply similar aids.

Syringe-filling device

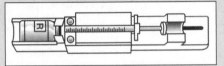

A syringe-filling device precisely measures insulin doses for a visually impaired person with diabetes. Designed for use with a disposable U-100 syringe and an insulin bottle, the device is set by the caregiver to accommodate the syringe's width. The patient then positions the plunger at the point determined by the dose and tightens the stop. When the device is set, they can draw up the precise dose ordered for each injection.

Drawbacks
The device has several drawbacks:
• It can't be used if insulin must be mixed or if doses vary.

• The settings must be checked and adjusted whenever the syringe size or type is changed.
• The screws must be checked regularly because they loosen with repeated use.

Syringe scale magnifier

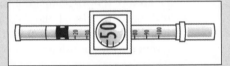

A syringe scale magnifier helps a visually impaired patient with diabetes read syringe markings, thereby enabling him to fill his own syringe. The plastic magnifier snaps onto the syringe barrel.

Drawbacks
This device may be impractical for a patient with arthritis who can't easily attach the magnifier to the syringe.

Be able to I.D. the candidate for I.M.

Children, elderly patients, or thin people may tolerate less than 2 ml. For some drugs, you may give I.M. injections using a Z-track technique or a needle-free injection system.

Giving an I.M. injection

You may be required to inject drugs intramuscularly, such as pain medications (opioids) or gold injections for arthritis.

Reflection before injection

Some situations will prevent I.M. administration of drugs. (See *Precautions for I.M. injections.*)

Precautions for I.M. injections

Before you give your patient an I.M. injection, remember these precautions:
• Don't give I.M. injections into inflamed, edematous, or irritated sites or sites with moles, birthmarks, scar tissue, or other lesions.
• I.M. injections may be contraindicated in patients who have impaired coagulation or conditions that hinder peripheral absorption, such as peripheral vascular disease, edema, and hypoperfusion, and during an acute myocardial infarction.
• Never give an I.M. injection into an immobile limb because the drug will absorb poorly and a sterile abscess could develop.

What you need

Prescribed drug, 3- to 5-ml syringe, 20G to 25G needle (lower gauge for a thicker drug) about 1″ to 3″ (2.5 to 7.5 cm) long depending on the site used and the amount of fat present ✳ clean gloves ✳ alcohol pads ✳ a small bandage

Sold separately

The needle may be packaged separately, or it may come attached to the syringe. Usually, you'll use a 1½″ to 2″ needle. Your technique and all equipment must be sterile.

Getting ready

• Verify the order on the patient's chart.
• Always look up the drug in the drug guide if you have not given the drug before and are not familiar with the purpose, dosage, contraindications, possible side effects, and nursing considerations.
• Check the MAR and drug allergies.
• Reconstitute the drug, if necessary; then check the drug's color, clarity, and expiration date.
• Draw the correct amount into the syringe.
• Confirm the patient's identity using at least two patient identifiers (not including the patient's room number).
• Explain the procedure to the patient.
• Wash your hands.

Muscling up

• If your patient is an adult, consider using the ventrogluteal, vastus lateralis, or deltoid muscle. (It is recommended to not use other sites due to the risk of complications with nerves and blood vessels that could be present.) (See *Locating I.M. injection sites*, page 250.)
• If your patient is an infant or a child, consider using the vastus lateralis muscle. (See *I.M. injection sites in infants and children*, page 251.)
• If your patient is elderly, additional points need to be considered. (See *I.M. injections in elderly patients*, page 252.)

Locating I.M. injection sites

The most common I.M. injection sites used in adults are discussed below.

Deltoid

Find the lower edge of the acromial process and the point on the lateral arm in line with the axilla. Insert the needle 1″ to 2″ (2.5 to 5 cm) below the acromial process, usually two or three fingerwidths, at a 90-degree angle or angled slightly toward the process. A typical injection is 0.5 ml with a range of 0.5 to 2 ml.

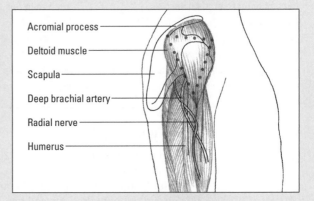

Acromial process

Deltoid muscle

Scapula

Deep brachial artery

Radial nerve

Humerus

Ventrogluteal

Locate the greater trochanter of the femur with the heel of your hand. Then spread your index and middle fingers from the anterior superior iliac spine to as far along the iliac crest as you can reach. Insert the needle between the two fingers at a 90-degree angle to the muscle. (Remove your fingers before inserting the needle.) A typical injection is 1 to 4 ml with a range of 1 to 5 ml.

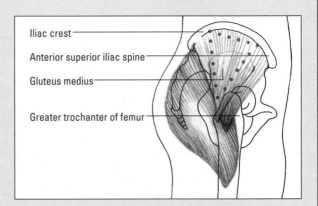

Iliac crest

Anterior superior iliac spine

Gluteus medius

Greater trochanter of femur

Vastus lateralis

Use the lateral muscle of the quadriceps group, from a handbreadth below the greater trochanter to a handbreadth above the knee. Insert the needle into the middle third of the muscle parallel to the surface on which the patient is lying. You may have to bunch the muscle before insertion. A typical injection is 1 to 4 ml with a range of 1 to 5 ml (1 to 3 ml for infants).

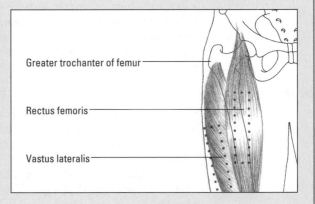

Greater trochanter of femur

Rectus femoris

Vastus lateralis

Ages and stages

I.M. injection sites in infants and children

When selecting the best site for a child's I.M. injection, consider the child's age, weight, and muscular development; the amount of subcutaneous fat over the injection site; the type of drug you're administering; and the drug's absorption rate.

Vastus lateralis and rectus femoris injections

For a child younger than age 3, you'll typically use the vastus lateralis or rectus femoris muscle for an I.M. injection. Constituting the largest muscle mass in this age-group, the vastus lateralis and rectus femoris have few major blood vessels and nerves.

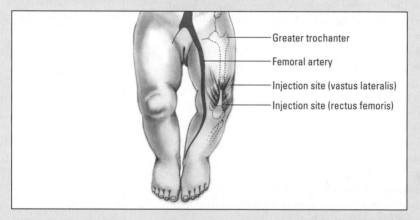

Greater trochanter

Femoral artery

Injection site (vastus lateralis)

Injection site (rectus femoris)

Ventrogluteal injections

For a child older than age 3 who has been walking for at least 1 year, you'll probably use the ventrogluteal muscle. These muscles are relatively free of major blood vessels and nerves.

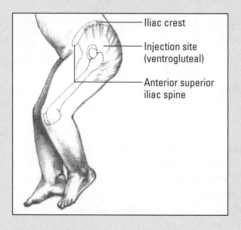

Iliac crest

Injection site (ventrogluteal)

Anterior superior iliac spine

How you do it

- Position and drape the patient so you have easy access to the chosen site. Locate the specific insertion site, and choose the proper needle angle.
- Check the injection site to make sure it has no lumps, depressions, redness, warmth, or bruising.
- Put on clean gloves.
- Clean the site with an alcohol pad, starting at the center of the site and spiraling outward about 2″ (5 cm). Let the skin air-dry.
- Remove the needle cover, and expel all air bubbles from the syringe.
- Urge the patient to relax the muscle that will receive the injection. A tense muscle increases pain and bleeding.
- With the thumb and index finger of your nondominant hand, gently stretch the skin taut at the injection site.
- Position the syringe at a 90-degree angle to the skin surface, with the needle a few inches away from the skin.
- Tell the patient that they will feel a prick, and then quickly thrust the needle into the muscle.

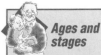

Ages and stages

I.M. injections in elderly patients

If your patient is elderly, consider using a shorter needle for I.M. injections. Also, because elderly people have less subcutaneous tissue and more fat around the hips, abdomen, and thighs, consider using the vastus lateralis or ventrogluteal area.

Seeing red? Stop!

- While supporting the syringe with your nondominant hand, use your dominant hand to aspirate for blood. (Check agency policy on this protocol.) If blood appears in the syringe, the needle is in a blood vessel. Withdraw it, discard it, and prepare another injection with a new syringe and fresh medication.
- If you aspirate no blood, then inject the drug slowly and steadily into the muscle, allowing it to distend and accept the drug gradually. You should feel little or no resistance.

Quickly yet gently

- After you've injected the drug, remove the needle quickly but gently, at a 90-degree angle.
- Using a gloved hand, immediately cover the injection site with an alcohol pad. Applying pressure is not recommended due to leakage and damage to the tissue.

If blood appears in the syringe, you've hit a blood vessel. Withdraw the needle, discard it, and try again with fresh medication.

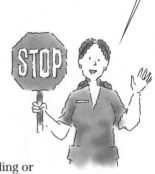

Inspection of injection

- Remove the alcohol pad, and inspect the site for bleeding or bruising. If bleeding continues, apply pressure. If a bruise develops, apply ice. Watch for adverse reactions at the site for 30 minutes after the time of injection.
- Discard all equipment according to standard precautions.
- Document the medication.

Practice pointers

• If your patient complains of pain and anxiety from repeated I.M. injections, numb the site with ice for several seconds before you give the injection.
• If you need to inject more than 5 ml of drug, split it between two different sites.

A pinch of gentleness

• If the patient is extremely thin, pinch the muscle gently to elevate it, so you won't push the needle completely through the muscle.
• For an infant or toddler, use a 25G to 27G, ½″ to 1″ needle. Also, don't exceed recommended volumes when giving the injection. (See *Adapting injections for children.*)
• If necessary, when giving an I.M. injection to a child younger than age 5, stand on the side opposite the vastus lateralis muscle and bend over them so your torso acts as a restraint.

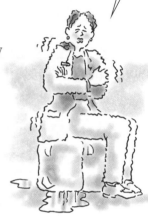

It may not be ideal, but it's one way to ice an injection site quickly.

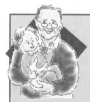

Ages and stages

Adapting injections for children

When giving an I.M. injection to a child, you'll need to adapt your approach to accommodate the child's age, the injection site, and the volume of drug you need to give. Use this table as a guide.

Deltoid	• Not recommended for children younger than age 3. • Can be used to give 0.5 ml or less in children ages 18 months to 3 years if no other site is available. • Give 0.5 ml or less in patients ages 3 to 15. • Give 1 ml or less in patients ages 16 to adult.
Gluteus maximus or ventrogluteal site	• Not recommended for children younger than age 3. • Can be used to give 1 ml or less in children ages 18 months to 3 years if no other site is available. • Give 1.5 ml or less in patients ages 4 to 6. • Give 2 ml or less in patients ages 7 to 15. • Give 2.5 ml or less in patients ages 16 to adult.
Vastus lateralis or rectus femoris	• Give 1 ml or less in children younger than age 3. • Give 1.5 ml or less in patients ages 3 to 6. • Give 2 ml or less in patients ages 7 to 15. • Give 2.5 ml or less in patients ages 16 to adult.

• Elderly patients have a higher risk of hematoma and may need direct pressure over the puncture site for a longer time than usual.

Remember to rotate

• Rotate sites if your patient needs repeated injections.
• Prevent complications associated with I.M. injections. (See *I.M. injection complications.*)

Giving a Z-track injection

If you need to give an irritating drug (such as iron dextran) or if you need to give an injection to an elderly patient with decreased muscle mass, use the Z-track method of I.M. administration. A Z-track injection is a method of displacing the tissues before you insert the needle for an I.M. injection. Afterward, restoring the tissues to their normal positions traps the drug inside the muscle.

What you need

Prescribed drug, syringe of appropriate size ✳ two needles (one of which should be 3″ [7.6 cm] long) ✳ alcohol pads clean gloves

Getting ready

• Verify the order on the patient's chart.
• Always look up the drug in the drug guide if you have not given the drug before and are not familiar with the purpose, dosage, contraindications, possible side effects, and nursing considerations.
• Check the MAR and drug allergies.
• Reconstitute the drug as needed. Check the drug's color, clarity, and expiration date.
• Draw the correct amount into the syringe.
• After drawing up the ordered dose, add 0.3 to 0.5 ml of air into the syringe. Then replace the original needle with a sterile one that's 3″ long.
• Confirm the patient's identity using at least two patient identifiers (not including the patient's room number).
• Explain the procedure to the patient.
• Wash your hands and put on gloves.

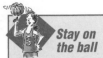

Stay on the ball

I.M. injection complications

Accidentally injecting concentrated or irritating medications into subcutaneous tissue or other areas where they can't be fully absorbed can cause sterile abscesses to develop.

In addition, failing to rotate sites in patients who require repeated injections can lead to deposits of unabsorbed medications. Such deposits can reduce the desired pharmacologic effect and may lead to abscess formation or tissue fibrosis.

You may give zee I.M. injection another way if necessaire, n'est pas?

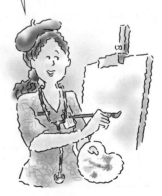

How you do it

- Select an injection site.
- Use an alcohol pad to clean the site, starting at the center and spiraling outward about 2″ (5 cm). Let the skin air-dry.

Here's the skinny

- Place the index finger of your nondominant hand on the injection site, and drag the skin about ½″ (1.3 cm) to one side.
- Insert the needle at a 90-degree angle into the site on which you originally placed your finger.
- Inject the drug, and withdraw the needle.
- Then release the skin, allowing the displaced layers to return to their original positions. (See *Displacing the skin for Z-track injection*.)

Practice pointers

- Never inject more than 5 ml into a single site using the Z-track method.

Displacing the skin for Z-track injection

Discomfort and tissue irritation may result from drug leakage into subcutaneous tissue. Displacing the skin helps prevent these problems.

By blocking the needle pathway after an injection, the Z-track technique allows I.M. injection while minimizing the risk of subcutaneous irritation and staining from such drugs as iron dextran.

How to do it

To begin, place your finger on the skin surface, and pull the skin and subcutaneous layers out of alignment with the underlying muscle, as shown below. You should move the skin about ½″ (1.5 cm).

Insert the needle at a 90-degree angle at the site where you initially placed your finger, as shown below. Inject the drug, and withdraw the needle.

Lastly, remove your finger from the skin surface, allowing the layers to return to their normal positions. The needle track (shown by the dotted line below) is now broken at the junction of each tissue layer, trapping the drug in the muscle.

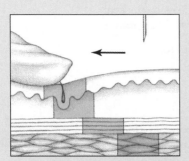 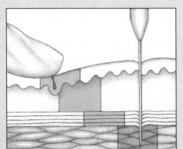 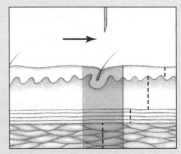

Here's a new message: Don't massage!

- Never massage a Z-track injection site because you could cause irritation or force the drug into subcutaneous tissue.
- To increase the rate of absorption, encourage such physical activity as walking.
- For subsequent injections, alternate sites.

> Walking is a good way to increase the rate of absorption after receiving a Z-track injection.

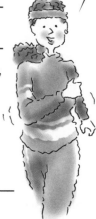

References

Berman, A., & Snyder, S. J. (2012). *Skills in clinical nursing* (7th ed.). Upper Saddle River, NJ: Pearson Education.

Berman, A., Snyder, S. J., & McKinney, D. S. (2011). *Nursing basics for clinical practice.* Upper Saddle River, NJ: Pearson Education.

Treas, L. S., & Wilkinson, J. M. (2014). *Basic nursing concepts, skills & reasoning.* Philadelphia, PA: F. A. Davis.

Quick quiz

1. When administering tablets or capsules by the oral route, you would:

A. assess the patient's ability to swallow before administering the drug.

B. give a drug that had been poured by someone else to save time.

C. return any unused opened or unwrapped drug to the patient's medication drawer to avoid unnecessary waste.

D. give a drug from a poorly labeled or an unlabeled bottle.

Answer: A. Before administering tablets or capsules by the oral route, assess the patient's ability to swallow to prevent aspiration.

2. When instilling eyedrops, instruct your patient to:

A. look down and away.

B. look up and away.

C. look straight ahead.

D. look up and directly at the dropper.

Answer: B. When instilling eyedrops, ask your patient to look up and away. Doing so moves the cornea away from the lower lid and minimizes the risk of touching the cornea with the dropper.

3. When choosing supplies for a nonretention enema, what size rectal tube would you select for a child younger than age 2?
   A.   #12 French
   B.   #14 French
   C.   #18 French
   D.   #26 French

Answer: A. For a child younger than age 2, select a #12 French rectal tube.

4. Which route of administration would you use if you wanted to inject a small amount of liquid drug (usually 0.5 ml or less) into the outer layers of a patient's skin?
   A.   I.D.
   B.   SubQ
   C.   I.M.
   D.   I.V.

Answer: A. An I.D. injection allows injection of a small amount of liquid drug (usually 0.5 ml or less) into the outer layers of a patient's skin.

5. Which statement *best* describes a Z-track injection?
   A.   It's a method of depositing a drug deep into muscle tissue that's richly supplied with blood.
   B.   It's a method of injecting a small amount of liquid drug (usually 0.5 to 2 ml) into the subcutaneous tissue beneath the patient's skin.
   C.   It's a method of displacing the tissues before you insert the needle for an I.M. injection.
   D.   It's a method of aligning the tissues before you insert the needle for a subcutaneous injection.

Answer: C. A Z-track injection is a method of displacing the tissues before you insert the needle for an I.M. injection. Afterward, restoring the tissues to their normal positions traps the drug inside the muscle.

Scoring

☆☆☆   If you answered all five questions correctly, sensational! Needleless to say, you're in the top of your class!

☆☆   If you answered three or four questions correctly, great! You absorbed the material well.

☆   If you answered fewer than three questions correctly, it looks like you might need a shot in the arm. Review the chapter, and you'll soon feel sharp!

I.V. therapy

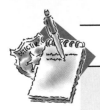

Just the facts

In this chapter, you'll learn:

♦ uses of I.V. therapy

♦ I.V. delivery methods

♦ I.V. infusion rates

♦ legal and professional standards governing the use of I.V. therapy

♦ patient teaching regarding I.V. therapy

♦ proper procedures for documenting I.V. therapy.

A look at I.V. therapy

One of your most important nursing responsibilities is to administer fluids, medications, and blood products to patients. In I.V. therapy, liquid solutions are introduced directly into the bloodstream.

I.V. therapy is used to:
- restore and maintain fluid and electrolyte balance
- provide medications and chemotherapeutic agents
- transfuse blood and blood products
- deliver parenteral nutrients and nutritional supplements.

Benefits of I.V. therapy

I.V. therapy has great benefits. For example, it can be used to administer fluids, drugs, nutrients, and other solutions when a patient can't take oral substances.

On target and fast

I.V. drug delivery also allows more accurate dosing. Because the entire amount of a drug given I.V. reaches the bloodstream immediately, the drug begins to act almost instantaneously.

Risks of I.V. therapy

Like other invasive procedures, I.V. therapy has its downside. Risks include:
- bleeding
- blood vessel damage
- infiltration (infusion of the I.V. solution into surrounding tissue rather than the blood vessel)
- infection
- overdose (because response to I.V. drugs is more rapid)
- incompatibility when drugs and I.V. solutions are mixed
- adverse or allergic responses to infused substances.

Strings attached

Patient activity can also be problematic. Simple tasks, such as transferring to a chair, ambulating, and washing oneself, can become complicated when the patient must cope with I.V. poles, I.V. lines, and dressings.

No such thing as a free lunch

Finally, I.V. therapy is more costly than oral, subcutaneous, or I.M. methods of delivering medications.

Fluids, electrolytes, and I.V. therapy

One of the primary objectives of I.V. therapy is to restore and maintain fluid and electrolyte balance. To understand how I.V. therapy works to restore fluid and electrolyte balance, let's first review some basics of fluids and electrolytes.

We're all wet (well mostly)

The human body is composed largely of liquid. These fluids account for about 60% of total body weight in an adult who weighs 155 lb (70.3 kg) and about 80% of total body weight in an infant.

Of solvents and solutes

Body fluids are composed of water (a solvent) and dissolved substances (solutes). The solutes in body fluids include electrolytes (such as sodium) and nonelectrolytes (such as proteins).

Fluid functions

What functions do body fluids provide? They:
- help regulate body temperature
- help transport nutrients throughout the body
- carry cellular waste products to excretion sites.

Aim for the optimum

When fluid levels are optimal, the body performs swimmingly; however, when fluid levels deviate from the acceptable range, organs and systems can quickly become congested.

Inside and outside

Body fluids exist in two major compartments: inside the cells and outside the cells. Normally, the distribution of fluids between the two compartments is constant. Fluid is classified by whether it's inside or outside:
• intracellular fluid (ICF)—the fluid inside the cells, which is about 55% of the total body fluid
• extracellular fluid (ECF)—accounts for the rest of the body fluid.

The ABCs of ECF

ECF occurs in two forms: interstitial fluid (ISF) and intravascular fluid. ISF surrounds each cell of the body; even bone cells are bathed in it. Intravascular fluid is blood plasma, the liquid component of blood. It surrounds red blood cells and accounts for most of the blood volume.

In an adult, about 5% of body fluid is intravascular ECF; about 15% is interstitial ECF. Part of that interstitial ECF is transcellular fluid, which includes cerebrospinal fluid and lymph. Transcellular fluid contains secretions from the salivary glands, pancreas, liver, and sweat glands.

It's a balancing act

Maintaining fluid balance in the body involves the kidneys, heart, liver, adrenal and pituitary glands, and nervous system. This balancing act is affected by:
• fluid volume
• distribution of fluids in the body
• concentration of solutes in the fluid.

You gain some, you lose some

Every day, the body gains and loses fluid. To maintain fluid balance, the gains must equal the losses. (See *Daily fluid gains and losses.*)

Hormones at work

Fluid volume and concentration are regulated by the interaction of two hormones: antidiuretic hormone (ADH) and aldosterone. ADH, sometimes referred to as the *water-conserving hormone*, affects fluid volume and concentration by regulating water retention. It's secreted

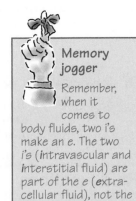

Memory jogger

Remember, when it comes to body fluids, two i's make an e. The two i's (intravascular and interstitial fluid) are part of the e (extracellular fluid), not the i (intracellular fluid).

Daily fluid gains and losses

Each day the body gains and loses fluid through several different processes. This illustration shows the main sites involved. The amounts shown apply to adults; infants exchange a greater amount of fluid than adults.

Note: Gastric, intestinal, pancreatic, and biliary secretions total about 8,200 ml. However, because they're almost completely reabsorbed, they aren't usually counted in daily fluid gains and losses.

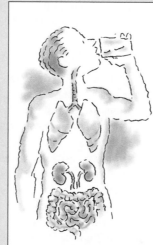

**Daily total intake —
2,400 to 3,200 ml**
- Liquids — 1,400 to 1,800 ml
- Water in foods (solid) — 700 to 1,000 ml
- Water of oxidation (combined water and oxygen in the respiratory system) —300 to 400 ml

**Daily total output —
2,400 to 3,200 ml**
- Lungs (respiration) — 600 to 800 ml
- Skin (perspiration) — 300 to 500 ml
- Kidneys (urine) — 1,400 to 1,800 ml
- Intestines (feces) — 100 ml

when plasma osmolarity increases or circulating blood volume decreases and blood pressure drops. Aldosterone acts to retain sodium and water. It's secreted when the serum sodium level is low, the potassium level is high, or the circulating volume of fluid decreases.

Water, I need water!!

The thirst mechanism (awareness of the desire to drink) also regulates water volume and participates with hormones in maintaining fluid balance. Thirst is experienced when water loss equals 2% of body weight or when osmolarity (solute concentration) increases. Drinking water restores plasma volume and dilutes ECF osmolarity.

Picking out the baseline

Nurses must anticipate changes in fluid balance that may take place during I.V. therapy. Therefore, it's important to establish the patient's baseline fluid status before starting fluid replacement therapy. During I.V. therapy, changes in fluid status alert the nurse to impending fluid imbalances. (See *Identifying fluid imbalances*, page 262.)

Identifying fluid imbalances

By carefully assessing a patient before and during I.V. therapy, you can identify fluid imbalances early—before serious complications develop. The following assessment findings and test results indicate fluid deficit or excess.

Fluid deficit
- Weight loss
- Increased, thready pulse rate
- Diminished blood pressure, commonly with orthostatic hypotension
- Decreased central venous pressure
- Sunken eyes, dry conjunctivae, decreased tearing
- Poor skin turgor (not a reliable sign in elderly patients)
- Pale, cool skin
- Poor capillary refill (more than 2 seconds)
- Lack of moisture in groin and axillae
- Thirst
- Decreased salivation
- Dry mouth
- Dry, cracked lips
- Furrows in tongue
- Difficulty forming words (patient needs to moisten mouth first)
- Mental status changes
- Weakness
- Diminished urine output
- Increased hematocrit
- Increased serum electrolyte levels
- Increased blood urea nitrogen (BUN) levels
- Increased serum osmolarity

Fluid excess
- Weight gain
- Elevated blood pressure
- Bounding pulse that isn't easily obliterated
- Jugular vein distention
- Increased respiratory rate
- Dyspnea
- Moist crackles or rhonchi on auscultation
- Edema of dependent body parts; sacral edema in patients on bed rest; edema of feet and ankles in ambulatory patients
- Generalized edema
- Puffy eyelids
- Periorbital edema
- Slow emptying of hand veins when the arm is raised
- Decreased hematocrit
- Decreased serum electrolyte levels
- Decreased BUN levels
- Reduced serum osmolarity

Electrolytes

Electrolytes are a major component of body fluid. There are six major electrolytes:

 sodium

potassium

 calcium

 chloride

 phosphorus

 magnesium.

You'll get a charge outta this

As the name implies, electrolytes are associated with electricity. These vital substances are chemical compounds that dissociate in solution into electrically charged particles called *ions*. Like wiring for the body, the electrical charges of ions conduct current that's necessary for normal cell function. (See *Understanding electrolytes*.)

Fluid and electrolyte balance

Fluids and electrolytes are usually discussed in tandem, especially where I.V. therapy is concerned, because fluid balance and electrolyte balance are interdependent. Any change in one alters the other, and any solution given I.V. can affect a patient's fluid and electrolyte balance.

Understanding electrolytes

Six major electrolytes play important roles in maintaining chemical balance: sodium, potassium, calcium, chloride, phosphorus, and magnesium. Electrolyte concentrations are expressed in milliequivalents per liter (mEq/L) and milligrams per deciliter (mg/dl).

Electrolyte	Principal functions	Signs and symptoms of imbalance
Calcium (Ca^{++}) • Major cation found in ECF of teeth and bones • Normal serum level: 8.9 to 10.1 mg/dl	• Enhances bone strength and durability (along with P) • Helps maintain cell membrane structure, function, and permeability • Affects activation, excitation, and contraction of cardiac and skeletal muscles • Participates in neurotransmitter release at synapses • Helps activate specific steps in blood coagulation • Activates serum complement in immune system function	*Hypocalcemia:* muscle tremor; muscle cramps; tetany; tonic-clonic seizures; paresthesia; bleeding; arrhythmias; hypotension; numbness or tingling in fingers, toes, and area surrounding the mouth *Hypercalcemia:* lethargy, headache, muscle flaccidity, nausea, vomiting, anorexia, constipation, hypertension, polyuria
Chloride (Cl$^-$) • Major anion found in ECF • Normal serum level: 96 to 106 mEq/L	• Maintains serum osmolarity (along with Na$^-$) • Combines with major cations to create important compounds, such as sodium chloride (NaCl), hydrogen chloride (HCl), potassium chloride (KCl), and calcium chloride (CaCl$_2$)	*Hypochloremia:* increased muscle excitability, tetany, decreased respirations *Hyperchloremia:* stupor; rapid, deep breathing; muscle weakness

(continued)

Understanding electrolytes *(continued)*

Electrolyte	Principal functions	Signs and symptoms of imbalance
Magnesium (Mg^{++}) • Major cation found in ICF (closely related to Ca^{++} and P) • Normal serum level: 1.5 to 2.5 mg/dl with 33% bound protein and remainder as free cations	• Activates intracellular enzymes; active in carbohydrate and protein metabolism • Acts on myoneural vasodilation • Facilitates Na$^-$ and K$^+$ movement across all membranes • Influences Ca^{++} levels	*Hypomagnesemia:* dizziness, confusion, seizures, tremor, leg and foot cramps, hyper-irritability, arrhythmias, vasomotor changes, anorexia, nausea *Hypermagnesemia:* drowsiness; lethargy; coma; arrhythmias; hypotension; vague neuro-muscular changes (such as tremor); vague GI symptoms (such as nausea); peripheral vasodilation; facial flushing; sense of warmth; slow, weak pulse
Phosphorus (P) • Major anion found in ICF • Normal serum phosphate level: 2.5 to 4.5 mg/dl	• Helps maintain bones and teeth • Helps maintain cell integrity • Plays a major role in acid–base balance (as a urinary buffer) • Promotes energy transfer to cells • Plays an essential role in muscle, red blood cell, and neurologic function	*Hypophosphatemia:* paresthesia (circumoral and peripheral), lethargy, speech defects (such as stuttering or stammering), muscle pain and tenderness *Hyperphosphatemia:* renal failure, vague neuroexcitability to tetany and seizures, arrhythmias and muscle twitching with sudden rise in phosphate level
Potassium (K$^+$) • Major cation in ICF • Normal serum level: 3.5 to 5.0 mEq/L	• Maintains cell electroneutrality • Maintains cell osmolarity • Assists in conduction of nerve impulses • Directly affects cardiac muscle contraction • Plays a major role in acid–base balance	*Hypokalemia:* decreased GI, skeletal muscle, and cardiac muscle function; decreased reflexes; rapid, weak, irregular pulse; muscle weakness or irritability; fatigue; decreased blood pressure; decreased bowel motility; paralytic ileus *Hyperkalemia:* muscle weakness; nausea; diarrhea; oliguria; paresthesia (altered sensation) of the face, tongue, hands, and feet
Sodium (Na$^+$) • Major cation in ECF • Normal serum level: 135 to 145 mEq/L	• Maintains appropriate ECF osmolarity • Influences water distribution (with Cl$^-$) • Affects concentration, excretion, and absorption of potassium and chloride • Helps regulate acid–base balance • Aids nerve- and muscle-fiber impulse transmission	*Hyponatremia:* muscle weakness, muscle twitching, decreased skin turgor, headache, tremor, seizures, coma *Hypernatremia:* thirst; fever; flushed skin; oliguria; disorientation; dry, sticky membranes

Electrolyte balance

Not all electrolytes are distributed evenly. The major intracellular electrolytes are:
- potassium
- phosphorus.
    The major extracellular electrolytes are:
- sodium
- chloride.
    ICF and ECF contain different electrolytes because the cell membranes separating the two compartments have selective permeability—that is, only certain ions can cross those membranes. Although ICF and ECF contain different solutes, the concentration levels of the two fluids are about equal when balance is maintained.

Extra (cellular) credit

The two ECF components—ISF and intravascular fluid (plasma)—have identical electrolyte compositions. Pores in the capillary walls allow electrolytes to move freely between the ISF and plasma, allowing for equal distribution of electrolytes in both substances.

The protein content of ISF and plasma differs, however. ISF doesn't contain proteins because protein molecules are too large to pass through capillary walls. Plasma has a high concentration of proteins.

Fluid movement

Fluid movement is another mechanism that regulates fluid and electrolyte balance.

Ebb and flow

Body fluids are in constant motion. Although separated by membranes, they continually move between the major fluid compartments. In addition to regulating fluid and electrolyte balance, this movement is how nutrients, waste products, and other substances get into and out of cells, organs, and systems.

Fluid movement is influenced by membrane permeability and colloid osmotic and hydrostatic pressures. Balance is maintained when solute and fluid molecules are distributed evenly on each side of the membrane. When this scale is tipped, these molecules are able to restore balance by crossing membranes as needed.

Solute and fluid molecules have several modes for moving through membranes. Solutes move between compartments mainly by:
- diffusion (passive transport)
- active transport.
    Fluids (such as water) move between compartments by:
- osmosis
- capillary filtration and reabsorption.

Passive is popular

Most solutes move by diffusion—that is, their molecules move from areas of higher concentration to areas of lower concentration. This change is referred to as "moving down the concentration gradient." The result is an equal distribution of solute molecules. Because diffusion doesn't require energy, it's considered a form of passive transport.

> Water moves by osmosis—flowing passively across a membrane from an area of higher concentration to one of lower concentration.

Moving against the gradient

By contrast, in active transport, molecules move from areas of lower concentration to areas of higher concentration. This change, referred to as "moving against the concentration gradient," requires energy in the form of adenosine triphosphate.

In active transport, molecules are moved by physiologic pumps. You're probably familiar with one active transport pump—the sodium-potassium pump. It moves sodium ions out of cells to the ECF and potassium ions into cells from the ECF. This pump balances sodium and potassium concentrations.

Oh, osmosis

Fluids (particularly water) move by osmosis. Movement of water is caused by the existence of a concentration gradient. Water flows passively across the membrane from an area of higher water concentration to an area of lower water concentration. This dilution process stops when the solute concentrations on both sides of the membrane are equal.

Osmosis between the ECF and the ICF depends on the osmolarity (concentration) of the compartments. Normally, the osmotic (pulling) pressures of ECF and ICF are equal.

Equal, yet imbalanced

Osmosis can create a fluid imbalance between the ECF and ICF compartments, despite equal concentrations of solute, if the concentrations aren't optimal. This imbalance can cause complications such as tissue edema.

Up against the capillary wall

Of all the vessels in the vascular system, only capillaries have walls thin enough to let solutes pass. Water and solutes move across capillary walls by two opposing processes:

 capillary filtration

 capillary reabsorption.

From high to low

Filtration is the movement of substances from an area of high hydrostatic pressure to an area of lower hydrostatic pressure. (Hydrostatic pressure is the pressure at any level on water at rest due to the weight of water above it.) Capillary filtration forces fluid and solutes through capillary wall pores and into the ISF.

Left unchecked, capillary filtration would cause plasma to move in only one direction—out of the capillaries. This movement would cause severe hypovolemia and shock.

Reabsorption to the rescue

Fortunately, capillary reabsorption keeps capillary filtration in check. During filtration, albumin (a protein that can't pass through capillary walls) remains behind in the diminishing volume of water. As the albumin concentration inside the capillaries increases, the albumin begins to draw water back in by osmosis. Water is thus reabsorbed by capillaries.

May the force be with you

The osmotic, or pulling, force of albumin in capillary reabsorption is called *colloid osmotic pressure* or *oncotic pressure*. As long as capillary blood pressure exceeds colloid osmotic pressure, water and diffusible solutes can leave the capillaries and circulate into the ISF. When capillary blood pressure falls below colloid osmotic pressure, water and diffusible solutes return to the capillaries.

Pressure points

In any capillary, blood pressure normally exceeds colloid osmotic pressure up to the vessel's midpoint, and then falls below colloid osmotic pressure along the rest of the vessel. That's why capillary filtration takes place along the first half of a capillary and reabsorption occurs along the second half. As long as capillary blood pressure and plasma albumin levels remain normal, no net movement of water occurs. Water is equally lost and gained in this process.

Correcting imbalances

The effect an I.V. solution has on fluid compartments depends on the solution's osmolarity compared with serum osmolarity.

Osmolarity at parity?

Osmolarity is the concentration of a solution. It's expressed in milliosmoles of solute per liter of solution (mOsm/L). Normally, serum has the same osmolarity as other body fluids, about 300 mOsm/L. A lower serum osmolarity suggests fluid overload; a higher serum osmolarity suggests hemoconcentration and dehydration.

Bring back the balance

The doctor may order I.V. solutions to maintain or restore fluid balance. (See *Understanding I.V. solutions*.) There are three basic types of I.V. solutions:

 isotonic

 hypotonic

 hypertonic. (See *Quick guide to I.V. solutions*.)

Isotonic solutions

An isotonic solution has the same osmolarity (or tonicity) as serum and other body fluids. Because the solution doesn't alter serum osmolarity, it stays where it's infused—inside the blood vessel (the intravascular compartment). The solution expands this compartment without pulling fluid from other compartments.

Understanding I.V. solutions

Solutions used for I.V. therapy may be isotonic, hypotonic, or hypertonic. The type you give a patient depends on whether you want to change or maintain his body fluid status.

Isotonic solution

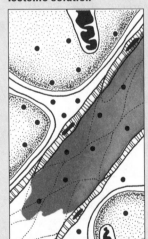

An isotonic solution has an osmolarity about equal to that of serum. Because it stays in the intravascular space, it expands the intravascular compartment.

Hypotonic solution

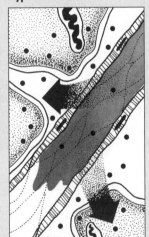

A hypotonic solution has an osmolarity lower than that of serum. It shifts fluid out of the intravascular compartment, hydrating the cells and the interstitial compartments.

Hypertonic solution

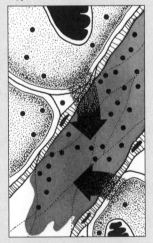

A hypertonic solution has an osmolarity higher than that of serum. It draws fluid into the intravascular compartment from the cells and the interstitial compartments.

Quick guide to I.V. solutions

A few common solutions can be used to illustrate the role of I.V. therapy in restoring and maintaining fluid and electrolyte balance. A solution is isotonic if its osmolarity falls within (or near) the normal range for serum (240 to 340 mOsm/L). A hypotonic solution has a lower osmolarity; a hypertonic solution, a higher osmolarity. This chart lists common examples of the three types of I.V. solutions and provides key considerations for administering them.

Solution	Examples	Nursing considerations
Isotonic	• Lactated Ringer's (275 mOsm/L) • Ringer's (275 mOsm/L) • Normal saline (308 mOsm/L) • Dextrose 5% in water (D$_5$W) (260 mOsm/L) • 5% albumin (308 mOsm/L) • Hetastarch (310 mOsm/L) • Normosol (295 mOsm/L)	• Because isotonic solutions expand the intravascular compartment, closely monitor the patient for signs of fluid overload, especially if he has hypertension or heart failure. • Because the liver converts lactate to bicarbonate, don't give lactated Ringer's solution if the patient's blood pH exceeds 7.5. • Avoid giving D$_5$W to a patient at risk for increased intracranial pressure (ICP) because it acts like a hypotonic solution. (Although usually considered isotonic, D$_5$W is actually isotonic only in the container. After administration, dextrose is quickly metabolized, leaving only water—a hypotonic fluid.)
Hypotonic	• Half-normal saline (154 mOsm/L) • 0.33% sodium chloride (103 mOsm/L) • Dextrose 2.5% in water (126 mOsm/L)	• Administer cautiously. Hypotonic solutions cause a fluid shift from blood vessels into cells. This shift could cause cardiovascular collapse from intravascular fluid depletion and increased ICP from fluid shift into brain cells. • Don't give hypotonic solutions to patients at risk for increased ICP from stroke, head trauma, or neurosurgery. • Don't give hypotonic solutions to patients at risk for third-space fluid shifts (abnormal fluid shifts into the interstitial compartment or a body cavity)—for example, patients suffering from burns, trauma, or low serum protein levels from malnutrition or liver disease.
Hypertonic	• Dextrose 5% in half-normal saline (406 mOsm/L) • Dextrose 5% in normal saline (560 mOsm/L) • Dextrose 5% in lactated Ringer's (575 mOsm/L) • 3% sodium chloride (1,025 mOsm/L) • 25% albumin (1,500 mOsm/L) • 7.5% sodium chloride (2,400 mOsm/L)	• Because hypertonic solutions greatly expand the intravascular compartment, administer them by I.V. pump and closely monitor the patient for circulatory overload. • Hypertonic solutions pull fluid from the intracellular compartment, so don't give them to a patient with a condition that causes cellular dehydration—for example, diabetic ketoacidosis. • Don't give hypertonic solutions to a patient with impaired heart or kidney function—his system can't handle the extra fluid.

One indication for an isotonic solution is hypotension due to hypovolemia. Common isotonic solutions include lactated Ringer's and normal saline.

Hypertonic solutions

A hypertonic solution has an osmolarity higher than serum osmolarity. When a patient receives a hypertonic I.V. solution, serum osmolarity initially increases, causing fluid to be pulled from the interstitial and intracellular compartments into the blood vessels.

> A hypertonic solution can be beneficial postoperatively because it helps reduce edema, stabilize blood pressure, and regulate urine output.

When, why, and how to get hyper

Hypertonic solutions may be ordered for patients postoperatively because the shift of fluid into the blood vessels caused by a hypertonic solution has several beneficial effects for these patients. For example, it:
• reduces the risk of edema
• stabilizes blood pressure
• regulates urine output.

Hypotonic solutions

A hypotonic solution has an osmolarity lower than serum osmolarity. When a patient receives a hypotonic solution, fluid shifts out of the blood vessels and into the cells and interstitial spaces, where osmolarity is higher. A hypotonic solution hydrates cells while reducing fluid in the circulatory system.

Hypotonic solutions may be ordered when diuretic therapy dehydrates cells. Other indications include hyperglycemic conditions, such as diabetic ketoacidosis and hyperosmolar hyperglycemic nonketotic syndrome. In these conditions, high serum glucose levels draw fluid out of cells.

Flood warning

Because hypotonic solutions flood cells, certain patients shouldn't receive them. For example, patients with cerebral edema or increased intracranial pressure shouldn't receive hypotonic solutions because the increased ECF can cause further edema and tissue damage.

Additional uses of I.V. therapy

In addition to restoring and maintaining fluid and electrolyte balance, I.V. therapy is used to administer drugs, transfuse blood and blood products, and deliver parenteral nutrition.

Drug administration

The I.V. route provides a rapid, effective way of administering medications. Commonly infused drugs include antibiotics; thrombolytics; histamine-receptor antagonists; and antineoplastic, cardiovascular, and anticonvulsant drugs.

Drugs may be delivered long-term by continuous infusion, over a short period, or directly as a single dose.

Blood administration

Your nursing responsibilities may include giving blood and blood components and monitoring patients receiving transfusion therapy. Blood products can be given through a peripheral or central I.V. line. Various blood products are given to:
• restore and maintain adequate circulatory volume
• prevent cardiogenic shock
• increase the blood's oxygen-carrying capacity
• maintain hemostasis.

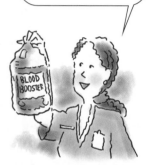

One of your responsibilities as a nurse is to administer blood and blood components and monitor transfusion therapy. So you gotta know your blood facts.

Parts of the whole

Whole blood is composed of cellular elements and plasma. Cellular elements include:
• erythrocytes (red blood cells)
• leukocytes (white blood cells)
• thrombocytes (platelets).

Each of these elements is packaged separately for transfusion. Plasma may be delivered intact or separated into several components that may be given to correct various deficiencies. Whole blood transfusions are unnecessary unless the patient has lost massive quantities of blood (25% to 30%) in a short period.

It may not be a gourmet meal, but TPN is packed with all the essential nutrients your patient needs.

Parenteral nutrition

Parenteral nutrition provides essential nutrients to the blood, organs, and cells by the I.V. route. It isn't the same as a seven-course meal in a fine restaurant, but parenteral nutrition can contain the essence of a balanced diet.

It isn't gourmet, but it has all you need . . .

Total parenteral nutrition (TPN) is customized for each patient. The ingredients in solutions developed for TPN are designed to meet a patient's energy and nutrient requirements, including:
• proteins
• carbohydrates

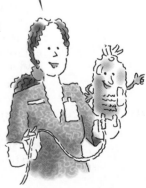

- fats
- electrolytes
- vitamins
- trace elements
- water.

Time for TPN?

TPN should be used only when the gastrointestinal (GI) tract is unable to absorb nutrients. A patient can receive TPN indefinitely; however, long-term TPN can cause liver damage.

A limited menu

Peripheral parenteral nutrition (PPN) is delivered by peripheral veins. PPN is used in limited nutritional therapy. The solution contains fewer nonprotein calories and lower amino acid concentrations than TPN solutions. It may also include lipid emulsions. A patient can receive PPN for approximately 3 weeks. It can be used to support the nutritional status of a patient who doesn't require total nutritional support. Complications associated with PPN include the risks of vein damage and infiltration.

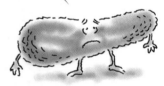

If your patient is receiving parenteral nutrition, please keep a close eye on my enzymes.

Tracking changes

When your patient is receiving parenteral nutrition, keep close track of changes in his fluid and electrolyte status and glucose levels. You'll also need to assess your patient's response to the nutrient solution to detect early signs of such complications as alterations in the pancreatic enzymes (lipase, amylase trypsin, and chymotrypsin), triglycerides, or albumin.

I.V. delivery

Depending in part on how concentrated an I.V. solution is, it may be delivered through a peripheral vein or a central vein. Usually, a low concentration solution is infused through a peripheral vein in the arm or hand; a more concentrated solution must be given through a central vein. (See *Veins used in I.V. therapy.*) Medications or fluids that may be administered centrally include:
- those with a pH less than 5 or greater than 9
- those with an osmolarity greater than 500 mOsm/L
- parenteral nutrition formulas containing more than 10% dextrose or more than 50% protein
- continuous vesicant chemotherapy (chemotherapy that's toxic to tissues).

Veins used in I.V. therapy

This illustration shows the veins commonly used for peripheral and central venous therapy.

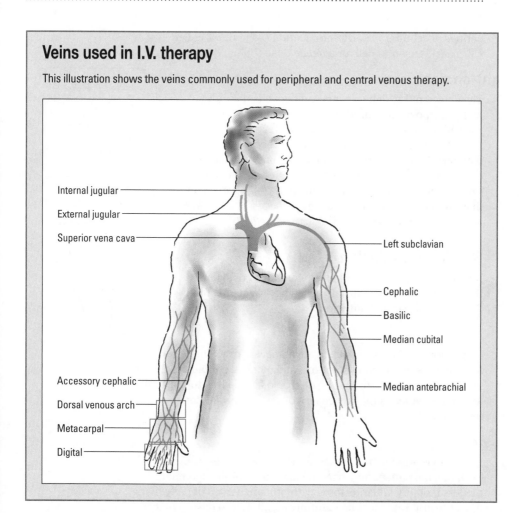

Internal jugular

External jugular

Superior vena cava

Left subclavian

Cephalic

Basilic

Median cubital

Accessory cephalic

Median antebrachial

Dorsal venous arch

Metacarpal

Digital

Delivery methods

There are three basic methods for delivering I.V. therapy:

 continuous infusion

 intermittent infusion

 direct injection.

Setting the terms

Continuous I.V. therapy allows you to give a carefully regulated amount of fluid over a prolonged period. In intermittent I.V. therapy, a solution (commonly a medication) is given for shorter periods at set intervals. Direct injection (sometimes called *I.V. push*) is used to deliver a single dose (bolus) of a drug.

Making the right choice

The choice of I.V. delivery method depends not only on the purpose and duration of therapy but also on the patient's condition, age, and health history.

At times, a patient may receive I.V. therapy by more than one delivery method. Also, variations of each delivery method may be used. Some therapies also require extra equipment. For example, in some long-term chemotherapy, an implanted central venous access device is needed. (See *Comparing I.V. delivery methods.*)

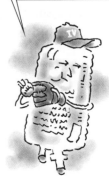

I always thought my delivery depended on my windup, pitch, and follow-through . . . boy, was I off base!

Continuous infusion

A continuous I.V. infusion helps maintain a constant therapeutic drug level. It's also used to provide I.V. fluid therapy or parenteral nutrition.

Upside . . .

Continuous I.V. infusion has its advantages. For example, less time is spent mixing solutions and hanging containers than with the intermittent method. You'll also handle less tubing and access the patient's I.V. device less often, decreasing the risk of infection.

. . . and downside

Continuous administration has some disadvantages, too. For example, the patient may become distressed if the equipment hinders mobility and interferes with other activities of daily living. Also, the drip rate must be carefully monitored to ensure that the I.V. fluid and medication don't infuse too rapidly or too slowly.

Intermittent infusion

The most common and flexible method of administering I.V. medications is by intermittent infusion.

On again, off again

In intermittent infusion, drugs are administered over a specified period at varying intervals, thereby maintaining therapeutic blood levels. A small volume (1 to 250 ml) may be delivered over several minutes or a few hours, depending on the infusion prescription. You can deliver an intermittent infusion through a primary line (the most common method) or a secondary line. The secondary line is usually connected or piggybacked into the primary line by way of a Y-site (a Y-shaped section of tubing with a self-sealing access port).

Comparing I.V. delivery methods

This chart lists the indications, advantages, and disadvantages of methods commonly used to administer I.V. medications.

Method and indications	Advantages	Disadvantages
Direct injection *Into a vein* • Generally doesn't involve an administration set and is commonly referred to as *I.V. push* • When a nonirritating drug with a low risk of immediate adverse reactions is required for a patient with no other I.V. needs (e.g., single injection of furosemide, a diuretic)	• Eliminates the risk of complications from an implanted (indwelling) venous access device • Eliminates the inconvenience of an indwelling venous access device	• Can only be given by a doctor or specially certified nurse • Requires venipuncture, which can cause patient anxiety • Requires two syringes—one to administer the medication and one to flush the vein after administration • Requires dilution of the medication before injection • Risks infiltration (puncture of the vein, allowing the solution to enter the surrounding tissue) from the steel needle • Makes it impossible to dilute the drug or interrupt delivery when irritation occurs
Through an existing infusion line • When the patient requires immediate high blood levels of a medication (e.g., regular insulin, dextrose 50%, atropine, or antihistamines) • In emergencies, when the drug must be given quickly for immediate effect	• Doesn't require time or authorization to perform venipuncture because the vein is already accessed • Doesn't require needle puncture, which can cause patient anxiety • Allows the use of an I.V. solution to test the patency of the venous access device before drug administration • Allows continued venous access in case of adverse reactions	• Carries the same inconveniences and complication risks as an indwelling venous access device
Intermittent infusion *Piggyback method* • Requires connecting a second administration set to a primary line • Commonly used with drugs given over short periods at varying intervals (e.g., antibiotics and gastric secretion inhibitors)	• Avoids multiple intramuscular injections • Permits repeated administration of drugs through a single I.V. line • Provides high drug blood levels for short periods	• May cause periods when the drug level becomes too low to be clinically effective (e.g., when peak and trough times aren't considered in the medication order)

(continued)

Comparing I.V. delivery methods *(continued)*

Method and indications	Advantages	Disadvantages
Intermittent infusion *(continued)* *Saline lock* • Allows for maintenance of venous access • When the patient requires constant venous access but not continuous infusion	• Provides venous access for patients with fluid restrictions • Allows better patient mobility between doses • Preserves veins by reducing frequent venipuncture • Lowers cost	• Requires close monitoring during administration so the device can be flushed on completion • Most commonly used in adults with peripheral I.V. access devices
Volume-control set • Has a medication chamber that allows it to deliver small doses over an extended period • When the patient requires a low volume of fluid	• Requires only one large-volume container and prevents fluid overload from runaway infusion	• May have high equipment costs • Carries a high contamination risk • Requires that the flow clamp be closed when the set empties (if set doesn't contain a membrane that blocks the air passage when it's empty)
Continuous infusion *Through primary line* • When continuous serum levels are needed • When consistent fluid levels are needed	• Maintains steady serum levels • Lowers the risk of rapid shock and vein irritation from a large volume of fluid diluting the drug	• Increases the risk of incompatibility with drugs administered by piggyback infusion • Restricts patient mobility when the patient is connected to an I.V. system • Increases the risk of undetected infiltration because slow infusion makes it difficult to see swelling in the area of infiltration
Through secondary line • Connected to a primary line • When the patient requires continuous infusion of two or more compatible admixtures administered at different rates • When there's a moderate to high chance of abruptly stopping one admixture without infusing the drug remaining in the I.V. tubing	• Permits the primary infusion and each secondary infusion to be given at different rates • Permits the primary line to be shut off and kept standing by to maintain venous access in case a secondary line must be abruptly stopped	• Eliminates the use of drugs with immediate incompatibility • Increases the risk of phlebitis or vein irritation from an increased number of drugs • Uses multiple I.V. systems (e.g., primary lines with secondary lines attached), which can create physical barriers to patient care and limit patient mobility, especially for those with electronic pumps or controllers

Direct injection

You might say that I.V. therapy by direct injection gets right to the point. A vein can be accessed directly for a single dose of a prescribed drug or solution. The needle is then removed when the bolus is completed. A bolus injection may also be administered through an intermittent infusion device that's already in place.

Administration sets

You need to choose the correct administration set for your patient's infusion. Your choice depends on the type of infusion to be provided, the infusion container, and whether you're using a volume-control device.

Vented and unvented

I.V. administration sets come in two forms: vented and unvented. The vented set is for containers that have no venting system (I.V. plastic bags and some bottles). Unvented bottles have their own venting system.

Other features and options

I.V. administration sets come with various other features as well, including ports for infusing secondary medications and filters for blocking microbes, irritants, or large particles. The tubing also varies. Some types are designed to enhance the proper functioning of devices that help regulate the infusion rate. Other tubing is used specifically for continuous or intermittent infusion or for infusing parenteral nutrition and blood.

Infusion rates

A key aspect of administering I.V. therapy is maintaining accurate infusion rates for the solutions. If an infusion runs too fast or too slow, your patient may suffer complications, such as phlebitis, infiltration, circulatory overload (possibly leading to heart failure and pulmonary edema), and adverse drug reactions.

Volume-control devices and the correct administration set help prevent such complications. You can help, too, by being familiar with all of the information in doctors' orders and being able to recognize incomplete or incorrectly written orders for I.V. therapy. (See *Reading an I.V. order,* page 278.)

Reading an I.V. order

Orders for I.V. therapy may be standardized for different illnesses and therapies or individualized for a particular patient. Some facility policies dictate an automatic stop order for I.V. fluids. For example, I.V. orders are good for 24 hours from the time they're written, unless otherwise specified.

It's complete
A complete order for I.V. therapy should specify:
• type and amount of solution
• additives and their concentrations (such as 10 mEq potassium chloride in 500 ml dextrose 5% in water)

• rate and volume of infusion
• duration of infusion.

When it isn't complete
If you find that an order isn't complete or if you think an I.V. order is inappropriate because of the patient's condition, consult the doctor.

Calculating infusion rates

There are two basic types of infusion rates available with I.V. administration sets: macrodrip and microdrip. Each set delivers a specific number of drops per milliliter (gtt/ml). Macrodrip delivers 10, 15, or 20 gtt/ml; microdrip delivers 60 gtt/ml. Regardless of the type of set you use, the formula for calculating infusion rates is the same. (See *Calculating infusion rates.*)

Regulating infusion rates

When a patient's condition requires you to maintain precise I.V. infusion rates, use an infusion control device, such as:
• clamps
• volumetric pumps.

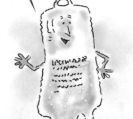

An infusion control device is an excellent way to regulate your patient's infusion rate, but you still need to monitor it and the device.

ml/hour or gtt/minute??

When you regulate the I.V. infusion rate with a clamp, the rate is usually measured in drops per minute (gtt/minute). If you use a pump, the infusion rate is measured in milliliters per hour (ml/hour).

I.V. clamps

You can regulate the infusion rate with two types of clamps: screw and roller. The screw clamp offers greater accuracy, but the roller clamp, used for standard fluid therapy, is faster and easier to manipulate. A third type, the slide clamp, can stop or start the infusion but can't regulate the rate.

Calculating infusion rates

When calculating the infusion rate (drops per minute) of I.V. solutions, remember that the number of drops required to deliver 1 ml varies with the type of administration set used and its manufacturer:
• Administration sets are of two types—macrodrip (the standard type) and microdrip. Macrodrip delivers 10, 15, or 20 gtt/ml; microdrip usually delivers 60 gtt/ml (see illustrations).

• Manufacturers calibrate their devices differently, so be sure to look for the "drop factor"—expressed in drops per milliliter or gtt/ml—in the packaging that accompanies the set you're using. (This packaging also has crucial information about such things as special infusions and blood transfusions.) When you know your device's drop factor, use the following formula to calculate specific infusion rates:

$$\frac{\text{volume of infusion (in milliliters)}}{\text{time of infusion (in minutes)}} \times \text{drop factor (in drops per milliliter)} = \text{infusion rate (in drops per minute)}$$

After you calculate the infusion rate for the set you're using, remove your watch or position your wrist so you can look at your watch and the drops at the same time. Next, adjust the clamp to achieve the ordered infusion rate and count the drops for 1 full minute. Readjust the clamp as necessary and count the drops for another minute. Keep adjusting the clamp and counting the drops until you have the correct rate.

Macrodrip

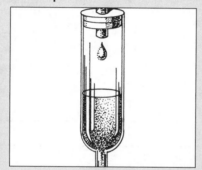

Microdrip

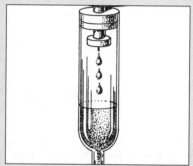

Pumps

New pumps are being developed all the time; be sure to attend instruction sessions to learn how to use them. On your unit, keep a file of instruction manuals (provided by the manufacturers) for each piece of equipment used.

Factor these in

When you're using a clamp for infusion regulation, you must monitor the infusion rate closely and adjust as needed. Such factors as vein spasm, vein pressure changes, patient movement, manipulations of the clamp, and bent or kinked tubing can cause the rate to vary markedly. For easy monitoring, use a time tape, which marks the prescribed solution level at hourly intervals. (See *Using a time tape*, page 280.)

Other factors that affect infusion rate include the type of I.V. fluid and its viscosity, the height of the infusion container, the type of administration set, and the size and position of the venous access device.

Using a time tape

Here's a simple way to monitor I.V. infusion rate: Attach a piece of tape or a preprinted strip to the I.V. container; then write hourly times on the tape or strip beginning with the time you hung the solution.

By comparing the actual time with the label time, you can quickly see if the rate needs to be adjusted. Remember that you should never increase I.V. infusion rates by more than 30% unless you first check with the doctor.

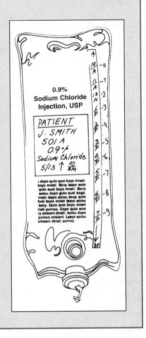

Checking infusion rates

Infusion rates can be fickle; you must check and adjust them regularly. The frequency with which you should check infusion rates depends on the patient's condition and age and the solution or medication being administered.

I'll be back!

Many nurses check the I.V. infusion rate every time they're in a patient's room and after each position change. Assess the infusion rate more frequently for some patients, such as:
• critically ill patients
• patients with conditions that might be exacerbated by fluid overload
• pediatric patients
• elderly patients
• patients receiving a drug that can cause tissue damage if infiltration occurs.

While you're there

When checking the infusion rate, inspect and palpate the I.V. insertion site, and ask the patient how it feels.

If the infusion rate slows, you can get it back on schedule by making slight adjustments. However, if the rate is off by more than 30%, consult the doctor.

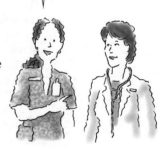

Minor (not major) adjustments

If the infusion rate slows significantly, you can usually get it back on schedule by adjusting the rate slightly. Don't make a major adjustment, though. If the rate must be increased by more than 30%, check with the doctor.

You should also time an infusion control device or rate minder for 1 to 2 hours per shift. (These devices have an error rate ranging from 2% to 10%.) Before using any infusion control device, become thoroughly familiar with its features. Attend instruction sessions and perform return demonstrations until you learn the system.

Professional and legal standards

Administering drugs and solutions to patients is one of the most legally significant tasks nurses perform. Unfortunately, the number of lawsuits directed against nurses who are involved in I.V. therapy is increasing. For example, a 1995 Missouri study reported a high incidence of errors involving I.V. solution administration in which wrong solutions were used or solutions were administered by an incorrect route. Many lawsuits centered on errors in infusion pump use.

Lawsuits may also result from administration of the wrong medication dosage, inappropriate placement of an I.V. line, and failure to monitor for adverse reactions, infiltration, dislodgment of I.V. equipment, or other mishaps.

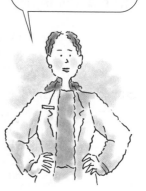

It's sobering to learn that a high percentage of lawsuits brought against nurses involve errors with I.V. administration.

Court cases involving I.V. therapy

Here are some examples of lawsuits involving I.V. therapy.

Versed verdict

In Los Angeles, a nurse administered midazolam (Versed) through a port in an I.V. line to an infant, leading to the infant's death. This nurse had never administered I.V. Versed to an infant or child before. A facility protocol prohibited the use of Versed on the pediatric floor. The manufacturer recommended a dosage of 0.1 mg/kg, and the infant weighed 9 kg. The hospital record indicated 5 mg had been administered. A settlement awarded the plaintiff $225,000.

Still accountable

In another Los Angeles case, continuous infusion of 145 mg of morphine over 18 hours led to a patient's death. The doctor failed to limit the amount to be infused. Nevertheless, the charge nurse and staff nurse were held accountable for failing to recognize a "gross overdose." The patient's widow and children were awarded more than $2 million for lost wages and general damages.

Syringe confusion

In Illinois, a nurse administered the wrong dose of lidocaine (Xylocaine). The order was for 100 mg; the nurse injected 2 g. The packaging caused confusion: the Xylocaine was provided in a 2-g syringe for mixing into an I.V. solution and in a 100-mg syringe for direct injection. The nurse accidentally used the 2-g syringe. However, information about previous overdose incidents from the Food and Drug Administration and medical literature had been available to the hospital.

Clamp error

In Ohio, a nurse failed to clamp a pump regulating the flow of an antibiotic through a central line to a child. This resulted in delivery of nearly seven times the prescribed dosage of gentamicin, causing the child to become totally deaf.

Infiltration injury

In Pennsylvania, an emergency department nurse misplaced an I.V. line, which infiltrated the patient's hand, resulting in reflex sympathetic dystrophy. The patient couldn't return to work and won a $702,000 award.

Striking a nerve

Several recent lawsuits have involved allegations that a nurse struck a patient's radial nerve during insertion of an I.V. line. Such injuries can cause compartment syndrome and may require emergency fasciotomy, skin grafts, and other surgery. Uncorrected compartment syndrome can progress to gangrene and amputation of fingers. One New York case involving finger amputation resulted in a $40 million jury verdict, which was later reduced to $5 million.

The bottom line is, live up to your professional standards and know your legal and ethical responsibilities to better serve your patients and protect yourself.

Listen up

When monitoring an I.V. line, listening to the patient is as important as monitoring the site, pump, and tubing. In the Tampa, Florida, case of *Frank v. Hillsborough County Hospital,* a patient's frequent complaints of pain were ignored. The patient suffered permanent nerve damage and later obtained an award of almost $60,000.

Know your responsibility

As a nurse, you have a legal and ethical responsibility to your patients. The good news is that if you honor

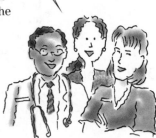

these duties and meet the appropriate standards of care, you'll be able to hold your own in court.

By becoming aware of professional standards and laws related to administering I.V. therapy, you can provide the best care for your patients and protect yourself legally. Professional and legal standards are defined by state nurse practice acts, federal regulations, and facility policies.

State nurse practice acts

Each state has a nurse practice act that broadly defines the legal scope of nursing practice. Your state's nurse practice act is the most important law affecting your nursing practice.

Know your limits

Every nurse is expected to care for patients within defined limits. If a nurse gives care beyond those limits, she becomes vulnerable to charges of violating her state nurse practice act. For a copy of your state nurse practice act, contact your state nurse's association or your state board of nursing or its Web site.

Many states' nurse practice acts don't specifically address scope of practice regarding I.V. therapy by registered nurses (RNs). However, many nurse practice acts do address whether licensed practical nurses (LPNs) or licensed vocational nurses (LVNs) can administer I.V. therapy. It's important for LPNs and LVNs as well as for the RNs who are supervising or training them to be familiar with this information.

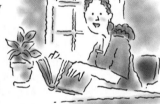

Become familiar with the scope and limitations of what you legally can and can't do regarding I.V. therapy in your state.

Federal regulations

The federal government issues regulations and establishes policies related to I.V. therapy administration. For example, it mandates adherence to standards of I.V. therapy practice for health care facilities so that they can be eligible to receive reimbursement under Medicare, Medicaid, and other programs.

Millions served

Medicare and Medicaid, the two major federal health care programs, serve about 75 million Americans. They're run by the Health Care Financing Administration (HCFA), which is part of the U.S. Department of Health and Human Services. HCFA formulates national Medicare policy, including policies related to I.V. therapy, but contracts with private insurance companies to oversee claims and make payment for services and supplies provided under Medicare. These agencies, in turn, enforce HCFA policy by accepting or denying claims for reimbursement. When reviewing claims, agencies may evaluate practices and quality of care—an important factor underlying the emphasis on proper documentation in health care.

Medicaid, which serves certain low-income people, is a state-federal partnership administered by a state agency. There are broad federal requirements for Medicaid, but states have a wide degree of flexibility to design their own programs.

> It's important to adhere to federal regulations and policies to ensure that your facility is eligible to receive reimbursement for federally funded programs.

One patient, many regulators

To be eligible for reimbursement, health care agencies must comply with the standards of a complex network of regulators. Consider, for example, a patient receiving I.V. medications at home with a reusable pump. This patient is primarily covered by Medicare with secondary Medicaid coverage. A variety of carriers, fiscal intermediaries, and agencies share responsibility for reimbursement and regulatory oversight of the patient's care:

• An insurance carrier contracts with Medicare to cover services such as refilling the pump.
• A separate insurance carrier (a durable medical equipment carrier designated by HCFA) covers administered drugs, the pump, and pump supplies.
• Another insurance carrier (called a *fiscal intermediary*) contracts with Medicare to cover preliminary in-hospital training of the patient in I.V. therapy techniques.
• A Medicaid agency also covers a portion of the patient's care.

Nursing documentation must be complete to meet the requirements of all these different agencies. The underlying (though unstated) philosophy of these agencies is that "if it isn't documented, it isn't done." The regulatory network is becoming more complicated as many Medicare and Medicaid patients are being covered by managed care organizations that have their own rules and procedures.

Facility policy

Every health care facility has I.V. therapy policies for nurses. Such policies are required to obtain accreditation from the Joint Commission on Accreditation of Healthcare Organizations (JCAHO) and other accrediting bodies. These policies can't go beyond what a state's nurse practice act permits, but they more specifically define your duties and responsibilities.

Awareness of facility policy is particularly important in rapidly developing areas of practice such as home care, where the intensity of service and patient needs is increasing dramatically. For example, home health nurses must be acutely aware of patient and family education policies because infusion systems are being used in the home 24 hours per day without the presence of full-time nursing staff.

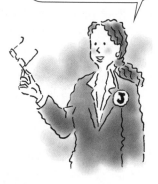

By complying with your facility's I.V. therapy policy, you help secure your facility's accreditation by JCAHO and other accrediting bodies.

INS—not just about immigration

The Infusion Nurses Society (INS) has developed a set of standards, the *Infusion Nursing Standards of Practice*, that are commonly used by committees developing facility policy. According to the INS, the goals of these standards are to "protect and preserve the patient's right to safe, quality care and protect the nurse who administers infusion therapy." These standards address all aspects of I.V. nursing. For more information, contact the INS at (781) 440-9408 or at http://www.ins1.org.

Documentation

You must document I.V. therapy for several reasons. Proper documentation provides:
• accurate description of care that can serve as legal protection (e.g., as evidence that a prescribed treatment was administered)
• mechanism for recording and retrieving information
• record for health care insurers of equipment and supplies used.

Translated, this means "document, document, document!"

Documenting initiation of I.V. therapy

When you initiate I.V. therapy, it's important to include specific information about where the I.V. was started, what kind of equipment was used, and what solution was infused. (See *Documenting I.V. therapy,* page 286.)

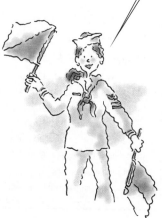

Take note!

Documenting I.V. therapy

Follow these tips to document your care when you perform I.V. site care or catheter removal or when you document I.V. infusion using a sequential system or on a flow sheet or an intake and output sheet.

I.V. site care

When you perform I.V. site care, document the following:
• date and time of the dressing change
• condition of the insertion site, noting signs of infection (redness and pain), infiltration (coolness, blanching, or edema), or thrombophlebitis (redness, firmness, pain, or edema)
• care given and the type of dressing applied
• patient education provided.
    If complications are present, document:
• name of the doctor notified
• time of the notification
• specific orders given
• your interventions
• patient's response.

I.V. catheter removal

When an I.V. catheter is removed, document the following:
• date and time of removal
• condition of the catheter tip
• condition of the site
• drainage at the puncture site
• samples of drainage and actual device tip sent to laboratory for culture, according to your facility policy
• site care given
• type of dressing applied
• patient education provided.

Sequential system

One way to document I.V. solutions throughout therapy is to number each container sequentially. For example, if a patient is to receive normal saline solution at 125 ml/hour (3,000 ml/day) on day 1, number the 1,000-ml containers as 1, 2, and 3. If another 3,000 ml is ordered on day 2, number those containers as 4, 5, and 6. This system may reduce administration errors. Also, check your facility's policy and procedures; some facilities require beginning the count

again if the type of fluid changes, whereas others keep the count sequential regardless of the type of fluid.

Flow sheets

Flow sheets highlight specific patient information according to preestablished parameters of nursing care. They have spaces for recording dates, times, and specific interventions. When you use an I.V. flow sheet, record:
• date
• infusion rate
• use of an electronic flow device or flow controller
• type of solution
• sequential solution container
• date and time of dressing and tubing changes.

Intake and output sheets

When you're documenting I.V. therapy on an intake and output sheet, follow these guidelines:
• If the patient is a child, note fluid levels on the I.V. containers hourly. If the patient is an adult, note these levels at least twice per shift.
• With children and critical care patients, record intake of all I.V. infusions, including fluids, medications, flush solutions, blood and blood products, and other infusates, every 1 to 2 hours.
• Document the total amount of each infusate and totals of all infusions at least every shift, so you can monitor fluid balance.
• Note output hourly or less often (but at least once each shift), depending on the patient's condition. Output includes urine, stool, vomitus, and gastric drainage. For an acutely ill or unstable patient, you may need to assess urine output every 15 minutes.
• Read fluid levels from the infusate containers or electronic volume-control device to estimate the amounts infused and the amounts remaining to be infused.

How to label an I.V. bag

When you place a label on an I.V. bag, be sure not to cover the name of the I.V. solution. To properly label an I.V. solution container, include (in addition to the time tape):
• patient's name, identification number, and room number
• date and time the container was hung
• any additives and their amounts
• rate at which the solution is to run
• sequential container number
• expiration date and time of infusion
• your name.

How to label a dressing

To label a new dressing over an I.V. site, include:
• date of insertion
• gauge and length of venipuncture device
• date and time of the dressing change
• your initials.

Forms, forms, forms

I.V. therapy may be documented on progress notes, a sequential system, a special I.V. therapy sheet or flow sheet, a nursing care plan on the patient's chart, or an intake and output sheet.

Label that dressing . . .

In addition to documentation in the patient's chart, you need to label the dressing on the catheter insertion site. Whenever you change the dressing, label the new one. (See *How to label a dressing*.)

. . . and the container

You should also label the fluid container and place a time tape on it. With a child, you may need to label the volume-control set as well. In labeling the container and the set, follow your facility's policy and procedures. (See *How to label an I.V. bag*.)

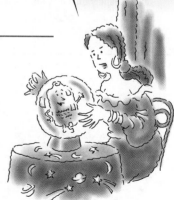

Be crystal clear when documenting how the I.V. site is maintained. I predict you will be a better nurse for doing so!

Documenting I.V. maintenance

It's equally important to document how the I.V site is maintained, including the conditions of the site; care that was provided; dressing, solution, tubing, or equipment changes you made; and teaching you provided. (See *Teaching about I.V. therapy*, page 288.)

Teacher's lounge

Teaching about I.V. therapy

Although you may be accustomed to I.V. therapy, many patients aren't. Your patient may be apprehensive about the procedure and concerned that his condition has worsened.

Teaching the patient and, when appropriate, members of his family will help him relax and take the mystery out of I.V. therapy.

Based on past experience

Begin by determining your patient's previous infusion experience, expectations, and knowledge of venipuncture and I.V. therapy. Then base your teaching on your findings.

Your teaching should include these steps:
• Describe the procedure. Tell the patient that I.V. means "inside the vein" and that a plastic catheter or needle will be placed in his vein.
• Explain that fluids containing certain nutrients or medications will flow from a bag or bottle through a length of tubing, and then through the catheter or needle into the vein.
• Tell the patient how long the catheter or needle may stay in place, and explain that the doctor will decide how much and what type of fluid and medication is needed.

The whole story

Give the patient as much information as possible. Consider providing pamphlets, sample catheters and I.V. equipment, slides, videotapes, and other appropriate information. Make sure you tell the whole story:
• Tell the patient they may feel transient pain as the needle goes in, the discomfort will stop when the catheter or needle is in place.

• Explain why I.V. therapy is needed and how the patient can help by holding still and not withdrawing if they feel pain when the needle is inserted.
• Explain that the I.V. fluids may feel cold at first, but the sensation should last only a few minutes.
• Instruct the patient to report any discomfort they feel after therapy begins.
• Explain activity restrictions such as those regarding bathing and ambulating.

Easing anxiety

Give the patient time to express concerns and fears, and take the time to provide reassurance. Also, encourage the patient to use stress-reduction techniques such as deep, slow breathing. Allow the patient and their family to participate in the patient's care as much as possible.

But did they get it?

Make sure you evaluate how well your patient and members of the patient's family understand your instruction. Evaluate their understanding while you're teaching and when you're done. You can do this by asking frequent questions and having them explain or demonstrate what you have taught.

Don't forget the paperwork

Document all your teaching in the patient's records. Note what you taught and how well the patient understood it.

References

Berman, A., & Snyder, S. J. (2012). *Skills in clinical nursing* (7th ed.). Upper Saddle River, NJ: Pearson Education.

Berman, A., Snyder, S. J., & McKinney, D. S. (2011). *Nursing basics for clinical practice.* Upper Saddle River, NJ: Pearson Education.

Treas, L. S., & Wilkinson, J. M. (2014). *Basic nursing concepts, skills & reasoning.* Philadelphia, PA: F. A. Davis.

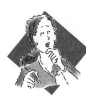

Quick quiz

1. The fluid located inside the cell is called:
   A. interstitial.
   B. intracellular.
   C. extracellular.
   D. internal.

Answer: B. The fluid inside the cells—about 55% of total body fluid—is called *intracellular fluid.* The rest is called *extracellular fluid.*

2. The major extracellular electrolytes are:
   A. sodium and chloride.
   B. potassium and phosphorus.
   C. potassium and sodium.
   D. phosphorus and chloride.

Answer: A. The major extracellular electrolytes are sodium and chloride.

3. An example of a hypertonic solution is:
   A. half-normal saline.
   B. 0.33% sodium chloride.
   C. dextrose 2.5% in water.
   D. dextrose 5% in half-normal saline.

Answer: D. Some examples of hypertonic solutions are dextrose 5% in half-normal saline (405 mOsm/L), dextrose 5% in normal saline (560 mOsm/L), and dextrose 5% in lactated Ringer's solution (527 mOsm/L).

4. When capillary blood pressure exceeds colloid osmotic pressure, which situation occurs?
   A. Water and diffusible solutes leave the capillaries and circulate into the interstitial fluid.
   B. Water and diffusible solutes return to the capillaries.

C.   No change occurs.

D.   Intake and output are affected.

Answer: A. When capillary blood pressure exceeds colloid osmotic pressure, water and diffusible solutes leave the capillaries and circulate into the interstitial fluid. When capillary blood pressure falls below colloid osmotic pressure, water and diffusible solutes return to the capillaries.

Scoring

☆☆☆   If you answered all four questions correctly, super! Your knowledge of I.V. therapy is diffuse.

☆☆   If you answered three questions correctly, bravo! You're no drip when it comes to I.V. therapy.

☆   If you answered fewer than three questions correctly, don't despair! Review the chapter for an infusion of I.V. know-how and try again.

Part III Physiologic needs

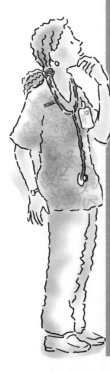

Part III.   Pharmacology...

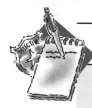

Oxygenation

Just the facts

In this chapter, you'll learn:

♦ components that make up the respiratory system

♦ processes involved in respiration

♦ principles of acid–base balance

♦ treatments for respiratory disorders.

A look at the respiratory system

The respiratory system includes the airways, lungs, bony thorax, respiratory muscles, and central nervous system. They work together to deliver oxygen to the bloodstream and remove excess carbon dioxide from the body. Knowing the basic structures and functions of the respiratory system will help you perform a comprehensive respiratory assessment and recognize any abnormalities. (See *A close look at the respiratory system*, page 294.)

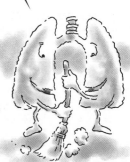

One of my main jobs is to get rid of excess carbon dioxide. Out the door with you now!

Airways and lungs

The airways are divided into the upper and lower airways. The upper airways include the nasopharynx (nose), oropharynx (mouth), laryngopharynx, and larynx. Their purpose is to warm, filter, and humidify inhaled air. They also help make sound and send air to the lower airways.

Flapped for your protection

The epiglottis is a flap of tissue that closes over the top of the larynx when the patient swallows. The epiglottis protects the patient from aspirating food or fluid into the lower airways.

A close look at the respiratory system

The major structures of the upper and lower airways are illustrated below. The alveolus, or *acinus,* is shown in the inset.

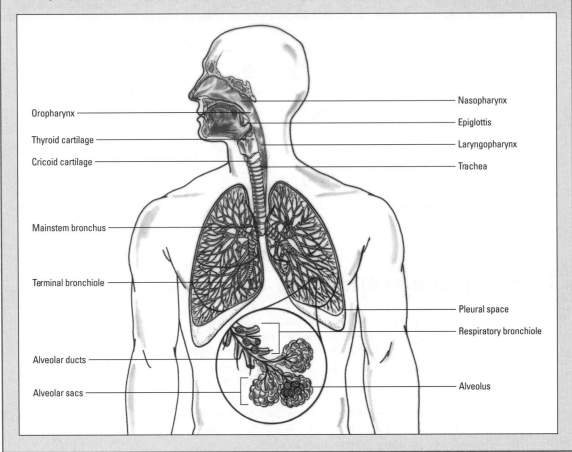

Oropharynx

Thyroid cartilage

Cricoid cartilage

Mainstem bronchus

Terminal bronchiole

Alveolar ducts

Alveolar sacs

Nasopharynx

Epiglottis

Laryngopharynx

Trachea

Pleural space

Respiratory bronchiole

Alveolus

Vocal point

The larynx is located at the top of the trachea and houses the vocal cords. It's the transition point between the upper and lower airways.

The lowdown on the lower airways

The lower airways begin with the trachea, which then divides into the right and left mainstem bronchi. The mainstem bronchi divide into the lobar bronchi, which are lined with mucus-producing ciliated epithelium, one of the lungs' major defense systems.

The lobar bronchi then divide into secondary bronchi, tertiary bronchi, terminal bronchioles, respiratory bronchioles, alveolar ducts and, finally, into the alveoli, the gas-exchange units of the lungs. An adult's lungs typically contain about 300 million alveoli.

> Hang tight! These lobar bronchi can get a little slippery from all that mucus in the lining.

Lungs and lobes

Each lung is wrapped in a lining called the *visceral pleura*. The right lung is larger and has three lobes: upper, middle, and lower. The left lung is smaller and has only an upper and a lower lobe.

Smooth moves

The lungs share space in the thoracic cavity with the heart and great vessels, the trachea, the esophagus, and the bronchi. All areas of the thoracic cavity that come in contact with the lungs are lined with parietal pleura.

A small amount of fluid fills the area between the two layers of the pleura. This pleural fluid allows the layers to slide smoothly over each other as the chest expands and contracts. The parietal pleura also contain nerve endings that transmit pain signals when inflammation occurs.

Thorax

The bony thorax includes the clavicles, sternum, scapula, 12 sets of ribs, and 12 thoracic vertebrae.

Rack of ribs

Ribs consist of bone and cartilage and allow the chest to expand and contract during each breath. All ribs attach to the thoracic vertebrae. The first seven ribs also attach directly to the sternum. The 8th, 9th, and 10th ribs attach to the cartilage of the preceding rib. The 11th and 12th ribs are called *floating ribs* because they don't attach to anything in the anterior thorax.

Respiratory muscles

The diaphragm and the external intercostal muscles are the primary muscles used in breathing. They contract when the patient inhales and relax when the patient exhales.

> Yes, sir, it's the respiratory muscle again. It is asking whether you can slow the breathing rate just a tad . . . something about too much carbon dioxide in the CSF. Shall I put them through?

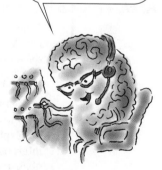

A close look at the mechanics of breathing

These illustrations show how mechanical forces, such as the movement of the diaphragm and intercostal muscles, produce a breath. A plus sign (+) indicates positive pressure, and a minus sign (−) indicates negative pressure.

At rest

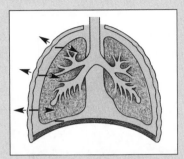

Inhalation

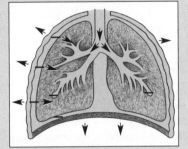

Exhalation

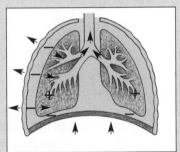

- Inspiratory muscles relax.
- Atmospheric pressure is maintained in the tracheobronchial tree.
- No air movement occurs.

- Inspiratory muscles contract.
- The diaphragm descends and flattens.
- Negative alveolar pressure is maintained.
- Air moves into the lungs.

- Inspiratory muscles relax, causing lungs to recoil to their resting size and position.
- The diaphragm ascends, returning to its resting position.
- Positive alveolar pressure is maintained.
- Air moves out of the lungs.

Message in a nerve

The respiratory center in the medulla initiates each breath by sending messages to the primary respiratory muscles over the phrenic nerve. Impulses from the phrenic nerve adjust the rate and depth of breathing, depending on the carbon dioxide and pH levels in the cerebrospinal fluid (CSF). (See *A close look at the mechanics of breathing*.)

Accessory to breathing

Other muscles, called *accessory muscles*, assist in breathing. Accessory inspiratory muscles include the trapezius, the sternocleidomastoid, and the scalene, which combine to elevate the scapula, clavicle, sternum, and upper ribs. That elevation expands the front-to-back diameter of the chest when use of the diaphragm and intercostal muscles isn't effective.

Expiration occurs when the diaphragm and external intercostal muscles relax. If the patient has an airway obstruction, he may also use the abdominal muscles and internal intercostal muscles to exhale.

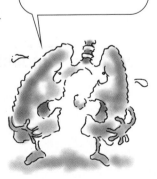

Where are the accessory muscles when you need them?!

Functions of the respiratory system

The functions of the respiratory system are respiration and ventilation to help maintain acid–base balance.

Respiration

Effective respiration requires gas exchange in the tissues (internal respiration) and in the lungs (external respiration). This exchange is vital to maintain adequate oxygenation and acid–base balance. Internal respiration occurs only through diffusion. External respiration occurs through three processes:

Ventilation (gas distribution into and out of the pulmonary airways)

Pulmonary perfusion (blood flow from the right side of the heart, through the pulmonary circulation, and into the left side of the heart)

Diffusion (gas movement from an area of greater to lesser concentration through a semipermeable membrane)

Ventilation

Adequate ventilation depends on the nervous, musculoskeletal, and pulmonary systems for the requisite lung pressure changes. Any dysfunction in these systems increases the work of breathing, diminishing its effectiveness.

Nervous system influence

Although ventilation is largely involuntary, individuals can control its rate and depth. Involuntary breathing results from neurogenic stimulation of the respiratory center in the medulla and the pons of the brainstem. The medulla controls the rate and depth of respiration; the pons moderates the rhythm of the switch from inspiration to expiration. Specialized neurovascular tissue alters these phases of the breathing process automatically and instantaneously.

A special response

When carbon dioxide in the blood diffuses into the CSF, specialized tissue in the respiratory center of the brainstem responds. At the same time, peripheral chemoreceptors in the aortic arch and the bifurcation

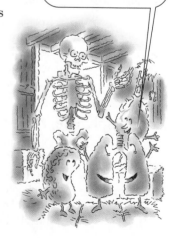

What do ya' say, guys? I bet with a little elbow grease and a couple more windows, we could turn this into the coolest respiration clubhouse!

of the carotid arteries respond to reduced oxygen levels in the blood. When the carbon dioxide level rises or the oxygen level falls noticeably, the respiratory center of the medulla initiates respiration.

Musculoskeletal influence

The adult thorax is a flexible structure—its shape can be altered by contracting the chest muscles. The medulla controls ventilation primarily by stimulating contraction of the diaphragm and the external intercostal, the major muscles of breathing.

I'm inspired!

The diaphragm descends to expand the length of the chest cavity, whereas the external intercostal contracts to expand the anteroposterior and lateral chest diameter. These actions produce changes in intrapulmonary pressure that cause inspiration.

Pulmonary influence

During inspiration, air flows through the right and left mainstem bronchi. The air flow continues into the increasingly smaller bronchi, then into bronchioles, alveolar ducts, alveolar sacs, and finally reaching the alveolar membrane. Many factors can alter airflow distribution, including air flow pattern, volume, and location of the functional reserve capacity (air retained in the alveoli that prevents their collapse during respiration); amount of intrapulmonary resistance; and presence of lung disease.

The path of least resistance

If disrupted, airflow distribution will follow the path of least resistance. For example, an intrapulmonary obstruction or forced inspiration will cause an uneven distribution of air.

Active, then passive

Normal breathing requires active inspiration and passive expiration. Forced breathing, as in cases of emphysema, demands active inspiration and expiration. It activates accessory muscles of respiration, which require additional oxygen to work, resulting in less efficient ventilation with an increased workload.

Noncompliance, resistance, fatigue—oh, my!

Other alterations in airflow, such as changes in compliance (dispensability of the lungs and thorax) and resistance (interference with airflow in the tracheobronchial tree), can also increase oxygen and energy demands and lead to respiratory muscle fatigue.

Just keep going. I'm sure we'll see the path of least resistance soon after the next bend in the road.

Pulmonary perfusion

Optimal pulmonary perfusion aids external respiration and promotes efficient alveolar gas exchange. However, factors that reduce blood flow, such as a cardiac output that's less than average (5 L/minute) and elevated pulmonary and systemic vascular resistance, can interfere with gas transport to the alveoli. Also, abnormal or insufficient hemoglobin (Hgb) picks up less oxygen than is needed for efficient gas exchange.

That's heavy

Gravity can affect oxygen and carbon dioxide transport by influencing pulmonary circulation. Gravity pulls more unoxygenated blood to the lower and middle lung lobes relative to the upper lobes, where most of the tidal volume also flows.

No uniformity

As a result, neither ventilation nor perfusion is uniform throughout the lung. Areas of the lung where perfusion and ventilation are similar have good ventilation-perfusion matching. In such areas, gas exchange is most efficient. Areas of the lung that demonstrate ventilation-perfusion inequality result in less efficient gas exchange.

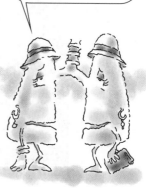

I wasn't aware of any dress code when I signed up for this job. What's all this business about ventilation and perfusion needing to match anyway?

Diffusion

In diffusion, molecules of oxygen and carbon dioxide move between the alveoli and the capillaries. Partial pressure (the pressure exerted by one gas in a mixture of gases) dictates the direction of movement, which is always from an area of greater concentration to one of lesser concentration.

Let's move it!

During diffusion, oxygen moves across the alveolar and capillary membranes, then dissolves in the plasma, and passes through the red blood cell (RBC) membrane. Carbon dioxide moves in the opposite direction. (See *Exchanging gases*, page 300.)

Spaces in between

Successful diffusion requires an intact alveolocapillary membrane. The alveolar epithelium and the capillary endothelium are composed of a single layer of cells. Between these layers are minute interstitial spaces filled with elastin and collagen.

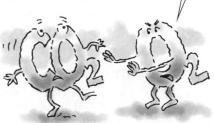

Where do you think you're going? Diffuse yourself in the opposite direction, buddy!

Exchanging gases

Gas exchange occurs very rapidly in the millions of tiny, thin-membraned alveoli within the respiratory units. Inside these air sacs, oxygen from inhaled air diffuses into the blood while carbon dioxide diffuses from the blood into the air and is exhaled. Blood then circulates throughout the body, delivering oxygen and picking up carbon dioxide. Lastly, the blood returns to the lungs to be oxygenated again.

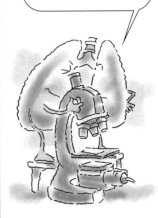

Boy, you're not kidding. Those gases whiz by so quickly. It's like, now you see it, now you don't!

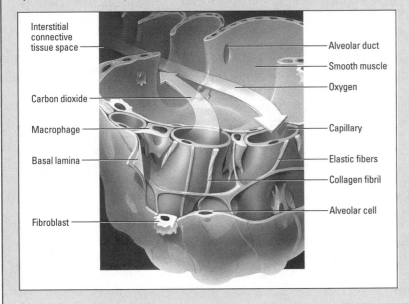

Interstitial connective tissue space

Carbon dioxide

Macrophage

Basal lamina

Fibroblast

Alveolar duct

Smooth muscle

Oxygen

Capillary

Elastic fibers

Collagen fibril

Alveolar cell

From the RBCs to the alveoli

Normally, oxygen and carbon dioxide move easily through all of these layers. Oxygen moves from the alveoli into the bloodstream, where it's taken up by Hgb in the RBCs. From there, it displaces carbon dioxide (the by-product of metabolism), which diffuses from the RBCs into the blood, and then it moves to the alveoli. Most transported oxygen binds with Hgb to form oxyhemoglobin while a small portion dissolves in the plasma (measurable as the partial pressure of oxygen in arterial blood).

Up and down

After oxygen binds to Hgb, the RBCs travel to the tissues. At this point, the blood cells contain more oxygen, and the tissue cells contain more carbon dioxide. Internal

They said to look for oxygen and carbon dioxide exchange in the tissues, but I don't see anything. Think it's a prank?

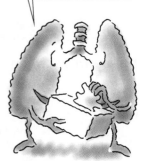

respiration occurs during cellular diffusion, as RBCs release oxygen and absorb carbon dioxide. The RBCs then transport carbon dioxide back to the lungs for removal during expiration.

Acid–base balance

The lungs help maintain acid–base balance in the body by maintaining external and internal respiration. Oxygen collected in the lungs is transported to the tissues by the circulatory system, which exchanges it for the carbon dioxide produced by cellular metabolism. Because carbon dioxide is 20 times more soluble than oxygen, it dissolves in the blood, where most of it forms bicarbonate (base) and smaller amounts form carbonic acid (acid).

And back again

The lungs control bicarbonate levels by converting bicarbonate to carbon dioxide and water for excretion. In response to signals from the medulla, the lungs can change the rate and depth of ventilation.

Maintaining the balance

Such changes maintain acid–base balance by adjusting the amount of carbon dioxide that's lost. For example, in metabolic alkalosis, which results from excess bicarbonate retention, the rate and depth of ventilation decrease so that carbon dioxide is retained. This increases carbonic acid levels. In metabolic acidosis (a condition resulting from excess acid retention or excess bicarbonate loss), the lungs increase the rate and depth of ventilation to exhale excess carbon dioxide, thereby reducing carbonic acid levels.

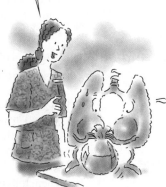

You're hyperventilating . . . just keep breathing slowly into the paper bag and you'll be OK.

Broken balance beam

A patient with inadequately functioning lungs can experience acid–base imbalances. For example, hypoventilation (reduced rate and depth of ventilation) of the lungs, which results in carbon dioxide retention, causes respiratory acidosis. Conversely, hyperventilation (increased rate and depth of ventilation) of the lungs leads to increased exhalation of carbon dioxide and will result in respiratory alkalosis.

Therapy for altered function

When altered respiratory function occurs, such nursing interventions as coughing and deep-breathing exercises, incentive spirometry, chest physiotherapy, and oxygen administration can enhance your patient's respiratory effort and improve oxygen status. Pulse oximetry allows you to monitor your patient's oxygen saturation. Surgical interventions, such as tracheostomy and chest tube insertion, can also improve oxygenation. Proper care of the patient during and after these procedures is vital.

Coughing exercises

Patients who are at risk for developing excess secretions should practice coughing exercises. However, patients who have recently had ear or eye surgery or repair of a hiatal or large abdominal hernia shouldn't do coughing exercises. Also, patients undergoing neurosurgery shouldn't practice coughing exercise postoperatively because intracranial pressure will rise.

If the patient's condition permits, instruct them to sit on the edge of the bed. Provide a small stool if their feet don't touch the floor. Instruct them to bend the legs and lean slightly forward.

Slow and deep

If the patient is scheduled for or recently has had chest or abdominal surgery, teach them how to splint the incision with a pillow before they cough.

In through the nose . . .

Instruct the patient to take a slow, deep breath; they should breathe in through the nose and concentrate on fully expanding the chest.

. . . and out through the mouth

Next, they should breathe out through the mouth and concentrate on feeling the chest sink downward and inward. Then they should take a second breath in the same manner.

Quick, grab the pillow. We have time for one good coughing session before the new CSI episode begins. Don't you just love Sweeps Week?

Once isn't enough

Then, tell them to take a third deep breath and hold it. They should then cough two or three times in a row. (Once isn't enough.) This coughing will clear the breathing passages. Encourage them to concentrate on feeling the diaphragm force out all the air in the chest. Then take three to five normal breaths, exhale slowly, and relax.

Say again?

Have the patient repeat this exercise at least once. After surgery, they will need to perform it at least every 2 hours to help keep the lungs free from secretions. Reassure the patient that the stitches are very strong and won't split during coughing.

Deep-breathing exercises

Advise the patient that performing deep-breathing exercises several times per hour helps keep the lungs fully expanded. To deep-breathe correctly, they must use the diaphragm and abdominal muscles—not just the chest muscles. Tell the patient to practice the following exercises two or three times per day before surgery.

Get comfortable

Have the patient lie on their back in a comfortable position with one hand on the chest and the other over the upper abdomen. Teach them to relax and bend their knees slightly.

Inhale deeply . . .

Instruct the patient to exhale normally. Close their mouth and inhale deeply through the nose, concentrating on feeling the abdomen rise. The chest shouldn't expand. They should hold their breath and count to five.

> Let's go over it again one more time. Exhale normally through your nose . . . close your mouth and inhale deeply through your nose . . .

. . . and then exhale

Next, have the patient purse their lips as though about to whistle and then exhale completely through the mouth, without letting the checks puff out. The ribs should sink downward and inward.

Rest and repeat

After resting several seconds, the patient should repeat the exercise 5 to 10 times. They should also do this exercise while lying on their side, sitting, standing, or turning in bed.

Incentive spirometry

Incentive spirometry involves using a breathing device to help the patient achieve maximal ventilation. The device measures the patient's inspiratory effort (flow rate) in cubic centimeters per second (cc/second). The device encourages the patient to take a deep breath and hold it for several seconds. This deep breath:

- increases lung volume
- boosts alveolar inflation
- promotes venous return
- loosens respiratory secretions.

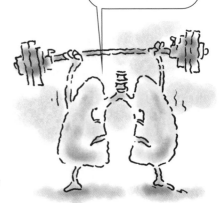

Any exercise that promises to get me back in shape is incentive enough for me.

Longer inflation, less collapse

This exercise also establishes alveolar hyperinflation for a longer time than is possible with a normal deep breath, thus preventing and reversing the alveolar collapse that causes atelectasis and pneumonitis.

What you see is what you get

Devices used for incentive spirometry provide a visual incentive to breathe deeply and encourage slow, sustained maximal inspiration. They can be divided into two types:

Flow incentive spirometer, used for patients at low risk for developing atelectasis

Volume incentive spirometer, used for patients at high risk for developing atelectasis (See *Types of spirometers.*)

Let's get some incentive or float

Flow incentive spirometers contain plastic floats, which rise according to the amount of air the patient pulls through the device when he inhales. Volume incentive spirometers are activated when the patient inhales a certain volume of air. The device then estimates the amount of air inhaled. This device measures lung inflation more precisely and helps you determine whether your patient is inhaling adequately.

You can use a flow incentive spirometer if your patient is at low risk for developing atelectasis—or a volume incentive device, which is more precise, if they are at higher risk.

Benefits

Incentive spirometry benefits the patient on prolonged bed rest, especially the postoperative patient who may regain his normal respiratory pattern slowly because of such predisposing factors as abdominal or thoracic surgery, advanced age, inactivity, obesity, smoking, and decreased ability to cough effectively and expel lung secretions.

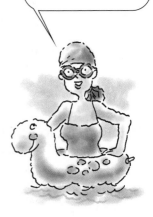

Types of spirometers

Spirometers can be volume incentive or flow incentive.

Volume incentive

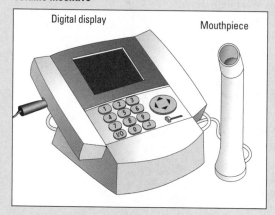

Digital display

Mouthpiece

Flow incentive

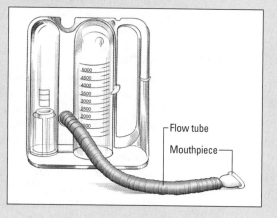

Flow tube

Mouthpiece

What you need

Flow or volume incentive spirometer, as indicated, with sterile disposable tube and mouthpiece (The tube and mouthpiece are sterile on first use and clean on subsequent uses.) ✳ stethoscope ✳ watch

Getting ready

• Assemble the ordered equipment at the patient's bedside.
• Remove the sterile flow tube and mouthpiece from the package, and attach them to the device.
• Set the flow rate or volume goal as determined by the doctor or respiratory therapist and based on the patient's preoperative performance.
• Explain the procedure to the patient, making sure that they understand the importance of performing incentive spirometry regularly to maintain alveolar inflation.

How you do it

• Help the patient into a comfortable sitting or semi-Fowler's position to promote optimal lung expansion. If you're using a flow incentive spirometer and the patient is unable to assume or maintain this position, they can perform the procedure in any position as long as the device remains upright. Tilting a flow incentive spirometer decreases the required patient effort and reduces the exercise's effectiveness.

Do you hear what I hear?

- Auscultate the patient's lungs to provide a baseline for comparison with posttreatment auscultation.
- Instruct the patient to exhale normally and then tell them to insert the mouthpiece and close the lips tightly around it because a weak seal may alter flow or volume readings.

Sustained but maximal

- Tell the patient to inhale as slowly and as deeply as possible. If they have difficulty with this step, tell them to suck as they would through a straw but more slowly. Ask the patient to retain the entire volume of air they inhaled for 3 seconds or, if you're using a device with a light indicator, until the light turns off. This deep breath creates sustained transpulmonary pressure near the end of inspiration and is sometimes called a *sustained maximal inspiration*.
- Tell the patient to remove the mouthpiece and exhale normally. Allow them to relax and take several normal breaths before attempting another breath with the spirometer. Repeat this sequence 5 to 10 times during every waking hour. Note tidal volumes.

Practice pointers

- Evaluate the patient's ability to cough effectively, and encourage coughing after each effort because deep lung inflation may loosen secretions and facilitate their removal. Observe any expectorated secretions.
- Auscultate the patient's lungs and compare findings with the first auscultation.

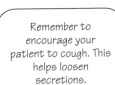

Just a quick listen before we begin with the incentive spirometry exercises. Don't worry, I remembered to warm up the stethoscope first.

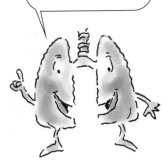

Remember to encourage your patient to cough. This helps loosen secretions.

Chest physiotherapy

Chest physiotherapy is usually performed with other treatments, such as suctioning, incentive spirometry, and administration of such medications as small-volume nebulizer aerosol treatments and expectorants.

Especially important for the bedridden patient, chest physiotherapy improves secretion clearance and ventilation and helps prevent or treat atelectasis and pneumonia, which can hinder recovery. Chest physiotherapy procedures include:

• percussion, which involves cupping the hands and fingers together and clapping them alternately over the patient's lung fields to loosen secretions (also achieved with the gentler technique of vibration)
• vibration, which can be used with percussion or as an alternative to it in a patient who's frail, in pain, or recovering from thoracic surgery or trauma
• postural drainage, which uses gravity to promote drainage of secretions from the lungs and bronchi into the trachea
• deep-breathing exercises, which help loosen secretions and promote more effective coughing
• coughing, which helps clear secretions in the lungs, bronchi, and trachea and prevents aspiration.

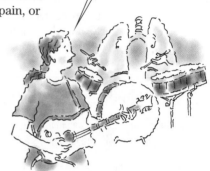

Enough with the percussion already! Let's start our next set with "Good Vibrations." Ready on the two . . . one, two . . .

What you need

Stethoscope ✳ pillows ✳ adjustable hospital bed ✳ emesis basin ✳ facial tissues ✳ suction equipment as needed ✳ equipment for oral care ✳ towel ✳ trash bag ✳ optional: sterile specimen container, supplemental oxygen

Getting ready

• Administer pain medication before the treatment as ordered, and teach the patient to splint his/her incision.
• Auscultate the lungs to determine baseline status, and check the doctor's order to determine which lung areas require treatment.
• Obtain pillows and a tilt board, if necessary.
• Don't schedule therapy immediately after a meal; wait 2 to 3 hours to reduce the risk of nausea and vomiting.
• Make sure the patient is adequately hydrated to facilitate removal of secretions.
• If ordered, administer bronchodilator and mist therapies before the treatment.
• Provide tissues, an emesis basin, and a cup for sputum.
• Set up suction equipment if the patient doesn't have an adequate cough to clear secretions.
• If they need oxygen therapy or are borderline hypoxemic without it, provide adequate flow rates of oxygen during therapy.

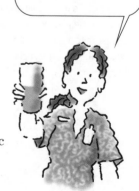

It's important that your patient is well hydrated before beginning chest physiotherapy to facilitate removal of secretions.

How you do it

- Position the patient as ordered. (The doctor usually determines a position sequence after auscultation and chest X-ray review.) Be sure to position the patient so drainage is always oriented toward larger, more central airways.
- If the patient has a localized condition, such as pneumonia in a specific lobe, expect to start with that area first to avoid infecting uninvolved areas. If the patient has a diffuse disorder, such as bronchiectasis, expect to start with the lower lobes and work toward the upper ones. (See *Positioning the patient for postural drainage.*)

Positioning the patient for postural drainage

Postural drainage is most commonly required for the lower lobes of the lung. These illustrations show various postural drainage positions and the lung areas affected by each position.

Lower lobes: Posterior basal segments

Elevate the foot of the bed 30 degrees. Have the patient lie prone with their head lowered. Position pillows under the chest and abdomen. Percuss the lower ribs on both sides of the spine.

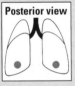
Posterior view

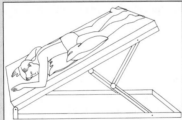

Lower lobes: Anterior basal segments

Elevate the foot of the bed 30 degrees. Instruct the patient to lie on their side with their head lowered. Then place pillows as shown. Percuss with a slightly cupped hand over the lower ribs just beneath the axilla. If an acutely ill patient has trouble breathing in this position, adjust the bed to an angle they can tolerate. Then begin percussion.

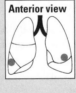
Anterior view

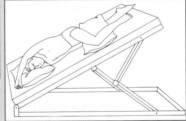

Lower lobes: Lateral basal segments

Elevate the foot of the bed 30 degrees. Instruct the patient to lie on his abdomen with the head lowered and the upper leg flexed over a pillow for support. Then have them rotate a quarter turn upward. Percuss the lower ribs on the uppermost portion of the lateral chest wall.

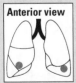
Anterior view

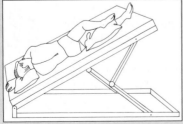

Lower lobes: Superior segments

With the bed flat, have the patient lie on their abdomen. Place two pillows under their hips. Percuss on both sides of the spine at the lower tip of the scapulae.

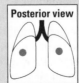
Posterior view

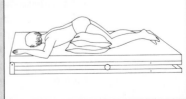

The percussion section

• Place your cupped hands against the patient's chest wall and rapidly flex and extend your wrists, generating a rhythmic, popping sound. (A hollow sound helps verify correct performance of the technique.) (See *Performing percussion and vibration*.)

• Percuss each segment for a minimum of 3 minutes. The vibrations you generate pass through the chest wall and help loosen secretions from the airways.

• Perform percussion throughout inspiration and expiration, and encourage the patient to take slow, deep breaths.

• Don't percuss over the spine, sternum, liver, kidneys, or the female patient's breasts *because you may cause trauma, especially in elderly patients.*

• Percussion is painless when done properly, and the impact is diminished by a cushion of air formed in the cupped palm. This technique requires practice.

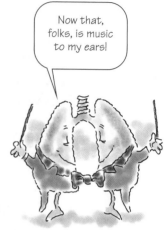

Now that, folks, is music to my ears!

Performing percussion and vibration

To perform *percussion*, hold your hands in a cupped shape, with fingers flexed and thumbs pressed tightly against your index fingers. Percuss each segment for 1 to 2 minutes by alternating your hands against the patient in a rhythmic manner. Listen for a hollow sound on percussion to verify correct technique.

To perform *vibration*, ask the patient to inhale deeply and then exhale slowly through pursed lips. During exhalation, firmly press your fingers and the palms of your hands against the chest wall. Tense your arm and shoulder muscles in an isometric contraction to send fine vibrations through the chest wall. Vibrate during five exhalations over each chest segment.

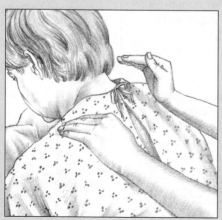

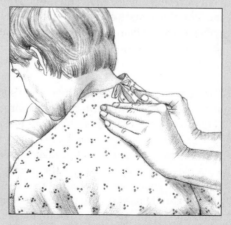

Vibration

- Ask the patient to inhale deeply and then exhale slowly through pursed lips.
- During exhalation, firmly press your fingers and the palms of your hands against the chest wall. Tense the muscles of your arms and shoulders in an isometric contraction to send fine vibrations through the chest wall.
- Repeat vibration for five exhalations over each chest segment.
- When the patient says "ah" on exhalation, you should hear a tremble in their voice.

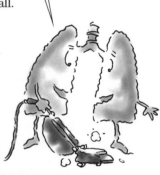

Percussion and vibration can help clean me out and make me feel brand new!

Practice pointers

- Evaluate the patient's tolerance for therapy, and make adjustments as needed. Watch for fatigue, and remember that the patient's ability to cough and breathe deeply diminishes as they tire.
- Assess for difficulty expectorating secretions. Use suction if the patient has an ineffective cough or a diminished gag reflex.
- Provide oral hygiene after therapy; secretions may taste foul or have an unpleasant odor.
- Be aware that postural drainage positions can cause nausea, dizziness, dyspnea, and hypoxemia.
- The patient with chronic bronchitis, bronchiectasis, or cystic fibrosis may need chest physiotherapy at home.

Oxygen therapy

In oxygen therapy, oxygen is delivered by mask, nasal prongs, nasal catheter, or transtracheal catheter to prevent or reverse hypoxemia and reduce the work of breathing. Possible causes of hypoxemia include emphysema, pneumonia, Guillain-Barré syndrome, heart failure, and myocardial infarction. (See *Oxygen delivery systems*.)

Geez, I've been waiting over an hour for the delivery truck to come and pick me up. Where is that guy?

Fully equipped

The equipment depends on the patient's age and condition as well as the required fraction of inspired oxygen (FIO_2). High-flow systems, such as a Venturi mask and ventilators, deliver a precisely controlled air-oxygen mixture. Low-flow systems, such as nasal prongs, a nasal catheter, a simple mask, a partial rebreather mask, and a non-rebreather mask, allow variation in the oxygen percentage delivered based on the patient's respiratory pattern. Children and infants don't tolerate masks. (See *Oxygen delivery in children*, page 313.)

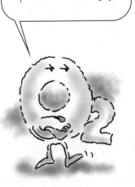

Oxygen delivery systems

Patients may receive oxygen through one of several administration systems, including a nasal cannula, a simple mask, a partial rebreather mask, a nonrebreather mask, a Venturi mask, a continuous positive airway pressure (CPAP) mask, aerosols, and transtracheal oxygen.

Nasal cannula

Oxygen is delivered in concentrations of less than 40% through a plastic cannula in the patient's nostrils.

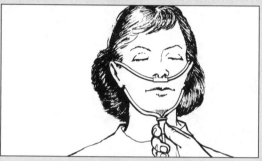

Simple mask

Oxygen flows through an entry port at the bottom of the mask and exits through large holes on the sides of the mask. It delivers oxygen in concentrations of 40% to 60%.

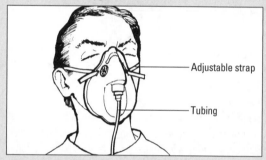

Adjustable strap

Tubing

Partial rebreather mask

The patient inspires oxygen from a reservoir bag along with atmospheric air and oxygen from the mask. The first third of exhaled tidal volume enters the bag; the rest exits the mask. Because air entering the reservoir bag comes from the trachea and bronchi, where no gas exchange occurs, the patient rebreathes the oxygenated air they just exhaled. Oxygen can be administered in concentrations of 40% to 60%.

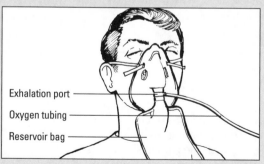

Exhalation port

Oxygen tubing

Reservoir bag

Nonrebreather mask

On inhalation, the one-way inspiratory valve opens, directing oxygen from a reservoir bag into the mask. On exhalation, gas exits the mask through the one-way expiratory valves and enters the atmosphere. The patient breathes air only from the bag. It delivers the highest possible oxygen concentration (60% to 90%) short of intubation and mechanical ventilation.

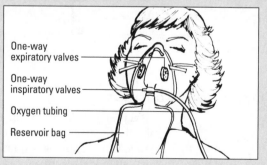

One-way
expiratory valves

One-way
inspiratory valves

Oxygen tubing

Reservoir bag

(continued)

Oxygen delivery systems (continued)

Venturi mask

The mask is connected to a Venturi device, which mixes a specific volume of air and oxygen. It delivers highly accurate oxygen concentration despite the patient's respiratory pattern.

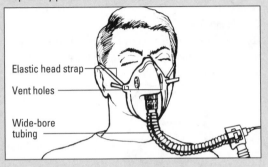

Aerosols

A face mask, hood, tent, or tracheostomy tube or collar is connected to wide-bore tubing that receives aerosolized oxygen from a jet nebulizer. It delivers high-humidity oxygen.

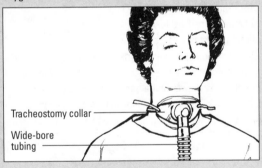

CPAP mask

This system allows the spontaneously breathing patient to receive CPAP with or without an artificial airway.

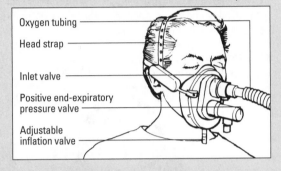

Transtracheal oxygen

The patient receives oxygen through a catheter inserted into the base of their neck in a simple outpatient procedure.

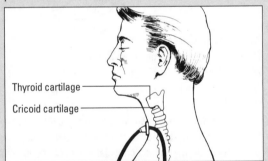

Compare and contrast

Nasal prongs deliver oxygen at flow rates ranging from 0.5 to 6 L/minute. Inexpensive and easy to use, the prongs permit talking, eating, and suctioning—interfering less with the patient's activities than other devices. Even so, the prongs may cause nasal drying and can't deliver high oxygen concentrations. In contrast, a nasal catheter can deliver low-flow oxygen at somewhat higher concentrations, but it isn't commonly used because of discomfort and drying of the mucous membranes.

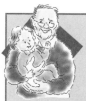

Ages and stages

Oxygen delivery in children

Oxygen delivery to children can be accomplished using an oxygen hood, a nasal cannula or prongs, or a mist tent.

Oxygen hood

Oxygen delivery to an infant is best tolerated by administering it through an oxygen hood, as shown below.

High as well as low concentrations of oxygen can be delivered by an oxygen hood. Remember not to allow the oxygen to flow directly on the infant's face. This cold stimulation can trigger the diving reflex, which results in bradycardia and shunting of blood to the central circulation. Older infants and children can also use a nasal cannula or nasal prongs.

Mist tent

For children beyond infancy, an oxygen tent or mist tent, shown below, is another option. The drawback is that the concentration of the oxygen within the tent is difficult to regulate.

Remember to remove all toys that may produce a spark, including those that are battery operated. Oxygen supports combustion, and the smallest spark can cause a fire.

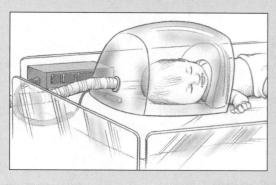

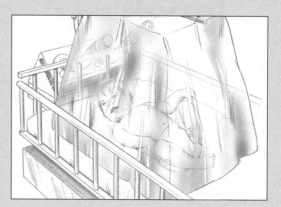

The big cover-up

Masks deliver up to 100% oxygen concentrations but can't be used to deliver controlled oxygen concentrations. In addition, they may fit poorly, causing discomfort, and must be removed to eat. Transtracheal oxygen catheters, used for patients requiring chronic oxygen therapy, permit highly efficient oxygen delivery and increased mobility with portable oxygen systems and avoid the adverse effects of nasal delivery systems. Even so, they may

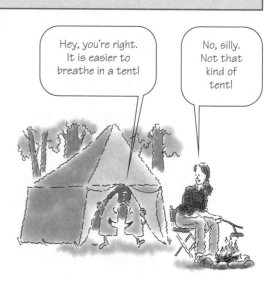

become a source of infection and require close monitoring and follow-up after insertion as well as daily maintenance care.

What you need

The equipment depends on the type of delivery system ordered by the doctor. Equipment includes selections from the following list: oxygen source (wall unit, cylinder, liquid tank, or concentrator) ✳ flow meter ✳ adapter (if using a wall unit) or a pressure reduction gauge (if using a cylinder) ✳ sterile humidity bottle and adapters ✳ sterile distilled water ✳ OXYGEN PRECAUTIONS sign ✳ appropriate oxygen delivery system (a nasal cannula, a simple mask, a partial rebreather mask, or a nonrebreather mask for low flow and variable oxygen concentrations; a Venturi mask; an aerosol mask; a T tube; or a tracheostomy collar) ✳ small diameter and large diameter connection tubing ✳ water-soluble lubricant ✳ gauze pads and tape (for oxygen masks) ✳ jet adapter for Venturi mask (if adding humidity) ✳ optional: oxygen analyzer

Getting ready

• Instruct the patient, their roommates, and visitors not to use improperly grounded radios, televisions, electric razors, or other equipment. Place an OXYGEN PRECAUTIONS sign on the outside of the patient's door.
• Perform a cardiopulmonary assessment, and check that a baseline arterial blood gas (ABG) or oximetry value has been obtained.

How you do it

• Check the patency of the patient's nostrils. (He may need a mask if they're blocked.) Consult the doctor if a change in administration route is necessary.
• Assemble the equipment, check the connections, and turn on the oxygen source. Make sure the humidifier bubbles and oxygen flows through the prongs, catheter, or mask.
• Set the flow rate as ordered. If necessary, have the respiratory care practitioner check the flow meter for accuracy.

Practice pointers

• Periodically perform a cardiopulmonary assessment on the patient receiving any form of oxygen therapy.

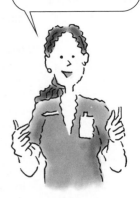

Don't forget basic position changes for patients on bed rest. Practice good skin care to prevent irritation and breakdown caused by oxygen devices.

To everything turn, turn, turn

- If the patient is on bed rest, change their position frequently to ensure adequate ventilation and circulation.
- Provide good skin care to prevent irritation and breakdown caused by the tubing, prongs, or mask.

To humidify or not to humidify . . .

- Be sure to humidify oxygen flow exceeding 3 L/minute to help prevent drying of mucous membranes. However, don't add humidity when using a Venturi mask because water can block the Venturi jets.
- Assess for signs of hypoxia, including decreased level of consciousness (LOC), tachycardia, arrhythmias, diaphoresis, restlessness, altered blood pressure or respiratory rate, clammy skin, and cyanosis. If these occur, notify the doctor, obtain a pulse oximetry reading, and check the oxygen delivery equipment to see whether it's malfunctioning. Be especially alert for changes in respiratory status when you change or discontinue oxygen therapy.

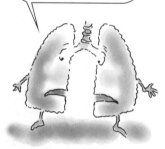

Be aware that too much oxygen can cause oxygen toxicity, with such symptoms as burning, substernal chest pain, and dyspnea.

Check those valves

- If your patient is using a nonrebreather mask, periodically check the valves to see that they're functioning properly. If the valves stick closed, the patient is inhaling carbon dioxide and not receiving adequate oxygen. Replace the mask, if necessary.
- If the patient receives high oxygen concentrations (exceeding 50%) for more than 24 hours, ask about symptoms of oxygen toxicity, such as burning, substernal chest pain, dyspnea, and dry cough. Atelectasis and pulmonary edema may also occur.

Take a deep breath and cough

- Encourage coughing and deep breathing to help prevent atelectasis. Frequently monitor ABG levels, pulse oximetry values, or both, and reduce oxygen concentrations as soon as ABG results or pulse oximetry values indicate it's feasible.
- Use a low flow rate if your patient has chronic pulmonary disease. However, do not use a simple face mask because low flow rates won't flush carbon dioxide from the mask and the patient will rebreathe carbon dioxide. Watch for alterations in LOC, heart rate, and respiratory rate.

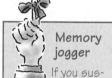

Memory jogger

If you suspect that your patient is becoming hypoxic, check for high, low, clammy, and blue:

↑ heart rate, respiratory rate, and restlessness

↓ level of consciousness

Clammy, diaphoretic skin

Blue coloring (cyanosis)

Go home with the flow

- If the patient needs oxygen at home, the doctor will order the flow rate, the number of hours per day to be used, and the conditions of use. Several types of delivery systems are available, including a tank, concentrator, and liquid oxygen system. The chosen system depends on the patient's needs and the availability and cost of each system. Make sure the patient can use the prescribed system safely and effectively. He'll need regular follow-up care to evaluate their response to therapy.

Pulse oximetry

Pulse oximetry is a noninvasive way to monitor your patient's oxygen saturation to determine how well the patient's lungs are delivering oxygen to their blood. It can be performed continuously or intermittently.

Light reading

In pulse oximetry, two diodes send red and infrared light through a pulsating arterial vascular bed such as the one in the fingertip. A photodetector slipped over the finger measures the transmitted light as it passes through the vascular bed, detects the relative amount of color absorbed by arterial blood, and calculates the exact mix of venous oxygen saturation without interference from surrounding venous blood, skin, connective tissue, or bone. (See *How oximetry works.*)

Symbolically speaking

Pulse oximetry usually denotes arterial saturation values with the symbol Spo_2. Invasively measured arterial oxygen saturation values, such as from ABG analysis, on the other hand, are denoted by the symbol Sao_2.

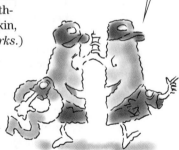

Pulse oximetry measures how well I deliver oxygen to the blood. I'd say I'm right on time, every time!

What you need

Pulse oximetry ✳ alcohol pads ✳ nail polish remover, if necessary

Getting ready

- Review the manufacturer's directions for assembling the oximeter.
- Select a finger for the test. Although the index finger is commonly used, a smaller finger may be selected if the patient's fingers are too large for the equipment.

How oximetry works

The pulse oximetry allows noninvasive monitoring of a patient's arterial oxygen saturation (Sa$_{O2}$) levels by measuring the absorption (amplitude) of light waves as they pass through areas of the body that are highly perfused by arterial blood. Oximetry also monitors pulse rate and amplitude.

Light-emitting diodes in a transducer (photodetector) attached to the patient's body (shown at right on the index finger) send red and infrared light beams through tissue. The photodetector records the relative amount of each color absorbed by arterial blood and transmits the data to a monitor, which displays the information with each heartbeat. If the Sa$_{O2}$ level or pulse rate varies from preset limits, the monitor triggers visual and audible alarms.

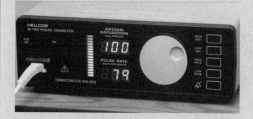

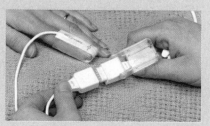

• Make sure the patient isn't wearing false fingernails, and remove any nail polish from the test finger.

How you do it

• Place the transducer (photodetector) probe over the patient's finger so that the light beam sensors oppose each other. If the patient has long fingernails, position the probe perpendicular to the finger, if possible, or clip the fingernail.

Be level with the heart

• Always position the patient's hand at heart level *to eliminate venous pulsations and promote accurate readings.* (See *Pediatric pulse oximetry.*)
• Turn on the power switch. If the device isn't working properly, a beep will sound, a display will light momentarily, and the pulse searchlight will flash. The Sp$_{O2}$ and pulse rate displays will show stationary zeroes. After four to six heartbeats, the Sp$_{O2}$ and the pulse rate displays will supply information with each heartbeat, and the pulse amplitude indicator will begin tracking the pulse.

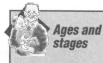

Ages and stages

Pediatric pulse oximetry

If you must monitor arterial oxygen saturation in a neonate or a small infant, wrap the oximeter's probe around the infant's foot so that light beams and detectors oppose each other. For a large infant, use a probe that fits on the great toe and secure it to the foot.

Practice pointers

If oximetry has been performed properly, readings are typically accurate. However, certain factors, such as a low body temperature and low blood pressure, may interfere with accuracy.

Detour over the bridge

• If the patient has compromised circulation in his extremities, you can place a photodetector across the bridge of the nose.
• If an automatic blood pressure cuff is used on the same extremity that's used for measuring SpO_2, the cuff will interfere with SpO_2 readings during inflation.

Problem solving

• Normal SpO_2 levels for pulse oximetry are 95% to 100% for adults and 93.8% to 100% by 1 hour after birth for healthy, full-term neonates. Lower levels may indicate hypoxemia, which warrants intervention. For such patients, the doctor should be notified. (See *Documenting pulse oximetry*.)

Tracheostomy care

Whether a tracheotomy is performed in an emergency situation or after careful preparation, as a permanent measure or as temporary therapy, tracheostomy care has identical goals:
• ensure airway patency by keeping the tube free from mucus buildup
• maintain mucous membrane and skin integrity
• prevent infection
• provide psychological support.

Simple, medium, and complex

The patient may have one of two types of tracheostomy tube:

An uncuffed tube, which may be plastic, polyvinyl chloride, or metal, comes in various sizes, lengths, and styles depending on the patient's needs. It allows air to flow freely around the tracheostomy tube and through the larynx, reducing the risk of tracheal damage.

A fenestrated tube allows speech to be possible through the upper airway when the external opening is

Take note!

Documenting pulse oximetry

In your notes, document the procedure, including the date, time, procedure type, oximetric measurement, and actions taken. Record the readings on appropriate flowcharts, if indicated.

capped and the cuff is deflated. Mechanical ventilation is possible with the inner cannula in place and the cuff inflated.

A cuffed tube is made of plastic or polyvinyl chloride and is disposable. The cuff and the tube won't separate accidentally inside the trachea because the cuff is bonded to the tube. Also, it doesn't require periodic deflating to lower pressure because cuff pressure is low and evenly distributed against the tracheal wall. Although cuffed tubes may cost more than other tubes, they reduce the risk of tracheal damage. (See *Comparing tracheostomy tubes*, page 320.)

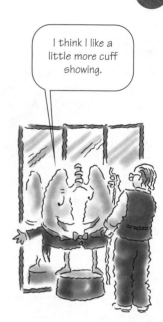

I think I like a little more cuff showing.

Keepin' it clean

Whichever tube is used, tracheostomy care should be performed using aseptic technique until the stoma has healed to prevent infection. For recently performed tracheotomies, use sterile gloves for all manipulations at the tracheostomy site. When the stoma has healed, clean gloves may be substituted for sterile ones.

What you need

For aseptic stoma and outer cannula care

Waterproof trash bag ✳ two sterile solution containers ✳ normal saline solution ✳ hydrogen peroxide ✳ sterile cotton-tipped applicators ✳ sterile 4″ × 4″ gauze pads ✳ sterile gloves ✳ prepackaged sterile tracheostomy dressing (or 4″ × 4″ gauze pad) ✳ equipment and supplies for suctioning and mouth care ✳ materials as needed for cuff procedures and for changing tracheostomy ties (see the following)

For aseptic inner cannula care

All of the preceding equipment plus a prepackaged commercial tracheostomy care set or sterile forceps ✳ sterile nylon brush ✳ sterile, 6″ (15.2 cm) pipe cleaners ✳ clean gloves ✳ a third sterile solution container ✳ disposable temporary inner cannula (for a patient on a ventilator)

Comparing tracheostomy tubes

Tracheostomy tubes are made of plastic or metal and come in uncuffed, cuffed, or fenestrated varieties. Tube selection depends on the patient's condition and the doctor's preference. Make sure you're familiar with the advantages and disadvantages of these commonly used tracheostomy tubes.

Uncuffed
(plastic or metal)

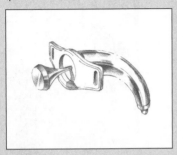

Plastic cuffed
(low pressure and high volume)

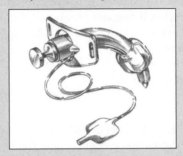

Fenestrated

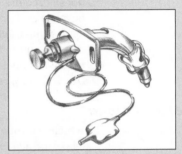

Advantages

• Free flow of air around tube and through larynx
• Reduced risk of tracheal damage
• Mechanical ventilation possible in patient with neuromuscular disease

Disadvantages

• Increased risk of aspiration in adults due to lack of cuff
• Adapter possibly needed for ventilation

Advantages

• Disposable
• Cuff bonded to tube (won't detach accidentally inside trachea)
• Low cuff pressure that's evenly distributed against tracheal wall (no need to deflate periodically to lower pressure)
• Reduced risk of tracheal damage

Disadvantages

• Possibly more expensive than other tubes

Advantages

• Speech possible through upper airway when external opening is capped and cuff is deflated
• Breathing by mechanical ventilation possible with inner cannula in place and cuff inflated
• Easy removal of inner cannula for cleaning

Disadvantages

• Possible occlusion of fenestration
• Possible dislodgment of inner cannula
• Cap removal necessary before inflating cuff

For changing tracheostomy ties
A 30″ (76.2 cm) length of tracheostomy twill tape or prepackaged disposable trach ties ✳ bandage scissors ✳ sterile gloves ✳ hemostat

For emergency tracheostomy tube replacement
Sterile tracheal dilator or sterile hemostat ✳ sterile obturator that fits the tracheostomy tube in use ✳ extra sterile tracheostomy tube and obturator in appropriate size ✳ suction equipment and supplies

In plain sight

Keep these supplies in full view in the patient's room at all times for easy access in case of an emergency. Consider taping an emergency sterile tracheostomy tube in a sterile wrapper to the head of the bed for easy access.

For cuff procedures

A 5- or 10-ml syringe ✳ padded hemostat ✳ stethoscope

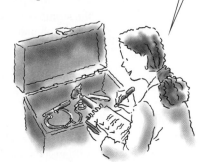

Sterile tracheal dilators . . . check. Sterile obturators . . . check. Sterile tracheostomy tubing . . . check. Suction equipment . . .

Getting ready

• Wash your hands, and assemble all equipment and supplies in the patient's room. Open the waterproof trash bag, and place it next to you *so that you can avoid reaching across the sterile field or the patient's stoma when discarding soiled items.*

Set the table

• Establish a sterile field near the patient's bed (usually on the overbed table), and place equipment and supplies on it. Pour normal saline solution, hydrogen peroxide, or a mixture of equal parts of both solutions into one of the sterile solution containers, then pour normal saline solution into the second sterile container for rinsing.

For the inner

• For inner cannula care, you may use a third sterile solution container to hold the gauze pads and cotton-tipped applicators saturated with cleaning solution. If you'll be replacing the disposable inner cannula, open the package containing the new inner cannula while maintaining sterile technique. Obtain or prepare new tracheostomy ties, if indicated.

How you do it

• Assess the patient's condition *to determine their need for care.*
• Explain the procedure to the patient even if they are unresponsive. Provide privacy.
• Place the patient in semi-Fowler's position (unless it's contraindicated) *to decrease abdominal pressure on the diaphragm and promote lung expansion.*
• Remove humidification or ventilation devices.
• Using sterile technique, suction the entire length of the tracheostomy tube *to clear the airway of any secretions that may hinder oxygenation.* (See "Tracheal suction," page 327.)
• Reconnect the patient to the humidifier or ventilator, if necessary.

Cleaning a stoma and outer cannula

• Put on sterile gloves if you aren't already wearing them.
• With your dominant hand, saturate a cotton-tipped applicator or sterile gauze pad with the cleaning solution. Squeeze out the excess liquid *to prevent accidental aspiration*. Then wipe the patient's neck under the tracheostomy tube flanges and twill tapes.
• Use more pads or cotton-tipped applicators to clean the stoma site and the tube's flanges. Wipe only once with each pad or applicator and then discard it *to prevent contamination of a clean area with a soiled pad*.
• Rinse debris and peroxide (if used) with one or more sterile 4″ × 4″ gauze pads dampened in normal saline solution. Dry the area thoroughly with additional sterile gauze pads, then apply a new sterile tracheostomy dressing.
• Remove and discard your gloves.

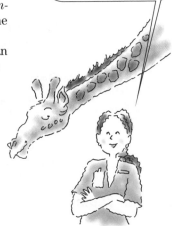

Can you imagine having to suction a patient with a trachea this long?

Cleaning a nondisposable inner cannula

• Put on sterile gloves.

Remove and discard

• Using your nondominant hand, remove and discard the patient's tracheostomy dressing. Then, with the same hand, disconnect the ventilator or humidification device and unlock the tracheostomy tube's inner cannula by rotating it counterclockwise. Place the inner cannula in the container of hydrogen peroxide.

Scrub a dub-dub

How do you agitate a cannula? Poke fun at its skinny neck and goofy socks. Thank you! I'll be here all week. Try the veal!

• Working quickly, use your dominant hand to scrub the cannula with the sterile nylon brush. If the brush doesn't slide easily into the cannula, use a sterile pipe cleaner.
• Immerse the cannula in the container of normal saline solution, and agitate it for about 10 seconds *to rinse it thoroughly*.
• Inspect the cannula for cleanliness. Repeat the cleaning process, if necessary. If it's clean, tap it gently against the inside edge of the sterile container *to remove excess liquid and prevent aspiration*. Don't dry the outer surface *because a thin film of moisture acts as a lubricant during insertion*.
• Reinsert the inner cannula into the patient's tracheostomy tube. Lock it in place, and then

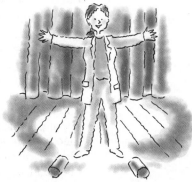

gently pull on it *to make sure it's positioned securely*. Reconnect the mechanical ventilator. Apply a new sterile tracheostomy dressing.
• If the patient can't tolerate being disconnected from the ventilator for the time it takes to clean the inner cannula, replace the existing inner cannula with a clean one and reattach the mechanical ventilator. Then clean the cannula just removed from the patient, and store it in a sterile container for the next time.

Caring for a disposable inner cannula
• Put on clean gloves.
• Using your dominant hand, remove the patient's inner cannula. After evaluating the secretions in the cannula, discard it properly.
• Pick up the new inner cannula, touching only the outer locking portion. Insert the cannula into the tracheostomy and, following the manufacturer's instructions, lock it securely.

Changing tracheostomy ties
• Obtain assistance from another nurse or a respiratory therapist *because of the risk of accidental tube expulsion during this procedure.* Patient movement or coughing can dislodge the tube.
• Wash your hands thoroughly, and put on sterile gloves if you aren't already wearing them.
• If you aren't using commercially packaged tracheostomy ties, prepare new ties from a 30″ (76.2 cm) length of twill tape by folding one end back 1″ (2.5 cm) on itself. Then, with the bandage scissors, cut a ½″ (1.3 cm) slit down the center of the tape from the folded edge.
• Prepare the other end of the tape the same way.

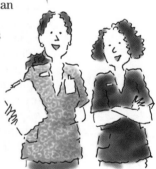

Always elicit the help of another nurse or a respiratory therapist before attempting to change tracheostomy ties.

Cut to order

• Hold both ends together and, using scissors, cut the resulting circle of tape so that one piece is approximately 10″ (25 cm) long and the other is about 20″ (51 cm) long.
• Help the patient into semi-Fowler's position, if possible.
• After your assistant puts on gloves, instruct her to hold the tracheostomy tube in place *to prevent its expulsion during replacement of the ties.* If you must perform the procedure without assistance, fasten the clean ties in place before removing the old ties *to prevent tube expulsion.*
• With the assistant's gloved fingers holding the tracheostomy tube in place, cut the soiled tracheostomy ties with the bandage scissors or untie them and discard the ties. Be careful not to cut the tube of the pilot balloon.

Thread and tie

- Thread the slit end of one new tie a short distance through the eye of one tracheostomy tube flange from the underside; use the hemostat, if needed, to pull the tie through. Then thread the other end of the tie completely through the slit end, and pull it taut so it loops firmly through the flange. *This avoids knots that can cause throat discomfort, tissue irritation, pressure, and necrosis at the patient's throat.*
- Fasten the second tie to the opposite flange in the same manner.

Know your knots

- Instruct the patient to flex their neck while you bring the ties around to the side, and tie them together with a square knot. *Flexion produces the same neck circumference as coughing and helps prevent an overly tight tie.* Instruct your assistant to place one finger under the tapes as you tie them *to ensure that they're tight enough to avoid slippage but loose enough to prevent choking or jugular vein constriction.*
- After securing the ties, cut off the excess tape with the scissors and instruct your assistant to release the tracheostomy tube.
- Make sure the patient is comfortable and can reach the call button easily.
- Check tracheostomy tie tension often on patients with traumatic injury, radical neck dissection, or cardiac failure *because neck diameter can increase from swelling and cause constriction.* Also check neonatal or restless patients frequently *because ties can loosen and cause tube dislodgment.*

Concluding tracheostomy care

- Replace the humidification device.
- Provide oral care as needed because the oral cavity can become dry and malodorous or develop sores from encrusted secretions.

Look closely

- Observe soiled dressings and suctioned secretions for amount, color, consistency, and odor.
- Properly clean or dispose of all equipment, supplies, solutions, and trash according to facility policy.
- Take off and discard your gloves.
- Make sure that the patient is comfortable.

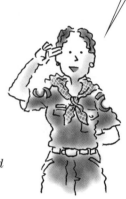

Be prepared by knowing the correct way to thread ties and secure knots. And always remember, patient safety first!

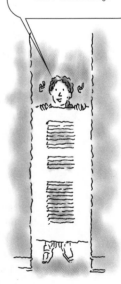

Take a lesson from teenage girls everywhere . . . Frequent dressing changes are, like, sooo necessary!

• Make sure all necessary supplies are readily available at the bedside.
• Repeat the procedure at least once every 8 hours or as needed. Change the dressing as often as necessary regardless of whether you also perform the entire cleaning procedure *because a wet dressing with exudate or secretions predisposes the patient to skin excoriation, breakdown, and infection.*

Deflating and inflating a tracheostomy cuff

• Read the cuff manufacturer's instructions *because cuff types and procedures vary widely.*
• Assess the patient's condition, explain the procedure to them, and be reassuring. Wash your hands thoroughly.

Sit up . . .

• Help the patient into semi-Fowler's position, if possible, or place them in a supine position *so secretions above the cuff site will be pushed up into their mouth if they are receiving positive-pressure ventilation.*

. . . and suction

• Suction the oropharyngeal cavity *to prevent pooled secretions from descending into the trachea after cuff deflation.*
• If a hemostat is present, release the padded hemostat clamping the cuff inflation tubing.

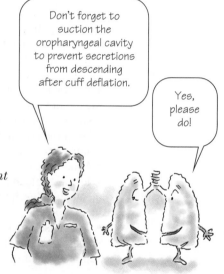

Don't forget to suction the oropharyngeal cavity to prevent secretions from descending after cuff deflation.

Yes, please do!

Slowly deflate . . .

• Insert a 5- or 10-ml syringe into the cuff pilot balloon, and very slowly withdraw all air from the cuff. Leave the syringe attached to the tubing for later reinflation of the cuff. *Slow deflation allows positive lung pressure to push secretions upward from the bronchi. Cuff deflation may also stimulate the patient's cough reflex, producing additional secretions.*
• Remove any ventilation device. Suction the lower airway through any existing tube *to remove all secretions.* Then reconnect the patient to the ventilation device.
• Maintain cuff deflation for the prescribed time. Observe the patient for adequate ventilation, and suction as necessary. If the patient has difficulty breathing, reinflate the cuff immediately by depressing the syringe plunger very slowly. Inject the least amount of air necessary to achieve an adequate tracheal seal.

... then pump back up

- If you're inflating the cuff using cuff pressure measurement, be careful not to exceed 25 mm Hg. Note the exact amount of air needed to inflate the cuff. If pressure exceeds 25 mm Hg, notify the doctor *because you may need to change to a larger size tube, use higher inflation pressures, or permit a larger air leak.* Recommended cuff pressure is about 18 mm Hg.
- After you have inflated the cuff, if the tubing doesn't have a one-way valve at the end, clamp the inflation line with a padded hemostat (to protect the tubing) and remove the syringe.

No sounds allowed

- Check for a minimal-leak cuff seal. You shouldn't feel air coming from the patient's mouth, nose, or tracheostomy site, and a conscious patient shouldn't be able to speak.
- Be alert for air leaks from the cuff itself. Suspect a leak if injection of air fails to inflate the cuff or increase cuff pressure, you're unable to inject the amount of air you withdrew, the patient can speak, ventilation fails to maintain adequate respiratory movement with pressures or volumes previously considered adequate, or air escapes during the ventilator's inspiratory cycle.
- Make sure the patient is comfortable.
- Properly clean or dispose of all equipment, supplies, and trash according to facility policy.
- Replenish any used supplies, and make sure all necessary emergency supplies are at the bedside.

> I suspect I have a leak!

Practice pointers

- Make sure the patient can easily reach the call button and communication aids.
- Keep appropriate equipment at the patient's bedside for immediate use in an emergency.
- Follow facility policy regarding the procedure if a tracheostomy tube is expelled or if the outer cannula becomes blocked. Use extreme caution when attempting to reinsert an expelled tracheostomy tube *because of the risk of tracheal trauma, perforation, compression, and asphyxiation.*

What not to do

- Refrain from changing tracheostomy ties unnecessarily during the immediate postoperative period before the stoma track is well formed (usually 4 days) *to avoid accidental dislodgment and expulsion of the tube.* Unless secretions or drainage is a problem, ties can be changed once per day.

Take note!

Documenting tracheostomy care

When you've finished performing tracheostomy care, record in your notes:
- date and time of the procedure
- type of procedure
- amount, consistency, color, and odor of secretions
- stoma and skin condition
- patient's respiratory status
- tracheostomy tube changes made by the doctor

- duration of cuff deflation
- amount of cuff inflation
- cuff pressure readings, with patient's body position during reading
- complications and nursing actions taken
- patient's tolerance of the procedure
- patient or family teaching provided.

Class time

- If the patient is being discharged with a tracheostomy, start self-care teaching as soon as they are receptive. Teach the patient how to change and clean the tube.
- Assess for complications, which can occur within the first 48 hours after tracheostomy tube insertion. Complications can include hemorrhage at the operative site, causing drowning; bleeding or edema in tracheal tissue, causing airway obstruction; aspiration of secretions; introduction of air into the pleural cavity, causing pneumothorax; hypoxia or acidosis, triggering cardiac arrest; and introduction of air into surrounding tissues, causing subcutaneous emphysema. (See *Documenting tracheostomy care*.)

Tracheal suction

Tracheal suction involves the removal of secretions from the trachea or bronchi by means of a catheter inserted through the mouth or nose, a tracheal stoma, a tracheostomy tube, or an endotracheal (ET) tube.

Say no to pneumonia

In addition to removing secretions, tracheal suctioning also stimulates cough reflex. This procedure helps maintain a patent airway to promote

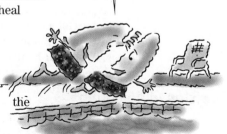

Sometimes, a pool can be fun—but not when it's a pool of secretions. Yuck!

the

optimal exchange of oxygen and carbon dioxide and to prevent pneumonia that results from pooling of secretions. Performed as frequently as the patient's condition warrants, tracheal suction calls for strict aseptic technique.

What you need

Oxygen source (wall or portable unit, and handheld resuscitation bag with a mask, 15-mm adapter, or positive end-expiratory pressure [PEEP] valve, if indicated) ✳ wall or portable suction apparatus ✳ collection container ✳ connecting tube ✳ suction catheter kit or a sterile suction catheter, one sterile glove, one clean glove, and a disposable sterile solution container ✳ gown ✳ mask ✳ goggles ✳ 1-L bottle of sterile water or normal saline solution ✳ sterile water-soluble lubricant (for nasal insertion) ✳ syringe for deflating the cuff of the ET or tracheostomy tube ✳ optional: sterile towel

Getting ready

• Choose the correct suction catheter. The diameter should be no larger than half the inside diameter of the tracheostomy or ET tube *to minimize hypoxia during suctioning.* (A #12 or #14 French catheter may be used for an 8-mm or larger tube.) Place the suction apparatus on the overbed table or bedside stand.
• Attach the collection container to the suction unit and the connecting tube to the collection container. Label and date the normal saline solution or sterile water. Put on gown, mask, and goggles.

How you do it

• Before suctioning, determine whether your facility requires a doctor's order and then obtain one, if necessary.
• Assess the patient's vital signs, breath sounds, and general appearance *to establish a baseline for comparison after suctioning.* Review the patient's ABG values and oxygen saturation levels, if they're available. If you'll be performing nasotracheal suctioning, check the patient's history for a deviated septum, nasal polyps, nasal obstruction, nasal trauma, epistaxis, or mucosal swelling.
• Wash your hands. Explain the procedure to the patient even if he's unresponsive.

Positioned to cough

• Unless contraindicated, place them in semi-Fowler's or high-Fowler's position *to promote lung expansion and productive coughing.*

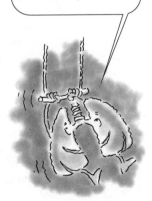

And now for my big finale . . . full-twisting double front layouts dismount from a high-Fowler's position.

• Using your nondominant hand, set the suction pressure according to facility policy. Typically, pressure may be set between 80 and 120 mm Hg or lower for pediatric patients. *Higher pressures may cause traumatic injury.* Occlude the suction port *to assess suction pressure.*

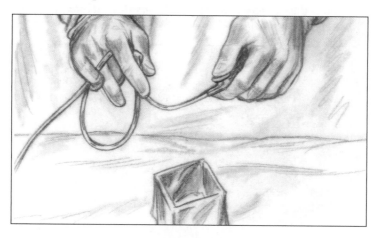

• Remove the top from the normal saline solution or water bottle.
• Open the package containing the sterile solution container.
• Using aseptic technique open the kit and put on gloves or open the suction catheter and gloves, placing the nonsterile glove on your nondominant hand and then the sterile glove on your dominant hand.
• Using your nondominant (nonsterile) hand, pour the normal saline solution or sterile water into the solution container.
• Place a small amount of lubricant on the sterile area *to facilitate passage of the catheter during nasotracheal suctioning.*
• Place a sterile towel over the patient's chest, if desired, *to provide an additional sterile area.*

One hand does this . . .

Using your dominant (sterile) hand, unwrap the catheter. Keep it coiled so it can't touch a nonsterile object. Using your other hand, attach the tubing to the catheter.

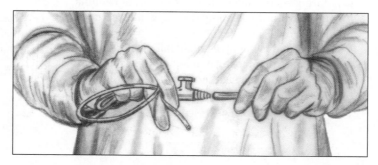

• Dip the catheter tip in the saline solution *to lubricate the outside of the catheter and reduce tissue trauma during insertion.*

• With the catheter tip in the solution, occlude the control valve with your nondominant thumb. Suction a small amount of solution through the catheter *to lubricate the inside of it and facilitate passage of secretions.*

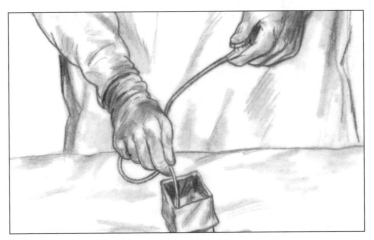

• For nasal insertion of the catheter, lubricate the tip of the catheter with the sterile, water-soluble lubricant *to reduce tissue trauma during insertion.*

• If the patient isn't intubated or is intubated but isn't receiving supplemental oxygen or aerosol, instruct them to take three to six deep breaths *to help minimize or prevent hypoxia during suctioning.*

Add oxygen?

• If the patient isn't intubated but is receiving oxygen, evaluate their need for preoxygenation. If indicated, instruct them to take three to six deep breaths while using the supplemental oxygen. (If needed, the patient may continue to receive supplemental oxygen during suctioning by leaving the nasal cannula in one nostril or by keeping the oxygen mask over the mouth.)

• If the patient is being mechanically ventilated, preoxygenate them using a handheld resuscitation bag, by adjusting the sigh mode on the ventilator, or by adjusting the F_{IO_2} to 0.1. To use the resuscitation

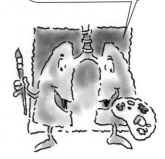

I paint a pretty good picture of the general suctioning procedure, don't I?

bag, set the oxygen flow meter at 15 L/minute, disconnect the patient from the ventilator, and deliver three to six breaths with the resuscitation bag.

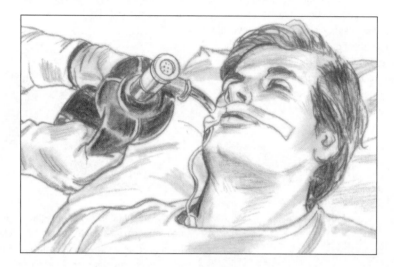

• If the patient is being maintained on PEEP, evaluate the need to use a resuscitation bag with a PEEP valve.

Nasotracheal insertion in a nonintubated patient
• Disconnect the oxygen from the patient, if applicable.
• Using your nondominant hand, raise the tip of the patient's nose *to straighten the passageway and facilitate catheter insertion.*
• Insert the catheter into the patient's nostril while gently rolling it between your fingers *to help it advance through the turbinate.*
• As the patient inhales, quickly advance the catheter as far as possible. *To avoid oxygen loss and tissue trauma,* don't apply suction during insertion.
• If the patient coughs as the catheter passes through the larynx, briefly hold the catheter still and then resume advancement when the patient inhales.

Insertion in an intubated patient
• If you're using a closed system, see *Closed tracheal suctioning,* page 332.
• Using your nonsterile hand, disconnect the patient from the ventilator.

Closed tracheal suctioning

The closed tracheal suction system can ease removal of secretions and reduce patient complications. Consisting of a sterile suction catheter in a clear plastic sleeve, the system permits the patient to remain connected to the ventilator during suctioning. As a result, the patient can maintain the tidal volume, oxygen concentration, and PEEP delivered by the ventilator while being suctioned, which reduces the occurrence of suction-induced hypoxemia.

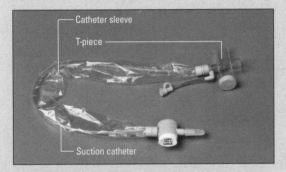

Another advantage of this system is a reduced risk of infection, even when the same catheter is used many times. Because the catheter remains in a protective sleeve, gloves aren't required; however, they're still recommended. The caregiver doesn't need to touch the catheter, and the ventilator circuit remains closed.

Implementation

To perform the procedure, gather a closed suction control valve, a T-piece to connect the artificial airway to the ventilator breathing circuit, and a catheter sleeve that encloses the catheter and has connections at each end for the control valve and the T-piece. Put on personal protective equipment, if you haven't already done so. Then follow these steps:

• Remove the closed suction system from its wrapping. Attach the control valve to the connecting tubing.
• Depress the thumb suction-control valve, and keep it depressed while setting the suction pressure to the desired level.
• Connect the T-piece to the ventilator breathing circuit, making sure that the irrigation port is closed; then connect the T-piece to the patient's endotracheal or tracheostomy tube (as shown below).

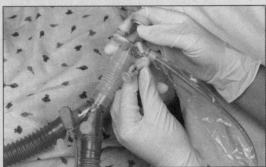

• With one hand keeping the T-piece parallel to the patient's chin, use the thumb and index finger of the other hand to advance the catheter through the tube and into the patient's tracheobronchial tree (as shown below). It may be necessary to retract the catheter sleeve gently as you advance the catheter.

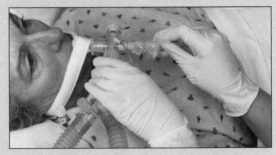

• While continuing to hold the T-piece and control valve, apply intermittent suction and withdraw the catheter until it reaches its fully extended length in the sleeve. Repeat the procedure as necessary.
• After you've finished suctioning, flush the catheter by maintaining suction while slowly introducing normal saline solution or sterile water into the irrigation port.
• Place the thumb control valve in the off position.
• Dispose of and replace the suction equipment and supplies according to facility policy.
• Change the closed suction system every 24 hours to minimize the risk of infection.

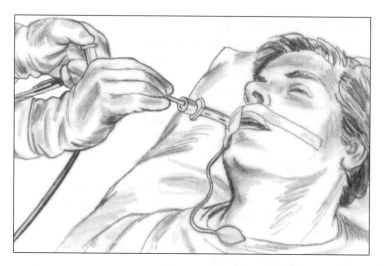

• Using your sterile hand, gently insert the suction catheter into the artificial airway. Advance the catheter, without applying suction, until you meet resistance. If the patient coughs, pause briefly and then resume advancement.

Suctioning the patient

• After inserting the catheter, apply suction intermittently by removing and replacing the thumb of your nondominant hand over the control valve. Simultaneously use your dominant hand to withdraw the catheter as you roll it between your thumb and forefinger. *This rotating motion prevents the catheter from pulling tissue into the tube as it exits, avoiding tissue trauma.* Never suction more than 10 seconds at a time *to prevent hypoxia.*

• If the patient is intubated, use your nondominant hand to stabilize the tip of the ET tube as you withdraw the catheter *to prevent mucous membrane irritation or accidental extubation.*

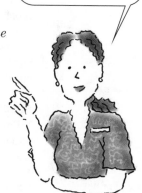

Remember, advance the catheter only while the patient inhales and never suction during insertion.

May the source be with you

• If applicable, resume oxygen delivery by reconnecting the source of oxygen or ventilation and hyperoxygenating the patient's lungs before continuing *to prevent or relieve hypoxia.*

• Observe the patient, and allow them to rest for a few minutes before the next suctioning.

Taking the secret out of secretions

• Observe the secretions. If they're thick, clear the catheter periodically by dipping the tip in the saline solution and applying suction. If the patient's heart rate and rhythm are being monitored, observe for arrhythmias. If they occur, stop suctioning and ventilate the patient.

• Patients who can't mobilize secretions effectively may need to perform tracheal suctioning after discharge.

After suctioning

• After suctioning, hyperoxygenate the patient being maintained on a ventilator with the handheld resuscitation bag by adjusting the F_{IO_2} to 0.1 or by using the ventilator's sigh mode.

• Readjust the F_{IO_2} and, for ventilated patients, the tidal volume to the ordered settings.

• After suctioning the lower airway, assess the patient's need for upper airway suctioning. If the cuff of the ET or tracheostomy tube is inflated, suction the upper airway before deflating the cuff with a syringe. Always change the catheter and sterile glove before resuctioning the lower airway *to avoid introducing microorganisms into the lower airway.*

• Discard the gloves, gown, mask, goggles, and catheter. Clear the connecting tubing by aspirating the remaining saline solution or water. Discard and replace suction equipment and supplies according to facility policy. Wash your hands.

• Auscultate the lungs bilaterally and take vital signs, if indicated, *to assess the procedure's effectiveness.*

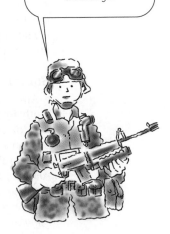

Ten hut! Let's mobilize those secretions now to avoid tracheal suctioning after discharge!

Practice pointers

• Raising the patient's nose into the sniffing position (if the patient's condition allows) helps align the larynx and pharynx and may facilitate passing the catheter during nasotracheal suctioning.

• Don't allow the collection container on the suction machine to become more than three-quarters full *to keep from damaging the machine.*

• Assess the patient for complications of tracheal suctioning. (See *Complications of tracheal suctioning,* page 335, for details.)

• Document the procedure according to facility policy. (See *Documenting tracheal suctioning,* page 335.)

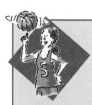

Stay on the ball

Complications of tracheal suctioning

Common complications of tracheal suctioning include:
• hypoxemia and dyspnea from removal of oxygen along with secretions
• altered respiratory patterns from anxiety
• cardiac arrhythmias from hypoxia and vagus nerve stimulation
• tracheal or bronchial trauma from traumatic or prolonged suctioning
• hypoxemia, arrhythmias, hypertension, and hypotension in patients with compromised cardiovascular or pulmonary status
• bleeding in patients with a history of nasopharyngeal bleeding, those receiv-ing anticoagulants, those who have undergone a recent tracheostomy, and those with blood dyscrasias
• further rise in intracranial pressure (ICP) in patients with increased ICP.

Rare complications
Rare complications of suctioning include laryngospasm and bronchospasm. If either occurs, disconnect the suction catheter from the connecting tubing and let the catheter act as an airway. Discuss with the doctor whether the patient should receive bronchodilators or lidocaine to reduce the risk of the complication.

Take note!

Documenting tracheal suctioning

In your notes, document:
• date and time of the procedure
• suctioning technique used
• reason for suctioning
• amount, color, consistency, and odor of secretions
• complications and nursing actions taken
• patient's tolerance of the procedure.

Thoracic drainage

Thoracic drainage uses gravity (and occasionally suction) to restore negative pressure, to remove material that collects in the pleural cavity, or to reexpand a partially or totally collapsed lung. An underwater seal in the drainage system allows air and fluid to escape from the pleural cavity but doesn't allow air to reenter.

Rare sighting

The system is a self-contained, disposable system that collects drainage, creates a water seal, and controls suction. (See *Closed chest drainage systems*, page 336.)

> I wonder whether an aquatic turtle works as well as an underwater seal in these situations.

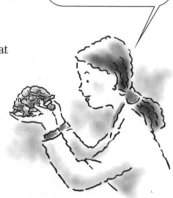

What you need

Closed chest drainage system (Pleur-evac, Argyle, or Thora-Klex system, which can function as a gravity drainage system or be connected to suction to enhance chest drainage) ✳ sterile distilled water

Closed chest drainage systems

One-piece, disposable plastic drainage systems, such as the Pleur-evac, contain three chambers. The drainage chamber is on the right and has three calibrated columns that display the amount of drainage collected. When the first column fills, drainage carries over into the second and, when that fills, into the third. The water-seal chamber is located in the center. The suction-control chamber on the left is filled with water to achieve various suction levels. Rubber diaphragms are provided at the rear of the device to change the water level or remove samples of drainage. A positive-pressure relief valve at the top of the water-seal chamber vents excess pressure into the atmosphere, preventing pressure buildup.

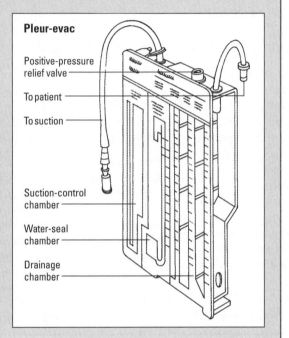

Pleur-evac

Positive-pressure relief valve

To patient

To suction

Suction-control chamber

Water-seal chamber

Drainage chamber

(usually 1 L) ✳ adhesive tape ✳ sterile clear plastic tubing ✳ bottle or system rack ✳ two rubber-tipped Kelly clamps ✳ sterile 50-ml catheter-tip syringe ✳ suction source, if ordered ✳ pain medication, if ordered

Getting ready

Check the doctor's order to determine the type of drainage system to be used and specific procedure details. If appropriate, request the drainage system and suction system from the central supply department. Collect the appropriate equipment, and take it to the patient's bedside.

How you do it

• Explain the procedure to the patient, and wash your hands.
• Maintain sterile technique throughout the entire procedure and whenever you make changes in the system or alter any of the connections *to avoid introducing pathogens into the pleural space.*

Setting up a commercially prepared disposable system

Open the packaged system, and place it on the floor in the rack supplied by the manufacturer *to avoid accidentally knocking it over or dislodging the components.* After the system is prepared, it may be hung from the side of the patient's bed.

> Keep it sterile to prevent pathogens from entering the pleural space.

Just add water

- Remove the plastic connector from the short tube attached to the water-seal chamber. Using a 50–ml catheter-tip syringe, instill sterile distilled water into the water-seal chamber until it reaches the 2–cm mark or the mark specified by the manufacturer.
- If suction is ordered, remove the cap (also called the *muffler* or *atmosphere vent cover*) on the suction-control chamber *to open the vent.* Next, instill sterile distilled water until it reaches the 20–cm mark or the ordered level, and recap the suction-control chamber.
- Using the long tube, connect the patient's chest tube to the closed drainage collection chamber. Secure the connection with tape.
- Connect the short tube on the drainage system to the suction source, and turn on the suction. Gentle bubbling should begin in the suction chamber, *indicating that the correct suction level has been reached.*

Managing closed chest underwater-seal drainage

- Repeatedly note the character, consistency, and amount of drainage in the drainage collection chamber.
- Mark the drainage level in the drainage collection chamber by noting the time and date at the drainage level on the chamber every 8 hours (or more often if there's a large amount of drainage).

> I don't know about you but, to me, gentle bubbling indicates pure relaxation!

Look for the level

- Check the water level in the water-seal chamber every 8 hours. If necessary, carefully add sterile distilled water until the level reaches the 2–cm mark indicated on the water-seal chamber of the commercial system.
- Check for fluctuation in the water-seal chamber as the patient breathes. Normal fluctuations of 2″ to 4″ (5 to 10 cm) reflect pressure changes in the pleural space during respiration. To check for

fluctuation when a suction system is being used, momentarily disconnect the suction system so the air vent is opened, and observe for fluctuation.

Bubbles, bubbles everywhere

• Check for intermittent bubbling in the water-seal chamber. Bubbling occurs normally when the system is removing air from the pleural cavity. If bubbling isn't readily apparent during quiet breathing, have the patient take a deep breath or cough. Absence of bubbling indicates that the pleural space has sealed.

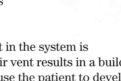

The amount of bubbling can tell you a lot about how efficiently air is being removed from the pleural cavity.

• Check the water level in the suction-control chamber. Detach the chamber from the suction source; when bubbling ceases, observe the water level. If necessary, add sterile distilled water to bring the level to the 20-cm line or as ordered.
• Check for gentle bubbling in the suction-control chamber *because it indicates that the proper suction level has been reached.* Vigorous bubbling in this chamber increases the rate of water evaporation.
• Periodically check that the air vent in the system is working properly. Occlusion of the air vent results in a buildup of pressure in the system that could cause the patient to develop a tension pneumothorax.

Always ready to clamp down

• Be sure to keep two rubber-tipped clamps at the bedside to clamp the chest tube if the system cracks or to locate an air leak in the system. (See *Clamping alert.*)
• Encourage the patient to cough frequently and breathe deeply *to help drain the pleural space and expand the lungs.*
• Tell him to sit upright *for optimal lung expansion* and to splint the insertion site while coughing *to minimize pain.*
• Check the rate and quality of the patient's respirations and auscultate his lungs periodically *to assess air exchange in the affected lung.* Diminished or absent breath sounds may indicate that the lung hasn't reexpanded.

Cause for alarm

• Tell the patient to report breathing difficulty immediately. Notify the doctor immediately if the patient

Stay on the ball

Clamping alert

Never leave a chest tube clamped for longer than 1 minute. Keeping it clamped too long may cause a tension pneumothorax from pressure that builds up when air and fluid can't escape.

develops cyanosis, rapid or shallow breathing, subcutaneous emphysema, chest pain, or excessive bleeding.
• Check the chest tube dressing at least every 8 hours. Palpate the area surrounding the dressing for crepitus or subcutaneous emphysema, which indicates that air is leaking into the subcutaneous tissue surrounding the insertion site. Change the dressing if necessary or according to facility policy.
• Give ordered pain medication as needed for comfort and to help with deep breathing and coughing.

Practice pointers

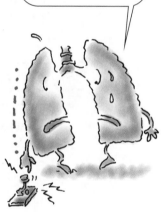

Alert the doctor immediately if the patient develops breathing difficulty or signs of complications.

• Avoid lifting the drainage system above the patient's chest *because fluid may flow back into the pleural space.*
• If excessive continuous bubbling is present in the water-seal chamber, especially if suction is being used, rule out a leak in the drainage system. Try to locate the leak by clamping the tube momentarily at various points along its length. Begin clamping at the tube's proximal end, and work down toward the drainage system, paying special attention to the seal around the connections. If a connection is loose, push it back together and tape it securely. *The bubbling will stop when a clamp is placed between the air leak and the water seal.* If you clamp along the tube's entire length and the bubbling doesn't stop, the drainage unit may be cracked and needs replacement.
• If the drainage collection chamber fills, replace it. To do this, double-clamp the tube close to the insertion site (use two clamps facing in opposite directions), exchange the system, remove the clamps, and retape the bottle connection.

If there's a crack

• If the commercially prepared system cracks, clamp the chest tube momentarily with the two rubber-tipped clamps at the bedside (placed there at the time of tube insertion). Place the clamps close to each other near the insertion site; they should face in opposite directions *to provide a more complete seal.* Observe the patient for altered respirations while the tube is clamped. Then replace the damaged equipment. (Prepare the new unit before clamping the tube.)

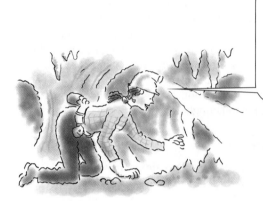

Investigate any excessive bubbling or suspected cracks promptly to rule out problems that can lead to tension pneumothorax.

• Tension pneumothorax may result from excessive accumulation of air, drainage, or both and eventually may exert pressure on the heart and aorta, causing a precipitous fall in cardiac output.

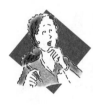

Quick quiz

1. When suctioning a patient, you should:
   A. apply suction intermittently as you insert the catheter.
   B. suction the patient for longer than 10 seconds at a time.
   C. oxygenate the patient's lungs before and after suctioning.
   D. apply suction continuously as you insert the catheter.

Answer: C. Oxygenate the patient before and after suctioning to reduce the risk of hypoxemia, avoid suctioning for longer than 10 seconds, and apply it intermittently as you withdraw the catheter.

2. To help the patient achieve maximal ventilation, use:
   A. an incentive spirometer.
   B. an MDI.
   C. a diskus.
   D. a turbo inhaler.

Answer: A. An incentive spirometer helps achieve maximal ventilation by inducing the patient to take a deep breath and hold it.

3. Which tube permits speech through the upper airway?
A. Uncuffed tube
B. Cuffed tube
C. Fenestrated tube
D. Two-piece tube

Answer: C. A fenestrated tube permits speech through the upper airway when you cap the external opening and deflate the cuff.

4. When performing chest physiotherapy, which of the following uses gravity to promote drainage of secretions?
A. Percussion
B. Postural drainage
C. Vibration
D. Deep-breathing exercises

Answer: B. Postural drainage uses gravity to promote drainage of secretions from the lungs and bronchi into the trachea.

Scoring

☆☆☆ If you answered all four questions correctly, congrats! Your brain is saturated with knowledge of oxygenation.

☆☆ If you answered three questions correctly, good job! Your knowledge of oxygenation is perfusing nicely.

☆ If you answered fewer than three questions correctly, don't despair! Take a deep breath to reoxygenate those tissues, and try again.

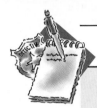

13

Self-care and hygiene

Just the facts

In this chapter, you'll learn:

♦ various methods for determining a patient's ability to perform activities of daily living

♦ factors that affect self-care

♦ ways that hygiene affects health

♦ common hygiene practices.

Learning about self-care and hygiene

Hygiene means performing practices that promote health through personal cleanliness. Those practices include bathing, cleaning and maintaining fingernails and toenails, shampooing and grooming hair, oral care, feeding, and toileting. Hygiene also refers to caring for assistive devices, including hearing aids, eyeglasses, contacts, and such dental appliances as dentures and removable dental bridges.

Many factors influence a person's hygiene practices and ability to perform them. A person's age, gender, personal preferences, socioeconomic status, and religious or cultural practices commonly affect his or her approach to self-care. Physical limitations, body image, or changes in health status can also affect a person's ability to attend to personal care needs. Nurses need to be mindful of how these factors affect self-care yet encourage patients to perform hygiene and self-care whenever possible.

> Hygiene practices can vary because of a person's age, gender, religion, culture, physical limitations, and changes in health.

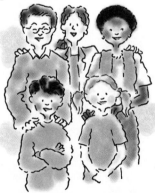

I want to do it myself!

The inability to perform self-care and attend to hygiene needs can be very embarrassing as well as frustrating for a patient, especially when they are an adult. A young child is accustomed to having an adult help with brushing teeth, combing hair, toileting, or bathing, but an older adult may feel a loss of dignity and independence when needing assistance.

I feel pretty, oh so pretty

The ability to independently perform self-care and hygiene procedures enhances a person's emotional well-being and health status. In fact, one of the goals of nursing is to help patients to learn or relearn self-care activities to achieve as much independence as possible with activities of daily living.

> Look, I did this all by myself! I feel great!

Normal self-care patterns

Daily self-care and hygiene routines are largely based on personal and cultural preferences. Many patients are accustomed to a morning routine of rising from sleep, then brushing their teeth, bathing, and dressing. Men may shave or trim facial hair and women may put on makeup as part of this routine.

Throwing a monkey wrench into the works

Illness and hospitalization can affect how and when these daily practices are carried out. Paying attention to a patient's usual routine schedule or what he considers normal self-care activity can help you determine which areas are problematic and when the patient needs your assistance. By doing so, you'll help the patient establish a routine that's as close to normal as possible.

A cool tool

The Katz index is a widely used tool for evaluating a patient's ability to perform daily personal care activities. The tool ranks a patient's ability to perform six functions:

bathing

dressing

toileting

transfer

continence

feeding. (See *Katz index of activities of daily living*, page 344.)

> I don't do mornings well . . . especially on weekends and holidays!

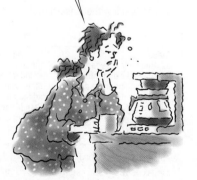

Katz index of activities of daily living

The Katz index of activities of daily living describes a patient's functional level at a specific point in time and objectively scores performance on a three-point scale.

Evaluation form   Name: *Harry Wilson*   Date: *January 14, 2006*

For each area of functioning listed below, check the description that applies. (The word "assistance" means supervision, direction, or personal assistance.)

Bathing: Sponge bath, tub bath, or shower

| ☑ Receives no assistance (gets into and out of tub by self if tub is the usual means of bathing) | ☐ Receives assistance in bathing only one part of the body (such as the back or a leg) | ○ Receives assistance in bathing more than one part of the body (or not bathed) |

Dressing: Gets clothes from closets and drawers, including underclothes and outer garments, and uses fasteners, including suspenders, if worn

| ☑ Gets clothes and gets completely dressed without assistance | ☐ Gets clothes and gets dressed without assistance except for tying shoes | ○ Receives assistance in getting clothes or in getting dressed or stays partly or completely undressed |

Toileting: Goes to the toilet room for bowel movement or urination, cleans self afterward, and arranges clothes

| ☑ Goes to toilet room, cleans self, and arranges clothes without assistance (may use an object for support, such as a cane, walker, or wheelchair, and may manage a night bedpan or commode, emptying it in the morning) | ○ Receives assistance in going to toilet room or in cleaning self or arranging clothes after elimination or in use of night bedpan or commode | ○ Doesn't go to toilet room for the elimination process |

Transfer

| ☑ Moves into and out of bed as well as into and out of chair without assistance (may use an object, such as a cane or walker, for support) | ○ Moves into or out of bed or chair with assistance | ○ Doesn't get out of bed |

Continence

| ☑ Controls urination and bowel movement completely by self | ☑ Has occasional accidents | ○ Supervision helps keep control of urination or bowel movement, a catheter is used, or patient is incontinent |

Feeding

| ☑ Feeds self without assistance | ☐ Feeds self except for assistance in cutting meat or buttering bread | ○ Receives assistance in feeding or is partly or completely fed through tubes or by I.V. fluids |

Index
☐ Indicates independence
○ Indicates dependence
Other: Dependent in at least two functions but not classifiable as C, D, E, or F

A: Independent in all six functions
B: Independent in all but one of these functions and one additional function
C: Independent in all but bathing and one additional function

D: Independent in all but bathing, dressing, and one additional function
E. Independent in all but bathing, dressing, toileting, and one additional function

F. Independent in all but bathing, dressing, toileting transferring, and one additional function
G. Dependent in all six functions

Evaluator: *B. James, RN*

Factors affecting self-care

Many factors can affect a patient's ability to perform self-care and hygiene, including:
- vision impairment
- activity intolerance or weakness from a past medical condition or a current illness
- mental impairment due to age or a psychiatric condition that alters cognitive ability
- pain or discomfort from surgery or disease
- neuromuscular impairment such as a stroke
- skeletal impairment, such as a fracture or joint replacement
- medically prescribed activity restriction such as a pregnant patient on bedrest
- therapeutic procedure that restrains physical activity, such as a cast application or an I.V. infusion that restricts his movement
- environmental barriers, such as financial restraints that may prevent the patient from affording shampoo, shaving supplies, or clean clothes or the resources to wash them
- psychological barriers such as a reluctance to ask for help.

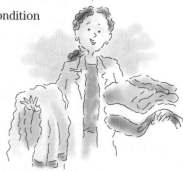

Hygiene and the body

Most hygiene practices help to maintain or restore healthy skin, mucous membranes, hair, and nails.

The integumentary system

The skin, also called the *integumentary system*, covers the internal structures of the body and protects them from the external world. Intact, healthy skin is important for preventing infection. Regular bathing removes excess oil, perspiration, and bacteria from the skin surface.

The skinny on skin

The skin is the body's largest organ and carries out several important functions, including:
- protecting the tissues from trauma and bacteria
- preventing the loss of water and electrolytes from the body
- sensing temperature, pain, touch, and pressure

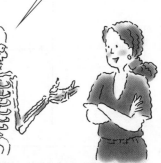

• regulating body temperature through sweat production and evaporation
• synthesizing vitamin D
• promoting wound repair by allowing cell replacement of surface wounds.

Layers of the skin

The skin consists of two distinct layers: the epidermis and the dermis. Subcutaneous tissue lies beneath these layers. The epidermis—the outer layer—is made of squamous epithelial tissue. It's thin and contains no blood vessels. The two major layers of the epidermis are the stratum corneum—the most superficial layer—and the deeper basal cell layer or stratum germinativum. (See *What's in your skin.*)

What's in your skin

This cross-section of the skin illustrates major skin structures.

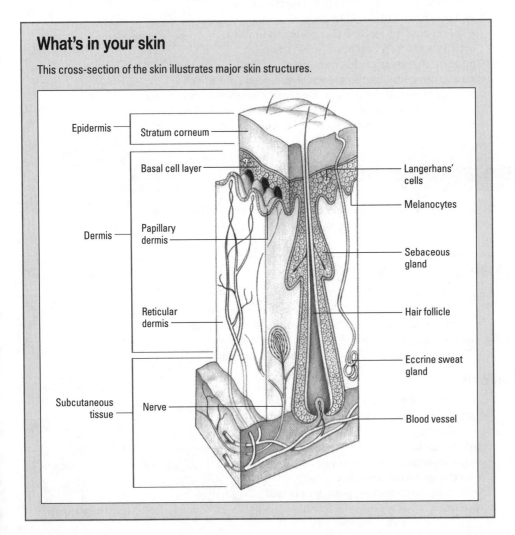

Migrant workers

The stratum corneum is made up of cells that form in the basal cell layer, then migrate to the skin's outer surface, and die as they reach the surface. However, because epidermal regeneration is continuous, new cells are constantly being produced.

Melon color's all the rage this season!

The basal cell layer contains melanocytes, which produce melanin and are responsible for skin color. Hormones, the environment, and heredity influence melanocyte production. Because melanocyte production is greater in some people than in others, skin color varies considerably.

> You don't need an oracle to understand how integral the matrix and connective tissue are to a person's dermis.

Laying it on thick

The dermis—the thick, deeper layer of the skin—consists of connective tissue and an extracellular material called *matrix*, which contributes to the skin's strength and pliability. Blood vessels, lymphatic vessels, nerves, and hair follicles are located in the dermis, as are sweat and sebaceous glands. Because it's well supplied with blood, the dermis delivers nutrition to the epidermis. In addition, wound healing and infection control take place in the dermis.

Give the glands a hand!

Sebaceous glands, found primarily in the skin of the scalp, face, upper body, and genital region, are part of the same structure that contains the hair follicles. Their main function is to produce sebum, which is secreted onto the skin or into the hair follicle to make the hair shiny and pliant.

There are two types of sweat glands:
- *Eccrine glands* are located over most of the body. In response to thermal stress, eccrine glands produce a watery fluid that helps regulate body temperature. Eccrine glands in the palms and soles secrete fluid in response to emotional stress.
- *Apocrine glands* secrete a milky substance and open into the hair follicle. They're located mainly in the axillae and the genital areas. Inadequate hygiene allows bacteria to break down the fluid causing body odor.

Hair

Hair is formed from keratin and produced by matrix cells in the dermal layer. Each hair lies in a hair follicle and receives nourishment from a papilla, a loop of capillaries at the base of the follicle. At the lower end of the hair shaft is the hair bulb. The hair bulb contains melanocytes, which determine hair color.

Each hair is attached at the base to a smooth muscle called the *arrector pili*. This muscle contracts during emotional stress or exposure to cold and elevates the hair, causing goose bumps.

Hair today, gone tomorrow

As a person ages, melanocyte function declines, producing light or gray hair, and the hair follicle itself becomes drier as sebaceous gland function decreases. Hair growth declines, so the amount of body hair decreases. Balding, which is genetically determined in younger individuals, occurs in many people as a normal result of aging.

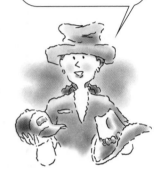

A person can't have too many hats . . . at least that's what Grandpa always says.

Nails

Nails are formed when epidermal cells are converted into hard plates of keratin. The nails are made up of the nail root (or nail matrix), nail plate, nail bed, lunula, nail folds, and cuticle.

What's on your plate?

The nail plate is the visible, hardened layer that covers the fingertip. The plate is clear with fine longitudinal ridges. The pink color results from blood vessels underlying vascular epithelial cells.

What is the matrix?

The nail matrix is the site of nail growth. It's protected by the cuticle. At the end of the matrix is the white, crescent-shaped area, the lunula, which extends beyond the cuticle.

Not hard as nails anymore

With age, nail growth slows and the nails become brittle and thin. Longitudinal ridges in the nail plate become more pronounced, making the nails prone to splitting. Also, the nails lose their luster and become yellowed.

Oral cavity

The mouth (also called the *buccal cavity* or *oral cavity*) contains glands that secrete saliva to moisten food for mechanical breakdown. Proper hygiene practices in the care of mucous membranes and teeth also contribute to optimal health.

Teeth

Teeth are considered accessory digestive organs. Upper teeth are anchored in the alveoli or sockets of the left and right maxillae; lower teeth, in the alveoli of the mandible. The tooth consists of enamel, dentin, and pulp.

Those pearly whites

All exposed surfaces of the teeth are covered with enamel, the hardest tissue of the body. Enamel protects the underlying layers from food acids, heat, and cold. It's shiny, hard, nonliving tissue that can't repair itself after being damaged.

Second hardest

Dentin is the second hardest tissue in the body. It's the yellow substance under tooth enamel. Millions of tiny canals contain nerve fibers and cells that form the dentin. Dentin has a slight flexibility that protects teeth from breaking during chewing.

Deep inside

Pulp is the innermost part of the tooth. It holds tiny nerves and blood vessels. The root canal is a conduit for nerve vessels between the tooth socket and the pulp area. A thin protective layer of cementum covers each tooth root. Cementum is similar to bone; it's alive and can repair itself.

Performing hygiene practices

Hygiene practices help maintain personal cleanliness and healthy integumentary structures. Most patients routinely perform bathing, shaving, brushing the teeth, shampooing, and caring for nails. Always ask the patient their personal hygiene practices before planning the care.

Giving a bed bath

A complete bed bath cleans the skin, stimulates circulation, provides mild exercise, and promotes comfort. Bathing also allows you to assess your patient's skin condition, joint mobility, and muscle strength. Depending on her overall condition and duration of hospitalization, your patient may have a complete or partial bath daily. A partial bath—including hands, face, axillae, back, genitalia, and anal region—may be more suitable than a complete bath for someone with dry, fragile skin or extreme weakness. It also can be given to supplement a complete bath when a patient has diaphoresis or incontinence.

Most people routinely perform bathing and other hygiene practices. I know I bathe as often as I can—purely for the health effects, of course!

What you need

Bath basin ✳ bath blanket ✳ soap ✳ towel ✳ washcloth ✳ skin lotion ✳ orangewood stick ✳ gloves ✳ deodorant ✳ optional: bath oil, perineal pad, abdominal (ABD) pad, and linen-saver pad

Getting ready

• Adjust the temperature of the patient's room, and close any doors or windows to prevent drafts.
• Determine the patient's preference for soap or other hygiene aids because some patients are allergic to soap or prefer bath oil or lotions. Assemble the equipment on an overbed table or bedside stand.

Can you help, please?

• Tell the patient you'll be giving them a bath, and provide privacy. If the patient's condition permits, encourage them to assist with bathing to provide exercise and promote independence.
• Fill the bath basin two-thirds full of warm water (about 115° F [46° C]), and bring it to the patient's bedside. If a bath thermometer isn't available, test the water temperature carefully with your elbow to avoid scalding or chilling the patient; the water should feel comfortably warm.
• If the bed will be changed after the bath, remove the top linen. If not, fanfold it to the foot of the bed.
• Raise the patient's bed to a comfortable working height to avoid back strain. Keep the side rail away from you raised. Offer him or her a bedpan or urinal.
• Put on gloves. Position the patient supine, if possible, and move the patient close to you.
• Remove the patient's gown and other articles, such as elastic stockings, elastic bandages, and restraints (as ordered). Cover her with a bath blanket *to provide warmth and privacy.*

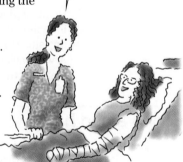

Try to get your patient to help with their bath. It's one way to provide exercise and promote independence.

How you do it

• Fold the washcloth into a mitt on your hand so there are no loose ends *because loose ends can cool quickly and drag across the patient, making her feel cold and uncomfortable.* (See *Making a washcloth mitt.*)

Chin up

• Place a towel under the patient's chin. To wash the face, begin with the eyes, working from the inner to the outer canthus without soap. Use a separate section of the washcloth for each eye to avoid spreading ocular infection.

Making a washcloth mitt

Follow these steps to fold a washcloth into a mitt so that there are no loose ends to drag across the patient's skin. Loose ends cool quickly and can chill the patient.

Fold the washcloth in thirds over your hand, as shown below.

Straighten the folded washcloth, as shown.

Fold the ends over your hand and tuck the loose ends of the washcloth over your palm.

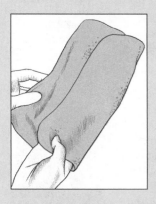
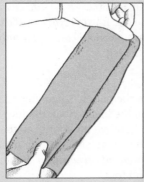
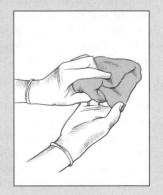

• If the patient tolerates soap, apply it to the cloth, and wash the rest of the face, ears, and neck, using firm, gentle strokes. Rinse thoroughly *because residual soap can cause itching and dryness*. Then dry the area thoroughly, taking special care in skin folds and creases. Observe the skin for irritation, scaling, or other abnormalities.

No tickling

• Turn down the bath blanket, and drape the patient's chest with a bath towel (uncover one side of the chest at a time, beginning with the far side). While washing, rinsing, and drying the chest and axillae, observe the patient's respirations. Use firm strokes to avoid tickling the patient. If the patient tolerates deodorant, apply it.
• Place a bath towel beneath the patient's arm farthest from you. Then bathe the arm, using long, smooth strokes and moving from wrist to shoulder *to stimulate venous circulation*.

Manicure anyone?

• If possible, soak the patient's hand in the basin *to remove dirt and soften nails*. Clean the patient's fingernails with the orangewood stick, if necessary. Observe the color of the hand

Observe the skin for irritation, scaling, or other abnormalities. Unfortunately, ladies, for most of us, wrinkles aren't abnormal—so they don't count!

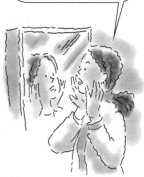

and nail beds *to assess peripheral circulation*. Follow the same procedure for the other arm and hand.

• Turn down the bath blanket to expose the patient's abdomen and groin, keeping a bath towel across the chest *to prevent chills*. Bathe, rinse, and dry the abdomen and groin while checking for abdominal distention or tenderness. Then turn back the bath blanket *to cover the patient's chest and abdomen*.

• Uncover the leg farthest from you, and place a bath towel under it. Use a bath sheet to cover the perineum. Flex this leg and bathe it, moving from ankle to hip *to stimulate venous circulation*. Don't massage the leg, however, *to avoid dislodging any existing thrombus, possibly causing a pulmonary embolus*. Rinse and dry the leg.

> Did I just hear someone say "foot soak"? Bring on the basin!

Ah, a foot soak!

• If possible, place a basin on the patient's bed, flex the leg at the knee, and place the foot in the basin. Soak the foot, and then wash and rinse it thoroughly. Remove the foot from the basin, dry it, and clean the toenails. Observe skin condition and color during cleaning *to assess peripheral circulation*. Repeat the procedure for the other leg and foot.

• Cover the patient with the bath blanket *to prevent chilling*. Then lower the bed and raise the side rails *to ensure patient safety while you change the bath water*.

No chill, thank you!

• When you return, roll the patient away from you, to her side or stomach, place a towel beneath her, and cover her *to prevent chilling*. Bathe, rinse, and dry her back and buttocks.

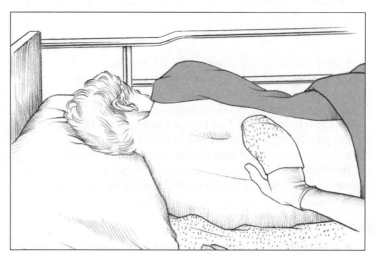

- Massage the patient's back with lotion, paying special attention to bony prominences. Check for redness, abrasions, and pressure ulcers. Do not massage reddened, bony prominences *because this can lead to further tissue damage.*
- Bathe the anal area from front *to back to avoid contaminating the perineum.* Rinse and dry the area well.

Remember front to back

- After lowering the bed and raising the side rails *to ensure the patient's safety,* change the bath water again. Then turn the patient on her back and bathe the genital area thoroughly but gently, using a different section of the washcloth for each downward stroke. Bathe from front to back, avoiding the anal area. Rinse thoroughly and pat dry.
- If applicable, perform indwelling urinary catheter care. Apply perineal pads or scrotal supports as needed.

Dressed to heal

- Dress the patient in a clean gown, and reapply elastic bandages, elastic stockings, or restraints removed before the bath.
- Remake the bed or change the linens, and remove the bath blanket.
- Place a bath towel beneath the patient's head *to catch loose hair,* and then brush and comb his or her hair.
- Return the bed to its original position, and make the patient comfortable.
- Carry soiled linens to the hamper with outstretched arms. *To avoid spreading microorganisms,* don't let soiled linens touch your clothing. Remove gloves.

Practice pointers

- Change the water as often as necessary *to keep it warm and clean.*
- Remove and dispose of gloves appropriately. Wash your hands.

Watch the powder puff

- Carefully dry creased skinfold areas—for example, under breasts; in the groin area; and between fingers, toes, and buttocks. Dust these areas lightly with powder after drying *to reduce friction.* Use powder sparingly *to avoid caking and irritation and provoking coughing in patients with respiratory disorders.*
- If the patient has very dry skin, use bath oil instead of soap. No rinsing is necessary. Warm the lotion before using it for back massage *because cold lotion can startle the patient and induce muscle tension and vasoconstriction.* (See "Providing back care," page 356.)

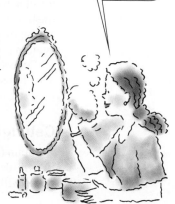

Remember, a little powder goes a long way.

- A bag bath involves the use of 8 to 10 premoistened, warmed, disposable cloths contained in a plastic bag or prepackaged pouch. The cloths contain a no-rinse surfactant instead of soap. Prior to use, the cloths are warmed in a microwave or a special warming unit supplied by the manufacturer. A separate cloth is used *to wash each part of the body.* A bag bath saves time compared to the conventional bed bath *because no rinsing is required.*
- To improve circulation, maintain joint mobility, and preserve muscle tone, move the body joints through their full range of motion during the bath.
- If the patient is incontinent, loosely tuck an ABD pad between their buttocks and place a linen-saver pad under them to absorb fecal drainage. Together, these pads will help prevent skin irritation and reduce the number of linen changes.

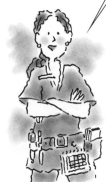

What will they think of next?! A bag bath comes in mighty handy when time is of the essence. It's another good hygiene tool!

Performing perineal care

Perineal care, which includes care of the external genitalia and the anal area, should be performed during the daily bath and, if necessary, at bedtime and after urination and bowel movements. The procedure promotes cleanliness and prevents infection. It also removes irritating and odorous secretions, such as smegma, a cheeselike substance that collects under the foreskin of the penis and on the inner surface of the labia. For the patient with perineal skin breakdown, frequent bathing followed by application of an ointment or cream aids healing.

Standard precautions must be followed when providing perineal care, with due consideration given to the patient's privacy.

It's important to maintain your patient's privacy during bath time. So, if you'll excuse us for a few minutes . . .

What you need

Gloves ✳ washcloths ✳ clean basin ✳ mild soap ✳ bath towel ✳ bath blanket ✳ toilet tissue ✳ linen-saver pad ✳ trash bag ✳ optional: bedpan, perineal bottle, antiseptic soap, petroleum jelly, zinc oxide cream, vitamin A and D ointment, and an ABD pad

Following genital or rectal surgery, you may need to use sterile supplies, including sterile gloves, gauze, and cotton balls.

Getting ready

- Obtain ointment or cream, as needed. Fill the basin two-thirds full with warm water. Also fill the perineal bottle with warm water, if needed.

- Assemble equipment at the patient's bedside, and provide privacy.
- Wash your hands thoroughly, put on gloves, and explain to the patient what you're about to do.

How you do it

- Adjust the bed to a comfortable working height *to prevent back strain*, and lower the head of the bed, if allowed. Lower the side rail closest to you.
- Provide privacy and help the patient to a supine position. Place a linen-saver pad under the patient's buttocks *to protect the bed from stains and moisture*.

Perineal care for the female patient

- *To minimize the patient's exposure and embarrassment*, place the bath blanket over her with corners head to foot and side to side. Wrap each leg with a side corner, tucking it under the hip. Then fold back the corner between the legs *to expose the perineum*.
- Ask the patient to bend her knees slightly and to spread her legs. Separate her labia with one hand and wash with the other, using gentle downward strokes from the front to the back of the perineum *to prevent intestinal organisms from contaminating the urethra or vagina*. Avoid the area around the anus, and use a clean section of washcloth for each stroke by folding each used section inward. *This prevents the spread of contaminated secretions or discharge*.

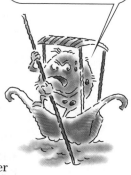

"Downward strokes . . . front to back . . . fold each section inward . . ." Yadda, yadda, yadda. Nurses—always coming up with some new scheme to ruin my good time!

Rinse and pat dry

- Using a clean washcloth, rinse thoroughly from front to back because soap residue can cause skin irritation. Pat the area dry with a bath towel because moisture can also cause skin irritation and discomfort.
- Apply ordered ointments or creams.
- Turn the patient on her side to Sims' position, if possible, *to expose the anal area*.
- Clean, rinse, and dry the anal area, starting at the posterior vaginal opening and wiping from front to back.
- Apply ordered ointments or creams.

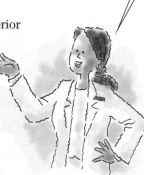

To minimize embarrassing a male patient when providing perineal care, drape his legs to ensure privacy and begin cleaning in a matter-of-fact way.

Perineal care for the male patient

- Drape the patient's legs to minimize exposure and embarrassment, and expose the genital area.
- Hold the shaft of the penis with one hand and wash with the other, beginning at the tip and working in a circular motion from the center to the periphery *to avoid*

introducing microorganisms into the urethra. Use a clean section of washcloth for each stroke to prevent the spread of contaminated secretions or discharge.
• Rinse thoroughly, using the same circular motion.

Retract and replace

• For the uncircumcised patient, gently retract the foreskin and clean beneath it. Rinse well but don't dry *because moisture provides lubrication and prevents friction when replacing the foreskin.* Replace the foreskin to avoid constriction of the penis, which causes edema and tissue damage.
• Wash the rest of the penis, using downward strokes toward the scrotum. Rinse well and pat dry with a bath towel.
• Clean the top and sides of the scrotum; rinse thoroughly and pat dry. Handle the scrotum gently *to avoid causing discomfort.*
• Turn the patient on his side. Clean the bottom of the scrotum and the anal area. Rinse well and pat dry.

After providing perineal care

• Reposition the patient and make him or her comfortable. Remove the bath blanket and linen-saver pad, and then replace the bed linens.
• Clean and return the basin and dispose of soiled articles, including gloves. Wash your hands.

Practice pointers

• Give perineal care in a matter-of-fact way *to minimize embarrassment.*
• If the patient is incontinent, first remove excess feces with toilet tissue. Then position him or her on a bedpan, and add a small amount of antiseptic soap to a perineal bottle *to eliminate odor.* Irrigate the perineal area *to remove any remaining fecal matter.*
• After cleaning the perineum, apply ointment or cream (petroleum jelly, zinc oxide cream, or vitamin A and D ointment) *to prevent skin breakdown by providing a barrier between the skin and excretions.*
• To reduce the number of linen changes, tuck an ABD pad between the patient's buttocks to absorb oozing feces.

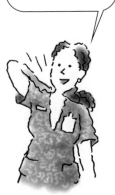

Everybody enjoys a gentle massage—or at least a pat on the back—from time to time.

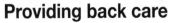

Providing back care

Regular bathing and massage of the neck, back, buttocks, and upper arms promotes patient relaxation and allows assessment of skin condition. Particularly important for the bedridden patient, massage causes cutaneous vasodilation, helping to prevent pressure ulcers caused by prolonged pressure on bony prominences or by perspiration. Although you can perform gentle back massage after a patient has a myocardial infarction, it may be contraindicated in those with rib fractures, surgical incisions, or other recent traumatic injury to the back.

What you need

Basin ✳ soap ✳ bath blanket ✳ bath towel ✳ washcloth ✳ back lotion with lanolin base ✳ gloves, if the patient has open lesions or has been incontinent ✳ optional: talcum powder

Getting ready

• Fill the basin two-thirds full with warm water. Place the lotion bottle in the basin to warm it. *Application of warmed lotion prevents chilling or startling the patient, thereby reducing muscle tension and vasoconstriction.*

> Application of warmed lotion prevents chilling or startling the patient.

How you do it

• Assemble the equipment at the patient's bedside.
• Explain the procedure to the patient and provide privacy. Ask them to tell you if you're applying too much or too little pressure.
• Adjust the bed to a comfortable working height and lower the head of the bed, if allowed. Wash your hands and put on gloves, if applicable. Lower the side rail closest to you.

Prone, look at a stone

• Place the patient in the prone position, if possible, or on their side. Position them along the edge of the bed nearest you *to prevent back strain.*
• Untie the patient's gown, and expose the back, shoulders, and buttocks. Then drape the patient with a bath blanket *to prevent chills and minimize exposure.* Place a bath towel next to or under their side *to protect bed linens from moisture.*

> While you're at it, you might want to check those bony prominences. Just a suggestion!

Make it into a mitt

• Fold the washcloth around your hand to form a mitt. This prevents the loose ends of the cloth from dripping water onto the patient and keeps the cloth warm longer.
• Work up a lather with soap. Using long, firm strokes, bathe the patient's back, beginning at the neck and shoulders and moving downward to the buttocks.

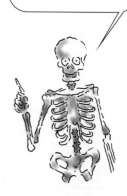

Rinse and dry

- Rinse and dry well *because moisture trapped between the buttocks can cause chafing and predispose the patient to pressure ulcers.*
- While giving back care, closely examine the patient's skin, especially the bony prominences of the shoulders, the scapulae, and the coccyx, for redness or abrasions.

Moisturize first, then massage

- Remove the warmed lotion bottle from the basin, and pour a small amount of lotion into your palm. Rub your hands together *to distribute the lotion.*
- Apply the lotion to the patient's back, using long, firm strokes. *The lotion reduces friction, making back massage easier.*
- Massage the patient's back, beginning at the base of the spine and moving upward to the shoulders. For a relaxing effect, massage slowly; for a stimulating effect, massage quickly. Alternate the three basic strokes: effleurage, friction, and pétrissage. (See *How to give a back massage.*) Add lotion as needed, keeping one hand on the patient's back *to avoid interrupting the massage.*

How to give a back massage

Three strokes commonly used during back massage are effleurage, friction, and pétrissage. Start with effleurage and then go on to friction and pétrissage. Perform each stroke at least six times before moving on to the next, and then repeat the whole series if desired.

When performing effleurage and friction, keep your hands parallel to the vertebrae to avoid tickling the patient. For all three strokes, maintain a regular rhythm and steady contact with the patient's back to help them relax.

Effleurage	**Friction**	**Pétrissage**
Using your palm, stroke from the buttocks up to the shoulders, over the upper arms, and back to the buttocks (as shown below). Use slightly less pressure on the downward strokes.	Use circular thumb strokes to move from buttocks to shoulders; then, using a smooth stroke, return to the buttocks (as shown below).	Using your thumb to oppose your fingers, knead and stroke half the back and upper arms, starting at the buttocks and moving toward the shoulder (as shown below). Then knead and stroke the other half of the back, rhythmically alternating your hands.

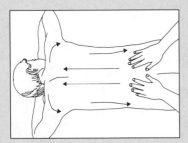 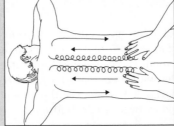 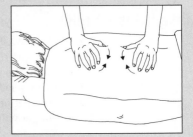

• Compress, squeeze, and lift the trapezius muscle *to help relax the patient.*
• Finish the massage by using long, firm strokes, and blot any excess lotion from the patient's back with a towel. Then retie the patient's gown and straighten or change the bed linens as needed.

When you're done

• Return the bed to its original position, and make the patient comfortable. Empty and clean the basin.
• Dispose of gloves, if used, and return equipment to the appropriate storage area. Wash your hands.

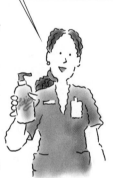

When providing a back massage, always choose an appropriate lotion and warm it in a basin of water first.

Practice pointers

• Before giving back care, assess the patient's body structure and skin condition and tailor the duration and intensity of the massage accordingly.
• If the patient has oily skin, substitute a talcum powder or lotion of the patient's choice. However, don't use powder if the patient has an endotracheal or tracheal tube in place *to avoid aspiration.*
• Don't massage the patient's legs unless ordered *because massage can dislodge the clot, causing an embolus.*
• Give special attention to bony prominences because pressure ulcers are common in these areas. Do not massage reddened, bony prominences.

Keep the powder and the lotion separate

• Avoid using powder and lotion together *because doing so may lead to skin maceration.*
• If you're giving back care at bedtime, have the patient ready for bed beforehand so the massage can help him fall asleep.
• Develop a turning schedule, and give back care at each position change.

For some people, it's wash and set once a week. For me, it's daily shampoos and a trip to the beauty salon every 5 weeks.

Performing hair care

Hair care includes combing, brushing, and shampooing. Combing and brushing stimulate scalp circulation, remove dead cells and debris, and distribute hair oils *to produce a healthy sheen.* Shampooing removes dirt and old oils and helps prevent skin irritation. Hair care also enhances self-esteem and body image.

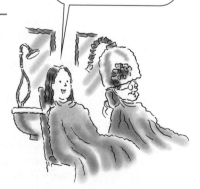

1 week for most

Frequency of hair care depends on the length and texture of the patient's hair, the duration of hospitalization, and the patient's condition. Usually, hair should be combed and brushed daily and shampooed according to the patient's normal routine. Typically, no more than 1 week should elapse between washings. Shampooing is contraindicated in patients with recent craniotomy, depressed skull fracture, conditions necessitating intracranial pressure monitoring, or other cranial involvement.

What you need

Comb and brush ✳ hand towel ✳ liquid shampoo (or mild soap, such as Castile) ✳ shampoo tray with tubing ✳ washcloth ✳ three bath towels ✳ two bath blankets ✳ cotton ✳ plastic shampoo basin ✳ two large pitchers or other large containers ✳ one small pitcher or beaker basin ✳ linen-saver pads ✳ gloves ✳ optional: hair conditioner or rinse, alcohol, oil, hair ties, footstool, drawsheet

The comb and brush should be clean. If necessary, wash them in hot, soapy water. The comb should have dull, even teeth to prevent scratching the scalp. The brush should have stiff bristles to enhance vigorous brushing and stimulation of circulation.

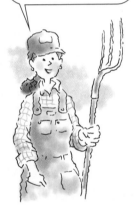

Make sure the comb and brush are clean and, perhaps, a little less pointy than a pitch fork.

Getting ready

Combing and brushing

• Tell the patient you're going to comb and brush their hair. If possible, encourage them to do it by themselves, assisting as needed.
• Recognize and apply principles regarding ethnic and cultural hair practices.
• Adjust the bed to a comfortable working height to prevent back strain. If the patient's condition allows, help them to a sitting position by raising the head of the bed.
• Provide privacy, and drape a bath towel over the patient's pillow and shoulders to catch loose hair and dirt. Put on gloves.

Shampooing a bedridden patient's hair

• Before shampooing the patient's hair, adjust room temperature and eliminate drafts to prevent chilling the patient. Next, obtain a shampoo tray or devise a trough, if necessary.
• Assemble the equipment on the patient's bedside stand.
• Cover the patient with a bath blanket. Then fanfold the linens to the foot of the bed, or remove them if they're scheduled to be changed.

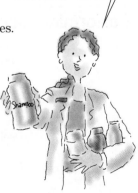

You need to gather more than just shampoo when you're shampooing a patient's hair!

- Fill large pitchers or containers with comfortably warm water and place them on the overbed table.
- Lower the head of the bed until it's horizontal, and remove the patient's pillow, if allowed. Lower the side rail closest to you.

A blanket buffer

- Fold the second bath blanket, and tuck it under the patient's shoulders to improve water drainage.
- Cover the bath blanket and the head of the bed with a linen-saver pad to protect them from moisture.
- Place a bath towel and linen-saver pad together, and position them around the patient's neck and over their shoulders *to protect the patient from moisture and to pad their neck against the pressure of the shampoo tray.*
- Place the shampoo tray under the patient's head with their neck in the U-shaped opening. Arrange the bath blanket and towel so the patient is comfortable.

Watch the waterway!

- Adjust the shampoo tray to carry wastewater away from the patient's head, and place the drainage tubing in the pail. Tuck a folded towel or drawsheet under the opposite side of the shampoo tray to promote drainage, if necessary. Put on gloves.

How you do it

Combing and brushing

- For short hair, comb and brush one side at a time. For long or curly hair, turn the patient's head away from you, and then part the hair down the middle from front to back. If the hair is tangled, rub alcohol or oil on the hair strands to loosen them. Comb and vigorously brush the hair on the side facing you. Then turn the patient's head, and comb and brush the opposite side.

Easy does it

- Part hair into small sections for easier handling. Comb one section at a time, working from the ends toward the scalp to remove tangles. Anchor each section of hair above the area being combed *to avoid hurting the patient.* After combing, brush vigorously. Avoid shaking the patient's head when brushing.

Braids, bangs, or barrettes?

- Style the hair as the patient prefers. Braiding long or curly hair helps prevent snarling. To braid, part

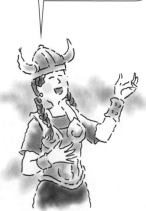

I usually let my braids hang freely so they don't interfere with the horns on my new Viking helmet. Think Wagner would approve?

hair down the middle of the scalp and begin braiding near the face. Don't braid too tightly *to avoid
patient discomfort.* Fasten the ends of the braids
with hair ties. Pin the braids across the top of the
patient's head or let them hang, as the patient desires,
*so the finished braids don't press against the
patient's scalp.*
• After styling the hair, carefully remove the towel by
folding it inward *to prevent loose hairs and debris from
falling onto the pillow or into the patient's bed.*

Shampooing a bedridden patient's hair
• Before shampooing, place cotton in the patient's ears
to prevent moisture from collecting in them.

One dip or two?

• Fill the small pitcher or beaker by dipping it into the
large pitcher. Carefully pour water over the patient's hair.
To avoid spills, don't overfill the shampoo tray.

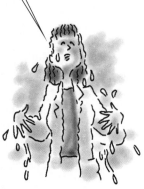

Shampooing a
bedridden patient's
hair is usually a fairly
simple procedure—a
little wet, but easy
enough.

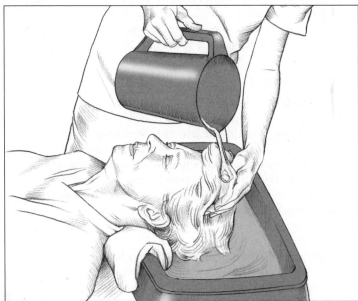

• Then, with your fingertips, rub shampoo into the patient's hair.
Massage the scalp well to emulsify hair oils. Vigorous rubbing
stimulates the scalp and also helps the patient relax. Do not hyper-
extend the neck or shake the head.
• Using the small pitcher or beaker, pour water over the patient's
hair until it's free of shampoo. Then reapply shampoo and rinse
again. Apply conditioner or a rinse, if desired.

It's a wrap!

• Remove the shampoo tray, and wrap the patient's hair in a towel. Remove the linen-saver pad from the bed, and return the bed to its original position.
• Dry the patient's hair by gently rubbing it with a towel. Then comb, brush, and style it.
• Remake the bed or change the linens, if needed, and remove the bath blanket.
• Reposition the patient comfortably.
• Remove and empty the pail. Clean the shampoo tray, and return it to storage. Remove pitchers from the bedside, and return the shampoo to the bedside stand.
• Remove your gloves. Wash your hands.

Practice pointers

• When giving hair care, check the patient's scalp carefully for signs of scalp disorders, head lice, or skin breakdown, particularly if the patient is bedridden. Make sure each patient has their own comb and brush to avoid cross-contamination.
• If you don't have a shampoo tray and can't devise a trough, place pillows under the patient's shoulders to elevate their head, and use a basin. Because a standard basin doesn't have a drainage spout, empty it frequently to prevent overflow.

Shaving a patient

Performed with a straight, safety, or electric razor, shaving is part of the male patient's usual daily care. In addition to reducing bacterial growth on the face, shaving promotes patient comfort by removing whiskers that can itch and irritate the skin and produce an unkempt appearance. Shaving may also promote positive self-esteem.

Do the electric slide

Because nicks and cuts are most common with use of a straight or safety razor, shaving with an electric razor is indicated for the patient with a clotting disorder or the patient undergoing anticoagulant therapy. Shaving may be contraindicated in the patient with a facial skin disorder or wound.

What you need
For a straight or safety razor
Shaving kit containing a straight razor and soap container or a safety razor ✳ gloves ✳ soap or

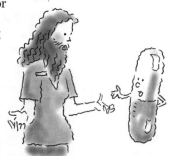

An unfortunate temporary adverse effect, I know! But, hey, look at the bright side . . . at least you'll get some firsthand experience with a straight razor and aftershave lotion.

shaving cream ✳ towel ✳ washcloth ✳ basin ✳ optional:
aftershave lotion, talcum powder

For an electric razor

Bath towel ✳ optional: precava and aftershave lotions, mirror, and
grounded three-pronged plug

Getting ready

• With a straight or a safety razor, make sure the blade is sharp,
clean, even, and rust-free. If necessary, insert a new blade securely
into the razor. A razor may be used more than once, but only by
the same patient. If the patient is bedridden, assemble the equipment on the bedside stand or overbed table; if he's ambulatory,
assemble it at the sink. When the patient is ready to shave, fill the
basin or sink with warm water.

Hey plug, you're grounded!

• If you're using an electric razor, check its cord for fraying or
other damage that could create an electrical hazard. If the razor
isn't double-insulated or battery operated, use a grounded three-
pronged plug. Examine the razor head for sharp edges and dirt.
Read the manufacturer's instructions, if available, and assemble
the equipment at the bedside.

A little privacy, please

• Tell the patient that you're going to shave him, and provide
privacy. Ask him to assist you as much as possible to promote his
independence.
• Unless contraindicated, place the conscious patient in
high-Fowler's or semi-Fowler's position. If the patient is
unconscious, elevate his head to prevent soap and water
from running behind it.
• Direct bright light onto the patient's face but not into
his eyes.

> Shaving involves
> the use of sharp
> instruments and the
> potential for blood
> exposure . . . don't
> forget the gloves!

How you do it

Using a straight or safety razor

• Drape a bath towel around the patient's shoulders, and tuck
it under his chin *to protect the bed from moisture and to
catch falling whiskers.*

Stay sharp as a razor's edge

• Put on gloves, and fill the basin with warm water. Using
the washcloth, wet the patient's entire beard with warm
water. Let the warm cloth soak the beard for at least
1 minute *to soften whiskers.*

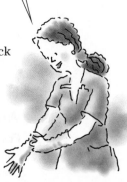

• Apply shaving cream to the beard. Or, if you're using soap, rub to form a lather.
• Gently stretch the patient's skin taut with one hand and shave with the other, holding the razor firmly. Ask the patient to puff his cheeks or turn his head, as necessary, to shave hard-to-reach areas.

Is Elvis in the house?

• Begin at the sideburns and work toward the chin using short, firm, downward strokes in the direction of hair growth *to reduce skin irritation and help prevent nicks and cuts.*

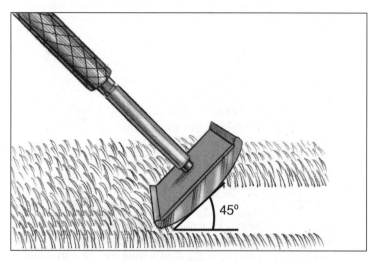

45°

• Rinse the razor often *to remove whiskers.* Apply more warm water or shaving cream to the face, as needed, *to maintain adequate lather.*

Smooth as a baby's bottom

• Shave across the chin and up the neck and throat. Use short, gentle strokes for the neck and the area around the nose and mouth *to avoid skin irritation.*
• Change the water, and rinse any remaining lather and whiskers from the patient's face. Then dry his face with a bath towel and, if the patient desires, apply aftershave lotion or talcum powder.
• Rinse the razor and basin, and then return the razor to its storage area.

Using an electric razor

• Plug in the razor and apply precava lotion, if available, to remove skin oils. If the razor head is adjustable, select the appropriate setting.

Done correctly, shaving should leave your patient's face smooth as a baby's bottom. And he may even want a little talcum powder to boot!

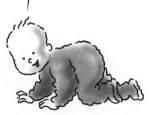

• Using a circular motion and pressing the razor firmly against the skin, shave each area of the patient's face until smooth.

Aqua Velva man?

• If the patient desires, apply talcum powder or aftershave lotion.
• Clean the razor head, and return the razor to its storage area.

Practice pointers

• If the patient is conscious, find out his usual shaving routine. Although shaving in the direction of hair growth is most common, the patient may prefer the opposite direction.

> Do you prefer a straight, safety, or electric razor? And do you usually go with or against the grain?

No borrowing allowed

• Don't interchange patients' shaving equipment *to prevent cross-contamination.*
• Shaving may be contraindicated if the patient is on anticoagulant therapy (e.g., after tissue plasminogen activator or heparin infusion). Check your facility's policy.

Performing foot care

Daily bathing of feet and regular trimming of toenails promotes cleanliness, prevents infection, stimulates peripheral circulation, and controls odor by removing debris from between toes and under toenails.

Put your foot down ... it's important!

Foot care is particularly important for bedridden patients and those especially susceptible to foot infection, such as patients with peripheral vascular disease, diabetes mellitus, poor nutritional status, arthritis, or a condition that impairs peripheral circulation. In such patients, proper foot care should include meticulous cleanliness and regular observation for signs of skin breakdown. (See *Foot care for diabetic patients.*)

What you need

Bath blanket * large basin * soap * towel * linen-saver pad * pillow * washcloth * orangewood stick * cotton-tipped applicator * cotton balls * lotion * water-absorbent powder * bath thermometer * gloves, if the patient has open lesions * optional: gauze pads and heel protectors

Foot care for diabetic patients

Because diabetes mellitus can reduce blood supply to the feet, normally minor foot injuries can lead to dangerous infection. When caring for a diabetic patient, keep these foot care guidelines in mind:
• Exercising the feet daily can help improve circulation. While the patient is sitting on the edge of the bed, ask them to point toes upward, then downward, 10 times. Then have make a circle with each foot 10 times.
• A diabetic patient's shoes must fit properly. Instruct the patient to break in new shoes gradually by increasing wearing time by 30 minutes each day. Also tell them to check old shoes frequently in case they develop rough spots in the lining.
• Tell the patient to wear clean socks daily and to avoid socks with holes; darned spots; or rough, irritating seams.
• Advise the patient to see a doctor if they have corns or calluses.

• Tell the patient to wear warm socks or slippers and to use extra blankets to avoid cold feet. The patient shouldn't use heating pads and hot water bottles because these can cause burns.
• Teach the patient to regularly inspect the skin on the feet for cuts; cracks; blisters; and red, swollen areas. Even slight cuts on the feet should receive a doctor's attention. As a first-aid measure, tell them to wash the cut thoroughly and apply a mild antiseptic. Urge the patient to avoid harsh antiseptics, such as iodine, because they can damage tissue.
• Advise the diabetic patient to avoid tight-fitting garments or activities that can decrease circulation. They should especially avoid sitting with their knees crossed, picking at sores or rough spots on their feet, walking barefoot, or applying adhesive tape to the skin on their feet.

Getting ready
• Fill the basin halfway with warm water. Test water temperature with a bath thermometer because patients with diminished peripheral sensation could burn their feet in excessively hot water (over 105° F [40.6° C]) without feeling any warning pain. If a bath thermometer isn't available, test the water by inserting your elbow. The water temperature should feel comfortably warm.
• Assemble equipment at the patient's bedside. Wash your hands, and put on gloves.

Remember that a patient with diminished peripheral sensation can burn their feet in hot water without feeling any warning pain. Always test bath water first.

Guaranteed to make them smile
• Tell the patient that you'll be washing their feet and providing foot and toenail care.
• Cover the patient with a bath blanket. Fanfold the top linen to the foot of the bed.
• Place a linen-saver pad and a towel under the patient's feet *to keep the bottom linen dry.* Then position the basin on the pad.

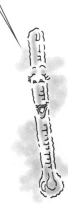

Positively pressure free
• Insert a pillow beneath the patient's knee *to provide support,* and cushion the rim of the basin with the edge of the towel *to prevent pressure.*

How you do it

• Immerse one foot in the basin, wash it with soap, and allow it to soak for about 10 minutes. *Soaking softens the skin and toenails, loosens debris under toenails, and comforts and refreshes the patient.*
• After soaking the foot, rinse it with a washcloth, remove it from the basin, and place it on the towel.

> If your patient's skin is dry, moisten it with lotion. If it's too moist, a pinch of water-absorbent powder between the toes should do the trick.

Soft-cloth touch

• Dry the foot thoroughly, especially between the toes, *to prevent skin breakdown.* Blot gently to dry *because harsh rubbing may damage the skin.*
• Empty the basin, refill it with warm water, and clean and soak the other foot.

Putting your best foot forward

• While the second foot is soaking, give the first one a pedicure. Using the cotton-tipped applicator, carefully clean the toenails. Using an orangewood stick, gently remove dirt beneath the toenails; avoid injuring subungual skin.
• Consult a podiatrist if nails need trimming.
• Rinse the foot that has been soaking, dry it thoroughly, and give it a pedicure.

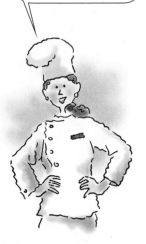

Test for doneness

• Apply lotion *to moisten dry skin* or lightly dust water absorbent powder between the toes *to absorb moisture.*
• Remove and clean all equipment. Dispose of gloves and wash your hands.

Practice pointers

• While providing foot care, observe the color, shape, and texture of the toenails. If you see redness, drying, cracking, blisters, discoloration, or other signs of traumatic injury, especially in patients with impaired peripheral circulation and/or diabetes, notify the doctor. *Because such patients are vulnerable to infection and gangrene, they need prompt treatment.*
• If a patient's toenail grows inward at the corners, tuck a wisp of cotton under it *to relieve pressure on the toe.* Consider referring ingrown toenails to a podiatrist.

> Redness, drying, cracking, blisters, discoloration, or any evidence of traumatic injury to the feet could be a sign of infection or gangrene.

WARNING!

Tailoring care to the bedridden patient

• When giving the bedridden patient foot care, perform range-of-motion exercises unless contraindicated *to stimulate circulation and prevent foot contractures and muscle atrophy.* Tuck folded 2″ × 2″ gauze pads between overlapping toes *to protect the skin from the toenails.* Apply heel protectors *to prevent skin breakdown.*

Performing mouth care

Given in the morning, at bedtime, or after meals, mouth care entails brushing and flossing the teeth and inspecting the mouth. Mouth care removes soft plaque deposits and calculus from the teeth, cleans and massages the gums, reduces mouth odor, and helps prevent infection. Patients' comfort and self-esteem are increased by freshening the patient's mouth. Appreciation of food is enhanced, thereby aiding appetite and nutrition.

A clean mouth is a healthy mouth and that means being able to enjoy eating all types of food.

A mouthful of attention

Although an ambulatory patient can usually perform mouth care alone, a bedridden patient may require partial or full assistance. A comatose patient requires use of suction equipment *to prevent aspiration during oral care.*

What you need

Towel or facial tissues ✳ emesis basin ✳ trash bag ✳ mouthwash ✳ toothbrush and toothpaste ✳ pitcher and glass ✳ drinking straw ✳ dental floss ✳ gloves ✳ dental floss holder, if available ✳ small mirror, if necessary ✳ optional: oral irrigating device

For the comatose or debilitated patient

Linen-saver pad ✳ bite block ✳ petroleum jelly ✳ hydrogen peroxide ✳ mineral oil ✳ cotton-tipped mouth swab ✳ along with a cotton-tipped mouth swab, suggest also including foam swab, which also may be used to cleanse oral tissues in a comatose patient ✳ oral suction equipment or gauze pads ✳ optional: mouth-care kit, tongue blade, 4″ × 4″ gauze pads, and adhesive tape

Getting ready

• Fill a pitcher with water, and bring it and other equipment to the patient's bedside.
• If you'll be using oral suction equipment, connect the tubing to the suction bottle and suction catheter, insert the plug into an outlet, and check for correct operation.

Dracula's nemesis

- If necessary, devise a bite block to protect yourself from being bitten during the procedure: Wrap a gauze pad over the end of a tongue blade, fold the edge in, and secure it with adhesive tape.
- Wash your hands thoroughly, put on gloves, explain the procedure to the patient, and provide privacy.

> Watch your patient closely to make sure they are flossing correctly and correct if necessary.

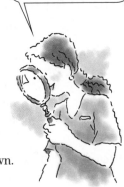

How you do it

- If the patient is bedridden but capable of self-care, encourage them to perform their own mouth care.
- If allowed, place the patient in Fowler's position. Place the overbed table in front of them, and arrange the equipment on it. Open the table and set up the built-in mirror, if available, or position a small mirror on the table.
- Drape a towel over the patient's chest to protect their gown. Tell them to floss teeth while looking into the mirror.

Inspecting the technique

- Observe the patient *to make sure they are flossing correctly,* and correct if necessary.
- Instruct them to wrap the floss around the second or third finger of each hand. Starting with the back teeth and without injuring the gums, they should insert the floss as far as possible into the space between each pair of teeth. Then they should clean the surfaces of adjacent teeth by pulling the floss up and down against the side of each tooth. After the patient flosses a pair of teeth, remind them to use a clean 1″ (2.5 cm) section of floss for the next pair.

After the floss

- After the patient flosses, mix mouthwash and water in a glass (or a mixture of half peroxide and half water), place a straw in it, and position the emesis basin nearby.
- Instruct brushing teeth and gums while looking into the mirror. Encourage rinsing frequently during brushing, a facial tissues to wipe the mouth.

> Don't forget the mouthwash!

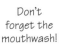

Performing mouth care

- If the patient is comatose or conscious but incapable of self-care, perform mouth care on him. If they wear dentures, clean them thoroughly. (See *Dealing with dentures.*) Some patients may benefit from using an oral irrigating device.

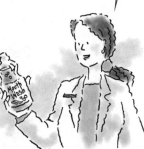

Stay on the ball

Dealing with dentures

Dentures require proper care to remove soft plaque deposits and calculus and to reduce mouth odor. Such care involves removing and rinsing dentures after meals, daily brushing and removal of tenacious deposits, and soaking in a commercial denture cleaner. Dentures must be removed from the comatose or presurgical patient to prevent possible airway obstruction.

Equipment and preparation

Start by assembling the following equipment at the patient's bedside: ✳ emesis basin ✳ labeled denture cup ✳ toothbrush or denture brush ✳ gloves ✳ toothpaste ✳ commercial denture cleaner ✳ paper towel ✳ cotton-tipped mouth swab and/or a foam swab mouthwash ✳ gauze ✳ optional: adhesive denture liner

Removing dentures

• Wash your hands and put on gloves.
• To remove a full upper denture, grasp the front and palatal surfaces of the denture with your thumb and forefinger. Position the index finger of your opposite hand over the upper border of the denture, and press to break the seal between denture and palate. Grasp the denture with gauze because saliva can make it slippery.
• To remove a full lower denture, grasp the front and lingual surfaces of the denture with your thumb and index finger and gently lift up.
• To remove partial dentures, first ask the patient or caregiver how the prosthesis is retained and how to remove it. If the partial denture is held in place with clips or snaps, then exert equal pressure on the border of each side of the denture. Avoid lifting the clasps, which can easily bend or break.

Oral and denture care

• After removing dentures, place them in a properly labeled denture cup. Add warm water and a commercial denture cleaner to remove stains and hardened deposits.

Follow package directions. Avoid soaking dentures in mouthwash containing alcohol because it may damage a soft liner.
• Instruct the patient to rinse with mouthwash to remove food particles and reduce mouth odor. Then stroke the palate, buccal surfaces, gums, and tongue with a soft toothbrush or cotton-tipped mouth swab to clean the mucosa and stimulate circulation. Check for irritated areas or sores because they may indicate a poorly fitting denture.
• Carry the denture cup, emesis basin, toothbrush, and toothpaste to the sink. After lining the basin with a paper towel, fill it with water to cushion the dentures in case you drop them. Hold the dentures over the basin, wet them with warm water, and apply toothpaste to a denture brush or long-bristled toothbrush. Clean the dentures using only moderate pressure to prevent scratches and using warm water to prevent distortion.
• Clean the denture cup, and place the dentures in it. Rinse the brush, and clean and dry the emesis basin. Return all equipment to the patient's bedside stand.

Wearing dentures

• If the patient desires, apply adhesive liner to the dentures. Moisten them with water, if necessary, to reduce friction and ease insertion.
• Encourage the patient to wears dentures to enhance appearance, facilitate eating and speaking, and prevent changes in the gum line that may affect denture fit.

Prepping the patient

- Raise the bed to a comfortable working height *to prevent back strain.* Then lower the head of the bed, and position the patient on their side, with the face extended over the edge of the pillow *to facilitate drainage and prevent fluid aspiration.*
- Arrange the equipment on the overbed table or bedside stand, including the oral suction equipment, if necessary. Turn on the machine. If a suction machine isn't available, wipe the inside of the patient's mouth frequently with a gauze pad.
- Place a linen-saver pad under the patient's chin and an emesis basin near their cheek *to absorb or catch drainage.*

Jellying up

- Lubricate the patient's lips with petroleum jelly *to prevent dryness and cracking.* Reapply lubricant, as needed, during oral care.
- If necessary, insert the bite block to hold the patient's mouth open during oral care. *Caution:* Never place your fingers in the patient's mouth.

Flossing and rinsing

- Using a dental floss holder, hold the floss against each tooth and direct it as close to the gum as possible without injuring the sensitive tissues around the tooth.
- After flossing the patient's teeth, mix mouthwash and water in a glass and place the straw in it.

Brushing them clean

- Wet the toothbrush with water. If necessary, use hot water *to soften the bristles.* Apply toothpaste.
- Brush the patient's lower teeth from the gum line up; the upper teeth, from the gum line down.

Covering all the angles

- Place the brush at a 45-degree angle to the gum line, and press the bristles gently into the gingival sulcus. Using short, gentle strokes *to prevent gum damage,* brush the buccal surfaces (toward the cheek) and the lingual surfaces (toward the tongue) of the bottom teeth; use just the tip of the brush for the lingual surfaces of the front teeth. Using the same technique, brush the buccal and lingual surfaces of the top teeth. Brush the biting surfaces of the bottom and top teeth using a back-and-forth motion.
- Hold the emesis basin steady under the patient's cheek, and wipe his mouth and cheeks with facial tissues as needed.

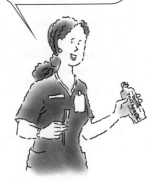

Follow the proper brushing technique, and use gentle strokes to prevent damaging tooth and gum surfaces.

Swabbing the deck clean

• After brushing the patient's teeth, dip a cotton-tipped mouth swab into the mouthwash solution (or a mixture of half peroxide and half water). Press the swab against the side of the glass to remove excess moisture. Gently stroke the gums, buccal surfaces, palate, and tongue *to clean the mucosa and stimulate circulation.*

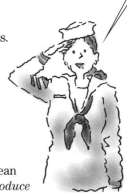

Aye, Sir ... Every good ensign knows that a cotton-tipped swab dipped in mouthwash is a good way to clean the mucosa and stimulate circulation ... Sir!

After mouth care

• Assess the patient's mouth for cleanliness and tooth and tissue condition.
• Rinse the toothbrush, and clean the emesis basin and glass.
• Empty and clean the suction bottle, if used, and place a clean suction catheter on the tubing.
• Return reusable equipment to the appropriate storage location, and discard disposable equipment in the trash bag. Remove gloves and wash your hands.

Practice pointers

• Use cotton-tipped mouth swabs and/or foam swab to clean the teeth of a patient with sensitive gums. *These swabs produce less friction than a toothbrush; however, they don't clean as well.*
• If your patient is breathing through his mouth or receiving oxygen therapy, moisten his mouth and lips regularly with mineral oil or water.

Making an unoccupied bed

Although considered routine, daily changing and periodic straightening of bed linens promotes patient comfort and prevents skin breakdown. When preceded by hand washing, performed using clean technique, and followed by proper handling and disposal of soiled linens, this procedure helps control nosocomial (hospital acquired) infections.

What you need

Two sheets (one fitted, if available) ✳ pillowcase ✳ bedspread ✳ gloves ✳ optional: bath blanket, laundry bag, linen-saver pads, and drawsheet

Getting ready

• Obtain clean linen, which should be folded in half lengthwise and then folded again. The bottom sheet should be folded so that the rough side of the hem is face down when placed on the bed *to help prevent skin irritation caused by the rough hem edge rubbing against the patient's heels.* The top sheet should be folded similarly so that the smooth side of the hem is face up when folded over the spread, *giving the bed a finished appearance and protecting the patient's skin.*

Vacating the premises

- Wash your hands thoroughly, put on gloves, and bring clean linen to the patient's bedside. If the patient is present, tell them that you're going to change the bed. Help them to a chair, if necessary.
- Move any furniture away from the bed *to provide ample working space.*
- Lower the head of the bed to make the mattress level and to ensure tight-fitting, wrinkle-free linens. Then raise the bed to a comfortable working height to prevent back strain. Make sure the wheels of the bed are locked.

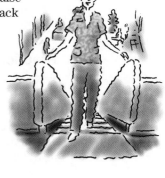

Do you think they'll give me an extra discount off the White Sale prices if I purchase enough sheets for the entire medical-surgical unit?

How you do it

- When stripping the bed, watch for any belongings that may have fallen among the linens.
- Remove the pillowcase and place it in the laundry bag, or use it, hooked over the back of a chair, as a laundry bag. Set the pillow aside.

It's in the bag

- Lift the mattress edge slightly and work around the bed, untucking the linens. If you plan to reuse the top linens, fold the top hem of the spread down to the bottom hem. Then pick up the hemmed corners, fold the spread into quarters, and hang it over the back of the chair. Otherwise, carefully remove and place the top linens in the laundry bag or pillowcase. *To avoid spreading microorganisms,* don't fan the linens, hold them against your clothing, or place them on the floor.
- Remove the soiled bottom linens, and place them in the laundry bag.

What do you think? Bed-in-a-bag patient hammocks . . . I think I may be on to something big!

Oops, it's sliding!

- If the mattress has slid downward, push it to the head of the bed. *Adjusting it after bed making loosens the linens.*
- Place the bottom sheet with its center fold in the middle of the mattress. For a fitted sheet, secure the top and bottom corners

over the mattress corners on the side of the bed nearest you. For a flat sheet, align the end of the sheet with the foot of the mattress, and miter the top corner *to keep the sheet firmly tucked under the mattress.*

Miter this

• To miter the corner, first tuck the top end of the sheet evenly under the mattress at the head of the bed. Then lift the side edge of the sheet about 12″ (30 cm) from the mattress corner and hold it at a right angle to the mattress. Tuck in the bottom edge of the sheet hanging below the mattress. Lastly, drop the top edge and tuck it under the mattress, as shown below.

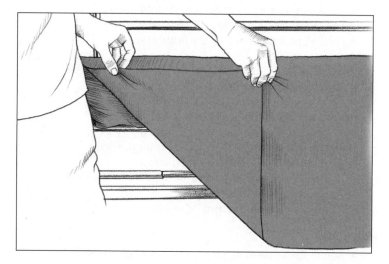

That's one "tuck," one "no-tuck"

• After tucking under one side of the bottom sheet, place the drawsheet (if needed) about 15″ (38 cm) from the top of the bed, with its center fold in the middle of the bed. Then tuck in the entire edge of the drawsheet on that side of the bed.

• Place the top sheet with its center fold in the middle of bed and its wide hem even with the top of the bed. Position the rough side of the hem face up *so that the smooth side shows after folding.* Allow enough sheet at the top of the bed to form a cuff over the spread.

• Place the spread over the top sheet with its center fold in the middle of the bed.

Heel and "toe"

• Make a 3″ (7.6 cm) toe pleat, or vertical tuck, in the top linens to allow room for the patient's feet and to prevent pressure that can cause discomfort, skin breakdown, and footdrop.

- Tuck the top sheet and spread under the foot of the mattress. Then miter the bottom corners.
- Move to the opposite side of the bed, and repeat the procedure.

Who "taut" you how to do that?

- After fitting all corners of the bottom sheet or tucking them under the mattress, pull the sheet at an angle from the head toward the foot of the bed. *Pulling the sheet tightens the linens, making the bottom sheet taut and wrinkle-free and promoting patient comfort.*
- Fold the top sheet over the spread at the head of the bed *to form a cuff and give the bed a finished appearance.* When making an open bed, fanfold the top linens to the foot of the bed. If a linen-saver pad is needed, place it on top of the bottom sheets.

> You don't have to go to finishing school to give a bed a finished look!

"Seams" like a good plan

- Slip the pillow into a clean case, tucking in the corners. Then place the pillow with its seam toward the top of the bed *to prevent it from rubbing against the patient's neck, causing irritation,* and its open edge facing away from the door *to give the bed a finished appearance.*
- Lower the bed, making sure the wheels remained locked *to ensure the patient's safety.*
- Assist the patient in returning to bed.

Getting carried away

- Return furniture to its proper place, and place the call button within the patient's easy reach. Carry away soiled linens in outstretched arms *to avoid contaminating your clothing.*
- After disposing of the linens, remove gloves if used and wash your hands thoroughly *to prevent the spread of microorganisms.*

> A simple demonstration of what *not* to do with soiled bed linens . . . and what I'll be wearing to this year's Halloween party.

Practice pointers

- Because a hospital mattress is usually covered with plastic to protect it and to facilitate cleaning between patients, a flat bottom sheet tends to loosen and become untucked. Use a fitted sheet, if available, to prevent this.
- If a fitted sheet isn't available, the top corners of a flat sheet may be tied together under the top of the mattress to prevent the sheet from becoming dislodged.
- A bath blanket placed on top of the mattress, under the bottom sheet, helps to absorb moisture and prevent dislodgment of the bottom sheet.

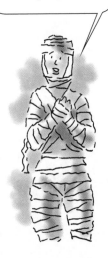

Making an occupied bed

For the bedridden patient, daily linen changes promote comfort and help prevent skin breakdown and nosocomial infection. Such changes necessitate the use of side rails to prevent the patient from rolling out of bed and, depending on the patient's condition, the use of a turning sheet to move them from side to side.

It takes two, baby

Making an occupied bed may require more than one person. It also entails loosening the bottom sheet on one side and fanfolding it to the center of the mattress instead of loosening the bottom sheet on both sides and removing it, as in an unoccupied bed. Also, the foundation of the bed must be made before the top sheet is applied instead of both the foundation and top being made on one side before being completed on the other side.

What you need

Two sheets (one fitted, if available) ✳ pillowcase ✳ one or two drawsheets ✳ spread ✳ one or two bath blankets ✳ gloves ✳ sheepskin or other comfort-enhancing device, as needed ✳ optional: laundry bag and linen-saver pad

Getting ready

• Obtain clean linen and make sure it's folded properly, as for an unoccupied bed.

Keep it clean

• Wash your hands, put on gloves, and bring clean linen to the patient's room.
• Identify the patient and tell them you'll be changing his bed linens. Explain how he can help if they are able, adjusting the plan according to their abilities and needs. Provide privacy.
• Move any furniture away from the bed *to ensure ample working space.*

Raising the bar

• Raise the side rail on the far side of the bed *to prevent falls.* Adjust the bed to a comfortable working height *to prevent back strain.* Make sure the wheels are locked.
• If allowed, lower the head of the bed to ensure tight-fitting, wrinkle-free linens.

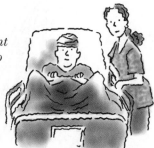

Tell the patient that you'll be changing the bed linens, and explain how they can help if they are able.

How you do it

- When stripping the bed, watch for belongings among the linens.
- Cover the patient with a bath blanket *to avoid exposure and provide warmth and privacy*. Then fanfold the top sheet and spread from beneath the bath blanket, and bring them back over the blanket.

Gather ye linens

- Loosen the top linens at the foot of the bed, and remove them separately. If reusing the top linens, fold each piece and hang it over the back of the chair. Otherwise, place it in the laundry bag. *To avoid dispersing microorganisms*, don't fan the linens, hold them against your clothing, or place them on the floor.
- If the mattress slides down when the head of the bed is raised, pull it up again. *Adjusting the mattress after the bed is made loosens the linens*. If the patient is able, ask them to grasp the head of the bed and pull with you; otherwise, ask a coworker to help you.

Roll 'em, roll 'em, roll 'em

- Roll the patient to the far side of the bed, and turn the pillow lengthwise under their head *to support the neck*. Ask the patient to help (if they can) by grasping the far side rail as they turn *so that they are positioned at the far side of the bed*.
- Loosen the soiled bottom linens on the side of the bed nearest you. Then roll the linens toward the patient's back in the middle of the bed, as shown below.

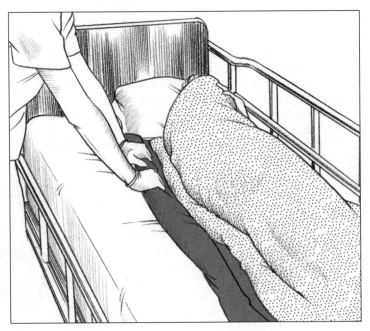

• Place a clean bottom sheet on the bed, with its center fold in the middle of the mattress. For a fitted sheet, secure the top and bottom corners over the side of the mattress nearest you. For a flat sheet, place its end even with the foot of the mattress. Miter the top corner as you would for an unoccupied bed *to keep linens firmly tucked under the mattress, preventing wrinkling.*

A center fold

• Fanfold the remaining clean bottom sheet toward the patient, and place the drawsheet, if needed, about 15″ (38 cm) from the top of the bed, with its center fold in the middle of the mattress. Tuck in the entire edge of the drawsheet on the side nearest you. Fanfold the remaining drawsheet toward the patient. Make sure the edge faces away from you.
• If necessary, position a linen-saver pad on the drawsheet *to absorb excretions or surgical drainage*, and fanfold it toward the patient.
• Raise the other side rail, and roll the patient to the clean side of the bed.

Loosen and remove

• Move to the unfinished side of the bed and lower the side rail nearest you. Then loosen and remove the soiled bottom linens separately and place them in the laundry bag.
• Pull the clean bottom sheet taut. Secure the fitted sheet or place the end of a flat sheet even with the foot of the bed, and miter the top corner. Pull the drawsheet taut and tuck it in. Unfold and smooth the linen-saver pad, if used.
• Assist the patient to the supine position, if their condition permits.
• Remove the soiled pillowcase, and place it in the laundry bag. Then slip the pillow into a clean pillowcase, tucking its corners well into the case *to ensure a smooth fit.* Place the pillow beneath the patient's head, with its seam toward the top of the bed *to prevent it from rubbing against the patient's neck, causing irritation.* Place the pillow's open edge away from the door *to give the bed a finished appearance.*

No "cuff" links

• Unfold the clean top sheet over the patient with the rough side of the hem facing away from the bed *to avoid irritating the patient's skin.* Allow enough sheets to form a cuff over the spread.

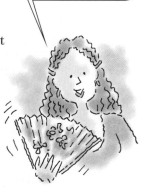

Just getting in a little backstage fanfolding practice while waiting for my big aria in *Aida*. Oh, there's my cue . . .

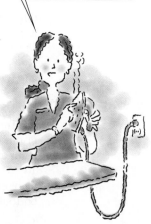

Now, for a truly finished appearance, you could always pull out the old iron and steam those wrinkles away.

• Remove the bath blanket from beneath the sheet, and center the spread over the top sheet.

Be kind to your patient's feet

• Make a 3″ (7.6 cm) toe pleat, or vertical tuck, in the top linens to allow room for the patient's feet and prevent pressure that can cause discomfort, skin breakdown, and footdrop.
• Tuck the top sheet and spread under the foot of the bed, and miter the bottom corners. Fold the top sheet over the spread *to give the bed a finished appearance*.

Lock and load

• Raise the head of the bed to a comfortable position, make sure both side rails are raised, and then lower the bed and lock its wheels *to ensure the patient's safety*. Assess the patient's body alignment and his mental and emotional status.
• Place the call button within the patient's easy reach. Remove the laundry bag from the room.
• Remove and discard gloves and wash your hands *to prevent the spread of nosocomial infections*.

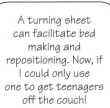

Remember the golden rule . . . Do unto your patient's feet as you would have them do unto yours (or something along those lines)!

Practice pointers

• Use a fitted sheet, when available, because a flat sheet slips out from under the mattress easily, especially if the mattress is plastic-coated.
• Prevent the patient from sliding down in bed by tucking a tightly rolled pillow under the top linens at the foot of the bed.
• For the diaphoretic or bedridden patient, fold a bath blanket in half lengthwise and place it between the bottom sheet and the plastic mattress cover; the blanket acts as a cushion and helps absorb moisture. *To help prevent sheet burns on the heels and bony prominences*, center a bath blanket or sheepskin over the bottom sheet, and tuck the blanket under the mattress.

A turning sheet can facilitate bed making and repositioning. Now, if I could only use one to get teenagers off the couch!

To every sheet, turn, turn

• If the patient can't help you move or turn him, devise a turning sheet to facilitate bed making and repositioning. To do so, first fold a drawsheet or bath blanket and place it under the patient's buttocks. Make sure the sheet extends from

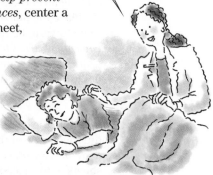

the shoulders to the knees so that it supports most of the patient's weight. Roll the sides of the sheet to form handles as close to the patient as possible. Next, ask a coworker to help you lift and move the patient. When lifting a patient, make sure both rolled handles are equidistant from the patient, lift at the same time, and don't drag the patient because this can promote back injury for the nurse. With one person holding each side of the sheet, you can move the patient without wrinkling the bottom linens.

Turn the tables on him

- If you can't get help and must turn the patient yourself, stand at the side of the bed. Turn the patient toward the rail, and, if they are able, ask them to grasp the opposite rolled edge of the turning sheet. Pull the rolled edge carefully toward you and turn the patient.

Reference

Berman, A., & Snyder, S. (2012). *Kozier & Erb's fundamentals of nursing: concepts, process, and practice* (9th ed.). Upper Saddle River, NJ: Pearson.

Quick quiz

1. When giving a back massage, which stroke uses alternating kneading and stroking of the patient's back and upper arms?
  A. Pétrissage
  B. Massage
  C. Effleurage
  D. Tapotement

Answer: A. Pétrissage involves using alternating kneading and stroking maneuvers on the patient's back and upper arms.

2. When performing personal hygiene on a female patient, it's important to wash the genital area in what direction?
  A. Back to front
  B. Side to side
  C. In a circular motion
  D. Front to back

Answer: D. It's best to wash the female genital area from the front to back to avoid contaminating the urethral orifice with fecal material from the anal area.

3. Which of the following is the correct position to perform mouth care on a comatose patient?

    A.   Semi-Fowler's
    B.   Side-lying
    C.   Prone
    D.   Supine

Answer: B. The side-lying position with the head of the bed lowered will help water and debris drain from the patient's mouth and prevent aspiration.

4. When providing morning care to a patient, which of the following is the correct direction for washing the patient's eye?

    A.   Outer canthus to inner canthus
    B.   Lower canthus to upper canthus
    C.   Inner canthus to outer canthus
    D.   Upper canthus to lower canthus

Answer: C. The eye should be cleaned from the inner canthus to the outer canthus.

Scoring

✳✳✳ If you answered all four questions correctly, congratulations! You really cleaned up!

✳✳ If you answered three questions correctly, great! You're fundamentally prepared to take care of yourself.

✳ If you answered fewer than three questions correctly, don't despair! Just review the chapter and you'll be a whiz at patient care in no time.

Mobility, activity, and exercise

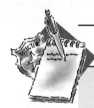

Just the facts

In this chapter, you'll learn:

♦ factors that affect musculoskeletal functioning

♦ proper patient positioning

♦ use of alignment and pressure-reducing devices

♦ methods of transferring a patient

♦ crutch walking and walker use

♦ ways to perform range-of-motion exercises.

A look at mobility, activity, and exercise

Mobility is defined as an individual's ability to move within, and interact with, the environment and the ability to move from one location to another. A patient's mobility or ability to move and be active affects not only his physical but also his emotional well-being. Mobility is essential to an individual's independence. Many older adults experience loss of mobility, along with functional loss and a lowered activity level. However, younger patients can also be affected by immobility from prolonged bed rest due to the physical restraints secondary to fractures or traction or from loss of strength due to illness.

Actively active

Activity keeps the mind and body active. Musculoskeletal inactivity or immobility adversely affects all body systems. Exercise—even passive range-of-motion (ROM) exercises— helps prevent muscle atrophy, prevent muscle contractures, and maintain circulation. Exercise increases muscle strength, tone, and mass. It also enhances the condition of other body systems.

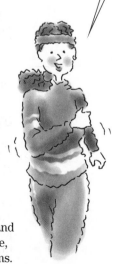

It's all about mobility. Another 30 minutes of mobility and I'm finished!

A look at the musculoskeletal system

Muscles, bones, joints, tendons, and ligaments give the human body its shape and ability to be mobile, perform such activities as those of daily living, and exercise. The three main components of the musculoskeletal system are:

 bones

 joints

 muscles.

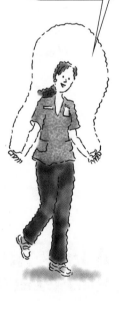

Exercise helps maintain circulation.

Bones

The 206 bones of the skeleton form the body's framework, supporting and protecting organs and tissues. The bones also serve as storage sites for minerals and contain bone marrow, the primary site for blood production. (See *A close look at the skeletal system.*)

Joints

The junction of two or more bones is called a *joint*. Joints stabilize the bones and allow a specific type of movement. The two types of joints are:

 nonsynovial

 synovial.

Nonsynovial

In nonsynovial joints, the bones are connected by fibrous tissue, also called *cartilage*. The bones may be immovable, such as the sutures in the skull, or slightly movable, such as the vertebrae.

Synovial

Synovial joints move freely; the bones are separate from each other and meet in a cavity filled with synovial fluid, a lubricant. In synovial joints, a layer of resilient cartilage covers the surfaces of opposing bones. This cartilage cushions the bones and allows full joint movement by making the surfaces of the bones smooth. These joints are surrounded by a fibrous capsule that stabilizes the joint structures. The capsule also surrounds the joint's ligaments— the tough, fibrous bands that join one bone to another.

A close look at the skeletal system

Of the 206 bones in the human skeletal system, 80 form the axial skeleton (skull, facial bones, vertebrae, ribs, sternum, and hyoid bone) and 126 form the appendicular skeleton (arms, legs, shoulders, and pelvis). Shown here are the body's major bones.

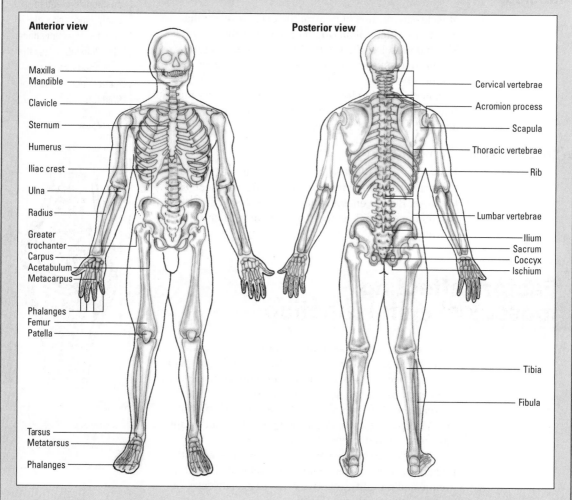

Anterior view

Maxilla
Mandible
Clavicle
Sternum
Humerus
Iliac crest
Ulna
Radius
Greater trochanter
Carpus
Acetabulum
Metacarpus
Phalanges
Femur
Patella
Tarsus
Metatarsus
Phalanges

Posterior view

Cervical vertebrae
Acromion process
Scapula
Thoracic vertebrae
Rib
Lumbar vertebrae
Ilium
Sacrum
Coccyx
Ischium
Tibia
Fibula

Popular joints

Synovial joints come in several types, including ball-and-socket joints and hinge joints. Ball-and-socket joints—the shoulders and hips being the only examples of this type—enable flexion, extension, adduction, and abduction. These joints also rotate in their sockets and are assessed by their degree of internal and external rotation. Hinge joints, such as the knee and elbow, typically move in flexion and extension only. (See *Synovial joint.*)

Muscles

Muscles are groups of contractile cells or fibers that effect movement of an organ or a part of the body. Skeletal muscles, the focus of this chapter, contract and produce skeletal movement when they receive a stimulus from the central nervous system (CNS). The CNS is responsible for involuntary and voluntary muscle function. Tendons, the tough fibrous portions of muscle, attach the muscles to bone.

Where would we be without bursae?

Bursae are sacs filled with friction-reducing synovial fluid; they're located in areas of high friction such as the knee. Bursae enable adjacent muscles or muscles and tendons to glide smoothly over each other during movement.

Factors affecting musculoskeletal function

When an individual has limited mobility and movement, his health can deteriorate and multiple complications can occur. The signs and symptoms of inactivity, commonly described as *disuse syndrome*, can include decreased muscle strength and tone, lack of coordination, altered gait, falls, decreased joint flexibility, pain on movement, and decreased activity tolerance.

Lifestyle and habits can affect a person's mobility. Regular exercise helps maintain musculoskeletal functioning and mobility. Inactivity due to age, disease, or trauma can alter that mobility.

Major or minor trauma

Anything that interferes with bone resiliency and strength or muscle strength may impair the musculoskeletal system's capacity to assist mobility. Trauma can result in injury to tendons, ligaments, joints, bones, or muscles. This damage can be minor or major and can affect mobility for a short time or for a longer time if it involves a dislocated joint, broken bone, torn tendons, or joint replacement.

Synovial joint

Normally, bones fit together. Cartilage—a smooth, fibrous tissue—cushions the end of each bone, and synovial fluid fills the joint space. This fluid lubricates the joint and eases movement, much as the brake fluid functions in a car.

Joint capsule

Cartilage

Bone

Joint space filled with synovial fluid

Such diseases as rheumatoid arthritis (RA), osteoporosis, gout, and osteoarthritis can also limit mobility. Bone tumors can cause pain and may require amputation of the affected limbs.

The nerves have it

Any disorder that impairs the nervous system's ability to control movement of the muscles and coordination hinders mobility. Such diseases as muscular dystrophy, Parkinson's disease, and multiple sclerosis slowly erode and destroy the patient's capacity for coordinated movement.

Two or four

Brain or spinal cord injuries can result in a severed or severely damaged spinal cord, causing paralysis below the injury. Decreased motor and sensory function to the legs is referred to as *paraplegia* and paralysis of the arms and the legs is called *quadriplegia.*

O_2 needed

Oxygen is needed for the muscles to function properly. Any disease that limits the oxygen supply affects muscle contraction and movement. Lung conditions reduce the amount of oxygen delivered to the cells, including skeletal muscles.

Ouch! That hurts!

Activity intolerance may be associated with pain or edema. Alternatively, the patient's activity may be severely restricted by such conditions as fractures requiring skeletal traction, RA, vertebral fractures, neurogenic arthropathy, Paget's disease, muscular dystrophy, and other disorders.

Treating immobility

Impaired physical mobility is related to many musculoskeletal disorders that involve joint inflammation as well as fractures, bone disorders, and other disorders that cause decreased mobility.

Proper positioning

Proper positioning and alignment and pressure-reducing devices help maintain correct body positioning and prevent complications that can occur with prolonged bed rest. (See *Positioning patients*, page 388.) When a patient is weak, in pain, frail, paralyzed, immobilized, or unconscious, they can't readily position and reposition themselves. Thus, your assistance to help or provide position changes may be needed. Assessing the skin and providing skin care before and after repositioning is also important.

Positioning patients

Dorsal recumbent position

In the dorsal recumbent (or *supine*) position, the patient is placed on their back with the knees slightly flexed. Place a pillow beneath the head for comfort. This position immobilizes the spine. It's commonly used for a spinal cord injury, urinary catheter insertion or, in women, a vaginal examination.

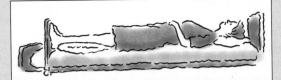

Semi-Fowler's position

For semi-Fowler's position, elevate the head of the bed to 30 degrees and raise the bed section under the patient's knees, flexing the knees slightly. This position promotes drainage, cardiac output, and ventilation. It also prevents aspiration of food and secretions. Like Fowler's position, it's commonly used for a patient who has a head injury, increased intracranial pressure, or dyspnea; has undergone abdominal surgery, cranial surgery, thyroidectomy, or eye surgery; or is vomiting.

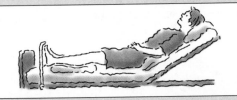

Prone position

The prone position is used to promote gas exchange and enable examination of the back. It's accomplished by placing the patient on their stomach with the head turned to one side and positioning the arms at the side or above the head. Make sure that the legs are extended. This position is commonly used for immobilization, acute respiratory distress syndrome, and after lumbar puncture or a myelogram.

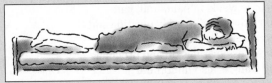

Lateral position

The lateral (or *side-lying*) position promotes safety and prevents atelectasis, pressure ulcers, and aspiration of food and secretions. Place the patient on their side, with the weight supported mostly by the lateral aspect of the lower scapula and the lower ilium. Support this position by placing pillows as needed. This position is commonly used for administering an enema or a suppository and for a patient who has undergone abdominal surgery, is in a coma, or has pressure ulcers.

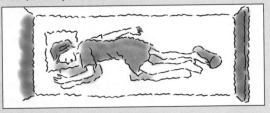

Sims' position

Also called a *semi-prone position*, Sims' position enables examination of the back and rectum and can help prevent atelectasis and pressure ulcers. Position the patient on their side with a small pillow placed beneath the head. Flex one knee toward the abdomen, with the other knee only slightly flexed. Place one arm behind the body and the other in a comfortable position. Support the patient in this position with pillows as needed. Sims' position is commonly used for a patient who has sustained rectal injuries or is in a coma.

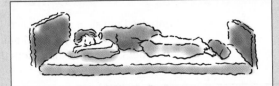

Change is good

Frequent position changes help prevent muscle discomfort, damage to superficial nerves and blood vessels, prolonged pressure resulting in pressure ulcers, and muscle contractures.

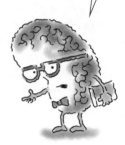

A disorder affecting the nervous system can impair a person's ability to coordinate movement.

Using alignment and pressure-reducing devices

Alignment and pressure-reducing devices include protective boots to protect the heels and help prevent skin breakdown and footdrop; abduction pillows to help prevent internal hip rotation after femoral fracture, hip fracture, or surgery; trochanter rolls to help prevent external hip rotation; and hand rolls to help prevent hand contractures. Several of these devices—protective boots, trochanter rolls, and hand rolls—are especially useful when caring for patients who have a loss of sensation, mobility, or consciousness or following a neuromuscular incident such as stroke.

What you need

Protective boots ✳ abduction pillow ✳ trochanter rolls ✳ hand rolls (See *Common preventive devices*, page 390.)

Getting ready

If you're using a device that's available in different sizes, select the appropriate size for the patient.

How you do it

• Explain the purpose and steps of the procedure to the patient.

Applying a protective boot

• Open the slit on the superior surface of the boot. Then place the patient's foot in the boot and fasten the ankle and foot straps. If the patient is positioned laterally, you may apply the boot only to the bottom foot and support the flexed top foot with a pillow.
• If appropriate, insert the other foot in the second boot.
• Position the patient's legs in alignment *to prevent strain on hip ligaments and pressure on bony prominences.*

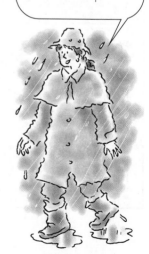

Yeah, these boots protect my feet, but they aren't the protective boots we're talking about here. Those protect the heels and prevent skin breakdown and foot drop.

Common preventive devices

These illustrations show different devices used to reduce pressure or help maintain positioning, depending on the patient's needs.

Protective boot

The protective boot prevents footdrop and skin breakdown. Some protective boots are made of soft material that cradles the heel to prevent pressure on the heel. Other models consist of aluminum frames with fleece lining and toe extensions that protect the toes and prevent hip adduction. High-topped sneakers may be used to help prevent footdrop, but they don't prevent external hip rotation or heel pressure.

Abduction pillow

The abduction pillow prevents internal hip rotation. It's a wedge-shaped piece of sponge rubber with lateral indentations for the patient's thighs. Its straps wrap around the thighs to maintain correct positioning. Although a properly shaped bed pillow may temporarily substitute for the commercial abduction pillow, it's difficult to apply and fails to maintain the correct lateral alignment.

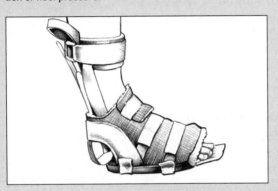

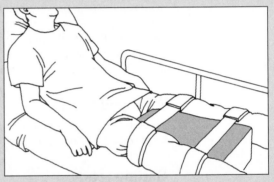

Trochanter roll

The trochanter roll prevents external hip rotation. The commercial trochanter roll is made of sponge rubber, but you can also improvise one from a rolled blanket or towel.

Hand roll

The hand roll prevents hand contractures. It's available in hard and soft materials and is held in place by fixed or adjustable straps. It can be improvised from a rolled washcloth secured with roller gauze and adhesive tape.

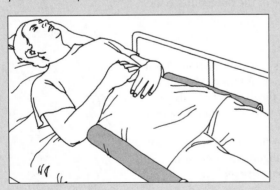

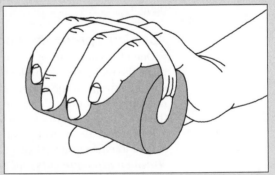

Applying an abduction pillow

• Place the patient in a supine position and put the pillow between his legs. Slide the pillow toward the groin so that it touches his legs all along their length.
• Place the upper part of both legs in the pillow's lateral indentations, and secure the straps *to prevent the pillow from slipping.*

Applying a trochanter roll

• Place one roll on the outside of the thigh from the iliac crest to midthigh. Then place another roll along the other thigh. Make sure neither roll extends as far as the knee *to avoid peroneal nerve compression and palsy, which can lead to footdrop.*
• If you've fashioned trochanter rolls from a towel or rolled sheet, leave several inches unrolled and tuck this part under the patient's thigh *to hold the device in place and maintain the patient's position.*

Applying a hand roll

• Place one roll in the patient's hand. *This will help maintain the neutral position.* Then secure the strap, if present, or apply roller gauze and secure with hypoallergenic or adhesive tape.
• Place another roll in the other hand.
• Remember that the use of assistive devices doesn't preclude regularly scheduled patient positioning, ROM exercises, and skin care.
• Contractures and pressure ulcers may occur with the use of a hand roll and, possibly, with other assistive devices. *To avoid these problems,* remove a soft hand roll every 4 hours (every 2 hours if the patient has hand spasticity); remove a hard hand roll every 2 hours.

Ambulating patients

Many patient care activities require you to push, pull, lift, and carry. By using proper body mechanics, you can avoid your own musculoskeletal injury and fatigue and reduce the risk of injuring patients.

Using proper body mechanics

Correct body mechanics can be summed up in three principles:

Keep a low center of gravity by flexing the hips and knees instead of bending at the waist to distribute weight evenly between the upper and lower body and maintain balance.

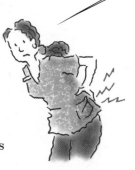

Spare your back. Know the proper way to lift, push, pull, and carry!

✌ Create a wide base of support by spreading your feet apart to provide lateral stability and lower your body's center of gravity.

🖐 Maintain proper body alignment and keep your body's center of gravity directly over the base of support by moving your feet rather than twisting and bending at the waist.

Do it right

In addition to the three basic principles, follow the directions below to push, pull, stoop, lift, and carry correctly.

Pushing and pulling correctly

• Stand close to the object, and place one foot slightly ahead of the other, as in a walking position. Tighten your leg muscles and set your pelvis by simultaneously contracting your abdominal and gluteal muscles.
• To push, place your hands on the object and flex your elbows. Lean into the object by shifting weight from your back leg to your front leg, and apply smooth, continuous pressure.
• To pull, grasp the object and flex your elbows. Lean away from the object by shifting weight from your front leg to your back leg. Pull smoothly, avoiding sudden, jerky movements.
• After you've started to move the object, keep it in motion; *stopping and starting uses more energy.*

Stooping correctly

• Stand with your feet 10″ to 12″ (25 to 30 cm) apart and one foot slightly ahead of the other *to widen the base of support.*
• Lower yourself by flexing your knees, and place more weight on the front foot than on the back foot. Keep your upper body straight by not bending at the waist.
• To stand up again, straighten your knees and keep your back straight.

Lifting and carrying correctly

• Assume the stooping position directly in front of the object *to minimize back flexion and avoid spinal rotation when lifting.*
• Grasp the object, and tighten your abdominal muscles.
• Stand up by straightening your knees, using your leg and hip muscles. Always keep your back straight *to maintain a fixed center of gravity.*
• Carry the object close to your body at waist height—near the body's center of gravity—*to avoid straining your back muscles.* (See *Transfer tips.*)

Transfer from bed to stretcher

Transfer from bed to stretcher, one of the most common transfers, can require the help of one or more coworkers, depending on the patient's size and condition and the primary nurse's physical ability. Techniques for achieving this transfer include the straight lift, carry lift, lift sheet, and sliding board.

What you need

Stretcher ✳ sliding board or lift sheet, if necessary

Getting ready

Adjust the bed to the same height as the stretcher.

How you do it

• Tell the patient that you're going to move them from the bed to the stretcher, and place them in the supine position.
• Instruct team members to remove watches and rings. *This will prevent scratching the patient during transfer.*

Four-person straight lift

• Place the stretcher parallel to the bed, and lock the wheels of both *to ensure patient safety.*

Get into position

• Stand at the center of the stretcher and have another team member stand at the patient's head. The two other team members should stand next to the bed on the other side— one at the center and the other at the patient's feet.
• Slide your arms, palms up, under the patient while the other team members do the same. In this position, you and the team member directly opposite to you support the patient's buttocks and hips; the team member at the head of the bed supports the patient's head and shoulders; and the one at the foot supports the patient's legs and feet.

One, two, three

• On a count of three, you and your team members lift the patient several inches, move them onto the stretcher, and slide your arms out from under them. Keep movements smooth *to minimize patient discomfort and avoid muscle strain by team members.*
• Position the patient comfortably on the stretcher, apply safety straps, and raise and secure the side rails.

Transfer tips

When transferring a patient or performing other care activities, remember these tips:
• Wear shoes with low heels, flexible nonslip soles, and closed backs to promote correct body alignment, facilitate proper body mechanics, and prevent accidents.
• When possible, pull rather than push an object because elbow flexors are stronger than extensors.
• When doing heavy lifting or moving, remember to use assistive or mechanical devices, if available, or obtain assistance from coworkers; know your limitations and use sound judgment.

Four-person carry lift
- Place the stretcher perpendicular to the bed, with the head of the stretcher at the foot of the bed. Lock the bed and the stretcher wheels *to ensure patient safety.*
- Raise the bed to a comfortable working height.

Top to bottom, tallest to shortest
- Line up all four team members on the same side of the bed as the stretcher. Place the tallest member at the patient's head and the shortest at their feet. The member at the patient's head is the team leader and gives the lift signals.
- Assume the team leader role and tell the team members to flex their knees and slide their hands, palms up, under the patient until they rest securely on their upper arms.
- Make sure the patient is adequately supported at the head and shoulders, buttocks and hips, and legs and feet.

Reduce the strain
- On a count of three, the team members straighten their knees and roll the patient onto his side, against their chests. *This reduces strain on the team members and allows them to hold the patient for several minutes if necessary.*
- Together, the team members step back, with the member supporting the feet moving the farthest.

On the count of three
- The team members move forward to the stretcher's edge and, on a count of three, lower the patient onto the stretcher by bending at the knees and sliding their arms out from under the patient.
- Position the patient comfortably on the stretcher, apply safety straps, and raise and secure the side rails.

Four-person lift sheet transfer
- Position the bed, stretcher, and team members for the straight lift.

Make it close to the patient
- Instruct the team to hold the edges of the sheet under the patient, grasping them close to the patient *to obtain a firm grip, provide stability, and spare the patient feelings of instability.*

One smooth, continuous motion
- On a count of three, the team members lift or slide the patient onto the stretcher in one smooth, continuous motion *to avoid muscle strain and minimize patient discomfort.*
- Position the patient comfortably on the stretcher, apply safety straps, and raise and secure the side rails.

Sliding-board transfer

• Place the stretcher parallel to the bed, and lock the wheels of both *to ensure patient safety.*
• Stand next to the bed, and instruct a coworker to stand next to the stretcher.
• Reach over the patient, and pull the far side of the bed sheet toward you *to turn the patient slightly on his side.*

Bridging the gap

• Instruct your coworker to place the sliding board beneath the patient, making sure the board bridges the gap between the stretcher and the bed.
• Ease the patient onto the sliding board, and release the sheet.

Making the transfer

• Instruct your coworker to grasp the near side of the sheet at the patient's hips and shoulders and to pull them onto the stretcher in a smooth, continuous motion. Then have her reach over the patient, grasp the far side of the sheet, and logroll the patient toward her.

Getting the patient settled

• Remove the sliding board as your coworker returns the patient to the supine position.
• Position the patient comfortably on the stretcher, apply safety straps, and raise and secure the side rails.

Special circumstances

If the patient is obese

• When transferring from the bed to the stretcher, lift and move the obese patient, in increments, to the edge of the bed. Then rest for a few seconds, and lift them onto the stretcher.
• Depending on the patient's size and condition, lift sheet transfer can require two to seven people.
• If available, consider using a mechanical lift to transfer the patient. (See *Using a mechanical lift*, page 396.)

If the patient can bear weight

• Two or three coworkers can perform a transfer if the patient can bear weight on their arms or legs. One can support the buttocks and guide the patient, another can stabilize the stretcher by leaning over it and guiding the patient into position and a third can transfer any attached equipment. If a team member isn't available

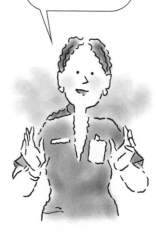

Make sure you apply safety straps and secure the side rails after any patient transfer.

Using a mechanical lift

After placing the patient in the supine position in the center of the sling, position the hydraulic lift above them (as shown below). Then attach the chains to the hooks on the sling.

Turn the lift handle clockwise to raise the patient to the sitting position. If they are positioned properly, continue to raise them until they are suspended just above the bed.

After positioning the patient above the wheelchair, turn the lift handle counterclockwise to lower them onto the seat. When the chains become slack, stop turning and unhook the sling from the lift.

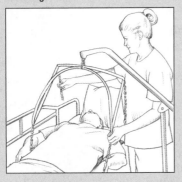
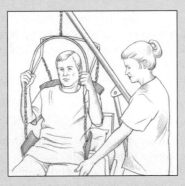
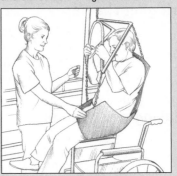

to guide equipment, move I.V. lines and other tubing first *to make sure they're out of the way and not in danger of pulling loose*, or disconnect the tubes if possible.

If the patient is light

- Three coworkers can perform the carry lift if the patient is light, but no matter how many team members are present, one must stabilize the patient's head if they can't support it themselves, have cervical instability or injury, or has undergone surgery.
- Document the time and type of transfer in your notes. Complete other required forms as necessary.

> Sure, this looks easy. A lift sheet transfer is nothing like this. It takes at least two people and can take up to seven, depending on the size of the patient.

Transfer from bed to wheelchair

For a patient with diminished or absent lower body sensation or one-sided weakness, immobility, or injury, transfer from bed to wheelchair may require partial support to full assistance—initially by at least two persons. After transfer, proper positioning helps prevent excessive pressure on bony prominences, which predisposes the patient to skin breakdown.

What you need

Wheelchair with locks (or sturdy chair) ✳ pajama bottoms (or robe) ✳ shoes or slippers with nonslip soles ✳ optional: transfer board if appropriate

Getting ready

• Explain the procedure to the patient and demonstrate the patient's role. (See *Teaching the patient to use a transfer board*, page 398.)
• Place the wheelchair parallel to the bed, facing the foot of the bed, and lock its wheels. Make sure the bed wheels are also locked. Raise the footrests *to avoid interfering with the transfer.*

Check the vitals

• Check the patient's pulse rate and blood pressure when they are in a supine position *to obtain a baseline.* Assist the patient with putting on pajama bottoms and slippers or shoes with nonslip soles *to prevent falls.*

How you do it

• Raise the head of the bed, and allow the patient to rest briefly *to adjust to posture changes.* Then bring him to the dangling position. Recheck his pulse rate and blood pressure if you suspect cardiovascular instability, and don't proceed until they're stabilized *to prevent falls.*

Out of the bed . . .

• Tell the patient to move toward the edge of the bed and, if possible, to place feet flat on the floor. Stand in front of the patient, blocking the toes with your feet and their knees with yours *to prevent the knees from buckling.*
• Flex your knees slightly, place your arms around the patient's waist, and tell them to place their hands on the edge of the bed. Avoid bending at your waist *to prevent back strain.*
• Ask the patient to push off the bed and to support as much of their own weight as possible. At the same time, straighten your knees and hips, raising the patient as you straighten your body.
• Supporting the patient as needed, pivot toward the wheelchair, keeping your knees next to his. Tell them to grasp the farthest armrest of the wheelchair with their closest hand.

. . . and into the chair

• Help the patient lower themselves into the wheelchair by flexing your hips and knees but not your back. Instruct the patient to reach back and grasp the other wheelchair armrest as they sit *to avoid abrupt contact with the seat.* Fasten the seat belt *to prevent*

Teacher's lounge

Teaching the patient to use a transfer board

For the patient who can't stand, a transfer board allows safe transfer from bed to wheelchair. To help the patient perform this transfer, take these steps:

Explain the procedure to the patient, and then demonstrate it. They may eventually become proficient enough to transfer with or without supervision.

Help the patient put on pajama bottoms or a robe and shoes or slippers.

Angle the wheelchair slightly facing the foot of the bed. Lock the wheels, and remove the armrest closest to the patient. Make sure the bed is flat, and adjust its height so that it's level with the wheelchair seat.

Assist the patient to a sitting position on the edge of the bed, with feet resting on the floor. Make sure the front edge of the wheelchair seat is aligned with the back of the patient's knees (as shown below left). Depending on the patient, they may find it easier to transfer to an even surface or to a slightly lower surface.

Ask the patient to lean away from the wheelchair while you slide one end of the transfer board under him.

Then place the other end of the transfer board on the wheelchair seat, and help the patient return to the upright position.

Stand in front of the patient to prevent them from sliding forward. Tell them to push down with both arms, lifting the buttocks up and onto the transfer board. Have them repeat this maneuver, edging along the board, until seated in the wheelchair. If they can't use their arms to help with the transfer, stand in front of the patient, put your arms around them, and—if they can—have the patient put their arms around you. Gradually slide them across the board until safely in the chair (as shown below right).

When the patient is in the chair fasten a seat belt, if necessary, to prevent falls.

Then remove the transfer board, replace the wheelchair armrest, and reposition the patient in the chair.

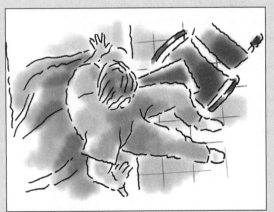

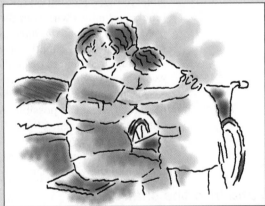

falls and, if necessary, check pulse rate and blood pressure *to assess cardiovascular stability.* If the pulse rate is 20 beats or more above baseline, stay with the patient and monitor them closely until the rate returns to normal *because they are experiencing orthostatic hypotension.*

Position, position, position

- If the patient can't position correctly, help them move their buttocks against the back of the chair *so that the ischial tuberosities, not the sacrum, provide the base of support.*
- Place the patient's feet flat on the footrests, pointed straight ahead.
- Position the knees and hips with the correct amount of flexion and in appropriate alignment.
- If appropriate, use elevating leg rests to flex the patient's hips at more than 90 degrees; *this position relieves pressure on the popliteal space and places more weight on the ischial tuberosities.*
- Position the patient's arms on the wheelchair's armrests with shoulders abducted, elbows slightly flexed, forearms pronated, and wrists and hands in the neutral position.
- If necessary, support or elevate their hands and forearms with a pillow *to prevent dependent edema.*
- If the patient starts to fall during transfer, ease them to the closest surface. Never stretch to finish the transfer. *Doing so can cause loss of balance, falls, muscle strain, and other injuries to you and the patient.*

Compensating for weakness

- If the patient has one-sided weakness, follow the preceding steps, but place the wheelchair on his unaffected side. Instruct them to pivot and bear as much weight as possible on the unaffected side. Support the affected side *because the patient will tend to lean to this side.* If the patient is hemiplegic, use pillows to support the affected side *to prevent slumping in the wheelchair.*

Crutch walking

Crutches remove weight from one or both legs, enabling the patient to support himself with his hands and arms. Typically prescribed for a patient with lower extremity injury or weakness, crutches require balance, stamina, and upper body strength for successful use. Crutch selection and walking gait depend on the patient's condition. A patient who can't use crutches may be able to use a walker.

What you need

Crutches with axillary pads, handgrips, and rubber suction tips ✳ optional: walking belt

Getting ready

• After choosing the appropriate crutches, adjust their height with the patient standing or, if necessary, recumbent. (See *Selecting and fitting a crutch*.)
• Consult with the patient's doctor and physical therapist *to coordinate rehabilitation orders and teaching.*

How you do it

• Describe the gait you'll teach and the reason for your choice. Then demonstrate the gait as necessary. Have the patient give a return demonstration.
• Place a walking belt around the patient's waist, if necessary, *to help prevent falls.* Tell the patient to position the crutches and shift his weight from side to side. Then place them in front of a full-length mirror *to facilitate learning and coordination.*

Four point

• Teach the four-point gait to the patient who can bear weight on both legs. Although this is the safest gait *because three points are always in contact with the floor,* it requires greater coordination than others *because of the constant weight shifting.* Use this sequence: right crutch, left foot, left crutch, right foot. Suggest counting *to help develop rhythm,* and make sure each short step is of equal length. If the patient gains proficiency at this gait, teach them the faster two-point gait.

Three point

• Teach the three-point gait to the patient who can bear only partial or no weight on one leg. Instruct them to advance both crutches 6″ to 8″ (15 to 20 cm) along with the involved leg. Then tell them to bring the uninvolved leg forward and to bear the bulk of the weight on the crutches but some of it on the involved leg, if possible. Stress the importance of taking steps of equal length and duration with no pauses.
• Teach the swing-to or swing-through gaits—the fastest gaits—to the patient with complete paralysis of the hips and legs. Instruct them to advance both crutches simultaneously and to swing the legs parallel to (swing-to) or beyond (swing-through) the crutches.

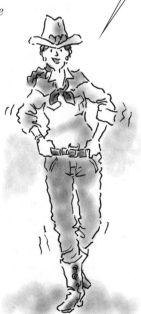

We aren't talking about the two-step here . . . this is all about the three-point gait.

Selecting and fitting a crutch

When fitting a patient for a crutch, selecting the right type of crutch is the first step. Three types of crutches are commonly used:

✌ Standard aluminum or wooden crutches are used by the patient with a sprain, strain, or cast. They require stamina and upper body strength.

✌ Aluminum forearm crutches are used by the paraplegic or other patient using the swing-through gait. They have a collar that fits around the forearm and a horizontal handgrip that provides support.

✌ Platform crutches are used by the arthritic patient who has an upper extremity deficit that prevents weight bearing through the wrist. They provide padded surfaces for the upper extremities.

The right fit

If the patient is using a standard aluminum or wooden crutch, it must be fit properly. To fit the crutch to the patient, position the crutch so that it extends from a point 4″ to 6″ (10 to 15 cm) to the side and 4″ to 6″ in front of the patient's feet to 1½″ to 2″ (4 to 5 cm) below the axillae (about the width of two fingers). Then adjust the handgrips so that the patient's elbows are flexed at a 15-degree angle when they are standing with the crutches in the resting position.

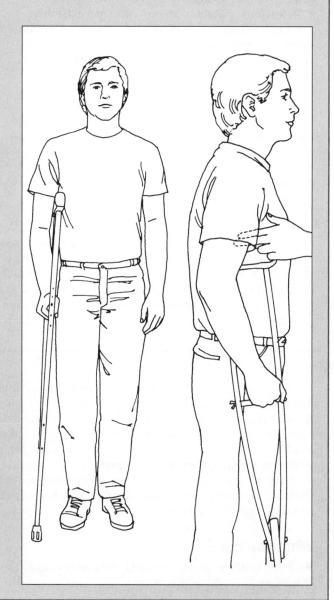

• To teach the patient who uses crutches to get up from a chair, tell them to hold both crutches in one hand, with the tips resting firmly on the floor. Then instruct them to push up from the chair with the free hand, supporting themselves with the crutches.

• To sit down, the patient reverses the process: Instruct them to support themselves with the crutches in one hand and lower themselves with the other.

• To teach the patient to ascend stairs using the three-point gait, tell them to lead with the uninvolved leg and follow with both the crutches and the involved leg. To descend stairs, they should lead with the crutches and the involved leg and follow with the good leg.

Memory jogger

To help your patient using the three-point gait to climb stairs, teach them to remember "The good goes up; the bad goes down." **Going up,** they should lead with the uninvolved leg, and **going down,** they should lead with the involved leg and the crutches.

Two point

• Teach the two-point gait to the patient with weak legs but good coordination and arm strength. This is the most natural crutch-walking gait *because it mimics walking, with alternating swings of the arms and legs.* Instruct the patient to advance the right crutch and left foot simultaneously followed by the left crutch and right foot.

Arms and shoulders

• Encourage arm- and shoulder-strengthening exercises *to pre-pare the patient for crutch walking.* If possible, consult physical therapy to teach the patient two techniques—one fast and one slow—and teach the patient to alternate between them *to prevent excessive muscle fatigue and enable an easier transition to walking.*

Using a walker

A walker consists of a metal frame with handgrips and four legs that buttresses the patient on three sides; one side remains open. *Because this device provides greater stability and security than other ambulatory aids,* it's recommended for the patient with insufficient strength and balance to use crutches or a cane or with weakness requiring frequent rest periods.

Attachments for standard walkers and modified walkers help meet special needs. For example, a walker may have a platform added to support an injured arm.

What you need

Walker ✳ platform or wheel attachments, as necessary (see *Types of walkers.*)

Types of walkers

Various types of walkers are available. The standard walker is used by the patient with unilateral or bilateral weakness or an inability to bear weight on one leg. It requires arm strength and balance. Platform attachments may be added to a standard walker for the patient with arthritic arms or a casted arm who can't bear weight directly on the hand, wrist, or forearm.

Got wheels

With the doctor's approval, wheels may be placed on the front legs of the standard walker to allow the extremely weak or poorly coordinated patient to roll the device forward, instead of lifting it. The rolling walker—used by the patient with very weak legs—has four wheels and may also have a seat. However, wheels aren't commonly applied because they pose a safety hazard.

Stair walker

The stair walker—used by the patient who must navigate stairs without bilateral hand rails—requires good arm strength and balance. Its extra set of handles extends toward the patient on the open side.

Reciprocation proclamation

The reciprocal walker—used by the patient with very weak arms—allows one side to be advanced ahead of the other.

Getting ready

• Obtain the appropriate walker with the advice of a physical therapist, and adjust it to the patient's height: The patient's elbows should be flexed at a 15-degree angle when standing comfortably within the walker with their hands on the grips.
• To adjust the walker, turn it upside down, and change the leg length by pushing in the button on each shaft and releasing it when the leg is in the correct position.
• Make sure the walker is level before the patient attempts to use it.

How you do it

• Help the patient stand within the walker, and instruct them to hold the handgrips firmly and equally. Stand behind the patient, closer to the involved leg.
• If the patient has one-sided leg weakness, tell them to advance the walker 6″ to 8″ (15 to 20 cm), step forward with the involved leg, and follow with the uninvolved leg, supporting themselves on their arms. Encourage them to take equal strides. If they have equal strength in both legs, instruct them to advance the walker 6″ to 8″ and step forward with either leg. If they can't use one leg, tell them to advance the walker 6″ to 8″ and swing onto it, supporting their weight on their arms.

Teacher's lounge

Teaching safe use of a walker

To teach a patient how to sit down and get up safely using a walker, follow the steps outlined here.

Sitting down

• First, tell the patient to stand with the back of the stronger leg against the front of the chair, the weaker leg slightly off the floor, and the walker directly in front.
• Tell them to grasp the armrests on the chair one arm at a time while supporting most of the weight on the stronger leg. (In the illustrations below, the patient has left leg weakness.)
• Tell the patient to lower themselves into the chair and slide backward. After seated, they should place the walker beside the chair.

Getting up

• After bringing the walker to the front of the chair, tell the patient to slide forward in the chair. Placing the back of his stronger leg against the seat, they should then advance the weaker leg.
• Next, with both hands on the armrests, the patient can push themselves to a standing position. Supporting themselves with the stronger leg and the opposite hand, the patient should grasp the walker's handgrip with the free hand.
• Then the patient should grasp the free handgrip with the other hand.

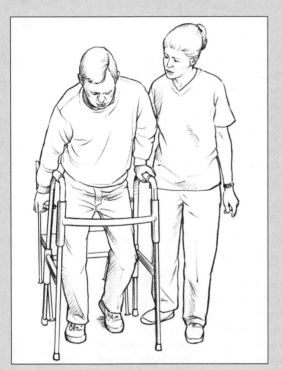
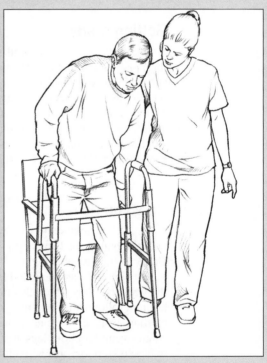

Two-point gait

- If the patient is using a reciprocal walker, teach them the two-point gait. Instruct the patient to stand with their weight evenly distributed between the legs and the walker. Stand behind the patient, slightly to one side. Tell them to advance simultaneously with the walker's right side and their left foot. Then have the patient advance the walker's left side and their right foot.

Four-point gait

- If the patient is using a reciprocal walker, also instruct them on the four-point gait. Instruct the patient to evenly distribute their weight between the legs and the walker. Stand behind the patient and slightly to one side. Have them move the right side of the walker forward. Then have the patient move their left foot forward. Next, instruct them to move the left side of the walker forward. Lastly, have them move the right foot forward.
- If the patient is using a wheeled or stair walker, reinforce the physical therapist's instructions. Stress the need for caution when using a stair walker.
- Teach the patient how to sit down and get up from a chair safely. (See *Teaching safe use of a walker.*)
- If the patient starts to fall, support their hips and shoulders *to help him maintain an upright position if possible.* If unsuccessful, ease them slowly to the closest surface—bed, floor, or chair.

Helping patients exercise

Exercise maintains or increases muscle strength and endurance and helps maintain cardiopulmonary function. *Because an immobilized patient may not be able to perform these exercises by himself,* learning how to assist a patient in exercise is an essential part of proper care and health promotion.

Passive then active

Passive ROM exercises help prevent deterioration of the muscles and tissues of a patient who can't independently perform exercise. Later, as this type of patient gains strength and no longer needs passive exercise, they can perform isometric or active ROM exercises.

Passive ROM exercises

Passive ROM exercises improve or maintain joint mobility and help prevent contractures. Performed by a nurse, a physical

> Passive ROM exercises help prevent deterioration of muscles and tissues. Later, the patient may be able to perform isometric or active ROM exercises.

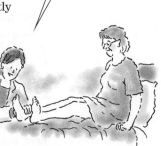

therapist, or a caregiver of the patient's choosing, these exercises are indicated for the patient with temporary or permanent loss of mobility, sensation, or consciousness. Passive ROM exercises require recognition of the patient's limits of motion and support of all joints during movement.

Just say no

Passive ROM exercises are contraindicated in patients with septic joints, acute thrombophlebitis, severe arthritic joint inflammation, or recent trauma with possible hidden fractures or internal injuries.

Equal opportunity exercises

The exercises discussed here treat all joints, but they don't have to be performed in the order given or all at once. You can schedule them over the course of a day, whenever the patient is in the most convenient position. Remember to perform all exercises slowly, gently, and to the end of the normal ROM or to the point of pain but no further. (See *Types of joint motion.*)

Getting ready

• Determine the joints that need ROM exercises, and consult the doctor or physical therapist about limitations or precautions for specific exercises.
• Before you begin, raise the bed to a comfortable working height.

How you do it

Use the following steps to perform ROM on the patient's neck, shoulder, elbow, forearm, wrist, fingers and thumb, hip and knee, ankle, and toes.

Exercising the neck

• Support the patient's head with your hands and extend the neck, flex the chin to the chest, and tilt the head laterally toward each shoulder.
• Rotate the head from right to left.

Exercising the shoulder

• Support the patient's arm in an extended, neutral position; then extend the forearm and flex it back. Abduct the arm outward from the side of the body, and adduct it back to the side.
• Rotate the patient's shoulder so that the arm crosses midline, and bend the elbow so that the hand touches the opposite shoulder and then the mattress of the bed for complete internal rotation.
• Return the shoulder to a neutral position and, with the elbow bent, push the arm backward so that the back of the hand touches the mattress for complete external rotation.

Types of joint motion

These illustrations show various areas of the body and what types of movements their joints allow.

Circumduction

Moving in a circular manner

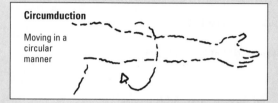

Flexion
Bending, decreasing the joint angle

Extension
Straightening, increasing the joint angle

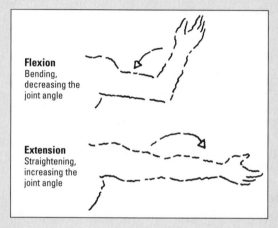

Abduction
Moving away from midline

Adduction
Moving toward midline

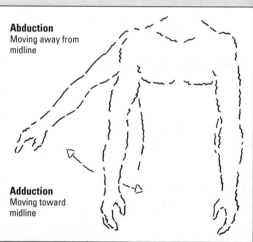

Retraction and protraction
Moving backward and forward

Pronation
Turning downward

Supination
Turning upward

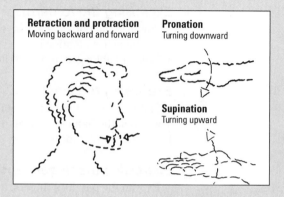

Internal rotation
Turning toward midline

External rotation
Turning away from midline

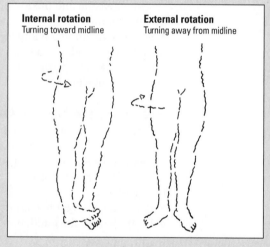

Eversion
Turning outward

Inversion
Turning inward

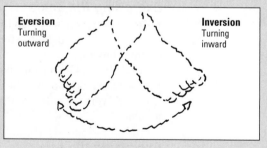

Exercising the elbow

• Place the patient's arm at the side with palm facing up.
• Flex and extend the arm at the elbow.

Exercising the forearm

• Stabilize the patient's elbow, and then twist the hand to bring the palm up (supination).
• Twist it back again to bring the palm down (pronation).

Exercising the wrist

• Stabilize the patient's forearm, and flex and extend the wrist. Then rock the hand sideways for lateral flexion, and rotate the hand in a circular motion.

Exercising the fingers and thumb

• Extend the patient's fingers, and then flex the hand into a fist; repeat extension and flexion of each joint of each finger and thumb separately.
• Spread two adjoining fingers apart (abduction), and then bring them together (adduction).
• Oppose each fingertip to the thumb, and rotate the thumb and each finger in a circle.

Exercising the hip and knee

• Extend the patient's leg, and then bend the hip and knee toward the chest, allowing full joint flexion.
• Next, move the straight leg sideways, out and away from the other leg (abduction), and then back, over, and across it (adduction).
• Rotate the straight leg internally toward the midline, then externally away from the midline.

Exercising the ankle

• Bend the patient's foot so that the toes push upward (dorsiflexion), and then bend the foot so that the toes push downward (plantar flexion).
• Rotate the ankle in a circular motion.
• Invert the ankle so that the sole of the foot faces his midline, and then evert the ankle so that the sole faces away from the midline.

Exercising the toes

• Flex the patient's toes toward the sole, and then extend them back toward the top of his foot.
• Spread two adjoining toes apart (abduction), and bring them together (adduction).

Time is of the essence

• Joints *begin to stiffen within 24 hours of disuse,* therefore, passive ROM exercises should be started as soon as possible, and performed at least once per shift, particularly while bathing or turning the patient. Use proper body mechanics, and repeat each exercise at least three times.

Get the family involved

• If the disabled patient requires long-term rehabilitation after discharge, consult a physical therapist, and teach a family member or caregiver to perform passive ROM exercises. (See *Documenting passive ROM exercises.*)

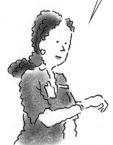

Start passive ROM exercises as soon as possible, and perform them at least once per shift.

Isometric and active ROM exercises

Patients on prolonged bed rest or with limited activity without profound weakness can also be taught to perform ROM exercises on their own (called *active ROM*) or they may benefit from isometric exercises. (See *Learning about isometric exercises,* page 410.)

Take note!

Documenting passive ROM exercises

To document passive ROM exercises, include in your notes:
• which joints were exercised
• patient's tolerance of the exercises
• edema or pressure areas
• pain from the exercises
• ROM limitation.

Learning about isometric exercises

A patient can strengthen and increase muscle tone by contracting muscles against resistance (from other muscles or from a stationary object, such as a bed or wall) without joint movement. These exercises require only a comfortable position—standing, sitting, or lying down—and proper body alignment. For each exercise, instruct the patient to hold each contraction for 2 to 5 seconds and to repeat it three to four times daily, below peak contraction level for the first week and at peak level thereafter.

Neck rotators

The patient places the heel of the hand above one ear. Then push the head toward the hand as forcefully as possible, without moving the head, neck, or arm. The patient repeats the exercise on the other side.

Neck flexors

The patient places both palms on the forehead. Without moving the neck, push the head forward while resisting with the palms.

Neck extensors

The patient clasps the fingers behind the head, and then pushes the head against the clasped hands without moving the neck.

Shoulder elevators

Holding the right arm straight down at the side, the patient grasps the right wrist with the left hand. They then try to shrug the right shoulder, but prevent it from moving by holding the arm in place. Repeat this exercise, alternating arms.

Shoulder, chest, and scapular musculature

The patient places the right fist in the left palm and raises both arms to shoulder height. They push the fist into the palm as forcefully as possible without moving either arm. Then, with the arms in the same position, clasp the fingers and try to pull the hands apart. Repeat the pattern, beginning with the left fist in the right palm.

Elbow flexors and extensors

With the right elbow bent 90 degrees and the right palm facing upward, the patient places the left fist against the right palm. Then try to bend the right elbow further while resisting with the left fist. Repeat the pattern, bending the left elbow.

Abdomen

The patient assumes a sitting position and bends slightly forward, with the hands in front of the middle of the thighs. They try to bend forward further, resisting by pressing the palms against the thighs.

Alternatively, in the supine position, clasp the hands behind the head. Then raise the shoulders about 1″ (2.5 cm), holding this position for a few seconds.

Back extensors

In a sitting position, the patient bends forward and places the hands under the buttocks. They try to stand up, resisting with both hands.

Hip abductors

While standing, the patient squeezes the inner thighs together as tightly as possible. Placing a pillow between the knees supplies resistance and increases the effectiveness of this exercise.

Hip extensors

The patient squeezes the buttocks together as tightly as possible.

Knee extensors

The patient straightens the knee fully. Then vigorously tightens the muscle above the knee so that it moves the kneecap upward. Repeat this exercise, alternating legs.

Ankle flexors and extensors

The patient pulls the toes upward, holding briefly. Then pushes them down as far as possible, again holding briefly.

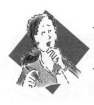

Quick quiz

1. Exercises performed without any effort by the patient are called:
A. strengthening exercises.
B. easy exercises.
C. active ROM exercises.
D. passive ROM exercises.

Answer: D. Passive ROM exercises are performed to test muscle tone and if the patient can't do active ROM exercises.

2. Your patient can't move his right arm toward the midline, so you document this as impaired:
A. supination.
B. abduction.
C. adduction.
D. eversion.

Answer: C. Adduction is the ability to move a limb toward the midline.

3. Which patient position requires that the head of the bed be elevated to 45 degrees?
A. Fowler's
B. Sims'
C. Prone
D. Semi-Fowler's

Answer: A. In Fowler's position the head of the bed is elevated to 45 degrees and the bed section under the patient's knees is also raised to flex the knees slightly.

4. Which gait should you teach a patient who can bear weight on both legs?
A. Three point
B. Four point
C. Two point
D. Five point

Answer: B. Teach the four-point gait to the patient who can bear weight on both legs.

Scoring

☆☆☆ If you answered all four questions correctly, wonderful! Your knowledge of mobility, activity, and exercise is going strong.

☆☆ If you answered three questions correctly, great! Your brain exercises are really paying off.

☆ If you answered fewer than three questions correctly, don't fret! Do some extra ROM (reading on mobility) and try again!

15

Skin integrity and wound healing

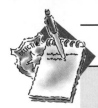

Just the facts

In this chapter, you'll learn:

♦ layers and functions of skin

♦ types of wounds

♦ phases of wound healing

♦ ways to classify wounds according to age, depth, and color

♦ basic wound care assessment and treatment

♦ pressure ulcer prevention, care, and treatment.

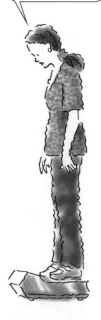

The skin accounts for about 6 to 8 pounds of a person's body weight!

A look at the skin

The skin, or *integumentary system*, is the largest organ in the body. It accounts for about 6 to 8 lb (2.5 to 3.5 kg) of a person's body weight and has a surface area of more than 20 square feet. The thickest skin is located on the hands and the soles of the feet; the thinnest skin, around the eyes and over the tympanic membranes in the ears.

The skin you're in

Skin is made up of distinct layers that function as a single unit. The outermost layer, which is actually a layer of dead cells, is completely replaced every 4 to 6 weeks by cells that migrate to the surface from the layers beneath. The living cells in the skin receive oxygen and nutrients through an extensive network of small blood vessels. In fact, every square inch of skin contains more than 158 blood vessels!

Up close and personal

Skin protects the body by acting as a barrier between internal structures and the external world. Skin also stands between each of us and the social world around us, so it's no wonder that the condition and characteristics of a person's skin influence how he feels about himself. When a person has healthy skin—unblemished skin with good tone (firmness) and color—he feels better about himself. Skin also reflects the body's general physical health. For example, if blood oxygen levels are low, skin may look bluish, and skin appears flushed or red if a person has a fever.

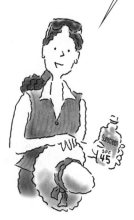

Bad burns from UV rays are wounds, too. Make sure you wear sunscreen and protect your skin!

Surgery, accidents, or sun

Any damage to the skin is considered a wound. Wounds can result from planned events, such as surgery, or unplanned events, including accidents such as a fall from a bike, and exposure to the environment, such as the damage caused by ultraviolet (UV) rays in sunlight.

Layers of the skin

Skin has two main layers: the *epidermis* and the *dermis*, which function as one interrelated unit. A layer of subcutaneous fatty connective tissue, sometimes called the *hypodermis*, lies beneath these layers. Five structural networks, which are stabilized by hair and sweat gland ducts, exist within the epidermis and dermis:

- collagen fibers
- elastic fibers
- small blood vessels
- nerve fibrils
- lymphatics.

Epidermis

The epidermis is the outermost of the skin's two main layers. It varies in thickness from about 0.1-mm thick on the eyelids to as much as 1-mm thick on the palms and soles. The epidermis is slightly acidic, with an average pH of 5.5. This is a really important point as the skin's acidity is protective and when altered may lead to skin breakdown. Covering the epidermis is the keratinized epithelium, a layer of cells that migrate up from the underlying dermis and die upon reaching the surface. These cells are continuously generated and replaced. The keratinized epithelium is supported by the dermis and underlying connective tissue.

In living color

The epidermis also contains melanocytes (cells that produce the brown pigment melanin), which give skin

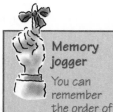

Memory jogger

You can remember the order of the skin's layers by thinking of the prefix **epi-**, which means "upon." Therefore, the **epi**dermis is upon, or on top of, the dermis.

and hair their colors. The more melanin produced by melanocytes, the darker the skin. Skin color varies from one person to the next, but it can also vary from one area of skin on the body to another. The hypothalamus regulates melanin production by secreting melanocyte-stimulating hormone.

Layer upon layer

The epidermis is divided into five distinct layers. Each layer's name reflects its structure or its function. Here's a look at them from the outside in:

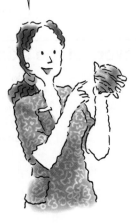

Just like this onion, your skin has a lot of layers.

The *stratum corneum* (horny layer) is the superficial layer of dead skin cells—the skin layer that's in contact with the environment. It has an acid mantle that helps protect the body from some fungi and bacteria. Cells in this layer are shed daily and replaced with cells from the layer beneath it, the stratum lucidum. In such diseases as eczema and psoriasis, the stratum corneum may become abnormally thick and irritate skin structures and peripheral nerves.

The *stratum lucidum* (clear layer) is a single layer of cells that forms a transitional boundary between the stratum corneum above and stratum granulosum below. This layer is most evident in areas where skin is thickest, as on the soles of the feet. It appears to be absent in areas where skin is especially thin, as on the eyelids. Although cells in this layer lack active nuclei, this is an area of intense enzyme activity that prepares cells for the stratum corneum.

The *stratum granulosum* (granular layer) is one to five cells thick and is characterized by flat cells with active nuclei. Experts believe this layer aids keratin formation.

The *stratum spinosum* is the area in which cells begin to flatten as they migrate toward the skin surface.

The *stratum basale* or *stratum germinativum* is only one cell thick and is the only layer of the epidermis in which cells undergo mitosis to form new cells. The stratum basale forms the dermoepidermal junction—the area where the epidermis and dermis are connected. Protrusions of this layer (called *rete pegs* or *epidermal ridges*) extend down into the dermis where they're surrounded by vascularized dermal papillae. This unique structure supports the epidermis and facilitates the exchange of fluids and cells between the skin layers.

Structural supports: Collagen and elastin

Normally, skin returns to its original position after it's pulled on due to the actions of the connective tissues collagen and elastin—two key components of skin. Collagen and elastin work together to support the dermis and give skin its physical characteristics.

Collagen

Collagen fibers form tightly woven networks in the papillary layer of the dermis. These fibers are relatively inextensible and nonelastic and, therefore, give the dermis high tensile strength. In addition, collagen constitutes approximately 70% of the skin's dry weight and is the skin's principal structural body protein.

Elastin

Elastin is made up of wavy fibers that intertwine with collagen in horizontal arrangements at the lower dermis and vertical arrangements at the epidermal margin. Elastin makes skin pliable and is the structural protein that enables extensibility in the dermis.

Seeing the effects of age

As a person ages, collagen and elastin fibers break down and the fine lines and wrinkles that are associated with aging develop. Extensive exposure to sunlight accelerates this breakdown process. Deep wrinkles are caused by changes in facial muscles. Over time, laughing, crying, smiling, and frowning cause facial muscles to thicken and eventually cause wrinkles in the overlying skin.

Memory jogger

To remember the five layers of the epidermis, think, "Contiguous Layers Generate Skin Barriers." In other words, the epidermis consists of the stratum:

Corneum

Lucidum

Granulosum

Spinosum

Basale.

Dermis

The dermis—the thick, deeper layer of skin—is composed of collagen and elastin fibers and an extracellular matrix, which contributes to skin's strength and pliability. Collagen fibers give skin its strength, and elastin fibers provide elasticity. The meshing of collagen and elastin determines the skin's physical characteristics. (See *Structural supports: Collagen and elastin*.)

In addition, the dermis contains:
• blood vessels and lymphatic vessels, which transport oxygen and nutrients to cells and remove waste products
• nerve fibers and hair follicles, which contribute to skin sensation, temperature regulation, and excretion and absorption through the skin
• fibroblast cells, which are important in the production of collagen and elastin.

Laying it on thick

The dermis is composed of two layers of connective tissue:

The *papillary dermis*, the outermost layer, is composed of collagen and reticular fibers, which are important in healing wounds. Capillaries in the papillary dermis carry the nourishment needed for metabolic activity.

The *reticular dermis* is the innermost layer. It's formed by thick networks of collagen bundles that anchor it to the subcutaneous tissue and underlying support structures, such as fasciae, muscle, and bone.

Sebaceous and sweat glands

Although sebaceous glands and sweat glands appear to originate in the dermis, they're actually appendages of the epidermis that extend downward into the dermis.

Give the glands a hand!

Sebaceous glands, found primarily in the skin of the scalp, face, upper body, and genital region, are part of the same structure that contains hair follicles. These saclike glands produce sebum, a fatty substance that lubricates and softens the skin.

Don't sweat it

Sweat glands are tightly coiled tubular glands; the average person has roughly 2.6 million of them. They're present throughout the body in varying amounts. The palms and soles have many, but the external ear, lip margins, nail beds, and glans penis have none.

The secreting portion of the sweat gland originates in the dermis and the outlet is on the surface of the skin. The sympathetic nervous system regulates the production of sweat, which, in turn, helps control body temperature.

There are two types of sweat glands:

Eccrine glands are active at birth and are found throughout the body. They're most dense on the palms, soles of the feet, and forehead. These glands connect to the skin's surface through pores and produce sweat that lacks proteins and fatty acids. Eccrine glands are smaller than apocrine glands.

Apocrine glands begin to function at puberty. These glands open into hair follicles; therefore, most are found in areas where hair typically grows, such as the scalp, groin, and axillary region. The coiled secreting portion of the gland lies deep in the dermis (deeper than eccrine glands), and a duct connects it to the upper portion of the hair follicle. The sweat produced by apocrine glands contains water, sodium, chloride, proteins, and fatty acids. It's thicker than the sweat produced by eccrine glands and has a milky white or yellowish tinge. (See *Oh no, B.O.!*)

Oh no, B.O.!

The sweat produced by apocrine glands contains the same water, sodium, and chloride found in the sweat produced by eccrine glands. However, it also contains proteins and fatty acids. The unpleasant odor associated with sweat comes from the interaction of bacteria with these proteins and fatty acids.

Subcutaneous tissue

The subcutaneous tissue, or *hypodermis*, is a subdermal (below the skin) layer of loose connective tissue that contains major blood vessels, lymph vessels, and nerves. Subcutaneous tissue:
• has a high proportion of fat cells and contains fewer small blood vessels than the dermis
• varies in thickness depending on body type and location
• constitutes 15% to 20% of a man's weight; 20% to 25% of a woman's weight
• insulates the body
• absorbs shocks to the skeletal system
• helps skin move easily over underlying structures.

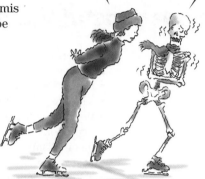

Are you cold?

Well, you would be, too, without any subcutaneous tissue!

Blood supply

The skin receives its blood supply through vessels that originate in the underlying muscle tissue. Here, arteries branch into smaller vessels, which then branch into the network of capillaries that permeate the dermis and subcutaneous tissue.

The thin and thinner of it

Within the vascular system, only capillaries have walls thin enough (typically only a single layer of endothelial cells) to let solutes pass through. These thin walls allow nutrients and oxygen to pass from the bloodstream into the interstitial space around skin cells. At the same time, waste products pass into the capillaries and are carried away. The pressure of arterial blood entering the capillaries is approximately 30 mm Hg. The pressure of venous blood leaving the capillaries is approximately 10 mm Hg. This 20 mm Hg difference in pressure within the capillaries is quite low when compared with the pressure found in the larger arteries in the body (85 to 100 mm Hg), which is known as *blood pressure*.

Lymphatic system

The skin's lymphatic system helps remove waste products from the dermis.

Go with the flow

Lymphatic vessels, or *lymphatics* for short, are similar to capillaries in that they're thin-walled, permeable vessels. However, lymphatics aren't part of the blood circulatory system. Instead, the lymphatics belong to a separate system that removes proteins, large waste products, and excess fluids from the interstitial spaces in skin and transports them to the venous circulation. The lymphatics merge into two main trunks—the thoracic duct and the right lymphatic duct—which empty into the junction of the subclavian and internal jugular veins.

Functions of the skin

Skin performs or participates in a host of vital functions, including:
- protection of internal structures
- sensory perception
- thermoregulation
- excretion
- metabolism
- absorption
- social communication.

Damage to skin impairs its ability to carry out these important functions. Let's take a closer look at each.

Protection

Skin acts as a physical barrier to microorganisms and foreign matter, protecting the body against infection. It also protects underlying tissue and structures from mechanical injury. Consider the feet for a moment. As a person walks or runs, the soles of the feet withstand a tremendous amount of force, yet the underlying tissue and bone structures remain unharmed.

The skin also helps maintain a stable environment inside the body by preventing the loss of water, electrolytes, proteins, and other substances. Any damage (any wound) jeopardizes this protection. However, when damaged, skin goes into repair mode to restore full protection by stepping up the normal process of cell replacement.

I think my nerve endings are working just fine. My sensory perception tells me I'm freezing!

Sensory perception

Nerve endings in the skin allow a person literally to touch the world around him. Sensory nerve fibers originate in the nerve roots along the spine and supply specific areas of the skin known as *dermatomes*. Dermatomes are used to document sensory function. This same network helps a person avoid injury by making him aware of pain, pressure, heat, and cold.

Just sensational

Sensory nerves exist throughout the skin; however, some areas are more sensitive than others—for example, the fingertips are more sensitive than the back. Sensation allows us to identify potential dangers and avoid injury. Any loss or reduction of sensation, local or general, increases the chance of injury.

Thermoregulation

Thermoregulation, or control of body temperature, involves the concerted effort of nerves, blood vessels, and eccrine glands in the dermis.

Warming up

When skin is exposed to cold or internal body temperature falls, blood vessels constrict, reducing blood flow and thereby conserving body heat.

Cooling down

Similarly, if skin becomes too hot or internal body temperature rises, small arteries within the skin dilate, increasing the blood flow, and sweat production increases to promote cooling.

Excretion

Unlikely as it may seem at first, the skin is an excretory organ. Excretion through the skin plays an important role in thermoregulation, electrolyte balance, and hydration. In addition, sebum excretion helps maintain the skin's integrity and suppleness.

Water works

Through its more than two million pores, skin efficiently transmits trace amounts of water and body wastes to the environment. At the same time, it prevents dehydration by ensuring that the body doesn't lose too much water. Sweat carries water and salt to the skin surface, where it evaporates, aiding thermoregulation and electrolyte balance. In addition, a small amount of water evaporates directly from the skin itself each day. A normal adult loses about 500 ml of water per day this way. While the skin is busy regulating fluids that are leaving the body, it's equally busy preventing unwanted or dangerous fluids from entering the body.

Metabolism

Skin also helps maintain the mineralization of bones and teeth. A photochemical reaction in the skin produces vitamin D, which is crucial to the metabolism of calcium and phosphate. These minerals, in turn, play a central role in the health of bones and teeth.

Let the sun shine in

When skin is exposed to sunlight—the UV spectrum in sunlight, to be specific—vitamin D is synthesized in a photochemical reaction. Keep in mind, however, that although some sunlight works wonders, overexposure to UV light causes skin damage that reduces its ability to function properly.

Absorption

Some drugs and, unfortunately, some toxic substances—for example, pesticides—can be absorbed directly through the skin and into the bloodstream. This process has been used to treat certain disorders via skin patch drug delivery systems. One of the best known examples of this method is the patch used in some nicotine withdrawal programs. However, today, this technology is also used to administer some forms of hormone replacement therapy, nitroglycerin, and some pain medications.

Social communication

A commonly overlooked but important function of the skin is its role in self-esteem development and social communication. Every time a person looks in the mirror, he decides whether he likes what he sees. Although bone structure, body type, teeth, and hair (or lack thereof!) all have an impact, the condition and characteristics of skin can have the greatest impact on a person's self-esteem. Ask any teenager with acne. If a person likes what he sees, self-esteem rises; if he doesn't, it sags.

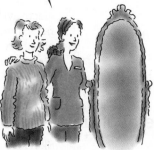

Skin is very important to self-esteem and social communication. Remember that when you're treating patients.

What you see

Virtually every interpersonal exchange includes the nonverbal languages of facial expression and body posture. Level of self-esteem and skin characteristics, which are visible at all times, have an impact on how a person communicates verbally and non-verbally and how a listener receives the person communicating.

Because the physical characteristics of skin are so closely linked to self-perception, there has been a proliferation of skin care products and surgical techniques offered to keep skin looking young and healthy.

A look at wound healing

Any break in the skin is considered a wound. Wounds can result from a planned event, such as surgery, or from an unexpected event, such as an accident, trauma, or exposure to pressure, heat, sun, or chemicals. Tissue damage in wounds varies widely, from a superficial break in the epithelium to deep trauma that involves the muscle and bone.

A "clean" wound is a wound produced by surgery. A wound is described as "dirty" if it may contain bacteria or debris. Trauma typically produces dirty wounds. The rate of recovery is influenced by the extent and type of damage incurred as well as other intrinsic factors, such as patient circulation, nutrition, hydration, and the presence of a chronic illness. However, regardless of the cause of a wound, the healing process is similar in all cases.

Types of wound healing

Wounds are classified by the way the wound closes. A wound can close by primary intention, secondary intention, or tertiary intention.

Primary intention

Primary healing involves re-epithelialization, in which the skin's outer layer grows closed. Cells grow in from the margins of the wound and out from epithelial cells lining the hair follicles and sweat glands.

Just a scratch

Wounds that heal through primary intention are, most commonly, superficial wounds that involve only the epidermis and don't involve the loss of tissue—a first-degree burn, for example. However, a wound that has well-approximated edges (edges that can be pulled together to meet neatly), such as a surgical incision, also heals through primary intention. Because there's no loss of tissue and little risk of infection, the healing process is predictable. These wounds usually heal in 4 to 14 days and result in minimal scarring.

Secondary intention

A wound that involves some degree of tissue loss heals by secondary intention. The edges of these wounds can't

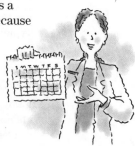

Wounds that heal by primary intention usually do so within 4 to 14 days.

be easily approximated, and the wound itself is described as *partial thickness* or *full thickness*, depending on its depth:
• Partial-thickness wounds extend through the epidermis and into, but not through, the dermis.
• Full-thickness wounds extend through the epidermis and dermis and may involve subcutaneous tissue, muscle, and possibly, bone.

Getting under the skin

During healing, wounds that heal by secondary intention fill with granulation tissue, a scar forms, and re-epithelialization occurs, primarily from the wound edges. Pressure ulcers, burns, dehisced surgical wounds, and traumatic injuries are examples of this type of wound. These wounds also take longer to heal, result in scarring, and have a higher rate of complications, such as the development of an infection, than wounds that heal by primary intention.

Tertiary intention

When a wound is intentionally kept open to allow edema or infection to resolve or to permit removal of exudate, the wound heals by tertiary intention or *delayed primary intention*. These wounds result in more scarring than wounds that heal by primary intention but less than wounds that heal by secondary intention.

Phases of wound healing

The healing process is the same for all wounds, whether the cause is mechanical, chemical, or thermal.

Don't let it phase you

Health care professionals discuss the process of wound healing in four specific phases:
• hemostasis
• inflammation
• proliferation
• maturation.

Although this categorization is useful, it's important to remember that healing rarely occurs in this strict order. Typically, the phases of wound healing overlap. (See *how wounds heal*.)

> C'mon, guys! We've got to begin the process of cleaning and healing the wound!

Hemostasis

Immediately after an injury, the body releases chemical mediators and intercellular messengers called *growth factors* that begin the process of cleaning and healing the wound.

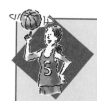

Stay on the ball

How wounds heal

The healing process begins at the instant of injury and proceeds through a repair "cascade," as outlined here.

1. When tissue is damaged, serotonin, histamine, prostaglandins, and blood from the injured vessels fill the area. Blood platelets form a clot, and fibrin in the clot binds the wound edges together.

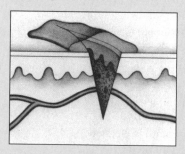

2. Lymphocytes initiate the inflammatory response, increasing capillary permeability. Wound edges swell; white blood cells from surrounding vessels move in and ingest bacteria and cellular debris, demolishing the clot. Redness, warmth, swelling, pain, and loss of function may occur.

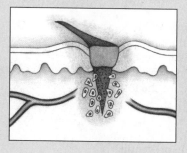

3. Adjacent healthy tissue supplies blood, nutrients, fibroblasts, proteins, and other building materials needed to form soft, pink, and highly vascular granulation tissue, which begins to bridge the area. Inflammation may decrease, or signs and symptoms of infection (increased swelling, increased pain, fever, and pus-filled discharge) may develop.

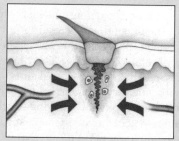

4. Fibroblasts in the granulation tissue secrete collagen, a glue-like substance. Collagen fibers criss-cross the area, forming scar tissue.

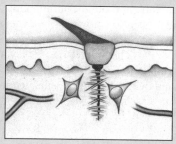

5. Meanwhile, epithelial cells at the wound edge multiply and migrate toward the wound center. A new layer of surface cells replaces the layer that was destroyed. New, healthy tissue or granulation tissue (if the blood supply is inadequate) appears.

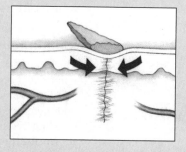

6. Damaged tissue (including lymphatics, blood vessels, and stromal matrices) regenerates. Collagen fibers shorten, and the scar diminishes in size. Scar size may decrease and normal function return or the scar may hypertrophy, leading to the formation of a keloid and the development of contractures.

Slow that flow!

When blood vessels are damaged, the small muscles in the walls of the vessels contract (vasoconstriction), reducing the flow of blood to the injury and minimizing blood loss. Vasoconstriction can last as long as 30 minutes.

Next, blood leaking from the inflamed, dilated, or broken vessels begins to coagulate. Collagen fibers in the wall of the damaged blood vessels activate the platelets in the blood in the wound. Aided by the action of prostaglandins, the platelets enlarge and stick together to form a temporary plug in the blood vessel, which helps prevent further bleeding. The platelets also release additional vasoconstrictors such as serotonin, which help prevent further blood loss. Thrombin forms in a cascade of events stimulated by the platelets, and a clot forms to close the small vessels and stop the bleeding.

This initial phase of wound healing occurs almost immediately after the injury occurs and works quickly (within minutes) in small wounds. It's less effective in stopping the bleeding in larger wounds.

Inflammation

The inflammatory phase is a defense mechanism and a crucial component of the healing process. (See *Understanding the inflammatory response.*) During this phase, the wound is cleaned and the process of rebuilding begins. This phase is marked by swelling, redness, and heat at the wound site.

During the inflammatory phase, vascular permeability increases, permitting serous fluid carrying small amounts of cell and plasma protein to accumulate in the tissue around the wound (edema). The accumulation of fluid causes the damaged tissue to appear swollen, red, and warm to the touch.

Seek and destroy

During the early phase of the inflammatory process, neutrophils (one type of white blood cell [WBC]) enter the wound. The primary role of neutrophils is *phagocytosis* or the removal and destruction of bacteria and other contaminants.

As neutrophil infiltration slows, monocytes appear. Monocytes are converted into activated macrophages and continue the job of cleaning the wound. The macrophages play a key role early in the process of granulation and re-epithelialization by producing growth factors and by attracting the cells needed for the formation of new blood vessels and collagen.

Telling time

The inflammatory phase of healing is important in preventing wound infection. The process is negatively influenced if the

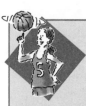

Understanding the inflammatory response

This flowchart outlines the sequence of events in the inflammatory process.

⬇

Microorganisms invade damaged tissue.

⬇

Basophils release heparin, and histamine and kinin production occurs.

⬇

Vasodilation occurs along with increased capillary permeability.

⬇

Blood flow increases to the affected tissues and fluid collects within them.

⬇

Neutrophils flock to the invasion site to engulf and destroy microorganisms from dying cells.

⬇

This repairs the tissue.

patient has a systemic condition that suppresses his immune system or if he's undergoing immunosuppressive therapy. In clean wounds, the inflammatory response lasts from 3 to 6 days. In dirty or infected wounds, the response can last much longer.

Proliferation

During the proliferation phase of the healing process, the body:
• fills the wound with connective tissue (granulation)
• contracts the wound edges (contraction)
• covers the wound with epithelium (epithelialization).

Presto change-o!

All wounds go through the proliferation phase, which begins on day 3 and lasts until about day 21, but it takes much longer in wounds with extensive tissue loss. Although phases overlap, wound granulation generally starts when the inflammatory response is complete. As the inflammatory phase subsides, the wound drainage (exudate) begins to decrease.

The proliferation phase involves regeneration of blood vessels (angiogenesis) and the formation of connective or granulation tissue, which is fragile and can bleed easily. The development of granulation tissue requires an adequate supply of blood and nutrients. Endothelial cells in blood vessels in surrounding tissue reconstruct damaged or destroyed vessels by first migrating and then proliferating to form new capillary beds. As the beds form, this area of the wound takes on a red, granular appearance. This tissue is a good defense against contaminants, but it's also quite fragile and bleeds easily.

I'm your local fibroblast and I'm here to build support to these cells.

The rebuilding process

During the proliferation phase, growth factors prompt fibroblasts to migrate to the wound. Fibroblasts are the most common cell in connective tissue. They're responsible for making fibers and ground substance—also known as *extracellular matrix*—which provides support to cells. At first, fibroblasts populate just the margins of the wound but, later, they spread over the entire wound surface.

Fibroblasts have the important task of synthesizing collagen fibers that, in turn, produce keratinocyte, a growth factor needed for re-epithelialization. This process necessitates a delicate balance of collagen synthesis and lysis (making new and removing old). If the process yields too much collagen, increased scarring results. If the process yields too little collagen, scar tissue is weak and easily ruptured. Because fibroblasts require a supply of oxygen to perform their important role, capillary bed regeneration is crucial to the process.

Pulling it all together

As healing progresses, myofibroblasts and the newly formed collagen fibers contract, pulling the wound edges toward each other. Contraction reduces the amount of granulation tissue needed to fill the wound, thereby speeding the healing process. (See *Contraction versus contracture.*)

Complete healing occurs only after epithelial cells have completely covered the surface of the wound. As this occurs, keratinocytes switch from a migrating mode to a differentiating mode. The epidermis thickens and becomes differentiated, and the wound is closed. Any remaining scab comes off and the new epidermis is toughened by the production of keratin, which also returns the skin to its original color.

Maturation

The final phase of wound healing is maturation, which is marked by shrinking and strengthening of the scar. This is a gradual, transitional phase of healing that can continue for months or even years after the wound have closed.

Contraction versus contracture

Contraction and contracture occur during the wound healing process. Although they have mechanisms in common, it's important to understand how contraction and contracture differ.

Contraction

Contraction, a desirable process that takes place during healing, occurs when the edges of a wound pull toward the center of the wound to close it. Contraction continues to close the wound until tension in the surrounding skin causes it to slow and then stop.

Contracture

Contracture is an undesirable process and a common complication of burn scarring. Typically, contracture occurs after healing is complete. Contracture involves an inordinate amount of pulling or shortening of tissue, resulting in an area of tissue with only limited ability to move. It's especially problematic over joints, which may be pulled to a flexed position. Stretching is the only way to overcome contracture, and patients typically require physical therapy.

During this phase, fibroblasts leave the site of the wound, vascularization is reduced, the scar shrinks and becomes pale, and the mature scar forms. If the wound involved extensive tissue destruction, the scar won't contain hair, sweat, or sebaceous glands.

The wound gradually gains tensile strength. In primary intention wounds, tissues will achieve approximately 30% to 50% of their original strength between days 1 and 14. When fully healed, tissue will achieve, at best, approximately 80% of its original strength. Scar tissue will always be less elastic than the surrounding skin.

Factors that affect wound healing

The healing process is affected by many factors. The most important influences include:
- nutrition
- oxygenation
- infection
- age
- chronic health conditions
- medications
- smoking.

Nutrition

Proper nutrition is arguably the most important factor affecting wound healing. Unfortunately, malnutrition is a common finding among patients with wounds. For older adults, the problem is more pervasive.

Poor nutrition prolongs hospitalization and increases the risk of medical complications, with the severity of complications being directly related to the severity of the malnutrition. In older patients, malnutrition is known to increase the risk of pressure ulcers and delay wound healing. It may also contribute to poor tensile strength in healing wounds, with an associated increase in the risk of wound dehiscence.

> Good nutrition is key when it comes to getting well.

Protein is key

Protein is critical for wounds to heal properly. In fact, a person needs to double the recommended dietary allowance of protein (from 0.8 g/kg/day to 1.6 g/kg/day) before tissue even begins to heal. If a significant amount of body weight has been lost in connection with the injury, as much as 50% of the lost weight must be regained before healing will begin. A patient who lacks protein reserves heals slowly, if at all, and a patient who's borderline malnourished can easily become malnourished under this demand.

The body needs protein to form collagen during the proliferation phase. Without adequate protein, collagen formation is reduced or delayed and the healing process slows. Studies of malnourished patients indicate that they have lower levels of serum albumin, which results in slower oxygen diffusion and, in turn, a reduction in the ability of neutrophils to kill bacteria. Wound exudate alone can contain up to 100 g of protein per day.

Other necessary nutrients

Fatty acids (lipids) are used in cell structures and play a role in the inflammatory process. Also, vitamins C, B complex, A, and E and the minerals iron, copper, zinc, and calcium are important in the healing process. A zinc deficiency adversely affects the proliferation phase by slowing the rate of epithelialization and decreasing the strength of collagen produced—and, thus, the strength of the wound.

In addition to protein and zinc, collagen synthesis requires supplies of carbohydrates and fat. Collagen cross-linking requires adequate amounts of vitamins A and C, iron, and copper. Vitamin C, iron, and zinc are important for developing tensile strength during the maturation phase of wound healing.

> Proper wound healing depends on a blend of nutrients, including protein, fatty acids, vitamins, and minerals.

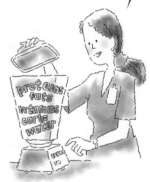

Oxygenation

Healing depends on a regular supply of oxygen. For example, oxygen is critical for leukocytes to destroy bacteria and fibroblasts to stimulate collagen synthesis. If the supply is hindered by poor blood flow to the area of the wound or if the patient's ability to take in adequate oxygen is impaired, the result is the same—impaired healing.

Possible causes of inadequate blood flow to the area of the wound include pressure, arterial occlusion, or prolonged vasoconstriction, possibly associated with such medical conditions as peripheral vascular disease and atherosclerosis. Possible causes of a lower than systemic blood oxygenation include:
- inadequate oxygen intake
- hypothermia or hyperthermia
- anemia
- alkalemia
- other medical conditions such as chronic obstructive pulmonary disease.

Infection

An infection can affect wound healing or be a complication of the healing process. Infection can be systemic or localized in the wound. A systemic infection, such as pneumonia or tuberculosis, increases the patient's metabolism and thus consumes the fluids, nutrients, and oxygen the body needs for healing.

Keeping it local

A localized infection in the wound itself is more common. Remember, any break in the skin allows bacteria to enter. The infection may occur as part of the injury or may develop later in the healing process. For example, when the inflammatory phase lingers, wound healing is delayed and metabolic by-products of bacterial ingestion accumulate in the wound. This buildup interferes with the formation of new blood vessels and the synthesis of collagen. Infection can also occur in a wound that has been healing normally. This situation happens especially in larger wounds involving extensive tissue damage. New or increased pain, redness, heat, and drainage are signs of a new infection. In any case, healing can't progress until the cause of infection is addressed.

In patients in long-term care facilities, infection may result from fecal contamination. Fecal incontinence affects 20% of long-term care patients and is associated with increased mortality. Typically, those affected are patients with poorer overall health.

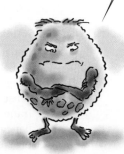

If there's a break in skin, I'll be sure to find it. Infections are my specialty.

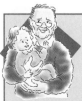

Ages and stages

Effects of aging on wound healing

These factors impede wound healing in older adults:
- slower turnover rate in epidermal cells
- poorer oxygenation at the wound due to increasingly fragile capillaries and a reduction in skin vascularization
- altered nutrition and fluid intake resulting from physical changes that can accompany aging, such as reduced saliva production, a declining sense of smell and taste, and decreased stomach motility
- altered nutrition and fluid intake attributable to troubling personal or social issues, such as loose-fitting dentures, financial concerns, eating alone after the death of a spouse, and problems preparing or obtaining food
- impaired function of the respiratory or immune systems
- reduced dermal and subcutaneous mass leading to an increased risk of chronic pressure ulcers
- healed wounds that lack tensile strength and are prone to reinjury.

Age

Skin changes that occur with aging cause a prolonged healing time in elderly patients. Although delayed healing is partially due to physiologic changes, it's also complicated by other problems associated with aging, such as poor nutrition and hydration, the presence of a chronic condition, and the use of multiple medications. (See *Effects of aging on wound healing*.)

Chronic health conditions

Respiratory problems, atherosclerosis, diabetes, and malignancies can increase the risk of wounds and interfere with wound healing. These conditions can interfere with systemic and peripheral oxygenation and nutrition, which affect healing.

Getting complicated

Impaired circulation, a common problem for patients with diabetes and other disorders, can cause tissue hypoxia (lack of oxygen). Neuropathy associated with diabetes reduces ability to sense pressure. As a result, patients with diabetes may experience trauma, especially to the feet, without realizing it. Insulin dependency can impair leukocyte function, which adversely affects cell proliferation.

Hemiplegia and quadriplegia involve the breakdown of muscle tissue and reduction in the padding around the large bones of the lower body. Because a patient with one of these conditions lacks sensation, he's at risk for developing chronic pressure ulcers.

Night and day shifts

Normally, a healthy person shifts position every 15 minutes or so, even during sleep. This shifting prevents tissue damage due to ischemia. Anything that impairs the ability to sense pressure, including spinal cord lesions, the use of pain medications, and cognitive impairment, puts the patient at risk (because the patient can't feel the growing discomfort of pressure and respond to it).

Other conditions that can delay healing include dehydration, end-stage renal disease, liver disease, thyroid disease, heart failure, peripheral vascular disease, and vasculitis and other collagen vascular disorders.

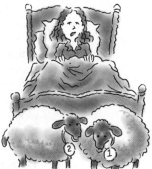

I think I've been shifting every 15 seconds! Time to try alternate measures . . .

Medications

Any medication that reduces a patient's movement, circulation, or metabolic function, such as sedatives and tranquilizers, has the potential to inhibit the patient's ability to sense and respond to pressure. Also, because movement promotes adequate oxygenation, lack of motion means that peripheral blood delivers less oxygen to the extremities than it should. This decrease in oxygen is especially problematic for older adults. Remember, oxygen is important; without it, the healing process slows and the potential for complications rises.

Interruptions!

Some medications, such as steroids and chemotherapeutic agents, reduce the body's ability to mount an appropriate inflammatory response. This reduction in response interrupts the inflammatory phase of healing and can dramatically lengthen healing time, especially in a patient with a compromised immune system such as one with AIDS. The use of antibiotics for long periods may place the patient at greater risk for developing an infection, which can affect wound healing.

Smoking

Carbon monoxide, a component of cigarette smoke, binds to the hemoglobin in blood in the place of oxygen. This binding significantly reduces the amount of oxygen circulating in the bloodstream, which can impede wound healing. To some extent, this reaction also occurs in people regularly exposed to secondhand smoke.

Complications of wound healing

The most common complications associated with wound healing are:
- hemorrhage
- dehiscence and evisceration
- infection
- fistula formation.

Hemorrhage

Internal hemorrhage (bleeding) can result in the formation of a hematoma—a blood clot that solidifies to form a hard lump under the skin. Hematomas are commonly found around bruises.

External hemorrhage is visible bleeding from the wound. External bleeding during healing isn't unusual because the newly developed blood vessels are fragile and rupture easily. This is one reason a wound needs to be protected by a dressing. However, each time the new blood vessels suffer damage, healing is delayed while repairs are made.

Dehiscence and evisceration

Dehiscence is a separation of skin and tissue layers. It's most likely to occur 3 to 11 days after the injury was sustained and may follow surgery. Evisceration is similar but involves protrusion of underlying visceral organs as well. (See *Recognizing dehiscence and evisceration*.)

Dehiscence and evisceration may constitute a surgical emergency, especially if they involve an abdominal wound. If a wound opens without evisceration, it may need to heal by secondary intention. Poor nutrition and advanced age are two factors that increase a patient's risk of dehiscence and evisceration.

Infection

Infection is a relatively common complication of wound healing that should be addressed promptly. Infection can lead to a bacterial infection that spreads to surrounding tissue. Signs that infection may be at work include:
- redness and warmth of the margins and tissue around the wound
- fever
- edema
- pain (or a sudden increase in pain)

Recognizing dehiscence and evisceration

In wound dehiscence (top), the layers of a wound separate. In evisceration (bottom), the viscera (in this case, a bowel loop) protrude through the wound.

Wound dehiscence

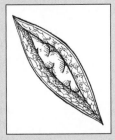

Evisceration of bowel loop

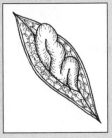

- pus
- increase in exudate or a change in its color
- odor
- discoloration of granulation tissue
- further wound breakdown or lack of progress toward healing.

Fistula formation

A fistula is an abnormal passage between two organs or between an organ and the skin. In a wound, it may appear as undermining or a sinus tract (tunneling) in the skin around the wound. If a sinus tract is present, it's important to determine its extent and direction.

Wound classification

The words you choose to describe your observations of a specific wound have to communicate the same meaning to other members of the health care team, insurance companies, regulators, the patient's family and, ultimately, the patient himself. This is a tall order when you consider that even wound care experts debate the descriptive phrases they use. *Slough* or *eschar? Undermining* or *tunneling?* How much drainage is *moderate?* Is the color green or yellow? Does the drainage have an odor?

The best way to classify wounds is to use the basic system described here, which focuses on three categories of fundamental characteristics:

 wound age

 wound depth (extent of tissue loss)

 wound color

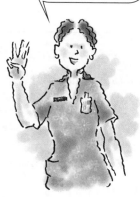

When it comes to classifying wounds, the magic number is 3—age, depth, and color.

Wound age

When determining the age of a wound, you need to first determine if the wound is acute or chronic. However, this determination can present a problem if you adhere solely to a time line. For instance, just how long is it before an acute wound becomes a chronic wound?

A different way of thinking

Rather than base your determination solely on time, consider a wound an acute wound if it's new or making progress as expected and a chronic wound any wound that isn't healing in a timely fashion. The main idea is that, in a chronic wound, healing has slowed or stopped and the wound is no longer getting smaller and shallower. Even if the wound bed appears healthy, red, and moist, if healing fails to progress, consider it a chronic wound.

More bad than good

Chronic wounds don't heal as easily as acute wounds. The drainage in chronic wounds contains a greater amount of destructive enzymes, and fibroblasts—the cells that function as the architects in wound healing—seem to lose their "oomph." They're less effective at producing collagen, divide less often, and send fewer signals to other cells telling them to divide and fill the wound. In other words, the wound changes from one that's vigorous and ready to heal, to one that's downright lazy!

Wound depth

Wound depth is another fundamental characteristic used to classify wounds. In your assessment, record wound depth as partial thickness or full thickness. (See *Classifying wound depth*.)

Classifying wound depth

Wounds are classified as partial thickness or full thickness according to the depth of the wound. Partial-thickness wounds involve only the epidermis or extend into the dermis but not through it. Full-thickness wounds extend through the dermis into tissues beneath and may expose adipose tissue, muscle, or bone. These diagrams illustrate the relative depth of both classifications.

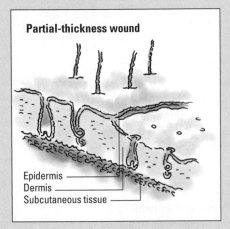

Partial-thickness wound

Epidermis
Dermis
Subcutaneous tissue

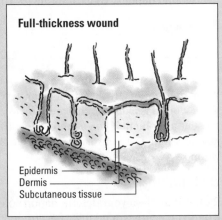

Full-thickness wound

Epidermis
Dermis
Subcutaneous tissue

Partial thickness

Partial-thickness wounds normally heal very quickly because they involve only the epidermal layer of the skin or extend through the epidermis into (but not through) the dermis. The dermis remains at least partially intact to generate the new epidermis needed to close the wound. Partial-thickness wounds are also less susceptible to infection because part of the body's first level of defense (the skin) is still intact. These wounds tend to be painful, however, and need protection from the air to reduce pain and decrease the risk of infection.

Full thickness

Full-thickness wounds penetrate completely through the skin into underlying tissues. The wound may expose adipose tissue (fat), muscle, tendon, or bone. In the abdomen, you may see adipose tissue or omentum (the covering of the bowel). If the omentum is penetrated, the bowel may protrude through the wound (evisceration). Granulation tissue may be visible if the wound has started to heal.

Full-thickness wounds heal by granulation and contraction, which require more body resources and more time than the healing of partial-thickness wounds. When assessing a full-thickness wound, report the depth as well as the length and width of the wound.

The added pressure of pressure ulcers

In the case of pressure ulcers, wound depth allows you to stage the ulcer according to the classification system developed by the National Pressure Ulcer Advisory Panel (NPUAP).

Wound color

Wounds are also classified by the color of the wound bed. Wound color helps the wound care team determine whether debridement is appropriate. (See *Tailoring wound care to wound color*, page 436.)

Be picky about wound bed color! Only red will do, and the best shade is red—not pale pink or grayish red. There are literally thousands of words to describe colors; however, you can simplify your assessment by sticking to the red-yellow-black classification system. This system is a useful tool for developing effective wound care management plans.

Red means you're ahead

If the wound bed is red (the color of healthy granulation tissue), the wound is healthy and normal healing is under way. When a wound begins to heal, a layer of pale pink granulation tissue covers the wound bed. As this layer thickens, it becomes red.

Tailoring wound care to wound color

With any wound, you can promote healing by keeping the wound moist, clean, and free from debris. For open wounds, using wound color can guide the specific management approach to aid healing.

Wound color	Management technique
Red	• Cover the wound, keep it moist and clean, and protect it from trauma. • Use a transparent dressing (such as Tegaderm or OPSITE), a hydrogel, foam, or hydrocolloid dressing over partial-thickness wounds to insulate and protect the wound.
Yellow	• Clean the wound and remove the yellow layer. • Cover the wound with a moisture-retentive dressing, such as a hydrogel or foam dressing, or a moist gauze dressing with or without a debriding enzyme. • Consider pulsatile lavage.
Black	• Debride the wound as ordered. Use an enzyme product (such as Collagenase Santyl), conservative sharp debridement, or pulsatile lavage. • For wounds with inadequate blood supply and noninfected heel ulcers, don't debride. Keep them clean and dry.

Mellow yellow

If the wound bed is yellow, beware! A yellow color in the wound bed may be a film of fibrin on the tissue. Fibrin is a sticky substance that normally acts as glue in tissue rebuilding. However, if the wound is unhealthy or too dry, fibrin builds up into a layer that can't be rinsed off and may require debridement. Tissue that has recently died due to ischemia or infection may also be yellow and must be debrided. Necrotic tissue in a wound bed that is yellow, gray, green, or tan; is adherent to the wound bed; and is dry or moist, is usually identified as slough.

Black = debridement

If the wound bed is black, be alarmed. A black wound bed signals necrosis (tissue death). Eschar (dead, avascular tissue) covers the wound, slowing the healing process and providing microorganisms with a site in which to proliferate. When eschar covers a wound, accurate assessment of wound depth is difficult and should be deferred until eschar is removed.

> Black may be best when it comes to cocktail parties, but watch out for black when it comes to the wound bed. A black wound signals necrosis.

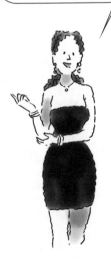

Ischemia exceptions

Typically, debridement is indicated for black wounds; however, ulcers caused by ischemia (damage due to inadequate blood supply) and uninfected heel pressure ulcers are exceptions. Ischemic wounds won't heal until blood supply is improved, and they're less likely to become infected if kept dry. The wound can be debrided and kept moist after blood supply is reestablished. (The body can then fend off infection and heal the wound.)

Multicolored wounds

If you note two or even all three colors in a wound, classify the wound according to the least healthy color present. For example, if your patient's wound appears both red and yellow, classify it as a yellow wound.

Wound assessment

Gathering information about a wound requires you to use almost all of your senses. Be sure to assess drainage, the wound bed, and patient pain. Assess the wound bed and the surrounding skin only after they've been cleaned. As you perform your assessment, remember that it doesn't matter what method you use to record your observations, it's just important to be consistent.

Components of a complete wound assessment

As you assess the wound, record information about:

> **Anatomic location**
> **Size**
> **Tunneling and undermining**
> **Characteristics of wound bed**
> **Wound edges**
> **Periwound skin**
> **Drainage / exudates**
>> **Amount**
>> **Consistency**
>> **Color**
>> **Odor**
> **Extent of tissue loss**

Okay, we already talked about the last item, extent of tissue loss. Now, let's move on to the next assessment parameter.

Anatomic location

Identifying the location of the wound is important because location can assist you in determining the etiology of the wound. Is it a pressure point, on the lower extremity, in the gluteal cleft, on the bottom of the foot? All of these locations suggest etiology.

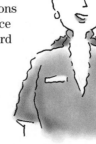

Record as much information about the wound as possible.

Size
Get out your ruler

The most common method of measuring wound dimensions is to use a tape measure. Make sure it's a disposable device to prevent contamination and cross-contamination. Record the length of the wound at the longest point in a head to toe direction and record the width as the longest measurement perpendicular (at a right angle) to your length measurement. (See *Measuring a wound.*)

Be sure to record any observed areas of discoloration of the intact skin around the wound opening separately—not as part of the wound bed. Record all measurements in centimeters.

Trace the wound

Another way to measure the wound is to use wound tracing (in which wound margins are traced on a sheet of clear plastic). You use the tracing to calculate an approximate wound area. This method provides only a rough estimate but is simple and fairly quick.

Photography

Photography may be used to document wound progress but has Health Insurance Portability and Accountability Act (HIPAA) and Health Information Technology for Clinical and Economic Health (HITECH) Act implications. Obtaining informed consent and maintaining safe storage of the photographs are required.

How deep

To measure the depth of the wound, you'll need a cotton-tipped swab. Gently insert the cotton-tipped swab into the deepest portion of the wound and then carefully mark the probe where it meets the edge of the skin. Remove the applicator and measure the distance from your mark to the end to determine depth.

Tunneling and undermining

It's also important to measure tunneling, or sinus tracts (extensions of the wound bed into adjacent tissue), and undermining (areas of the wound bed that extend under the skin). Measure these features just as you would the depth. Carefully insert a cotton-tipped swab to the bottom of the tunnel or to the end of the undermined area; then mark the stick and measure the distance from your mark to the end of the swab. If a tunnel is large, palpate it with a gloved finger rather than a swab because you can sense the end of the tunnel better with your finger.

> Make sure you measure tunneling of the wound.

Characteristics of wound bed

The type of tissue in the ulcer base determines the potential for healing and the type of treatment. Know how to identify necrotic tissue, granulation tissue, and epithelial tissue.

Measuring a wound

When measuring a wound, first determine the longest distance across the open area of the wound—in a head to toe direction. In this photograph, note the line used to illustrate this length.

A wound's width is simply the longest distance across the wound at a right angle to the length. Note the relationship of length and width in the photograph. Also, note the area of reddened, intact skin and white macerated skin. These areas would be measured and recorded as surrounding erythema and maceration—not as part of the wound itself. In this full-thickness ischial pressure ulcer, you would also record a depth and note areas of tunneling or undermining.

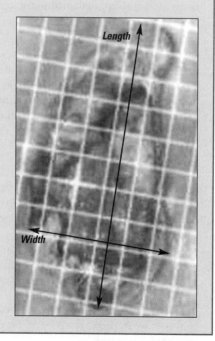

Necrotic tissue (nonviable)

Necrotic tissue may appear as a moist yellow or gray area of tissue that's separating from viable tissue. When dry, necrotic tissue appears as thick, hard, and leathery black eschar. Slough tissue appears as yellow/tan/gray tissue and is dry or moist, may be adherent or stringy in the base of the wound. Areas of necrotic or devitalized tissue may mask underlying abscesses and collections of fluid. Before the ulcer can begin to heal, necrotic tissue, drainage, and metabolic wastes must be removed from the wound.

Granulation tissue

Granulation tissue appears as beefy red, bumpy, shiny tissue in the base of the ulcer. As it heals, a full-thickness ulcer develops more and more granulation tissue. Such factors as tissue oxygenation, tissue hydration, and nutrition can alter the color and quality of granulation tissue.

Let's talk about "beefy red"

A wound that is red is healthy, but if you touch the wound and it bleeds easily (tissue is friable), this usually indicates excess bacteria (a bioburden) in the wound. Bioburden is not "infection" but an over-colonization of bacteria in the wound bed and can often be treated with topical antimicrobials.

Epithelial tissue

Epithelialization is the regeneration of epidermis across the ulcer surface. It appears as pale or dark pink skin, first becoming evident at ulcer borders in full-thickness wounds and as islands around hair follicles in partial-thickness wounds. Wound healing can be assessed and quantified by the percentage of surface covered by new epithelium.

Wound edges

Edges should be attached, moist, even, or flushed with wound base to enhance epithelialization. Premature "closure" of wound edge may be identified by rolled edges (epibole) and/or dry and thickened edges.

When assessing wound edges, you'll want to see skin that's smooth—not rolled—and tightly adherent to the wound bed. Rolled skin may indicate that the wound bed is too dry. Loose skin at the edges may indicate additional shearing injury (separation of skin layers), possibly due to a rough transfer or repositioning. In this case, improve transfer and repositioning techniques to prevent recurrence.

Periwound skin

Rainbow connections

In the past, sailors used the color of the sky to predict danger at sea. In a similar fashion, the color of the skin around the wound can alert you to impending problems that can impede healing:
• White skin indicates maceration, or too much moisture, and signals the need for a protective barrier around the wound and a more absorbent dressing (plus keep the dressing in the wound and off the skin).
• Red skin can indicate inflammation, injury (e.g., tape burn, excessive pressure, or chemical exposure), or infection. Remember that inflammation is healthy only during the inflammatory phase of healing—not after!
• Purple skin can indicate bruising, one sign of trauma.

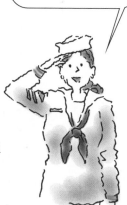

Just like sailors who use the color of the sky to predict weather, you can use wound and skin color to alert you to potential problems.

Let your fingers do the talking

Your fingers are invaluable tools you may be taking for granted. During your assessment of the area around the wound, your fingers will tell you much. For example, gently probe the tissue around the wound bed to determine if it's soft or hard (indurated). Indurated tissue, even in the absence of erythema (redness), is one indication of infection.

Similarly, if your patient has dark skin, it may be impossible to see color cues. Again, your fingers can help. Probe the area around the wound bed and compare the feel with surrounding healthy skin. A tender area of skin that appears shiny and feels hard may indicate inflammation in such a patient.

Drainage/exudates

The wound bed should be moist but not overly moist. Moisture allows the cells and chemicals needed for healing to move about the wound surface.

To begin collecting information about wound drainage, inspect the dressing as you remove it and record answers to such questions as:
• Is the drainage well contained, or is it oozing from the edges? If it's oozing, consider using a more absorbent dressing.
• In the case of an occlusive dressing, were the dressing edges well sealed? (A hydrocolloid in the gluteal cleft area becomes a greenhouse for bacteria if the edges are loose.) If the patient has fecal incontinence, it's even more important to note the seal status.

Drainage descriptors

This chart provides terminology that you can use to describe the color and consistency of wound drainage.

Description	Color and consistency
Serous	• Clear or light yellow • Thin and watery
Sanguineous	• Red (with fresh blood) • Thin
Serosanguineous	• Pink to light red • Thin • Watery
Purulent	• Creamy yellow, green, white, or tan • Thick and opaque

• Is the dressing saturated or dry?
• How much drainage is there: a scant, moderate, or large amount? Is there an odor?
• What are the color and consistency of the drainage? (See *Drainage descriptors*.)

Skipping the swab?

Also consider the texture of the drainage. If the drainage has a thick, creamy texture, the wound contains an excessive amount of bacteria. However, this doesn't necessarily mean a clinically significant infection is present. Document the characteristics of the drainage. Drainage might be creamy because it contains WBCs that have killed bacteria. The drainage is also contaminated with surface bacteria that naturally live in moist environments on the human body.

Because of this bacterial colonization, swab cultures are not the best way to identify wound infections. Nonetheless, some doctors still order swab cultures because they're easy to collect and inexpensive.

The Levine method is a suggested method:
• Cleanse wound with normal saline solution (NSS) and blot dry with sterile gauze.

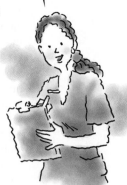

You need to be able to describe wound drainage.

- Identify a healthy area of wound about 1 cm^2.
- Moisten the swab with nonpreserved NSS.
- Press on the wound area, rotating the swab (apply enough pressure to elicit tissue fluid).
- When tip of swab is saturated, break the tip (if needed) and insert into container using sterile technique.

Punch biopsy of tissue or needle aspiration of fluid may also be used. These methods require more skill but are more likely to reveal accurate results.

Fish out of water

In dry wound beds, cells involved in healing, which normally exist in a fluid environment, are a bit like fish in a desert—they can't move. WBCs can't fight infection, enzymes like collagenase can't break down dead material, and macrophages can't carry away debris. The wound edges curl up to preserve moisture remaining in the edge and epithelial cells (new skin cells) fail to grow over and cover the wound. Healing grinds to a halt and necrotic tissue builds up.

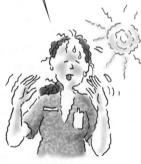

I'm no fish, but I can't go very far without moisture and neither can proper wound healing.

Flood watch

Too much moisture poses a different problem. It floods the wound and spills out onto the skin, where the constant moisture causes the death of skin cells.

Odor

If kept clean, a noninfected wound usually produces little, if any, odor. (One exception is the odor normally present under a hydrocolloid dressing that develops as a by-product of the degradation process.) A newly detected odor might be a sign of infection; record it in your findings and report it to the doctor. When documenting wound odor, it's important to include when the odor was noted and whether it went away with wound cleaning.

Odor eaters

If an odor develops, it can present an embarrassing or otherwise uncomfortable situation for the patient as well as his family, guests, and roommate. If you notice an odor, or if your patient says he notices one, use an odor eliminator. Odor eliminators differ from air fresheners in that they aren't scents that mask odors but rather compounds that bind with, and neutralize, the molecules responsible for the odor.

Pain

In addition to the wound characteristics, we always need to be assessing pain. You'll want to note not only pain associated with the injury itself but also pain associated with healing and with therapies employed to promote healing. To fully understand your patient's pain, talk with him and ask about the level of pain on a scale of 0 to 10, with 10 being the worst pain he has ever experienced. Then watch to see how he responds to pain and the therapies provided. As always, remember to record your findings.

Listen and learn

If your patient is conscious and can communicate, have him rate his pain before and during each dressing change. If your notes reveal that his pain is higher before the dressing change, it may indicate an impending infection, even before any other signs appear.

If your patient says the dressing change itself is painful, you might consider administering pain medication before the procedure or changing the dressing technique. However, remember to document this pain and report it to the doctor. Less painful methods of removing dead tissue exist but, if the patient's pain isn't documented and communicated, wet-to-dry debridement orders may stand and the patient may suffer unnecessary discomfort.

Useful tips for removal

In general, when removing adherent dressings, it's less painful if you soak the dressing or, over intact skin, use an adhesive remover. Also, keep the skin taut. Press down on the skin to release the dressing rather than just pulling the dressing off. Pull the dressing gently toward the wound using your index finger to gently release the skin from the adhesive.

Treatment for wounds

Treating impaired skin integrity involves a range of procedures, from basic wound care and wound irrigation to surgical wound management and closed wound drain management.

Basic wound care

Basic wound care centers on cleaning and dressing the wound. Because open wounds are colonized (or contaminated) with bacteria, practice clean technique using clean, nonsterile gloves during wound care unless sterile dressing changes are specified. Always follow standard precautions.

The goal of wound cleaning is to remove debris and contaminants from the wound without damaging healthy tissue. The wound should be cleaned initially; repeat cleaning as needed and always before a new dressing is applied.

The basic purpose of a dressing, to provide an optimal environment in which the body can heal itself, should be considered before one is selected. Functions of a wound dressing include:

• protecting the wound from contamination and trauma
• providing compression if bleeding or swelling is anticipated
• applying medications
• absorbing drainage or debrided necrotic tissue
• filling the "dead space" in the wound
• protecting the skin surrounding the wound.

The cardinal rule is to keep moist tissue moist and the surrounding skin dry. Ideally, a dressing should keep the wound moist, absorb drainage or debris, conform to the wound, and be adhesive to surrounding skin yet be easily removable. It should also be user-friendly, require minimal changes, decrease the need for a secondary dressing layer, and be cost-effective and comfortable for the patient.

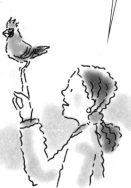

The cardinal rule of wound care is to keep moist tissue moist and dry tissue dry.

What you need

Hypoallergenic tape or elastic netting ✳ overbed table ✳ piston-type irrigating system ✳ two pairs of gloves ✳ cleaning solution (such as NSS) as ordered ✳ sterile 4″ × 4″ gauze pads ✳ selected topical dressing ✳ linen-saver pads ✳ impervious plastic trash bag ✳ disposable wound-measuring device

Getting ready

• Assemble the equipment at the patient's bedside. Use clean or sterile technique, depending on facility policy and wound care orders.
• Cut tape into strips for securing dressings. Loosen lids on cleaning solutions and medications *for easy removal.*
• Attach an impervious plastic trash bag to the overbed table *to hold used dressings and refuse.*
• Before any dressing change, wash your hands and review the principles of standard precautions.
• Provide privacy, and explain the procedure to the patient *to allay fears and promote cooperation.*

How you do it

• Position the patient in a way that maximizes comfort while allowing easy access to the wound site.
• Cover bed linens with a linen-saver pad *to prevent soiling.*

Cleaning the wound

- Open the cleaning solution container and carefully pour cleaning solution onto the opened plastic package of 4 × 4s or into a bowl *to avoid splashing*. (The bowl may be clean or sterile, depending on facility policy).
- Open other supplies as needed.
- Put on gloves.
- Gently roll or lift an edge of the soiled dressing *to obtain a starting point*. Support adjacent skin while gently releasing the soiled dressing from the skin. When possible, remove the dressing in the direction of hair growth. Assess the existing dressing for drainage, color, amount, and odor.
- Discard the soiled dressing and your contaminated gloves in the impervious plastic trash bag *to avoid contaminating the clean or sterile field*.
- Put on a clean pair of gloves (sterile or nonsterile, depending on facility policy or the wound care order).
- Inspect the wound. Note the color, amount, and odor of drainage and necrotic debris.
- Fold a sterile 4″ × 4″ gauze pad into quarters and grasp it with your fingers. Make sure the folded edge faces outward.
- Alternatively, use a wound cleanser in a spray-gun bottle.

Circles on the skin

- When cleaning, be sure to move from the least-contaminated area to the most-contaminated area. For a linear-shaped wound, such as an incision, gently wipe from top to bottom in one motion, starting directly over the wound and moving outward. For an open wound, such as a pressure ulcer, gently wipe in concentric circles, again starting directly over the wound and moving outward. Use a separate gauze pad each time the wound is cleaned.
- Discard the gauze pad in the plastic trash bag.
- Using a clean gauze pad for each wiping motion, repeat the procedure until you've cleaned the entire wound.
- Dry the wound with 4″ × 4″ gauze pads, using the same procedure as for cleaning. Discard the used gauze pads in the plastic trash bag.

Go back to the basics—measure the wound!

- Measure the perimeter of the wound with a disposable wound-measuring device (e.g., a square, transparent card with concentric circles arranged in bull's-eye fashion and bordered with a straight-edge ruler). Measure the longest length in a head to toe direction and the widest width.
- Measure the depth of a full-thickness wound.

Testing for tunneling
• Gently probe the wound bed and edges with your finger or a flexible probe *to assess for wound tunneling or undermining.* Tunneling usually signals wound extension along fascial planes. Gauge tunnel depth by determining how far you can insert your finger or the cotton-tipped applicator.
• Next, reassess the condition of the skin and wound. Note the character of the clean wound bed and the surrounding skin.
• If you observe adherent necrotic material, notify a wound care specialist or a doctor *to ensure appropriate debridement.*

Applying a dressing
• Prepare to apply the appropriate topical dressing if ordered. Instructions for applying topical moist saline gauze, hydrocolloid, transparent, alginate, foam, and hydrogel dressings follow. (See *Choosing a wound dressing*, page 448.) For other dressings or topical agents, follow your facility's protocol or the manufacturer's instructions.

Moist saline gauze dressing
• Moisten the gauze dressing with NSS. Wring out excess fluid.
• Open the gauze pad completely (often termed *fluffing*) and gently place the dressing into the wound. *To separate surfaces within the wound,* gently guide the gauze between opposing wound surfaces. *To avoid damage to tissues,* lightly fill the space—don't pack the gauze tightly.
• *To protect the surrounding skin from moisture,* apply a sealant or barrier.
• Change the dressing often enough to keep the wound moist.

Hydrocolloid dressing
• Choose a clean, dry, presized dressing, or cut one to overlap the wound by about 1″ (2.5 cm). Remove the dressing from its package, pull the release paper from the adherent side of the dressing, and apply the dressing to the wound. Hold the dressing in place with your hand *because the warmth will mold the dressing to the skin.*

Smooth operator

• As you apply the dressing, carefully smooth out wrinkles and avoid stretching the dressing.
• If the dressing's edges need to be secured with tape, apply a skin sealant to the intact skin around the wound. After the area is dry, tape the dressing to the skin. *The sealant protects the skin from tape burns and skin stripping and promotes tape adherence.* Avoid using tension or pressure when applying the tape.

Choosing a wound dressing

The patient's needs and wound characteristics determine which type of dressing to use on a wound. Think of dressings as maintaining moisture, donating moisture, or absorbing moisture.

Maintaining moisture
Gauze dressings
Made of absorptive cotton or synthetic fabric, gauze dressings are permeable to water, water vapor, and oxygen and may be impregnated with hydrogel or another agent. When uncertain about which dressing to use, you may apply a gauze dressing moistened in saline solution until a wound specialist recommends definitive treatment.

Hydrocolloid dressings
Hydrocolloid dressings are adhesive, moldable wafers made of a carbohydrate-based material and usually have waterproof backings. They're impermeable to oxygen, water, and water vapor, and most have some absorptive properties.

Transparent film dressings
Transparent film dressings are clear, adherent, and nonabsorptive. These polymer-based dressings are permeable to oxygen and water vapor but not to water. Their transparency allows visual inspection. Because they can't absorb drainage, they're used on partial-thickness wounds with minimal exudate.

Absorbing moisture
Alginate dressings
Made from seaweed, alginate dressings are nonwoven, absorptive dressings available as soft sterile pads or ropes. They absorb excessive exudate and may be used on infected wounds. As these dressings absorb exudate, many turn into a gel that keeps the wound bed moist and promotes healing. When exudate is no longer excessive, switch to another type of dressing.

Hydrofiber
These dressings are made of synthetic material and resemble alginates in shape, size, and absorbency. They absorb excessive exudate and may be used on infected wounds.

Foam dressings
Foam dressings are spongelike polymer dressings that may be impregnated or coated with other materials. Foams are adhesive or nonadhesive and bordered or nonbordered and are used when absorption is needed.

Donating moisture
Hydrogel dressings
Most hydrogels are primarily water-based. They're available as a gel in a tube, as flexible sheets, gel impregnated gauze pads, and as saturated gauze packing strips. They may have a cooling effect, which eases pain, and are used when the wound needs moisture.

- Remove your gloves and discard them in the impervious plastic trash bag. Dispose of refuse according to facility policy, and wash your hands.
- Change a hydrocolloid dressing every 2 to 7 days as necessary; change it immediately if the patient complains of pain, the dressing no longer adheres, or leakage occurs. Remember, hydrocolloids are occlusive and provide a barrier when intact. If drainage is leaking out, then bacteria can go in!

Transparent dressing
- Clean and dry the wound as described earlier.
- Select a dressing to overlap the wound by 1″ to 2″ (2.5 to 5 cm).

• Gently lay the dressing over the wound; avoid wrinkling the dressing. *To prevent shearing force,* don't stretch the dressing over the wound. Press firmly on the edges of the dressing *to promote adherence.* Although this type of dressing is self-adhesive, you may have to tape the edges *to prevent them from curling.*
• Change the dressing every 3 to 5 days, depending on the amount of drainage. If the seal is no longer secure or if accumulated tissue fluid extends beyond the edges of the wound and onto the surrounding skin, change the dressing. Occlusive dressings that are no longer secure or that are leaking on to the surrounding skin may cause a risk for infection or skin breakdown. The dressing should be monitored for dryness, intactness, and that it is secure.

Alginate/hydrofiber dressing

• Apply the alginate or hydrofiber dressing to the wound surface. Cover the area with a secondary dressing (such as gauze pads or transparent film) as ordered. Secure the dressing with tape or elastic netting.
• *Change* the dressing when strikethrough occurs (you can see the drainage outline on the secondary dressing). This means the alginate/hydrofiber has absorbed the maximum amount. When the drainage stops or the wound bed looks dry, stop using alginate/hydrofiber dressings.

Foam dressing

• Gently lay the foam dressing over the wound. But, if the wound is deep, then the dead space is not filled. Sometimes, foams are secondary dressings.
• Use tape, elastic netting, or gauze *to hold the dressing in place* if it is not bordered or adhesive.
• Change the dressing when the foam no longer absorbs the exudate and there is strikethrough on the top or edges of the dressing.

Hydrogel dressing

• Apply gel to the wound bed to cover the bed with a layer of gel.
• Cover partial thickness wounds with a secondary dressing (transparent film or a nonadherent dressing). For full-thickness wounds, use gel-impregnated gauze (4 × 4s or strip). If you do not have this available, apply gel over the wound bed and fill the dead space with fluffed, NSS moistened gauze.
• Change the dressing daily or as needed *to keep the wound bed moist.*
• If the hydrogel dressing you select comes in sheet form, cut the dressing to overlap the wound by 1″ (2.5 cm); then apply as you would a hydrocolloid dressing. Don't forget to protect the peri-wound skin with skin prep!

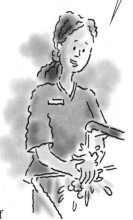

Make sure you wash your hands before and after each dressing change.

Practice pointers

- Be aware that infection may cause foul-smelling drainage, persistent pain, severe erythema, induration, and elevated skin and body temperatures. Advancing infection or cellulitis can lead to septicemia.
- Severe erythema may signal worsening cellulitis, which means the offending organisms have invaded the tissue and are no longer localized.

Wound irrigation

Irrigation cleans tissues and flushes cell debris and drainage from an open wound. It also helps prevent premature surface healing over an abscess pocket or infected tract.

After irrigation, fill open wounds to absorb additional drainage. Always follow the standard precaution guidelines of the Centers for Disease Control and Prevention (CDC).

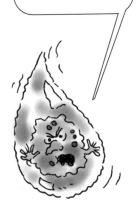

I'm a victim! I mean, there I was in my cozy wound with all my friends and then, the next thing I know, I'm floating in this giant emesis basin. Oh, the humiliation!

What you need

Waterproof trash bag ✳ linen-saver pad ✳ emesis basin ✳ clean gloves ✳ sterile gloves ✳ goggles ✳ gown, if indicated ✳ prescribed irrigant such as sterile NSS ✳ sterile water or NSS ✳ soft rubber or plastic catheter ✳ sterile container ✳ materials as needed for wound care ✳ sterile irrigation and dressing set ✳ commercial wound cleaner ✳ 35-ml piston syringe with 19G needle or catheter ✳ skin protectant wipe (skin sealant) or other protective skin barrier

Getting ready

- Assemble equipment in the patient's room. Check the expiration date on each sterile package and inspect for tears.
- Don't use any nonpreserved solution that has been open longer than 24 hours. As needed, dilute the prescribed irrigant to the correct proportions with sterile water or NSS. Allow the solution to reach room temperature, or warm it to 90° to 95° F (32.2° to 35° C).
- Open the waterproof trash bag and place it near the patient's bed. Form a cuff by turning down the top of the trash bag.

How you do it

- Check the doctor's order, assess the patient's condition, and identify allergies. Explain the procedure to the patient, provide

privacy, and position the patient correctly for the procedure. Place the linen-saver pad under the patient and place the emesis basin below the wound *so that the irrigating solution flows from the wound into the basin.*
• Wash your hands, and put on a gown and gloves.
• Remove the soiled dressing; then discard the dressing and gloves in the trash bag.
• Establish a clean or sterile field with all the equipment and supplies you'll need for wound irrigation and dressing. Pour the prescribed amount of irrigating solution into a clean or sterile container. Put on sterile gloves and a gown and goggles, if indicated. (See *Irrigating a deep wound,* page 452.)

From clean to dirty

• Fill the syringe with the irrigating solution and connect the catheter to the syringe. Gently instill a slow, steady stream of solution into the wound until the syringe empties. Make sure the solution flows from the clean to the dirty area of the wound *to prevent contamination of clean tissue by exudate.* Also make sure the solution reaches all areas of the wound.
• Refill the syringe, reconnect it to the catheter, and repeat the irrigation. Continue to irrigate the wound until you've administered the prescribed amount of solution or until the solution returns clear. Note the amount of solution administered. Then remove and discard the catheter and syringe in the waterproof trash bag.

Positioned for success

• Keep the patient positioned to allow further wound drainage into the basin.
• Clean the area around the wound with NSS and pat dry with gauze; wipe intact surrounding skin with a skin protectant wipe and allow it to dry.
• Fill the wound lightly if ordered, and apply a dressing.
• Remove and discard your gloves and gown.
• Make sure the patient is comfortable and wash your hands.
• Dispose of drainage, solutions, trash bag, and soiled equipment and supplies according to facility policy and CDC guidelines.

Practice pointers

• Try to coordinate wound irrigation with the doctor's visit *so that he can inspect the wound.*
• Irrigate with a bulb syringe if the wound is small or not particularly deep or if a piston syringe is unavailable. However, use a bulb syringe cautiously *because this type of syringe doesn't deliver enough pressure to adequately clean the wound and may increase the risk of aspirating drainage.*

Irrigating a deep wound

When preparing to irrigate a wound, attach a 19G needle or catheter to a 35-ml piston syringe. This setup delivers an irrigation pressure of 8 psi, which is effective in cleaning the wound and reducing the risk of trauma and wound infection. To prevent tissue damage or, in an abdominal wound, intestinal perforation, avoid forcing the needle or catheter into the wound.

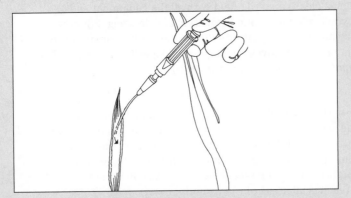

Irrigate the wound with gentle pressure until you have administered the prescribed amount and the solution returns clear. Allow the emesis basin to remain under the wound to collect any remaining drainage.

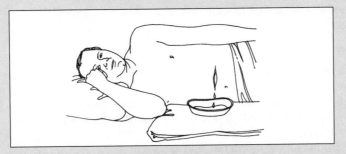

A syringe irrigation is another alternative. Where possible, direct the flow at right angle to the wound and allow the fluid to drain by gravity. Doing so requires careful positioning of the patient, either in bed or on a chair. The patient may need analgesia during the treatment.

   If irrigation isn't possible, gently swab away exudate before using antiseptic or saline solution to clean the wound (taking care not to push loose debris into the wound). Facility policy permitting, use sharp, sterile scissors to snip off loose dead tissue—never pull it off.

Surgical wound management

When caring for a surgical wound, you carry out procedures that help prevent infection by stopping pathogens from entering the wound. In addition to promoting patient comfort, such procedures protect the skin's surface from maceration and excoriation caused by contact with irritating drainage. They also allow you to measure wound drainage to monitor fluid and electrolyte balance.

The primary method used to manage a draining surgical wound is a dressing, negative pressure wound therapy, or a pouch. Usually, lightly seeping wounds with drains and wounds with minimal purulent drainage can be managed with dressings.

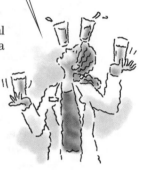

Infection-preventing procedures also allow you to monitor fluid and electrolyte imbalance.

What a lovely dress

Dressing a surgical wound calls for sterile technique and sterile supplies to prevent contamination. You may use the color of the wound to help determine which type of dressing to apply. Be sure to change the dressing often enough to keep the skin dry. Always follow standard precautions set by the CDC.

What you need

Waterproof trash bag ✳ clean gloves ✳ sterile gloves ✳ gown and face shield or goggles, if indicated ✳ sterile 4″ × 4″ gauze pads ✳ selected primary dressing(s)✳ sterile cotton-tipped applicators ✳ sterile dressing set ✳ topical medication, if ordered ✳ selected securing (adhesive or other tape, Montgomery straps, a fishnet tube elasticized dressing support, or a T-binder) ✳ skin protectant ✳ sterile NSS ✳ optional: forceps, nonadherent pads, collodion spray or acetone-free adhesive remover, graduated container.

For a wound with a drain

Sterile scissors ✳ sterile 4″ × 4″ gauze pads without cotton lining ✳ ostomy pouch or another collection pouch ✳ sterile precut tracheostomy pads or drain dressings ✳ adhesive tape (paper or silk tape if the patient is hypersensitive) ✳ surgical mask

Getting ready

• Ask the patient about allergies to tapes and dressings. Assemble all equipment in the patient's room. Check the expiration date on each sterile package, and inspect for tears.

• Open the waterproof trash bag, and place it near the patient's bed. Position the bag *to avoid reaching across the sterile field or the wound when disposing of soiled articles.* Form a cuff by turning down the top of the trash bag *to provide a wide opening and to prevent contamination of instruments or gloves by touching the bag's edge.*

How you do it
• Explain the procedure to the patient *to allay his fears and ensure his cooperation.*

Removing the old dressing
• Check the doctor's order for specific wound care and medication instructions. Note the location of surgical drains *to avoid dislodging them during the procedure.*
• Assess the patient's condition.
• Provide privacy, and position the patient as necessary. *To avoid chilling him,* expose only the wound site.
• Wash your hands thoroughly. Put on a gown and a face shield, if necessary. Then put on clean gloves.

Go toward the wound
• Loosen the soiled dressing by holding the patient's skin and pulling the tape or dressing toward the wound *to protect the newly formed tissue and prevent stress on the incision.* Moisten the tape with acetone-free adhesive remover, if necessary, *to make the tape removal less painful (particularly if the skin is hairy).* Don't apply solvents to the incision *because they could contaminate the wound.*
• Slowly remove the soiled dressing. If the gauze adheres to the wound, loosen the gauze by moistening it with sterile NSS.
• Observe the dressing for the amount, type, color, and odor of drainage.
• Discard the dressing and gloves in the waterproof trash bag.

Caring for the wound
• Wash your hands. Establish a sterile field with all the equipment and supplies you'll need for suture line care and the dressing change. If the doctor has ordered ointment, squeeze the needed amount onto the sterile field. If you're using an antiseptic from an unsterile bottle, pour the antiseptic cleaning agent into a sterile container *so you won't contaminate your gloves.* Then put on sterile gloves.

No cotton balls, please!

• Saturate the sterile gauze pads with the prescribed cleaning agent. Avoid using cotton balls *because they may shed fibers in the wound, causing irritation, infection, or adhesion.*
• If ordered, obtain a wound culture; then proceed to clean the wound.
• Irrigate the wound, if ordered, using the specified solution.
• Pick up the moistened gauze pad or swab, and squeeze out the excess solution.

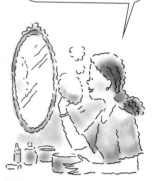

Cotton balls are great for taking off makeup but not so good for wound cleaning!

From top to bottom

• Working from the top of the incision, wipe once to the bottom and then discard the gauze pad. With a second moistened pad, wipe from top to bottom in a vertical path next to the incision (as shown below).

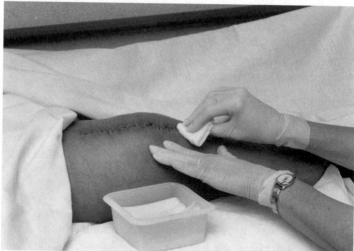

• Continue to work outward from the incision in lines running parallel to it. Always wipe from the clean area toward the less clean area (usually from top to bottom). Use each gauze pad or swab for only one stroke *to avoid tracking wound exudate and normal body flora from surrounding skin to the clean areas.* Remember that the suture line is cleaner than the adjacent skin and the top of the suture line is usually cleaner than the bottom *because more drainage collects at the bottom of the wound.*
• Use sterile, cotton-tipped applicators for efficient cleaning of tight-fitting wire sutures, deep and narrow wounds, and wounds with pockets. Remember to wipe only once with each applicator.

Watch out for the drain!

- If the patient has a surgical drain, clean the drain's surface last. *Because moist drainage promotes bacterial growth,* the drain is considered the most contaminated area. Clean the skin around the drain by wiping in half or full circles from the drain site outward.
- Clean all areas of the wound to wash away debris, pus, blood, and necrotic material. Try not to disturb sutures or irritate the incision. Clean to at least 1″ (2.5 cm) beyond the end of the new dressing. If you aren't applying a new dressing, clean to at least 2″ (5 cm) beyond the incision.

Line em up . . .

- Check to make sure the edges of the incision are lined up properly, and check for signs of infection (heat, redness, swelling, induration, and odor), dehiscence, and evisceration. If you observe such signs or if the patient reports pain at the wound site, notify the doctor.
- Wash skin surrounding the wound with normal saline, and pat dry using a sterile 4″ × 4″ gauze pad. Avoid oil-based soap *because it may interfere with pouch adherence.* Apply any prescribed topical medication.
- Apply a skin protectant if needed.

. . . and then apply the dressing

Applying a new gauze dressing

- Gently place sterile 4″ × 4″ gauze pads at the center of the wound, and move progressively outward to the edges of the wound site. Extend the gauze at least 1″ (2.5 cm) beyond the incision in each direction, and cover the wound evenly with enough sterile dressings (usually two or three layers) to absorb all drainage until the next dressing change. If ordered, pack the wound with gauze pads or strips folded to fit, using a sterile forceps. Avoid using cotton-lined gauze pads *because cotton fibers can adhere to the wound surface and cause complications.* Pack the wound, using the wet-to-damp method. Soak the packing material in solution and wring it out so that it's slightly moist *to provide a moist wound environment that absorbs debris and drainage.* However, removing the packing won't disrupt new tissue. Don't pack the wound tightly *because doing so will exert pressure and may damage the wound.* Use large absorbent dressings (abdominal pads also known as *ABDs*) to form outer layers, if needed, *to provide greater absorbency.*

• Secure the dressing's edges to the patient's skin with strips of tape *to maintain the sterility of the wound site* (as shown). Alternatively, secure the dressing with a T-binder or Montgomery straps *to prevent skin excoriation,* which may occur with repeated tape removal necessitated by frequent dressing changes.

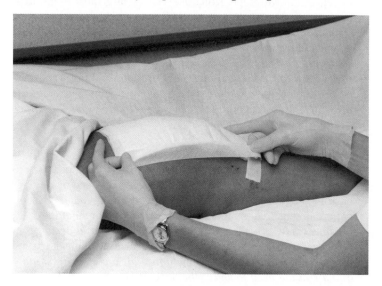

• Make sure the patient is comfortable.
• Properly dispose of the solutions and trash bag, and clean or discard soiled equipment and supplies according to your facility's policy.

Dressing a wound with a drain

• Use commercially precut gauze drain dressings or prepare a drain dressing by using sterile scissors to cut a slit in a sterile 4″ × 4″ gauze pad. Fold the pad in half; then cut inward from the center of the folded edge. Don't use a cotton-lined gauze pad *because cutting the gauze opens the lining and releases cotton fibers into the wound.* Prepare a second pad the same way.
• Gently press one drain dressing close to the skin around the drain so that the tubing fits into the slit. Press the second drain dressing around the drain from the opposite direction so that the two dressings encircle the tubing.
• Layer two to four uncut sterile 4″ × 4″ gauze pads or large absorbent dressings around the tubing as needed *to absorb expected drainage.* Tape the dressing in place, or use a T-binder or Montgomery straps.

Practice pointers

- If the patient has two wounds in the same area, cover each wound separately with layers of sterile 4″ × 4″ gauze pads. Then cover each site with a large absorbent dressing secured to the patient's skin with tape. Don't use a single large absorbent dressing to cover both sites *because drainage quickly saturates a pad, promoting cross-contamination.*
- When filling a wound, don't fill it too tightly *because doing so compresses adjacent capillaries and may prevent the wound edges from contracting.* Remember to "open and fluff" gauze before placing in wound. Avoid overlapping damp gauze or other dressing onto surrounding skin *because it macerates the intact tissue.*

A time saver

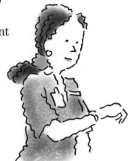

Using precut tracheostomy pads or drain dressings saves time.

- To save time when dressing a wound with a drain, use precut tracheostomy pads or drain dressings instead of custom-cut gauze pads to fit around the drain. If your patient is sensitive to adhesive tape, use paper or silk tape *because it's less likely to cause a skin reaction and peels off more easily than adhesive tape.* Use a surgical mask to cradle a chin or jawline dressing *to provide a secure dressing and avoid the need to shave the patient's hair.*
- If ordered, use a collodion spray or similar topical protectant instead of a gauze dressing. *This moisture- and contaminant-proof covering dries in a clear, impermeable film that leaves the wound visible for observation and avoids the friction caused by a dressing.*
- If a sump drain isn't adequately collecting wound secretions, reinforce it with an ostomy pouch or another collection bag. Use waterproof tape to strengthen a spot on the front of the pouch near the adhesive opening; then cut a small x in the tape. Feed the drain catheter into the pouch through the x cut. Seal the cut around the tubing with more waterproof tape; then connect the tubing to the suction pump. *This method frees the drainage port at the bottom of the pouch so you don't have to remove the tubing to empty the pouch.* If you use more than one collection pouch for a wound or wounds, record drainage volume separately for each pouch. Avoid using waterproof material over the dressing *because it reduces air circulation and promotes infection from accumulated heat and moisture.*

Not the first time!!

- *Because many doctors prefer to change the first postoperative dressing themselves to check the incision,* don't change the first dressing unless you have specific instructions to do so. If you have no such order and drainage comes through the dressings, reinforce the dressing with fresh sterile gauze. Request an order to change the dressing, or ask the doctor to change it as soon as possible. A reinforced dressing shouldn't remain in place longer than 24 hours *because it's an excellent medium for bacterial growth.*

Check and recheck!

• For the recent postoperative patient or a patient with complications, check the dressing every 15 to 30 minutes or as ordered. For the patient with a properly healing wound, check the dressing at least once every 8 hours.
• If the dressing becomes wet from the outside (e.g., from spilled drinking water), replace it as soon as possible *to prevent wound contamination.*
• If your patient will need wound care after discharge, provide appropriate teaching. If the patient will be doing self care, stress the importance of using clean technique, and teach how to examine the wound for signs of infection and other complications. Also demonstrate how to change dressings, and give written instructions for all procedures to be performed at home. If possible, have the patient do a return demonstration of the dressing change.

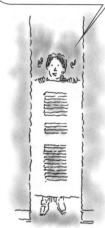

Don't perform the first dressing change unless you have specific instructions to do so.

Closed-wound drain management

Typically inserted during surgery in anticipation of substantial postoperative drainage, a closed-wound drain promotes healing and prevents swelling by suctioning the serosanguineous fluid that accumulates at the wound site. By removing this fluid, the closed-wound drain helps reduce the risk of infection and skin breakdown as well as the number of dressing changes. Hemovac and Jackson-Pratt closed drainage systems are most commonly used.

A closed-wound drain consists of perforated tubing connected to a portable vacuum unit. The distal end of the tubing lies within the wound and usually leaves the body from a site other than the primary suture line to preserve the integrity of the surgical wound. The tubing exit site is treated as an additional surgical wound; the drain is usually sutured to the skin.

If the wound produces heavy drainage, the closed-wound drain may be left in place for longer than 1 week. Drainage must be emptied and measured frequently to maintain maximum suction and prevent strain on the suture line.

Using a closed-wound drainage system

The portable closed-wound drainage system draws drainage from a wound site, such as the chest wall postmastectomy (shown at left), by means of a Y-tube. To empty the drainage, remove the plug and empty it into a graduated cylinder. To reestablish suction, compress the drainage unit against a firm surface to expel air and, while holding it down, replace the plug with your other hand (as shown in the center). The same principle is used for the Jackson-Pratt bulb drain (shown at right).

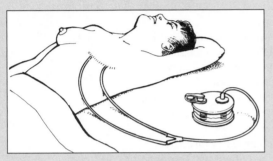 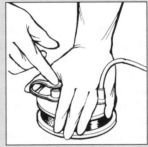 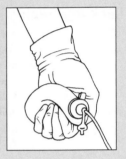

What you need

Graduated biohazard cylinder ✳ sterile laboratory container, if needed ✳ alcohol pads ✳ gloves ✳ gown ✳ face shield ✳ trash bag ✳ sterile gauze pads ✳ antiseptic cleaning agent ✳ prepackaged povidone-iodine swabs

Getting ready

• Check the doctor's order, and assess the patient's condition.
• Explain the procedure to the patient, provide privacy, and wash your hands.

How you do it

• Unclip the vacuum unit from the patient's bed or gown.
• Don clean gloves and using clean technique, release the vacuum by removing the spout plug on the collection chamber. The container expands completely as it draws in air. (See *Using a closed-wound drainage system.*)
• Empty the unit's contents into a graduated biohazard cylinder, and note the amount and appearance of the drainage. If diagnostic tests will be performed on the fluid specimen, pour the drainage directly into a sterile laboratory container, note the amount and appearance, and send it to the laboratory.
• Maintaining clean technique, use an alcohol pad to clean the unit's spout and plug.

• *To reestablish the vacuum that creates the drain's suction power,* fully compress the vacuum unit. With one hand holding the unit compressed to maintain the vacuum, replace the spout plug with your other hand.

No twist and shout!

• Check the patency of the equipment. Make sure the tubing is free from twists, kinks, and leaks *because the drainage system must be airtight to work properly.* The vacuum unit should remain compressed when you release manual pressure; rapid reinflation indicates an air leak. If reinflation occurs, recompress the unit and make sure the spout plug is secure.
• Secure the vacuum unit to the patient's gown. Fasten it below wound level *to promote drainage.* Don't apply tension on drainage tubing when fastening the unit *to avoid possible dislodgment.* Remove and discard your gloves and wash your hands thoroughly.

Be gentle

• Observe the sutures that secure the drain to the patient's skin; look for signs of pulling or tearing and for swelling or infection of surrounding skin. Gently clean the sutures with sterile gauze pads moistened with NSS or other solution as ordered.
• Properly dispose of drainage, solutions, and the trash bag, and clean or dispose of soiled equipment and supplies according to facility policy.

Practice pointers

• Empty the drain and measure its contents once during each shift if drainage has accumulated, more often if drainage is excessive. *Removing excess drainage maintains maximum suction and avoids straining the drain's suture line.*
• If the patient has more than one closed drain, number the drains *so you can record drainage from each site.*
• Document your care. (See *Documenting closed-wound drainage management.*)

Watch out!

• Be careful not to mistake chest tubes with water seal drainage devices for closed-wound drains *because the care of these devices differs from closed-wound drainage systems, and the vacuum of a chest tube should never be released.*

Take note!

Documenting closed-wound drainage management

Follow these tips when documenting your care of a closed-wound drainage unit. On the intake and output sheet, record drainage color, consistency, type, and amount. If the patient has more than one closed-wound drain, number the drains and record the information cited earlier separately for each drainage site.

Also record:
• the date and time you empty the drain
• appearance of the drain site
• presence of swelling or signs of infection
• equipment malfunction and consequent nursing action
• the patient's tolerance of the treatment.

A look at pressure ulcers

Pressure ulcers are a serious health problem. Although incidence figures vary widely because of differences in methodology, setting, and subjects, data gathered through 10 years of nationwide studies reveal that 10% to 15% of the general population suffers from chronic pressure ulcers. Although this finding is significant in itself, prevalence in some groups—such as patients with spinal cord injuries, patients in intensive care units, and nursing home residents—is shockingly higher.

At what cost?

Although prevalence statistics vary, what has become starkly evident are the costs associated with pressure ulcers—the cost in terms of suffering and diminished quality of life for patients, the cost to the health care industry in terms of resources consumed and manpower hours dedicated to managing the problem, and the very real monetary cost to individuals, health insurers, and government agencies.

The problem is so acute that many insurers and government agencies now track outcomes to discern whether specific interventions help treat pressure ulcers and to encourage prevention, early intervention, and closer monitoring by the health care industry. Because pressure ulcers are chronic conditions—they're hard to heal and tend to recur frequently—prevention and early intervention are critical for more effective management.

Island OASIS

Data collected from Outcome and Assessment Information Set (OASIS) forms provide a basis for relating these costs to clinical outcomes. The OASIS-B1 form is currently used by home health care agencies, as mandated by the Centers for Medicare and Medicaid Services.

The closer you get

Better disease management in pressure ulcer cases depends on closer collaboration among government agencies, insurers, and health care professionals. There's heartening evidence that this group effort is developing. All involved are paying closer attention to prevention and the effectiveness of interventions, and they're finding better methods of quantifying and disseminating results. Soon, pressure ulcers will be a reportable condition for the CDC. In addition, the health care objectives for the nation as a whole reflect a better understanding of the problem's severity. *Healthy People 2020* (a report of the nation's

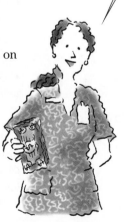

Pressure ulcers are costly—for the patient and the health care industry.

near-term health care goals) includes a goal of reducing the rate of pressure ulcers–related hospitalization by a 10% reduction in patients older than 65 years of age.

Causes

Chronic wounds are those that fail to heal in a timely manner, resist treatment, and tend to recur. Pressure ulcers are chronic wounds resulting from tissue death due to prolonged, irreversible ischemia brought on by compression of soft tissue.

If you want to get technical

Technically speaking, pressure ulcers are the clinical manifestation of localized tissue death due to lack of blood flow in areas under pressure.

Simplify, simplify!

Now, let's back up a bit to break down and better understand this description. First of all, different tissues have different tolerances for compression. Muscle and fat have comparatively low tolerances for pressure, whereas skin has a somewhat higher tolerance. All cells, regardless of tissue type, depend on blood circulation for the oxygen and nutrients they need. Tissue compression interferes with circulation, reducing or completely cutting off blood flow. The result, known as *ischemia*, is that cells fail to receive adequate supplies of oxygen and nutrients. Unless the pressure relents, cells eventually die. By the time inflammation signals impending necrosis on the surface of the skin, it's likely that necrosis has occurred in deeper tissues.

Location, location, location

Pressure ulcers are most common in areas where pressure compresses soft tissue over a bony prominence in the body—the tissue is pinched between the outer pressure and the hard underlying surface. The other three causal factors of skin breakdown are shear, friction, and moisture. Planning effective interventions for prevention and treatment requires a sound understanding of the etiology of pressure ulcers and addressing the four causal factors.

Pressure

Capillaries are connected to arteries and veins through intermediary vessels called *arterioles* and *venules*. In healthy individuals, capillary filling pressure is approximately 32 mm Hg where arterioles connect to capillaries and 12 mm Hg where capillaries connect to venules. Therefore, external pressure greater than capillary filling pressure can cause problems. In frail or ill people, capillary filling pressures may be much lower. External pressure that exceeds capillary perfusion pressure compresses blood vessels and causes ischemia in the tissues supplied by those vessels.

Tip of the iceberg

If the pressure continues long enough, capillaries collapse and thrombose, toxic metabolic by-products accumulate, and cells in nearby muscle and subcutaneous tissues begin to die. Muscle and fat are less tolerant of interruptions in blood flow than skin. Consequently, by the time signs of impending necrosis appear on the skin, underlying tissue has probably suffered substantial damage. Keep this "tip of the iceberg" effect in mind when assessing the size of a pressure ulcer. (See *Pressure points*.)

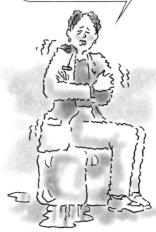

When assessing the size of a pressure ulcer, don't forget that it may just be the tip of the iceberg!

The pressure mounts

When external pressure exceeds venous capillary refill pressure (about 12 mm Hg), capillaries begin to leak. The resulting edema increases the amount of pressure on blood vessels, further impeding circulation. When interstitial pressure surpasses arterial intravascular pressure,

---

Pressure points

Pressure points are likely areas for ulcer formation. These illustrations show the areas at highest risk for ulcers when the patient is in different positions.

Sitting

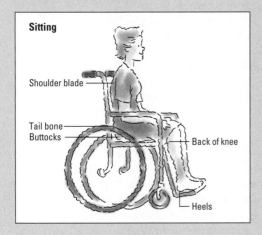

Shoulder blade

Tail bone
Buttocks

Back of knee

Heels

Lying

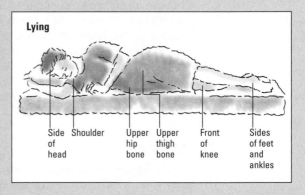

Side of head | Shoulder | Upper hip bone | Upper thigh bone | Front of knee | Sides of feet and ankles

blood is forced into nearby tissues (blanchable erythema). Continued capillary occlusion, lack of oxygen and nutrients, and buildup of toxic waste leads to necrosis of muscle, subcutaneous tissue and, ultimately, the dermis and epidermis.

Spreading the load

The force associated with any given pressure increases as the amount of body surface exposed to the pressure decreases. For example, the force exerted on the buttocks of a person lying in bed is about 70 mm Hg. However, when the same person sits on a hard surface, the force exerted on the ischial tuberosities can be as much as 300 mm Hg. Consequently, bony prominences are particularly susceptible to pressure ulcers. However, they aren't the only areas at risk. Ulcers can develop on any soft tissue subjected to prolonged pressure.

Between a bone and a hard place

When blood vessels, muscle, subcutaneous fat, and skin are compressed between a bone and an external surface—a bed or chair, for instance—pressure is exerted on the tissues from the external surface and the bone. In effect, the external surface produces pressure and the bone produces counterpressure. These opposing forces create a cone-shaped pressure gradient. (See *Understanding the pressure gradient.*) Although the pressure affects all tissues between these two points, tissues closest to the bony prominence suffer the greatest damage.

Understanding the pressure gradient

In this illustration, the V-shaped pressure gradient results from the upward force exerted by the supporting surface and the downward force of the bony prominence. Pressure is greatest on tissues at the apex of the gradient and lessens to the right and left of this point.

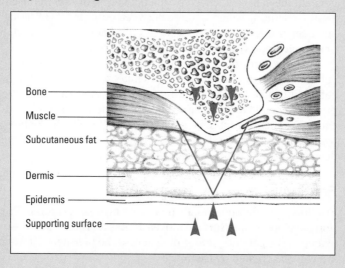

Bone

Muscle

Subcutaneous fat

Dermis

Epidermis

Supporting surface

Long-term lows are losers

Over time, pressure causes a growing discomfort that prompts a person to change position before tissue ischemia occurs. In ulcer formation, an inverse relationship exists between time and pressure. Typically, low pressure for long periods is far more damaging than high pressure for short periods. For example, a pressure of 70 mm Hg sustained for 2 hours or longer almost always causes irreversible tissue damage, whereas a pressure of 240 mm Hg can be endured for a short time with little or no tissue damage. Furthermore, after the time-pressure threshold for damage passes, damage continues even after the pressure stops. Although pressure ulcers can result from one period of sustained pressure, they're more likely to result from repeated ischemic events without adequate intervening time for recovery.

Shear

Shearing force intensifies the pressure's destructive effects. Shear is a mechanical force that runs parallel, rather than perpendicular, to an area of skin; deep tissues feel the brunt of the force.

The shear truth of it

Shearing force is most likely to develop during repositioning or when a patient slides down after being placed in high-Fowler's position. However, simply elevating the head of the bed increases shear and pressure in the sacral and coccygeal areas; gravity pulls the body down but the skin on the back resists the motion because of friction between the skin and the sheets. The result is that the skeleton (and attached tissues) actually slides somewhat beneath the skin (evidenced by the puckering of skin in the gluteal area), generating shearing force between outer layers of tissue and deeper layers. The force generated is enough to obstruct, tear, or stretch blood vessels. (See *Shearing force.*)

Shearing force reduces the length of time that tissue can endure a given pressure before ischemia or necrosis occurs. A sufficiently high level of shearing force can halve the amount of pressure needed to produce vascular occlusion. Research indicates that shearing force is responsible for the high incidence of triangular shaped sacral ulcers and the large areas of tunneling or deep sinus tracts beneath these ulcers.

Friction

Friction is another potentially damaging mechanical force. Friction develops as one surface moves across another surface—for example, the patient's skin sliding across the bedsheet. *Abrasions* are wounds created by friction.

Shearing force

Shear is a mechanical force parallel, rather than perpendicular, to an area of tissue. In this illustration, gravity pulls the body down the incline of the bed. The skeleton and attached tissues move, but the skin remains stationary, held in place by friction between the skin and the bed linen. The skeleton and attached tissues actually slide within the skin, causing skin to pucker in the gluteal area.

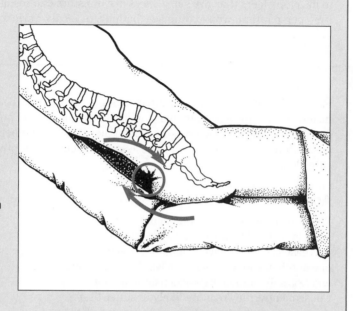

Those at particularly high risk for tissue damage due to friction include patients who have uncontrollable movements or spastic conditions, patients who wear braces or appliances that rub against the skin, and older patients. Friction is also a problem for patients who have trouble lifting themselves during repositioning. Rubbing against the sheet can result in an abrasion, which increases the potential for deeper tissue damage. Elevating the head of the bed, as discussed earlier, generates friction between the patient's skin and the bed linen as gravity tugs the patient's body downward. As the skeleton moves inside the skin, friction and shearing force combine to increase the risk of tissue damage in the sacral area. Such dry lubricants as cornstarch and adherent dressings with slippery backings can help reduce the impact of friction.

Excessive moisture

Prolonged exposure to moisture can waterlog, or *macerate*, skin. Maceration contributes to pressure ulcer formation by softening the connective tissue. Macerated epidermis erodes more easily, degenerates, and eventually sloughs off. In addition, damp skin adheres to bed linen more readily, making friction's effects

Prolonged exposure to moisture can waterlog, or macerate, skin, contributing to pressure ulcer formation.

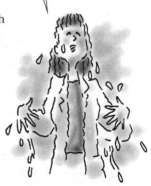

more profound. Consequently, moist skin is five times more likely to develop ulcers than dry skin. Excessive moisture can result from perspiration, wound drainage, bathing, or fecal or urinary incontinence.

Risk factors

Factors that increase the risk of developing pressure ulcers include advancing age, immobility, incontinence, infection, poor nutrition, and low blood pressure. High-risk patients, whether in an institution or at home, should be assessed regularly for pressure ulcers.

Age

With advancing age, the skin becomes more fragile as epidermal turnover slows, vascularization decreases, and skin layers adhere less securely to one another. Older adults have less lean body mass and less subcutaneous tissue cushioning bony areas. Consequently, they're more likely to suffer tissue damage due to friction, shear, and pressure. (See *Aging and skin function*.)

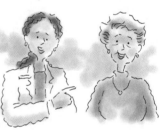

Older adults are more likely to suffer tissue damage due to friction, shear, and pressure.

An older adult can experience altered pain perception, which can increase the risk of pressure ulcer development. Other common problems include poor nutrition, poor hydration, and impaired respiratory or immune systems.

Immobility

Immobility may be the greatest risk factor for pressure ulcer development. The patient's ability to move in response to pressure sensations as well as the frequency with which his position is changed should always be considered in risk assessment.

Incontinence

Incontinence increases a patient's exposure to moisture and, over time, increases his risk of skin breakdown. Urinary and fecal incontinence create problems as a result of excessive moisture and chemical irritation. Due to pathogens in stools, fecal incontinence can cause more skin damage than urinary incontinence. Patients who have fecal and urinary incontinence have greater risk of skin breakdown from moisture. Feces contain both lipolytic and proteolytic enzymes which are inactivated

Ages and stages

Aging and skin function

Over time, skin loses its ability to function as efficiently or as effectively as it once did. As a result, the golden years of life place a person at greater risk for such injuries as pressure ulcers and tumors as well as various other skin conditions. This chart outlines the major changes that take place in the skin during the aging process and the implications of those changes for older people.

Change	Implications
50% reduction in the cell turnover rate in the stratum corneum (outermost layer) and a 20% reduction in dermal thickness	• Higher risk of infection because thinner skin is a less effective barrier to germs and allergens
Generalized reduction in dermal vascularization and an associated drop in blood flow to the skin	• Bruising more easily and increasing tendency of edema around wounds
Redistribution of subcutaneous tissue, which contains fewer fat cells in older people, to the stomach and thighs	• Risk of hyperthermia or hypothermia • Higher incidence of ischemia (cell damage resulting from too little oxygen reaching cells) in compressed tissue of bony areas
Flattening of papillae in the dermoepidermal junction (meeting of the epidermis and dermis), which reduces adhesion between layers	• Much higher incidence of shear and tear injuries
Drop in the number of Langerhans' cells (immune macrophages that attack invading germs) present in the skin	• Higher risk of infection • Slower sensitization response (redness, heat, discomfort), resulting in overuse of topical medications and more severe allergic reactions (because signs aren't evident early on)
50% decline in the number of fibroblasts and mast cells (cells that play a key role in the inflammatory response)	• Higher risk of infection
Marked reduction in the ability to sense pressure, heat, and cold, even though the same number of nerve endings in the skin are retained	• Higher incidence of pressure and thermal (hot and cold) damage to the skin • Higher incidence of ischemia (cell damage resulting from too little oxygen reaching cells) in compressed tissue • Higher incidence of skin tears
Significant decline in the number of sweat glands	• Difficulty with thermoregulation and increased risk of hyperthermia due to decreased production of sweat
Poorer absorption through the skin	• Risk of overdose of transdermal medications due to too frequent application
Reduction in the skin's ability to synthesize vitamin D	• Skin loses elasticity and wrinkles develop

during passage through the gastrointestinal tract. When the feces come into contact with the urine, the urea in the urine is converted into ammonia. Ammonia causes a shift in the pH of the skin and feces to alkalinity and this alkaline pH reactivates the enzymes in the feces.

Infection

Although the role of infection in pressure ulceration isn't fully understood, animal studies on the effects of pressure and infection indicate that compression encourages a localized increase in bacteria concentration. Bacteria injected into animals localized at the compression site, resulting in necrosis at lower pressures relative to the control group. Researchers concluded that compressed skin lowers local resistance to bacterial infection and that infection may reduce the pressure needed to cause tissue necrosis. Furthermore, researchers noted higher infection rates in pedicle flaps when denervation or loss of motor and sensory nerve function occurred. This may explain why neurologically impaired patients are more susceptible to infection and pressure ulceration.

Nutrition

Proper nutrition is vitally important to tissue integrity. A strong correlation exists between poor nutrition and pressure ulceration, yet nutrition is all too commonly overlooked during treatment.

Albumin acumen

Increased protein is required for the body to heal itself. Albumin is one of the key proteins in the body. A patient's serum albumin level is an important indicator of his protein levels. A subnormal serum albumin level is a late manifestation of protein deficiency. Normal serum albumin levels range from 3.5 to 5 g/dl. Serum albumin deficits are ranked as:
- mild—3 to 3.5 g/dl
- moderate—2.5 to 3 g/dl
- severe—less than 2.5 g/dl.

Pressure ulcer occurrence and severity are linked to malnutrition. One recent study found a direct correlation between pressure ulcer stage and degree of hypoalbuminemia (serum albumin level below 3.5 g/dl). Monitor the serum albumin levels of a high-risk patient and plan on nutritional intervention if he has hypoproteinemia.

Extra protein can help a patient's body heal itself. I think I need some extra healing so I'll help myself to another piece.

Blood pressure

Low arterial blood pressure is clearly linked to tissue ischemia, particularly in vascular patients. When blood pressure is low, the body shunts blood away from the peripheral vascular system that serves the skin and toward vital organs to ensure their health. As perfusion drops, the skin is less tolerant of sustained external pressure, and the risk of damage due to ischemia rises.

Assessing risk factors

Several assessment tools are available to help determine a patient's risk of developing pressure ulcers. Most are based on the work of Doreen Norton, who studied the pressure ulcer problem in Great Britain. Some years later, Gosnell and Braden developed a more refined scale based on data from independent studies.

Common denominators

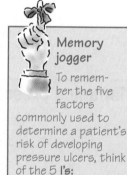

Most scales use the following factors to determine a patient's risk of developing pressure ulcers:
- immobility
- inactivity
- incontinence
- malnutrition
- impaired mental status or sensation.

Each category receives a value based on the patient's condition. The sum of these values determines the patient's score and level of risk. Scores for each category as well as the assessment as a whole guide the care team to develop appropriate interventions. Most health care facilities require an assessment score for every patient admitted.

The Braden scale

The Braden Pressure Sore Risk Assessment Scale is the most widely used scale. This tool scores etiologic factors that contribute to prolonged pressure as well as factors that contribute to diminished tissue tolerance for pressure. Factors scored in this assessment include sensory perception, moisture, activity, mobility, nutrition, and friction and shear. Each factor receives a score of 1 to 4, with the exception of friction and shear, which receives a score of 1 to 3. The highest possible score is 23; the lower the score, the higher the patient's risk of pressure ulceration. A score of 18 or lower denotes a risk of pressure ulcers.

In nursing home populations, most pressure ulcers develop during the 2 weeks immediately following admission, so early identification of at-risk patients is crucial. The Wound Ostomy &

Memory jogger

To remember the five factors commonly used to determine a patient's risk of developing pressure ulcers, think of the 5 I's:

Immobility

Inactivity

Incontinence

Improper nutrition (malnutrition)

Impaired mental status or sensation.

Continence Nurses Society (WOCN) Guidelines for Pressure Ulcer Prevention suggest we need to establish a risk assessment policy in all health care settings and to establish accuracy of assessments between/among nurses.

Long-term care (LTC)—on admission and daily for a week—and then quarterly or follow your facility policy

Acute care—on admission and daily on each shift

Long-term acute care (LTAC)—daily for first week, then weekly

Pressure ulcer prevention

Pressure ulcer prevention focuses on compensating for prevailing risk factors and addressing the underlying pathophysiology. When planning interventions, be sure to adopt a holistic approach and consider all of the patient's needs.

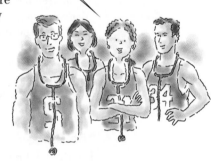

Overall assessment and scores for each category of pressure ulcer risk guide the team to develop appropriate interventions.

Managing pressure

Managing the intensity and duration of pressure is a fundamental goal in prevention, especially for the patient with mobility limitations. Frequent, careful repositioning helps the patient avoid the damaging repetitive pressure that can cause tissue ischemia and subsequent necrosis. When repositioning the patient, it's important to reduce the duration and the intensity of pressure.

Positioning

Any time that you reposition the patient, look for telltale areas of reddened skin and make sure the new position doesn't place weight on these areas. Avoid the use of donut-shaped supports or ring cushions that encircle the ischemic area because these can reduce blood flow to an even wider expanse of tissue. If the affected area is on an extremity, use pillows to support the limb and reduce pressure. As noted earlier, avoid raising the head of the bed more than 30 degrees to prevent tissue damage due to friction and shearing force.

Short stepping it

Inactivity increases a patient's risk of ulcer development. To the degree that the patient is physically able, encourage activity.

Start with a short step—help him out of bed and into a chair. As his tolerance improves, help him walk around the room and then down the hall.

Positioning a patient in bed

When the patient is on his side, never allow weight to rest directly on the greater trochanter of the femur. Instead, have the patient rest his weight on his buttock and use a pillow or foam wedge to maintain the position. This position ensures that no pressure is placed on the trochanter or sacrum. Also, a pillow placed between the knees or ankles minimizes the pressure exerted when one limb lies atop the other. (See *Repositioning a reclining patient.*)

Heel appeal

Heels present a particularly difficult challenge. Even with the aid of specially designed cushions, reducing the pressure on heels to below capillary refill pressure is almost impossible. Instead, suspend the patient's foot so the bony prominence

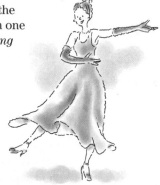

Ballroom dancing is great but not the right activity to start your patient on! Try something a little more elementary.

Repositioning a reclining patient

When repositioning a reclining patient, use the Rule of 30—that is, raise the head of the bed 30 degrees (as shown top right). Avoid raising the head of the bed more than 30 degrees to prevent the buildup of shearing pressure. When you must raise it more—at mealtimes, for instance—keep the periods brief.

As you reposition the patient from his left side to his right side, make sure his weight rests on his buttock, not his hip bone. Resting weight on his buttock reduces pressure on the trochanter and sacrum. The angle between the bed and an imaginary lateral line through his hips should be about 30 degrees. If needed, use pillows or a foam wedge to help the patient maintain the proper position (see illustration bottom right). Cushion pressure points, such as the knees and shoulders, with pillows as well.

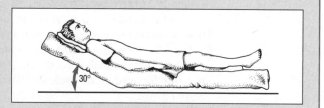

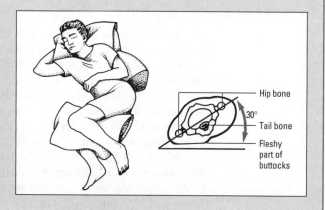

on the heel is under no pressure. A pillow or foam cushion under the patient's calves can permit a comfortable position while suspending the foot. Take care to avoid knee contraction, however. Use a heel pressure redistribution device if your facility has this product.

Positioning a seated patient

Unlikely as it seems, a patient is more likely to develop pressure ulcers from sitting than from reclining. Sitting tends to focus all of the patient's weight on the relatively small surface areas of the buttocks, thighs, and soles. Much of this weight is focused on the small area of tissue covering the ischial tuberosities. Proper posture and alignment help ensure that the weight of the patient's body is distributed as evenly as possible.

Posture perfect

Proper posture alone can significantly reduce the patient's risk of ulcers at the ankles, elbows, forearms, wrists, and knees. Explain proper posture to your patient, if necessary, as described here:
• Sit with back erect and against the back of the chair, thighs parallel to the floor, knees comfortably parted, and arms horizontal and supported by the arms of the chair. This posture distributes weight evenly over the available body surface area.
• Keep feet flat on the floor to protect the heels from focused pressure and distribute the weight of the legs over the largest available surface area—the soles.
• Avoid slouching, which causes shearing force and friction and places undue pressure on the sacrum and coccyx.
• Keep the thighs and arms parallel to ensure that weight is evenly distributed all along the thighs and forearms, instead of being focused on the ischial tuberosities and elbows, respectively.
• Part the knees to keep knees and ankles from rubbing together.

The comforts of home

If the patient likes to use an ottoman or footstool, check to see if his knees end up above the level of his hips. If so, it means that his weight has shifted from the back of his thighs to the ischial tuberosities—and that he needs to find a different footstool. The same problem—knees above hips—can occur if the chair itself is too short for the patient.

Patients at risk should reposition themselves every 15 minutes while sitting, if they can. Patients with spinal cord injuries can perform wheelchair pushups to intermittently relieve pressure on the buttocks and sacrum. This requires a fair amount of upper body strength, however, and some patients might not have the strength. Others may have injuries that preclude using this technique.

Pillows may be the most enduring support tools on the planet, but they're no longer the only options available. Today, people can choose from a vast array of support surfaces and cushioning aids. Special beds, mattresses, and seating options that employ foams, gels, water, and air as cushioning agents make it possible to tailor a comprehensive and personal system of supports for your patient.

Effective care depends on knowledge of the classes and types of products. In the course of your work, take time to learn as much as you can about these products. (See *Pressure redistribution devices*.)

False security

Be informed, but be cautious as well. Using these devices can instill a false sense of security. It's important to remember that as helpful as these devices may be, they aren't substitutes for attentive care. Patients require individual turning schedules, regardless of the equipment used, and this schedule depends on your assessment of the patient's tolerance for pressure.

Beds and mattresses

When we discuss horizontal support surfaces, we are, for the most part, talking about beds, mattresses, and mattress overlays. These products employ foams, gels, water, and air to minimize the pressure a patient experiences while lying in bed.

Pressure redistribution devices

Here are some special pads, mattresses, and beds that help redistribute pressure when a patient is confined to one position for long periods:

• Gel pads disperse pressure over a wide surface area.

• Water mattress or pads produce a wave effect that provides even distribution of body weight.

• Alternating-pressure air mattress involves alternating deflation and inflation of mattress tubes that changes areas of pressure.

• Foam mattress or pads, which must be a high-density foam, at least 3″ to 4″ (7.5 to 10 cm) thick, cushion skin, minimizing pressure. Solid foam is more effective than convoluted foam.

• Low-air-loss bed has a surface that consists of inflated air cushions. Each section is adjusted for optimal pressure relief for the patient's body size.

• Air-fluidized bed contains beads that move under an airflow to support the patient, thus reducing shearing force and friction and assist in redistributing pressure.

• Mechanical lifting device, including lift sheets and other devices, prevents shearing by lifting the patient rather than dragging him across the bed.

• Padding, including pillows, towels, and soft blankets, can reduce pressure in body hollows.

• Foot cradle lifts the bed linens to remove pressure over the feet.

Beds

There are specialty beds and mattresses that have low shear surfaces, may provide some air circulation, and have pressure redistribution properties. Beds that have the "turn assist" feature are to *assist* you with your turning. These beds *do not* turn the patient enough to provide pressure redistribution. There are other beds that do 30- to 60-degree turns and these beds are for pulmonary patients, *not* for pressure.

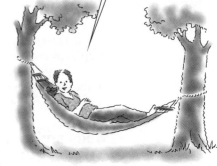

This is probably not the best for your patient in terms of support surfaces. Works fine for a quick nap for me though!

Palm reading

If the patient's weight completely compresses a mattress overlay, the overlay isn't helping. To make sure the patient isn't bottoming out, hand check whenever a new overlay is put into service or if you suspect an overlay is breaking down. To hand check an overlay, slide one hand—palm up and fingers outstretched—between the mattress overlay and the mattress. If you can feel the patient's body through the overlay, replace the overlay with a thicker one or add more air to the mattress.

Support aids for sitting

Products designed to help prevent pressure ulcers while sitting fall into two broad categories: products that pressure and products that ease repositioning.

Ambulatory and wheelchair-dependent patients should use seat cushions to distribute weight over the largest possible surface area. Wheelchair-dependent patients require an especially rugged seat cushion that can stand up to the rigors of daily use. In most instances, a good foam cushion 3″ to 4″ (7.5 to 10 cm) thick suffices. However, many wheelchair-seating clinics now use computers to create custom seating systems tailored to fit the physiology and needs of each patient. For patients with spinal cord injuries, the selection of wheelchair seating is based on pressure evaluation, lifestyle, postural stability, continence, and cost. Custom seats and cushions are more expensive; however, in this case, the added expense is justifiable. Encourage wheelchair patients to replace seat cushions as soon as their current one begins to deteriorate.

A position on repositioning

Repositioning is just as important when the patient is sitting as when he's reclining. For a patient requiring assistance, various devices are available. Such devices as overhead frames, trapezes, walkers, and canes can help the patient reposition himself as necessary. Health care personnel can help maneuver I.V. poles and other support equipment.

Managing skin integrity

An effective skin integrity management plan includes regular inspections for tissue breakdown, routine cleaning and moisturizing, and steps to protect the skin from incontinence, if this is an issue.

Inspecting the skin

The patient's skin should be routinely inspected for pressure areas, depending on the patient's assessed risk and his ability to tolerate pressure. Check for pallor and areas of redness—both signs of ischemia. Be aware that redness that occurs after the pressure is removed (called *reactive hyperemia*) is commonly the first external sign of ischemia due to pressure.

Cleaning the skin

Usually, cleaning with a gentle soap and warm water suffices for daily skin hygiene. Use a soft cloth to pat, rather than rub, the skin dry. Avoid scrubbing or the use of harsh cleaning agents.

Moisturizing the skin

Skin becomes dry, flaky, and less pliable when it loses moisture. Dry skin is more susceptible to ulceration. Avoid powder, especially in an elderly patient, because it can cause further drying of the skin. The number of skin moisturizing products available is truly staggering, so it shouldn't be hard to find one that the patient likes. The three categories of skin moisturizers are lotions, creams, and ointments.

Lotion notion

Lotions are dissolved powder crystals held in suspension by surfactants. Lotions have the highest water content and evaporate faster than any other type of moisturizer. Consequently, lotions must be applied more often. The high water content is why lotions feel cool as they're applied.

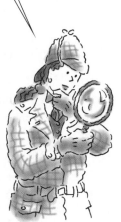

Effective management of skin integrity requires regular inspections as well as routine cleaning and moisturizing and protecting the skin from incontinence. It's elementary!

Cream regime

Creams are preparations of oil and water or water in oil. Water-in-oil creams are more moisturizing as they provide an oily barrier that reduces water loss from the stratum corneum, the outermost layer of the skin. Creams don't have to be applied as often as lotions; three or four applications per day should do the trick.

Ointment appointment

Ointments are preparations of oil in water (typically lanolin or petrolatum) and consequently are the best for skin protection against moisture. They're occlusive and effective as a skin protectant.

Protecting the skin

Although some moisture is good, too much is a problem. Waterlogged skin is easily eroded by friction and is more susceptible to irritants and bacteria colonization than dry skin. Close monitoring helps head off problems before they escalate.

Skin protection is particularly important if the patient is incontinent. Urine and feces introduce chemical irritants and bacteria as well as moisture, which can speed skin breakdown. To effectively manage incontinence, first determine the cause and then plan interventions that protect skin integrity while addressing the underlying problem.

In older adults, don't assume that incontinence is a normal part of aging. It isn't. Instead, consider factors that can precipitate incontinence, such as:
- fecal impaction and tube feeding (can cause diarrhea)
- reaction to a medication (can cause urinary incontinence)
- urinary tract infection
- mobility problems (can keep the patient from reaching the bathroom in time)
- confusion or embarrassment (can keep the patient from asking for a bedpan or help getting to the bathroom).

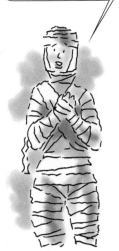

I wouldn't advise this method for protecting the skin. For your patient, determine the cause and plan interventions that protect skin integrity.

Lend a helping hand

Whether the underlying cause is reversible or not, encourage the patient to ask for help when he needs a bedpan or needs to go to the bathroom. Use incontinence collectors, adult briefs or underpads that wick and gel, and skin barriers, as appropriate, to minimize skin damage. Step up the frequency of inspections, cleaning, and moisturizing for these patients.

Assessing for pressure ulcers

Pressure ulcers can occur even with the best preventive measures. Effective treatment depends on a thorough assessment of the developing wound. Meaningful ulcer assessment requires a systematic, objective approach. In addition to the wound assessment parameters described in the beginning of the chapter, also document the ulcer history, including etiology, duration, and prior treatment.

On the border

Ulcer borders can provide clues to healing potential. Just as we discussed earlier, assess skin around the ulcer for:
- redness
- warmth
- induration or hardness
- swelling
- signs of infection.

Before you examine the ulcer, assess the patient's pain. In most cases, pressure ulcers cause some degree of pain; in some cases, pain is severe. Have the patient rate their pain on a verbal or visual analog scale of 0 to 10, with 0 representing no pain and 10 representing severe pain. Similarly, ask the patient whether the pain interferes with their ability to function normally and, if so, to what degree.

Location

Common locations for pressure ulcers include:
- sacrum
- coccyx
- ischial tuberosities
- greater trochanters
- elbows
- heels
- scapulae
- occipital bone
- sternum
- ribs
- iliac crests
- patellae
- lateral malleoli
- medial malleoli.

Bottoming out

Ulcers are more common on the lower half of the body because it has more major bony prominences and more body weight than the upper half of the body. Two thirds of pressure ulcers occur within the pelvic girdle.

Characteristics

Tissue involvement ranges from blanchable erythema to the deep destruction of tissue associated with a full-thickness wound. Pressure against tissue interrupts blood flow and causes pallor due to tissue ischemia. If prolonged, ischemia causes irreversible and extensive tissue damage.

Reactive hyperemia

Usually, reactive hyperemia is the first visible sign of ischemia. When the pressure causing ischemia is released, skin flushes red as blood rushes back into the tissue. This reddening is called *reactive hyperemia*, and it's due to a protective mechanism in the body that dilates vessels in the affected area to increase the blood flow and speed oxygen to starved tissues. Reactive hyperemia first appears as a bright flush that lasts about one half or three quarters as long as the ischemic period. If the applied pressure is too high for too long, reactive hyperemia fails to meet the demand for blood and tissue damage occurs.

Blanchable erythema

Blanchable erythema (redness) can signal imminent tissue damage. Erythema results from capillary dilation near the skin's surface. In the patient with pressure ulcers, the redness results from the release of ischemia-causing pressure. Blanchable erythema is redness that blanches—turns white—when pressed with a fingertip and then immediately turns red again when pressure is removed. Tissue exhibiting blanchable erythema usually resumes its normal color within 24 hours and suffers no long-term damage. However, the longer it takes for tissue to recover from finger pressure, the higher the patient's risk of developing pressure ulcers.

In dark-skinned patients, erythema is hard to discern. Use bright light and look for taut, shiny patches of skin with a purplish tinge. Also, assess carefully for localized heat, induration, or edema, which can be better indicators of ischemia than erythema.

Nonblanchable erythema

Nonblanchable erythema can be the first sign of tissue destruction. In high-risk patients, nonblanchable tissue can develop in as little as 2 hours. The redness associated with nonblanchable erythema is more intense and doesn't change when compressed with a finger. If recognized and treated early, nonblanchable erythema is reversible.

What you can't see

In many cases, the full extent of ulceration can't be determined by visual inspection because there may be extensive undermining along fascial planes. For example, tunneling can connect ulcers over the sacrum to ulcers over the trochanter of the femur or the ischial tuberosities. These cavities can contain extensive necrotic tissue.

Staging pressure ulcers

The most widely used system for staging pressure ulcers is the classification system developed by the NPUAP. This staging system defines four stages.

Now appearing on stage

Staging reflects the depth and extent of tissue involvement. Restaging isn't needed unless deeper layers of tissue are exposed by treatments such as debridement. Keep in mind that although staging is useful for classifying pressure ulcers, it's only one part of a comprehensive assessment. Ulcer characteristics and the condition of the surrounding skin provide equally important clues to the ulcer's prognosis. (See *Staging pressure ulcers*, pages 482 and 483.)

Mucosal pressure ulcers

Ulcers that occur related to medical devices often form on mucosal tissue (lips, nares, urinary meatal opening, tongue, etc.) cannot be staged with the pressure ulcer staging system. Mucous membranes do not have the same histologic structure as the skin. Classify these ulcers as partial or full thickness.

Reverse staging

When an ulcer develops and the tissue and structures are destroyed, they are not replaced during the healing process. Therefore, a stage IV pressure ulcer does not become a stage III as it becomes more shallow, then a II and then a I. This ulcer is a *healing stage IV or a healed stage IV*, period!

Stay on the ball

Staging pressure ulcers

You can use pressure ulcer characteristics gained from your assessment to stage the pressure ulcer, as described here. Staging reflects the anatomic depth of exposed tissue. Keep in mind that if the wound contains necrotic tissue, you won't be able to determine the stage until you can see the wound base.

Stage I

A stage I pressure ulcer is an area of skin with observable pressure-related changes when compared with an adjacent area or the same region on the other side of the body. This area presents clinically with persistent redness in patients with light skin or persistent red, blue, or purple in patients with darker skin. Indicators include a change in one or more of the following characteristics:

- skin temperature (warmth or coolness)
- tissue consistency (boggy or firm)
- sensation (pain or itching).

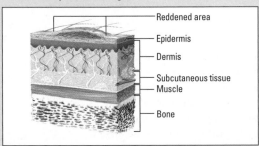

Stage II

A stage II pressure ulcer is a superficial partial-thickness wound that appears as an abrasion, a blister, or a shallow crater involving the epidermis and dermis.

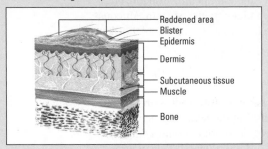

Stage III

A stage III pressure ulcer is a full-thickness wound with tissue damage or necrosis of subcutaneous tissue that can extend down to, but not through, underlying fasciae. The ulcer appears as a deep crater with or without undermining of adjacent tissue.

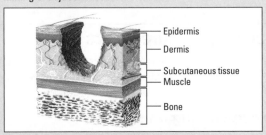

Stage IV

A stage IV pressure ulcer involves full-thickness skin loss with extensive damage, destruction, or necrosis to muscle, bone, and supporting structures (such as tendons and joint capsule). Undermining and sinus tracts may be present as well.

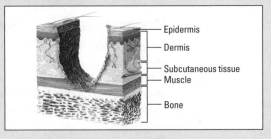

Staging pressure ulcers *(continued)*

Unstageable

This represents a full-thickness tissue loss in which actual depth of the ulcer is completely obscured by slough (yellow, tan, gray, green, or brown) and/or eschar (tan, brown or black) in the wound bed. The true depth cannot be determined until this tissue is removed, but we know it will be either a stage III or IV.

Suspected deep tissue injury—depth unknown

This purple or maroon localized area of discolored intact skin or blood-filled blister occurs due to damage of underlying soft tissue from pressure and/or *shear*. This area may be preceded by tissue that is painful, firm, mushy, boggy, warmer, or cooler as compared to adjacent tissue. Deep tissue injury may be difficult to detect in individuals with dark skin tones.

Treating pressure ulcers

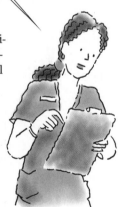

Topical agents can be used to treat some issues of wounds. Usually, cleaning, debriding, and dressings are part of treatment as well.

Treatment of pressure ulcers follows the four basic steps common to all wound care:
• Debride necrotic tissue and clean the wound to remove debris.
• Provide a moist wound-healing environment through the use of proper dressings.
• Protect the wound from further injury.
• Provide nutrition that's essential to wound healing.
    A key element in all pressure ulcer treatment plans is identifying and treating, when possible, the underlying pathophysiology. If the cause of the ulcer remains, existing ulcers don't heal and new ulcers develop.

That's so typical

Typically, wound care involves cleaning the wound, debriding necrotic tissue, and applying a dressing that keeps the wound bed moist. Topical agents are used to resolve various issues.

Patient education

Remember that the goal of patient education is to improve the outcome. For any care plan to succeed after the patient leaves the hospital, the patient or caregiver must understand the care plan, be physically capable of carrying it out at home, and perceive value in the information and the outcomes. Therefore, education and goal establishment should take into consideration the preferences and lifestyles of the patient and his family whenever possible.

Pressure ulcer do's and don'ts

With proper skin care and frequent position changes, patients and their caregivers can keep the patient's skin healthy—a crucial element in pressure ulcer prevention. Here are some important do's and don'ts to pass along to patients:

Do's

• Change position at least once every 2 hours while reclining. Follow a schedule. Lie on your right side, then your left side, then your back, then your stomach (if possible). Use pillows and pads for support. Make small position changes between the 2-hour changes.
• Check your skin for signs of pressure ulcers twice daily. Use a mirror to check areas you can't inspect directly, such as the shoulders, tailbone, hips, elbows, heels, and the back of the head. Report any breaks in the skin or changes in skin temperature to your doctor.
• Follow the prescribed exercise program, including range-of-motion exercises every 8 hours or as recommended.
• Eat a well-balanced diet, drink lots of fluids, and strive to maintain the recommended weight.

Don'ts

• Don't use commercial soaps or skin products that dry or irritate your skin—use oil-free lotions.
• Don't sleep on wrinkled bed sheets or tuck your covers tightly into the foot of your bed.

Teach the patient and his family how to prevent pressure ulcers and what to do when they occur. (See *Pressure ulcer do's and don'ts*.) Explain repositioning, and show them what a 30-degree laterally inclined position looks like. If the patient needs assistance with repositioning, make sure he knows the types of devices available and where to obtain them.

Mirror, mirror . . .

Show the patient how he can inspect his back and other areas using a mirror. If the patient can't do this, a family member can help. Make sure he understands the importance of inspecting skin over bony prominences for pressure-related damage every day.

If the patient needs to apply dressings at home, make sure he knows the proper ways to apply and remove them. Tell him where he can get supplies if he runs low.

Ensuring proper nutrition can be difficult, but the patient and his family need to know how important proper nutrition is to the healing process. Provide materials on nutrition and maintaining an ideal weight, as appropriate. Show them how to create an easy-to-read chart of care reminders for a wall at home.

> Teach the patient how to inspect his back and other areas using a mirror.

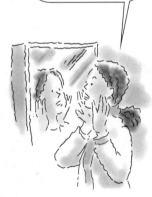

Pressure ulcers should be reassessed weekly. Measure progress by the reduction in necrotic tissue and drainage and the increase in granulation tissue and epithelial growth. Clean, vascularized pressure ulcers should show evidence of healing within 2 weeks. If they don't, and the patient has followed the guidelines for nutrition, repositioning, use of support surfaces, and wound care, it's time to reevaluate the care plan.

References

Association for Advancement in Wound Care. (2012). Pressure Ulcer Guidelines. Retrieved from http://aawconline.org/professional-resources/resources/

Baranoski, S., & Ayello, E. (2011). *Wound care essentials: Practice principles* (3rd ed.). Philadelphia, PA: Lippincott Williams & Wilkins.

Beitz, J. M. (2014). Providing quality skin and wound care for the bariatric patient: An overview of clinical challenges. *Ostomy Wound Management, 60*(1), 12–21.

Bryant, R. A., & Nix, D. P. (2011). *Acute and chronic wounds: Current management concepts* (4th ed.). St. Louis, MO: Mosby.

Doughty, D. (2012). Differential assessment of trunk wounds: Pressure ulceration versus incontinence associated dermatitis versus intertriginous dermatitis. *Ostomy Wound Management, 58*(4), 20–22.

European Pressure Ulcer Advisory Panel. (n.d.). Retrieved from http://www.epuap.org

Hurd, T. (2013). Evaluating the cost and benefits of innovations in chronic wound care products and practices [Supplement]. *Ostomy Wound Management,* 2–15.

Krasner, D. L., Rodeheaver, G. T., & Sibbald, R. G. (Eds.) (2012). *Chronic wound care: A clinical source book for healthcare professionals* (5th ed.). Wayne, PA: HMP Communications.

Langemo, D. K., Anderson, J., Hanson, D., Hunter, S., & Thompson, P. (2008). Measuring wound length, width, and area: Which technique? *Advances in Skin and Wound Care, 21,* 42–45.

LeBlanc, K., Baranoski, S., Christensen, D., Langemo, D., Sammon, M. A., Edwards, K., . . . Regan, M. (2013). International skin tear advisory panel: A tool kit to aid in the prevention, assessment, and treatment of skin tears using a simplified classification system. *Advances in Skin and Wound Care, 26*(10), 459–476.

National Pressure Ulcer Advisory Panel. (n.d.). Retrieved from http://www.npuap.org

National Pressure Ulcer Advisory Panel and European Pressure Ulcer Advisory Panel. (2009). *Prevention and treatment of pressure ulcers: Clinical practice guideline.* Washington, DC: National Pressure Ulcer Advisory Panel.

Sibbald, R. G., Krasner, D. L., & Woo, K. Y. (2011). Pressure ulcer staging revisited: Superficial skin changes & deep pressure ulcer framework. *Advances in Skin and Wound Care, 24*(12), 571–580.

U.S. Department of Health and Human Services. (n.d.). *LHI infographic gallery.* Retrieved from http://www.healthypeople.gov/2020/LHI/inforgraphicGallery.aspx

Wound, Ostomy, Continence Nurses Society. (2010). *Guideline for prevention and management of pressure ulcers.* Mt. Laurel, NJ: Author.

Quick quiz

1. The main functions of the skin include:

A.   support, nourishment, and sensation.

B.   protection, sensory perception, and temperature regulation.

C.   fluid transport, sensory perception, and aging regulation.

D.   support, protection, and communication.

Answer: B. The skin's main functions involve protection from injury, noxious chemicals, and bacterial invasion; sensory perception of touch, temperature, and pain; and regulation of body heat.

2. Which type of wound closes by primary intention?

A.   Second-degree burn

B.   Pressure ulcer

C.   Traumatic injury

D.   Surgical incision

Answer: D. A surgical incision is an example of a wound that closes by primary intention in which there's no deep tissue loss and the wound edges are well approximated.

3. Which wound bed color indicates normal, healthy granulation tissue?

A.   Red

B.   Yellow

C.   Tan

D.   Black

Answer: A. Red tissue indicates healthy granulation tissue.

4. Which intervention is most appropriate for preventing excessive heel pressure?

A.   Flexing the knees

B.   Placing a donut-shaped cushion under the feet

C.   Suspending the heels by placing a pillow under the calves

D.   Putting a pressure-reducing foam mattress under the heels

Answer: C. Suspending the heels using a pillow under the calves is the best way to protect heels from pressure ulceration.

Scoring

☆☆☆   If you answered all four questions correctly, superb! You have a lot of integrity when it comes to knowledge of skin and wounds.

☆☆   If you answered three questions correctly, great! You're holding up well under the pressure.

☆   If you answered fewer than three questions correctly, relax! Just take a load off, review the chapter, and try again.

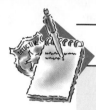

16

Comfort, rest, and sleep

Just the facts

In this chapter, you'll learn:

♦ sleep stages and circadian rhythms

♦ types of sleep disorders and their causes.

A look at comfort, rest, and sleep

Comfort is described as the absence of stress, which promotes rest, relaxation, and sleep. *Sleep* is a natural state of rest during which muscle movements and awareness of surroundings diminish. Sleep restores energy and well-being, enabling us to function optimally.

Sleep is of great importance and is essential to quality of life and well-being. Every patient along the continuum of age from infancy to elderly needs a restful sleep to enhance growth, healing, and general comfort. Not only does a person feel better with enough sleep but also during that time, the body does many important tasks such as processing new information. So, get some sleep nursing student.

Sleep disturbances can also have a direct impact on other family members' sleep patterns. For example, snoring may awaken the patient's spouse or prevent the spouse from falling asleep in the first place.

Primary or secondary

Sleep disorders may be primary or may arise secondary to a medical or psychiatric disorder, substance use, or environmental factors.

Medical conditions that can cause sleep disorders include Parkinson's disease, Huntington's disease, viral encephalitis, brain disease, thyroid disease, and hormonal imbalances.

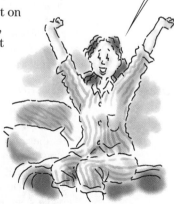

Sleep restores energy and well-being—two pretty important elements in my job!

A psychiatric disorder, such as depression or an anxiety disorder is the most common cause of chronic insomnia. High levels of stress may also contribute to sleep disorders.

Substances that can disrupt sleep include alcohol, caffeine, and prescription medications—most notably, antihistamines, corticosteroids, and central nervous system drugs. When a person uses substances seeming aiding in sleep, the opposite may happen. When someone has a lack of sleep, that person is oftentimes going to feel more stress and unhappiness, leading to a greater stress on relationships and family dynamics.

Sleep stages

Sleep occurs in five stages. With each stage, sleep becomes deeper and brain waves grow progressively larger and slower, as shown on electroencephalogram (EEG).

Stage 1

The lightest stage of sleep, stage 1, occurs as a person falls asleep. The muscles relax and brain waves are fast and irregular. Called *theta waves*, these spike-like waves have a low–medium amplitude and occur three to seven times per second. Stage 1 accounts for approximately 5% of an adult's total sleep time.

Stage 2

During stage 2, a relatively light stage of sleep, theta waves continue but become interspersed with sleep spindles (sudden increases in wave frequency) and K complexes (sudden increases in wave amplitude). Stage 2 makes up about 50% of total sleep time.

Stages 3 and 4

Stages 3 and 4 are the deepest stages of sleep. Delta waves—large, slow waves of high amplitude and low frequency—appear on the EEG. Stage 3 and stage 4 differ only in the percentage of delta waves seen; during stage 3, delta waves account for less than 50% of brain waves, whereas during stage 4, they account for more than 50%.

Conserve as you sleep

Arousing a sleeper from stage 3 or 4 is harder than during any other stage. Because these stages are marked by decreased body temperature and metabolism, researchers believe they function to conserve energy. They account for 10% to 20% of total sleep time.

As night fades into morning, stages 3 and 4 get progressively shorter. During the last few cycles of the sleep period, no delta-wave sleep occurs at all.

Stage 5

Stage 5 is a deep sleep called *rapid eye movement (REM) sleep.* During this stage, the sleeper shows darting eye movements, muscle twitching, and short, rapid brain waves resembling those seen during the waking state. (See *Sleep stages and brain waves.*)

REM sleep usually begins about 90 minutes after sleep onset. Over the course of the night, REM periods lengthen. Overall, REM sleep accounts for 20% to 25% of total sleep time.

Sleep stages and brain waves

Each sleep stage generates distinctive brain waves, as measured by EEG:
• During stage 1, which occurs as a person falls asleep, fast, irregular brain waves called *theta waves* appear on the EEG.
• During stage 2, theta waves are interspersed with wave phenomena called *sleep spindles* and *K complexes*.

• During stages 3 and 4, the EEG shows large, slow, high-amplitude waves, called *delta waves*.
• During stage 5, called *REM sleep*, short, rapid brain waves appear.

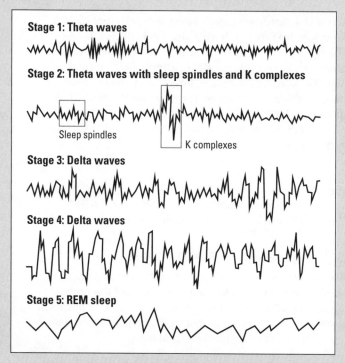

Stage 1: Theta waves

Stage 2: Theta waves with sleep spindles and K complexes
Sleep spindles
K complexes

Stage 3: Delta waves

Stage 4: Delta waves

Stage 5: REM sleep

To sleep, perchance to dream

Most story-like dreams take place during REM sleep. People awakened from REM sleep commonly report vivid dreams. In contrast, people awakened during stages 1 through 4 rarely report vivid dreams. Many people often wonder about the meanings of dreams. Multiple research studies have shown that dreams are a compilation of random thoughts that the brain attempts to interpret as real.

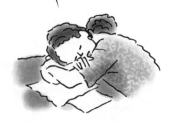

Sshhh! People awakened from REM sleep commonly report vivid dreams, and I'm in the middle of a good one!

Alternating sleep cycles

Throughout the night, REM (stage 5) and non-REM (NREM) (stages 1 through 4) sleep alternate in cycles of about 90 minutes each. Stages 3 and 4 occur during the first one third to first one half of the night. REM sleep increases toward the morning.

Functions of REM and NREM sleep

Scientists believe REM and NREM sleep serve different biological functions, although they don't know exactly what these functions are. REM sleep may stimulate brain growth or consolidate memory.

A person with a disturbed night's sleep is deprived of REM sleep. This patient is known to have a sleep debt. This missing sleep can be recouped usually during the next sleep period. The make-up sleep produces different EEG patterns from normal NREM sleep. If a patient experiences larger sleep debts, these losses cannot be so easily recouped. A person deprived of REM sleep tends to have longer REM cycles during the next sleep episode. These longer REM cycles are more intense, with more eye movements per minute.

Make-up sleep

Similarly, people deprived of NREM sleep have longer NREM sleep during the next sleep period—and the "make-up" NREM sleep produces different EEG patterns from normal NREM sleep.

Neurologic regulation of sleep stages

The various sleep stages are influenced by different parts of the brain. REM sleep is controlled by the pons (a part of the brain stem) and adjacent portions of the midbrain. Chemical stimulation of the pons may induce long periods of REM sleep, whereas damage to the pons may reduce or prevent REM sleep.

Paralysis and the pons

During REM sleep, neurons in the pons and midbrain that control muscle tone show various levels of activity: Some are active whereas others aren't. Reflecting this variable activity, certain body muscles remain inactive during REM sleep—especially those of the back, neck, arms, and legs. As a result, the sleeper is effectively paralyzed so he can't act out their dreams. However, if these regulatory neurons malfunction, the sleeper may be more active during dreams, thrashing about or becoming violent.

Baths and the basal forebrain

The basal forebrain, located in front of the hypothalamus, controls NREM sleep. Damage to this region of the brain may cause difficulty falling asleep or staying asleep. Some neurons in the basal forebrain are activated by heat, which may explain the sleep-promoting benefits of taking a warm bath in the evening.

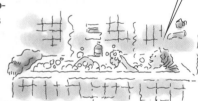

Ahhh. I can just feel the neurons in my basal forebrain getting happy!

Factors that affect sleep

Factors affecting sleep quality and quantity include the patient's age, lifestyle, sleep environment, and medication use.

Age

Amounts and patterns of sleep differ at each major stage of the life cycle. Both REM and NREM sleep periods decrease with age.

Neonates and toddlers

Neonates sleep the most, averaging 17 to 18 hours a day, with REM accounting for roughly one half of total sleep time.

Go to sleep-y, little baby

At first, a neonate sleeps in episodes of 3 to 4 hours. Gradually, by about age 3 or 4 months, he gets more sleep at night. A 6 month old typically sleeps 12 hours at night and naps 1 to 2 hours each day.

Toddlers sleep about 11 or 12 hours a night, with a 1- to 2-hour nap after lunch. Nap requirements vary, with some children taking naps up to age 5.

By age 5, children typically sleep 10 to 12 hours a day, with REM sleep accounting for about 20% of the total.

Tweens and teens

Preadolescents need about 10 hours of sleep. Adolescent requirements aren't well defined. Many teenagers get too little sleep because of their busy schedules and academic pressures.

Young adults

A typical young adult needs about 8 hours of sleep, although the requirement varies widely. Some young adults need as little as 6 or 7 hours, whereas others may need 9 or 10 hours to function optimally. Lifestyle choices make this group vulnerable to sleep disturbances.

Middle-aged adults

In middle-aged adults, sleep requirements may remain unchanged from those of the young adult years. Typical sleep disturbances during middle age may stem from hormonal changes in women, breathing-related disorders, and insomnia.

Elderly adults

Sleep problems are common among elderly adults. Besides taking longer to fall asleep, they spend less time in deep NREM sleep, so their sleep is more easily interrupted or fragmented. (See *Sleep requirements of elderly adults.*)

Bathroom breaks

Early awakening is also common in elderly adults and may result from an earlier rise in body temperature. Lastly, many seniors have trouble falling back to sleep after awakening to urinate. Patients who wake in the night to urinate should be encouraged to use night lights as a guide to prevent falls. The path to the bathroom should also be unencumbered.

Ages and stages

Sleep requirements of elderly adults

It's a common misconception that elderly adults need much less sleep than younger adults. On the contrary, sleep requirements increase in elderly people because they tend to get decreased amounts of deep sleep and suffer frequent sleep interruptions.

Travel, shift work, stress, and anxiety can greatly influence sleep. A person who travels through different time zones may suffer jet lag.

Lifestyle

Travel, shift work, stress, and anxiety can greatly influence sleep. A person who travels through different time zones may suffer jet lag, which is worse when traveling west to east. This person typically tries to sleep when they are not tired (traveling west to east) and tries to stay awake when it's daylight (traveling east to west).

Night-shift blues

In addition, up to 20% of night-shift workers experiences sleep problems resulting from disruption of the body's natural rhythms.

Environment

Sleep environment can greatly affect sleep quality. Environmental influences on sleep include noise, bright lights or sunlight, excessive activity, and an uncomfortable room temperature. When these influences are prominent, sleep can be difficult even for someone who's sleepy. Removing such stimuli produces an environment that's more conducive to sleeping.

Top 5 physical factors to sleepless nights:

 Bodily discomfort

 Noise

 Partner

 Room temperature

 Light levels

Hospital blues

Hospitalized patients commonly have trouble sleeping. First of all, they aren't in their own bed and the noises of everyday hospital routine can be disruptive. If they're in a special care unit, such as intensive and cardiac care, the bells and whistles of equipment can disturb sleep or prevent a patient from getting to sleep. In addition, the stress of hospitalization and the fear of a bad prognosis or new procedures can also disrupt routine sleeping patterns. Lastly, the routines of regular vital signs measurement, doctor visits, and medication regimens can also disrupt sleep.

Medications and substances

Medications of any kind may alter sleep patterns. Prescription drugs may cause somnolence (drowsiness) at inappropriate times; some may cause insomnia. Illicit drugs and other substances may also disturb established sleep patterns.

Alcohol

Alcohol's effect on sleep varies with the amount and time of consumption. In nonalcoholics, alcohol may have a sedative effect, increasing the amount of slow-wave sleep for the first 4 hours after sleep onset. After alcohol's effects wear off, sleep may be disrupted, with an increased amount of REM sleep and anxiety-causing dreams. Alcoholics may have trouble falling asleep and staying asleep. Many have REM sleep disturbances.

Withdrawal woes

During alcohol withdrawal, sleep deprivation is common. When sleep occurs, it's usually fragmented and accompanied by night-mares and anxiety-causing dreams.

No nite-nite

The most important symptoms of sleep disturbances are insomnia at night (the most common symptom) and sleepiness during waking hours. A thorough medical and psychological history should be obtained from a patient who complains of sleep problems. You may also need to question the family because the patient may be unaware of their sleep behavior.

Sometimes, a physical examination is also warranted. Because sleep disorders are commonly linked to mood disorders, psychological tests may be administered as well.

Common sleep disorders

Some of the most common sleep disorders include circadian rhythm disorders, breathing-related sleep disorders, narcolepsy, primary hypersomnia, and primary insomnia.

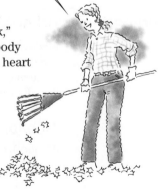

My circadian rhythms can help me adjust to disturbances like seasonal changes. Now if they could only help me enjoy raking these leaves!

Circadian rhythm disorders

Circadian refers to biological rhythms with a cycle of about 24 hours. (*Circadian* comes from the Latin phrase "circa diem," meaning "about a day.") The circadian rhythm functions as the body's internal "clock," regulating the 24-hour sleep-awake cycle and other body functions, such as body temperature, hormones, and heart rate. (See *Tick tock, it's the body clock.*)

The body's internal clock can reset itself to help a person adjust to such disturbances as seasonal changes, transitions to or from daylight savings time, or the start of a new workweek. However, it can't always overcome longer lasting disruptions resulting from shift work or jet lag.

Tick tock, it's the body clock

The human body has an internal "clock" that follows a 24-hour cycle of wakefulness and sleepiness. This clock runs on circadian rhythms, which are linked to nature's cycle of light and darkness.

Critical organs, such as the heart, liver, and kidneys, have their own "clocks" that work in a coordinated fashion with the body's master clock. Researchers know, for example, that certain cardiac events, such as heart attacks and sudden cardiac death, occur more commonly during specific times of the circadian cycle.

Lark versus owl

The body's clock keeps us alert during daylight hours and makes us sleepy when night falls. All of our physiologic functions are geared toward being active during the day and resting at night. The desire to sleep is strongest between 12 and 6 a.m.

Nonetheless, individual patterns of alertness vary, explaining why some people are relatively more alert during the day ("larks") while others are more alert at night ("night owls").

Mighty melatonin

The body's internal clock is regulated by melatonin, a hormone that causes sleepiness. Melatonin is secreted by the pineal gland, a structure located in the roof of the brain's third ventricle. Influenced by light, the pineal gland slows melatonin production during daylight hours to promote alertness and increases production when darkness falls, causing sleepiness.

With age, the body produces less melatonin. Not surprisingly, many elderly adults suffer from sleep disorders.

Breathing-related sleep disorders

Breathing-related sleep disorders are marked by abnormal breathing during sleep. Obstructive sleep apnea syndrome (OSAS) is the most common breathing-related sleep disorder. Other disorders in this category include central sleep apnea syndrome and central alveolar hypoventilation syndrome.

Breathing blockade

In OSAS, the upper airway becomes blocked during sleep, impeding airflow. With sleep apnea, reduced airway muscle tone and the pull of gravity in the supine position further limit airway size during sleep. As tissue collapse worsens, the airway may become completely obstructed.

With partial or complete airway obstruction, the patient struggles to breathe. Blockage of airflow lasts 10 seconds to 1 minute and arouses the patient from sleep as the brain responds to decreased blood oxygen levels. (However, arousal is commonly partial and goes unrecognized by the patient.)

Snoring, then silence

This pattern causes disturbed and fragmented sleep, with periods of loud snoring or gasping when the airway is partly open, alternating with silence when the airway is blocked. (However, not everyone who snores has OSAS.)

With arousal, the muscle tone of the tongue and airway tissues increases, causing the patient to awaken just enough to tighten the upper airway muscles and open the trachea. However, when they fall back to sleep, the tongue and soft tissue relax again—and the cycle begins anew. This cycle may be repeated hundreds of times each night.

Repetitive cycles of snoring, airway collapse, and arousal may lead to cardiovascular problems—high blood pressure, arrhythmias, and even myocardial infarction or stroke. In some high-risk patients, sleep apnea may lead to sudden death from respiratory arrest during sleep.

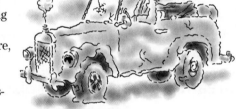

People with severe, untreated sleep apnea have two to three times the risk of motor vehicle accidents. That is, unless the car falls asleep first!

Drowsy, irritable, and indifferent

Frequent awakenings leave the patient sleepy during the day and can cause irritability or depression. The patient may suffer morning headaches, decreased mental functioning, and a reduced sex drive. People with severe, untreated sleep apnea have two to three times the risk of motor vehicle accidents. In addition, sleep apnea can lead to job disturbances as people fall asleep at work.

Narcolepsy

Narcolepsy is characterized by sudden, uncontrollable attacks of deep sleep lasting up to 20 minutes. These "sleep attacks" come on without warning and may be accompanied by paralysis and hallucinations. Although the brief sleep is refreshing, the urge to sleep soon returns.

Sleep paralysis and hallucinations typically occur during sleep onset (hypnagogic hallucinations) or during the transition from sleep to wakefulness (hypnopompic hallucinations). Mostly visual, these hallucinations are intense, dreamlike images commonly involving the immediate environment.

Confounding cataplexy

About 70% of patients with narcolepsy experience attacks of cataplexy—sudden loss of muscle tone and strength. (In more subtle forms of cateplexy, the patient's head may drop or his jaw may slacken.)

Cataplexy is commonly triggered by emotions—for example, the knees may buckle after the patient laughs, gets angry, or feels elated or surprised. Cataplexy typically lasts just a few seconds, and the patient remains alert during the episode. However, in severe cases, the patient falls down and becomes completely paralyzed for up to several minutes.

Narcoleptic sleep attacks may occur at any time of day. All too commonly, they occur during activities that call for undivided attention, such as driving.

Image problems

Besides causing accidents, narcolepsy can be disabling, impairing work performance and disrupting leisure activities and interpersonal relationships. Coworkers may perceive the patient as lazy; an employer may suspect him of illegal drug use. In one study, 24% of narcoleptic patients had to quit working and 18% had been fired because of the disease.

In children, narcolepsy impairs school performance and social relationships and invites ridicule from peers. Teenagers with the disorder are at increased risk for automobile accidents.

Primary hypersomnia

Primary hypersomnia is a condition of excessive sleepiness characterized by prolonged sleep periods at night or daytime sleep episodes occurring nearly every day. During long periods of drowsiness, the patient may exhibit automatic behavior, acting in a semi-controlled fashion. He may have trouble meeting morning obligations, commonly arriving late.

Symptomatic categories

Primary hypersomnia can be monosymptomatic or polysymptomatic:
• In the *monosymptomatic* form, the patient has isolated excessive daytime sleepiness unrelated to abnormal nocturnal awakenings.
• The *polysymptomatic* form involves abnormally long nighttime sleep and signs of sleep "drunkenness" (difficulty awakening completely, confusion, disorientation, poor motor coordination, and slowness) on awakening. Usually, the patient falls asleep easily at night and can stay asleep but seems out of sorts or even combative on awakening in the morning.

Primary insomnia

Many people believe that insomnia is a difficulty falling asleep. It is not limited to this disorder. Insomnia can also be defined as difficulty in remaining asleep for a sufficient period of time. Insomnia can be precipitated by stress, worry, environment, or any number of factors. (See *Factors contributing to insomnia*.)

Obsessing over insomnia

Insomnia can be acute or chronic. With chronic insomnia, the person may become preoccupied with getting enough sleep. The more he tries to sleep, the greater his sense of frustration and distress—and the more elusive sleep becomes.

Insomnia commonly leads to daytime drowsiness that causes poor concentration, memory impairments, difficulty coping with minor problems, and reduced ability to enjoy family and social relationships.

You don't snooze, you lose

Insomniacs are more than twice as likely as the general population to have a fatigue-related motor vehicle accident. Those who sleep fewer than 5 hours per night may have a higher death rate, too.

> **Factors contributing to insomnia**
>
> • reduced physical activity
> • chronic conditions
> • medications
> • neurologic diseases such as Alzheimer's
> • stress and lifestyle changes

Treatments for sleep disturbances

Various therapies can be used to treat sleep disorders, depending on the source of the disorder.

Asking the patient key questions in the assessment of this disorder may aid in treatment choices and possible referrals. (See *Key questions to ask about insomnia*.)

Breathing-related disorders

Treatments for breathing-related disorders such as OSAS include lifestyle changes, continuous positive airway pressure (CPAP), and dental devices.

Lifestyle changes

Lifestyle changes—especially weight loss—are used to treat OSAS. Weight loss reduces the amount of excess tissue in and around the airway. Decreasing the body mass index to 30 or less significantly reduces the frequency of obstructive sleep episodes. However, even small weight reductions can improve the patient's condition.

Key questions to ask about insomnia

When a patient complains of insomnia, ask the following questions:
• When did the problem begin?
• Do you have a medical or psychiatric illness that might affect your ability to sleep?
• What's your sleep environment like? Is it dark? Quiet? Bright? Noisy? Does it have a comfortable room temperature?
• What time do you usually go to bed?
• What time do you usually get up in the morning on weekdays? On weekends?

• Do you drink alcohol or smoke? Are you taking prescribed medications? Nonprescription preparations? Street drugs?
• What's your typical work schedule?
• How do you feel the day after a poor night's sleep?

Family inquiries

If possible, ask the patient's spouse or other family members if the patient snores or has unusual limb movements when he sleeps.

Supine isn't sublime

Sleeping on the side rather than in a supine (back-lying) position may reduce apneic episodes. Avoiding alcohol and sleeping pills can decrease the number and duration of these episodes.

Continuous positive airway pressure

CPAP therapy during sleep is the most common and effective treatment for OSAS. Positive pressure splints the airway open, preventing its collapse. The desired level of pressure varies with the type of CPAP device used. The patient wears either a full facial mask or a nasal mask.

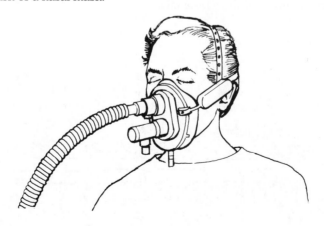

Dental devices

Oral appliances worn during sleep may help to relieve airway obstruction. However, they may be uncomfortable for some patients and may cause excessive salivation.

Insomnia

Treatments for insomnia include relaxation, sleep hygiene, behavioral interventions, cognitive therapy, alternative and complementary therapies, and medications.

Relaxation techniques

Because many insomniacs display high levels of physiologic and cognitive arousal (both at night and during the day), relaxation-based interventions may provide relief. Techniques that help deactivate the arousal system include progressive muscle relaxation, abdominal or deep breathing, biofeedback, and imagery training.

Sleep hygiene

For some patients, insomnia responds well to simple lifestyle changes, sometimes called *sleep hygiene*. Such changes include going to bed at the same time every night, optimizing sleeping conditions, and avoiding naps during the day. (See *Getting hygienic about sleep.*)

Behavioral interventions

Behavioral interventions aim to change maladaptive sleep habits, reduce autonomic arousal, and alter dysfunctional beliefs and attitudes. A wide range of behavioral techniques may be used to treat chronic primary insomnia.

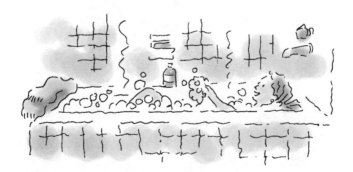

Getting hygienic about sleep

For most patients with insomnia, simple lifestyle measures—termed *sleep hygiene*—are used first. When teaching your patient about sleep hygiene, cover the following do's and don'ts.

Sleep-promoting measures
• Use the bed only for sleep and sex—not for reading, watching television, or working.
• Establish a regular bedtime and a regular time for getting up in the morning. Stick to these times even on weekends and on vacations.
• Exercise in the evening. Energy levels bottom out a few hours after exercise, promoting sleep at that time.
• Take a hot bath 90 minutes to 2 hours before bedtime to alter core body temperature and help you fall asleep more easily.
• During the 30 minutes before bedtime, do something relaxing, such as reading, meditating, or taking a leisurely walk.
• Keep the bedroom quiet, dark, relatively cool, and well ventilated.
• Eat dinner 4 to 5 hours before bedtime. At bedtime, a light snack (low

in sugar and calories) may promote sleep.
• Spend 30 minutes in the sun each day. (However, be sure to take precautions against overexposure.)
• If you don't fall asleep after 15 or 20 minutes, get up and go into another room. Read or perform a quiet activity, using dim lighting, until you feel sleepy.
• If your bed partner distracts you, consider moving to another bedroom or the sofa for a few nights. (One study showed that sleeping alone is more restful than sleeping with another person.)

What not to do
• Don't use the bedroom for work, reading, or watching television.
• Avoid large meals before bedtime.
• Don't look at the clock. Obsessing over time makes it harder to sleep.

• Avoid naps, especially in the evening.
• Don't drink a large amount of fluid after dinner or the need to urinate may disturb your sleep.
• Avoid exercising close to bedtime because this may make you more alert.
• Avoid alcohol and caffeine in the evening.
• Don't take a bath just before bedtime because this could increase your alertness.
• Don't engage in highly stimulating activities before bed, such as watching a frightening movie or playing competitive computer games.
• Quit smoking because nicotine's effects may contribute to sleep loss.
• Avoid tossing and turning in bed. Instead, get up and read or listen to relaxing music. However, don't watch television because it emits too bright a light.

Stimulus control
Stimulus control centers on the theory that insomnia represents a learned response to bedtime and bedroom cues.

Biofeedback
In biofeedback, the patient is connected to a device that measures brain waves and other body functions. Then they have given feedback so that they can learn to recognize certain states of tension or sleep stages—and either avoid or repeat these states voluntarily.

Sleep restriction
Sleep restriction creates a mild state of sleep deprivation, which may promote more rapid sleep onset and more "efficient" sleep. The patient limits the amount of time spent in bed in order to increase the percentage of time spent asleep.

Bedtime amendments

To maintain a consistent sleep-awake pattern, the patient usually alters his bedtime rather than his rising time. However, time in bed shouldn't be reduced to fewer than 5 hours per day. Naps aren't allowed (except in elderly adults).

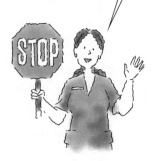

Unless the patient is elderly, sleep restriction means just say "No!" to naps!

Cognitive therapy

Cognitive therapy helps the patient identify his dysfunctional beliefs and attitudes about sleep (such as "I'll never fall asleep") and replace them with positive ones. Changing beliefs and attitudes can decrease the anticipatory anxiety that interferes with sleep. Cognitive therapy also focuses on actions intended to change behavior.

Alternative and complementary therapies

Alternative and complementary therapies that may be used to treat insomnia include acupressure, acupuncture, aromatherapy, massage, biofeedback, chiropractic, homeopathy, light and dark therapy, meditation, reflexology, visualization, and yoga.

A mouthful of electromagnetic waves

Another technique, low-energy emission therapy, delivers electromagnetic waves through a mouthpiece and may benefit some patients.

Supplements to sleep by

Some patients use herbal preparations (such as St. John's wort and chamomile), nutritional substances, and other nonprescription preparations to treat insomnia. However, few of such products have been demonstrated to be safe and effective.

Dietary supplements sometimes recommended for insomnia relief include vitamins B_6, B_{12}, and D. Some practitioners also recommend calcium and magnesium. Tryptophan may relieve insomnia in some patients, but the patient must be monitored for adverse effects. Melatonin may increase sleepiness and is currently undergoing clinical studies.

Pharmacologic options

If insomnia persists despite other measures, the doctor may recommend drug therapy. The most commonly prescribed drugs are short-acting sedative-hypnotics (primarily benzodiazepines), antidepressants, and antihistamines. (See *Pharmacologic therapy for sleep disorders*.)

Pharmacologic therapy for sleep disorders

This chart highlights several drugs used to treat sleep disorders. A patient with insomnia may receive a benzodiazepine, such as temazepam or triazolam; a nonbenzodiazepine such as eszopiclone; or a nonbenzodiazepine hypnotic such as zolpidem.

Drug	Adverse effects	Contraindications	Nursing interventions
Temazepam *(Restoril)*	• Dizziness • Drowsiness • Lethargy • Orthostatic hypotension	• Pregnancy	• Teach the patient about the drug's action, dosage, and adverse effects. • Instruct the patient not to take other medications unless the doctor approves. • Caution the patient not to drink alcohol, drive a motor vehicle, or operate machinery while under the influence of this drug. • Advise the patient to change position slowly to avoid dizziness. • Inform the patient that prolonged use isn't recommended.
Triazolam *(Halcion)*	• Dizziness • Drowsiness • Headache • Orthostatic hypotension • Rebound insomnia	• Concomitant ketoconazole (Nizoral) or itraconazole (Sporanox) therapy • Pregnancy	• Teach the patient about the drug's action, dosage, and adverse effects. • Tell the patient that rebound insomnia may occur after stopping this drug. • Teach safety measures to prevent injury. • Advise the patient to change positions slowly to avoid dizziness. • Inform the patient of the potential for physical and psychological dependence.
Zolpidem *(Ambien)*	• Abdominal pain • Daytime drowsiness • Dizziness • GI disturbances • Headache • Nightmares	• Breast-feeding • Hepatic impairment • Pregnancy	• Teach the patient about the drug's action, dosage, and adverse effects. • Advise them not to take the drug with or immediately after a meal. • Caution the patient against taking other medications unless the doctor approves. • Advise the patient not to drink alcohol, drive a motor vehicle, or operate machinery while under the influence of this drug. • Inform the patient that tolerance may occur if this drug is taken for more than a few weeks.
Eszopiclone *(Lunesta)*	• Dizziness • Drowsiness • Light-headedness • Difficulty with coordination • Unpleasant taste	• Pregnancy • Breast-feeding	• Teach the patient about the drug's action, dosage, and adverse effects. • Advise the patient not to drink alcohol, drive a motor vehicle, or operate machinery while under the influence of this drug. • Advise the patient to take the medication immediately before going to bed because it works very quickly.

Knockout pills

Sedative-hypnotics—usually temazepam (Restoril) and zolpidem (Ambien)—are commonly prescribed for short-term management of insomnia.

Prescription and nonprescription antihistamines can be used for short-term management of insomnia. Adverse effects include daytime sedation, cognitive impairment, and anticholinergic effects (e.g., dry mouth, constipation, and urine retention). Tolerance may also occur.

Antidepressants may be given in low dosages—especially if the patient has a related psychiatric disorder or a history of substance abuse. However, some antidepressants can exacerbate other disorders, such as mania and restless leg syndrome, so the patient should be monitored closely.

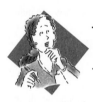

Quick quiz

1. Which condition is characteristic of REM sleep?
   A. Light sleep
   B. Paralysis of the muscles
   C. Restricted eye movements
   D. Nonvivid dreams

Answer: B. During REM sleep, many muscles are effectively paralyzed so the sleeper won't act out dreams. Eye movements are rapid.

2. Which part of the brain regulates NREM sleep?
   A. Pons
   B. Hypothalamus
   C. Basal forebrain
   D. Amygdala

Answer: C. The basal forebrain controls NREM sleep. The pons and midbrain control REM sleep.

3. What are questions to ask when taking a sleep history? (Select all that apply.)
   A. How many hours of sleep do you normally get per night?
   B. What size bed do you sleep on?
   C. What types of medications do you take before bed?
   D. What is your bedtime routine?
   E. What type of work do you do?

Answer: A, C, D, & E. Key questions about sleep patterns, sleep cycles, and outside influences may be helpful to determine the type of treatment or referral needed. The type of bed is not a key assessment question.

4. A patient may be assessed for a narcolepsy sleep disorder if the deep sleep attacks occur for which of the following time periods?

    A.   A period of up to 5 minutes.

    B.   A period of up to 10 minutes.

    C.   A period of up to 60 minutes.

    D.   A period of up to 20 minutes.

Answer: D. Narcolepsy is a sleep disorder in which the person has a sudden deep sleep episode lasting up to 20 minutes.

Scoring

☆☆☆ If you answered all four questions correctly, way to go! You're no slouch when it comes to sleeping.

   ☆☆ If you answered three questions correctly, good job! You're waking up to good sleep habits.

     ☆ If you answered fewer than three questions correctly, don't lose sleep over it! Take a nap, review the chapter, and try again.

Pain management

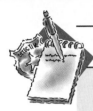

Just the facts

In this chapter, you'll learn:

♦ types of pain and theories that explain them

♦ effective ways to document pain assessment findings

♦ history and examination techniques for the patient with pain

♦ psychological characteristics of pain

♦ specific uses of pain medications

♦ physical therapies used in pain management

♦ roles of alternative and complementary therapies in relieving pain.

A look at pain

Pain is a perception that is complex in nature and helps to alert the body that a potential or real tissue damage is occurring. To put it succinctly, pain is whatever the patient says it is and it occurs whenever the patient says it does. When developing a plan for pain management with the patient, it is important that the nurse not only assess the physical manifestations of pain but also the subjective reports of pain as well.

Each patient reacts to pain differently because pain thresholds and tolerances vary from person to person. *Pain threshold* is a physiologic attribute that denotes the intensity of the stimulus needed to sense pain. *Pain tolerance* is a physiologic attribute that describes the amount of stimulus (duration and intensity) that the patient can endure before stating that they are in pain.

Reactions to pain vary from person to person and even within the same person at different times.

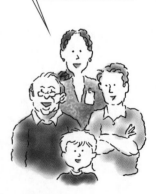

Beliefs about pain

Patients' attitudes, beliefs, expectations of themselves, coping resources, and beliefs about the health care system affect the entire spectrum of their pain behaviors.

Behavior and emotions are influenced by the interpretation as well as the facts of an event. This partly explains why patients may differ greatly in their beliefs about pain. Beliefs about pain are very individual. Each patient has different painful experience and therefore has different expectations about pain and painful experiences. Each individual copes with pain differently throughout life. Coping with pain is specific to each patient within each event of pain.

Coping

Patients' beliefs, judgments, and expectations about an event's consequences—and belief in their ability to influence the outcome—can affect their ability to function. That's because such beliefs, judgments, and expectations can influence mood directly and alter coping ability.

Patients with low back pain offer a good example. Many fail to comply with prescribed exercises. Their previous pain experience may foster a negative view of their abilities and an expectation of increased pain during exercise. These beliefs form a rationale for avoiding exercise.

Can you cope with these concepts?

Coping can be overt or covert; active or passive. *Overt* coping strategies include rest, drug therapy, and use of relaxation techniques. *Covert* coping strategies include distraction, reassuring oneself that the pain will diminish, seeking information, and solving problems.

Active coping strategies—efforts to function despite pain or to distract oneself from pain—lead to adaptive functioning. *Passive* coping strategies—restricting one's activities and depending on others for help in pain control—lead to greater pain and depression. (See *Encouraging active pain-coping strategies*, page 508.)

Attention

Pain can change the way the patient processes pain-related and other information by focusing attention on bodily signals. As these signals change, they may assume these changes mean that the underlying disease is getting worse and, as a result, may report increased pain.

In contrast, a patient who doesn't attribute symptoms to worsening disease tends to report less pain, even if their disease actually is progressing.

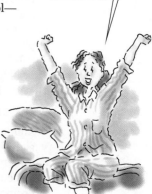

Rest and relaxation techniques can help patients cope with their pain.

Encouraging active pain-coping strategies

The patient's strategy for coping with pain may be active or passive. *Active* strategies include attempts to function despite pain. *Passive* strategies include relying on others for help in pain control.

If possible, steer the patient toward active coping strategies. A patient who uses active coping strategies tends to experience less pain and increased pain tolerance than one who uses passive strategies.

One strategy doesn't fit all

Even so, keep in mind that one particular active coping strategy isn't necessarily better than another. What's more, a given strategy may be helpful in one situation or for one patient but not helpful in a different situation or for another patient.

Likewise, certain strategies may help at one time but prove ineffective in other situations.

Out-of-control thoughts

The most important feature of poor coping seems to be "catastrophizing"—thinking extremely negative thoughts about one's plight rather than choosing poorly among active coping strategies.

If the patient falls into this trap, teach them that imagining more positive outcomes may help reduce his pain.

Too little feedback

Beliefs and expectations about a disease are hard to change. Patients tend to avoid experiences that might invalidate their beliefs and guide their behavior in keeping with their beliefs. Commonly, health professionals refrain from challenging patients about irrational beliefs and excessively restrictive activities. In doing so, they fail to give patients valuable corrective feedback.

Physical links to pain

Just as physical factors can affect a patient's psychological condition, psychological factors can affect their mood, coping ability, and nociception (sensation of pain).

Cognitive interpretations and affective arousal may influence physiology by increasing autonomic sympathetic nervous system (SNS) arousal and promoting endogenous opioid (endorphin) production.

Autonomic arousal

Thinking about pain and stress can increase muscle tension, especially in already painful areas. Chronic and excessive SNS arousal is a precursor to increased skeletal muscle tone. It may set the stage for hyperactive and persistent muscle contractions, which promote muscle spasms and pain.

Arousing sympathy

Patients who exaggerate the significance of their problems or focus on them too closely may influence sympathetic arousal. This predisposes them to further injury and can complicate recovery in other ways.

How thoughts affect endorphins

Studies show that thoughts can influence the concentration of endorphins available to control pain. Research results indicate that:
• a patient's feelings of self-efficacy predicted their pain tolerance; those with high self-efficacy had greater levels of endorphins (See *Self-efficacy and arthritis pain*.)
• naloxone (Narcan), an opioid antagonist, blocked the pain relieving effects of cognitive coping (which demonstrates how thoughts can directly affect endorphins and that self-efficacy may influence pain perception at least partially through endogenous opioids)
• lower concentrations of endorphins were associated with learned helplessness.

Pain assessment

To ensure that the patient receives effective pain relief, you must conduct a thorough and accurate pain assessment. That's a tall order because pain is so subjective.

Pain is influenced not just by physical pathology but by cultural and social factors, expectations, mood, and perceptions of control. What's more, you and the patient may have dramatically different pain thresholds and tolerances, expectations about pain, and ways of expressing pain. Many times a person's coping mechanism for the pain may be to try to ignore the pain. This patient may report moderate pain when asked but laugh with visitors or appear not in pain. Not all patients cry out or shed tears with pain. Some patients may be quiet and reserved wanting no visitors; others may be coping by trying to focus on something else. Even in the absence of visible injury, you as a nurse are not to question the presence of pain.

The patient knows best

Pain is *always* what the person says it is. You are not the judge or jury. To keep your pain assessment on track, keep in mind the first principle of pain assessment: Pain is whatever the patient says it is, occurring whenever he says it does. The patient's self-report

Self-efficacy and arthritis pain

Research suggests that feelings of self-efficacy can directly affect the physiology of pain. In one study, researchers provided stress management treatments to patients with rheumatoid arthritis. The autoimmune disorder, which may result from impaired suppressor T-cell functioning, causes inflammation of synovial membranes. Among the symptoms are joint pain and stiffness.

A boost to T cells
The study found that patients with increased feelings of self-efficacy had greater levels of suppressor T cells. Self-efficacy levels also related directly to the degree of pain and joint impairment the patients experienced.

of the presence and severity of pain is the most accurate, reliable means of pain assessment. If the patient reports pain, respect what he says and act promptly to assess and control it.

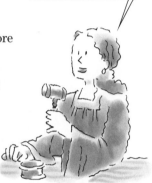

A nurse should never judge a patient's level of pain—pain is always what the person says it is.

Pain threshold and tolerance

Pain threshold refers to the intensity of the stimulus a person needs to sense pain. *Pain tolerance* is the duration and intensity of pain that a person tolerates before openly expressing pain. Tolerance has a strong psychological component. Identifying pain threshold and tolerance are crucial to pain assessment and the development of a pain management plan.

Even so, remember that pain threshold and tolerance vary widely among patients. They may even fluctuate in the same patient as circumstances change.

Differentiating types of pain

Pain falls into three broad categories—acute pain, chronic nonmalignant pain (also called *chronic persistent pain*), and cancer pain.

Acute pain

Acute pain comes on suddenly—for instance, after trauma, surgery, or an acute disease—and lasts from a few days to a few weeks. Typically, it's sharp, intense, and easily localized. It causes a withdrawal reflex and may trigger involuntary bodily reactions, such as sweating, fast heart and respiratory rates, and elevated blood pressure. (See *Acute pain: A sympathetic response.*)

Acute pain: A sympathetic response

In acute pain, certain involuntary (autonomic) reflexes may occur. Acute pain causes the sympathetic branch of the autonomic nervous system (ANS) to trigger the release of epinephrine and other catecholamines. These substances, in turn, cause physiologic reactions such as those seen in the fight-or-flight response.

It'll get your attention
Sympathetic activation directs immediate attention to the injury site. This attention promotes reflexive withdrawal and fosters other actions that prevent further damage and enhance healing. For example, if you place your hand on a hot stove, the ANS immediately generates a reflex withdrawal that jerks your hand away and minimizes tissue damage.

Differentiating acute and chronic pain

Acute pain may cause certain physiologic and behavioral changes that you won't observe in a patient with chronic pain.

Type of pain	Physiologic evidence	Behavioral evidence
Acute	• Increased respirations • Increased pulse • Increased blood pressure • Dilated pupils • Diaphoresis	• Restlessness • Distraction • Worry • Distress
Chronic	• Normal respirations, pulse, blood pressure, and pupil size • No diaphoresis	• Reduced or absent physical activity • Despair, depression • Hopelessness

Acute pain may be constant (as in a burn), intermittent (as in a muscle strain that hurts only with activity), or both (as in an abdominal incision that hurts a little at rest and a lot with movement or coughing). It can also be prolonged or recurrent. (See *Differentiating acute and chronic pain.*)

So long now

Prolonged acute pain can last days to weeks. Usually, it results from tissue injury and inflammation (as from a sprain or surgery) and subsides gradually.

At the injury site, release or synthesis of chemicals heightens sensitivity in nearby tissues. This hypersensitivity, called *hyperalgesia*, is normal. In fact, tenderness and tissue hypersensitivity help protect the injury site and prevent further damage.

Over and over again

Recurrent acute pain refers to brief painful episodes that recur at variable intervals. Examples include sickle cell vaso-occlusive crisis and migraine headache.

In migraine headache and some other recurrent conditions, pain serves no apparent useful purpose—no protective action can be taken and tissue damage can't be prevented. However, in others, such as sickle cell disease, acute pain encourages the person to seek medical treatment.

Chronic nonmalignant pain

Pain is considered chronic when it lasts beyond the normal time expected for an injury to heal or an illness to resolve. Many experts define chronic nonmalignant pain as pain lasting 6 months or longer that may continue during the patient's lifetime. Although it sometimes begins as acute pain, more typically, it starts slowly and builds gradually. Unlike acute pain, chronic pain isn't protective and doesn't warn of significant tissue damage.

Chronic nonmalignant pain is unrelated to cancer. This type of pain affects more people than any other type—roughly 100 million Americans. Causes of chronic pain include nerve damage, such as in brain injury, tumor growth, or unexplained and abnormal responses to tissue injury by the central nervous system (CNS). It can cause serious disability (as in arthritis or avascular necrosis), or it may be related to poorly understood disorders such as fibromyalgia and complex regional pain syndrome. Neuropathic pain is one type of chronic pain. (See *Understanding neuropathic pain.*)

Many experts define chronic nonmalignant pain as pain lasting 6 months or longer that may continue during the patient's lifetime.

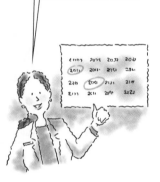

Understanding neuropathic pain

Commonly described as tingling, burning, or shooting, neuropathic pain is a puzzling type of chronic pain generated by the nerves. It commonly has no apparent cause and responds poorly to standard pain treatment.

We don't know the precise mechanism of neuropathic pain. Possibly, the peripheral nervous system has experienced damage that injures sensory neurons, causing continuous depolarization and pain transmission. Alternatively, it could result from repeated noxious stimuli that cause hypersensitivity and excitement in the spinal cord that results in chronic neuropathy in which a normally harmless stimuli causes pain.

The limb is gone, but the pain remains

Phantom pain syndrome is one example of neuropathic pain. This condition occurs when an arm or a leg has been removed but the brain still gets pain messages from the nerves that originally carried the limb's impulses. The nerves seem to misfire, causing pain.

Types of neuropathic pain

Neuropathic pain can involve peripheral or central pain.

Peripheral pain can occur as:
• *polyneuropathy*, which is pain felt along the peripheral nerves, as in diabetic neuropathy

• *mononeuropathy*, which is pain associated with an established injury and felt along the nerve, as in trigeminal neuralgia.

Central neuropathic pain also comes in two varieties:
• *sympathetic pain*, which results from dysfunction of the autonomic nervous system
• *deafferentation pain*, which is marked by elimination of sensory (afferent) impulses, as from damage to the central or peripheral nervous system (as in phantom limb pain).

High cost of chronic pain

Chronic pain may be severe enough to limit a patient's ability and desire to participate in career, family life, and even activities of daily living. If it's severe or intractable, the patient may experience decreased function, pain behaviors, depression, opioid dependence, "doctor shopping," and suicide.

Assessment obstacles

You may find pain assessment especially difficult in a patient with chronic pain. Over time, the autonomic nervous system (ANS) adapts to pain, so the patient may lack typical autonomic responses, such as dilated pupils, increased blood pressure, and fast heart and respiratory rates. Also, their facial expression may not suggest pain. They may sleep periodically and shift their attention away from the pain. Regardless, don't let the lack of outward signs lead you to conclude that they aren't in pain.

Cancer pain

Pain from cancer is more than just pain. You must assess for suffering and quality of life in addition to presence of pain. Cancer pain is a complex problem. It may result from the disease itself or from treatment. About 70% to 90% of patients with advanced cancer experience pain. Although cancer pain can be treated with oral medications, only one third of patients with cancer pain achieve satisfactory relief.

Sometimes, pain results from the pressure of a tumor impinging on organs, bones, nerves, or blood vessels. In other cases, limitations in activities of daily living may lead to muscle aches.

Don't treat me like that!

These cancer treatments may cause pain:
• chemotherapy, radiation, or drugs used to offset the impact of these therapies on blood counts and infection risk (such as mouth sores; peripheral neuropathy; and abdominal, bone, or joint pain from chemotherapy agents)
• surgery
• biopsies
• blood withdrawal
• lumbar punctures.

JCAHO pain management standards

In 2000, the Joint Commission on Accreditation of Healthcare Organizations (JCAHO) issued new standards for pain assessment, management, and documentation. These standards require health care workers to ask patients about pain when they're admitted to a JCAHO-accredited facility. Any patient who reports pain must be assessed further by licensed personnel. Facility policies must identify a standard pain screening tool to be used for all patients able to use it.

If you work in a JCAHO-accredited facility, check policies and procedures for information on which screening tool to use, how often to assess pain, and which pain level warrants further assessment and action. (In many facilities, this level is 4 or higher on a scale of 0 to 10.)

> According to JCAHO, good clinical practice dictates that any patient who reports pain must be assessed further by licensed personnel.

The fifth vital sign

Pain is commonly called the fifth vital sign because pain assessment scores must be monitored and recorded regularly—and at least as vigilantly as you monitor and record vital signs. To meet JCAHO standards, you must record pain assessment data in a way that promotes reassessment.

JCAHO standards also mandate that health care facilities plan and support activities and resources that assure pain recognition and use of appropriate interventions. These activities include:
• initial pain assessment
• regular reassessment of pain
• education of health care workers about pain assessment and management
• development of quality improvement plans that address pain assessment and reassessment.

Pain assessment tools

When a patient is admitted, ask them if they currently are in pain or have ongoing problems with pain. If they have ongoing pain, find out if they have an effective treatment plan. If so, continue with this plan if possible. If they do not have such a plan, use an assessment tool, such as a pain rating scale, to further assess the pain.

Pain rating scales

Pain rating scales quantify pain intensity—one of pain's most subjective aspects. These scales offer several advantages over semistructured and unstructured patient interviews:
• They're easier to administer.
• They take less time.
• They can uncover concerns that warrant a more thorough investigation.
• When used before and after a pain control intervention, they can help determine if the intervention was effective.

All shapes and sizes

Pain rating scales come in many varieties. When choosing an appropriate scale for your patient, consider his visual acuity, age, reading ability, and level of understanding.

Pain intensity rating scale

You can evaluate pain in a nonverbal manner for pediatric patients age 3 and older or for adult patients with language difficulties. One common pain rating scale consists of six faces with expressions ranging from happy and smiling to sad and teary.

Putting a face on pain

To use a pain intensity rating scale, tell the patient that each face represents a person with progressively worse pain. Ask them to choose the face that best represents how they feel. Explain that although the last face has tears, they can choose this face even if they are not crying. (See *Using a pain intensity rating scale.*)

Visual analog scale

The visual analog scale is a horizontal line, 10 cm (3⅞") long, with word descriptors at each end: "no pain" on one end and "pain as bad as it can be" on the other. The scale may also be used vertically.

Drawing the line on pain

Ask the patient to place a mark along the line to indicate the intensity of the pain. Then measure the line in millimeters up to his mark. This measurement represents the patient's pain rating. Be aware that this scale may be too abstract for some patients to use. (See *Visual analog scale.*)

Visual analog scale

To use the visual analog scale, ask the patient to place a line across the scale to indicate their current level of pain. The pain rating is determined by measuring the distance, in millimeters, from "no pain" to their marking.

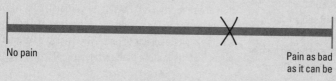

No pain   Pain as bad as it can be

Using a pain intensity rating scale

A pediatric patient or an adult patient with language difficulties may not be able to express the pain they are feeling. In such instances, use the pain intensity scale below. Ask your patient to choose the face that best represents the severity of the pain, on a scale from 0 to 5.

0

1

2

3

4

5

Numerical rating scale

The numerical rating scale is perhaps the most commonly used pain rating scale. Simply ask the patient to rate their pain on a scale from 0 to 10, with 0 representing no pain and 10 representing the worst pain imaginable. Instead of giving a verbal rating, the patient can use a horizontal or vertical line consisting of descriptive words and numbers.

Although most patients find the numerical rating scale quick and easy to use, it may be too abstract for some patients. The numerical rating scale may also be frustrating to the patient who has pain and hurts but pain is not unbearable. Many patients have the belief that in order to request pain medication, they have to be suffering. It is up to the nurse to offer pain medication on a regular basis, regardless of the number. The number should be used to assess pain management and not to judge whether a person needs to be medicated. (See *Using the numerical rating scale.*)

Verbal descriptor scale

With the verbal descriptor scale, the patient chooses a description of their pain from a list of adjectives, such as "none," "annoying," "uncomfortable," "dreadful," "horrible," and "agonizing."

Using the numerical rating scale

A numerical rating scale (NRS) can help the patient quantify their pain. Have them choose a number from 0 (indicating no pain) to 10 (indicating the worst pain imaginable) to reflect their current pain level. The patient can either circle the number on the scale itself or verbally state the number that best describes the pain.

No pain   0   1   2   3   4   5   6   7   8   9   10   Pain as bad as it can be

Not as simple as it sounds

To be on the safe side, don't assume that your patient knows how to use the scale. Provide teaching and then verify that they understand what you've taught. Be sure to document your teaching and your method of evaluating their understanding.

Work toward a comfort goal

Help the patient establish a comfort goal—a numerical pain level that will enable them to perform self-care activities, such as ambulation, coughing, and deep breathing. Usually, a level of 3 or less on a 0-to-10 scale is an adequate comfort level.

If the patient chooses a comfort goal of 4 or higher, teach them that unrelieved pain can damage their health. Discuss concerns they may have about using analgesics and clear up misconceptions such as those related to addiction.

When to evaluate the pain management plan

If the patient rates the pain as 10, he's experiencing severe pain—a sign that the pain management plan is ineffective. Consult with the doctor about increasing the analgesic dose or adding another analgesic.

When to use a vertical scale instead

Like some children, many adults who speak languages that are read from right to left (or vertically) may have trouble with the NRS because it's horizontal. They may find a vertical scale easier to use. When using a vertical scale, place 0 at the bottom of the scale and 10 at the top.

Like the numerical rating scale, the verbal descriptor scale is quick and easy, but it does have drawbacks:
- It limits the patient's choices.
- Patients tend to choose moderate rather than extreme descriptors.
- Some patients may not understand all the adjectives.

Overall pain assessment tools

Overall pain assessment tools evaluate pain in multiple dimensions, providing a wider range of information. These tools are time-consuming and may be more practical for outpatient use. Still, you might want to use one for a hospitalized patient with hard-to-control chronic pain. Be sure to document the patient's pain according to your facility policy. (See *Documenting pain assessment findings*.)

Take note!

Documenting pain assessment findings

Be sure to document baseline pain assessment findings so that you and other team members can use them for later comparison. You may want to use a standardized documentation form such as the pain assessment guide mentioned earlier.

If the patient has unrelieved pain, you'll need to conduct frequent assessments. To make pain assessment findings more visible, consider using a graphic sheet that lets you document pain severity next to vital signs.

Pain assessment flow sheet
A pain assessment flow sheet provides a convenient way to track the patient's pain level and response to interventions over time. On a typical flow sheet, you record information about the patient's pain severity rating, therapeutic interventions, effects of each intervention, and adverse effects of treatments (such as nausea and sedation).

A pain assessment flow sheet is useful inside and outside the hospital. After discharge, the patient and his family may want to use the flow sheet along with a pain diary in which the patient records their activities, pain intensity, and pain interventions. The diary can reveal the extent to which pain management measures and activities affect the pain level.

Analgesic infusion flow sheet
If the patient is receiving an analgesic infusion, you may use an analgesic infusion flow sheet to speed documentation and track their progress. Information to record on the flow sheet includes the:
- medication name and dosage
- date and time of each dose
- concentration of dose
- volume infused and volume remaining.

Oral medication flow sheet
An oral medication flow sheet can be a valuable tool for:
- patients who will receive analgesics after discharge
- home care patients with pain caused by progressive illness
- patients with chronic nonmalignant pain.

History and physical examination

Accurate pain assessment yields information that serves as the basis for an individualized pain management plan. For a patient with acute pain, a brief assessment may be adequate to formulate an appropriate plan.

However, a patient with chronic pain may require a thorough assessment that evaluates physical and psychosocial factors. Still, even the best history and examination techniques may not produce the definitive findings needed to make a precise diagnosis and clearly identify the origin of chronic pain. Usually, history and physical findings help the doctor interpret the results of diagnostic tests.

Patient history

Assessment begins with the patient interview. If they have acute pain from a traumatic injury, the interview may last for mere seconds. If they have chronic pain, it may be lengthy.

When interviewing a patient with chronic pain, try to elicit information that sheds light on his thoughts, feelings, behaviors, and physiologic responses to pain. Also find out about the environmental stimuli that can alter his response to pain. With a patient who is experiencing chronic pain, their lifestyle most likely has been affected by the pain. Find out if there are any activities that the person used to enjoy doing that are now impossible because of the pain.

Let's talk about your pain.

Play the match game

During the interview, assess the cognitive, affective, and behavioral components of the patient's pain experience. Doing so can help you later when working with the patient to develop pain management goals. Also ask questions to determine how the pain affects their mental state, relationships, and work performance.

Pain characteristics

Question the patient about these characteristics of his pain:
• *onset and duration*—when did the pain begin? Did it come on suddenly or gradually? Is it intermittent or continuous? How often does it occur? How long does it last? Is it prolonged or recurrent?
• *location*—ask the patient to point to the painful parts of the body or to mark these areas on a diagram. Be sure to assess each pain site separately.

• *intensity*—using a pain rating scale, ask the patient to quantify the intensity of the pain at its worst and at its best.

• *quality*—ask the patient what the pain feels like, in their own words. Does it have a burning quality? Is it knifelike? Do they feel pressure? Throbbing? Soreness?

• *relieving factors*—does anything help relieve the pain, such as a certain position or heat or cold applications? Besides helping to pinpoint the cause of the pain, the answers may aid in developing a pain management plan.

• *aggravating factors*—what seems to trigger the pain? What makes it worse? Does it get worse when the patient moves or changes position?

You may find the provoke, quality, radiate, severity, and time (PQRST) technique valuable when assessing pain. Each letter stands for a crucial aspect of pain to explore.

Medical and surgical history

The patient's medical history may offer clues to the source of pain or a condition that may exacerbate it. Ask them to list all of their past medical conditions, even those that have been resolved. Also question them about previous surgeries.

Past experience with pain

Explore the patient's experiences with pain. If they experienced significant pain in the past, they may have anticipatory fear of future pain—especially if they received inadequate pain relief.

Play "20 Questions"

Ask the patient which previous treatments—pharmacologic and otherwise—they tried, and find out which treatments helped and which didn't. Keep in mind that nonpharmacologic treatments include physical and occupational therapy, acupuncture, hypnosis, meditation, biofeedback, heat and cold therapy, transcutaneous nerve stimulation, and psychological counseling.

Drug history

Obtain a complete list of the patient's medications. (Many medications can alter the effectiveness of analgesics.) Besides prescribed drugs, ask if they take over-the-counter preparations, vitamins, nutritional supplements, or herbal or homemade remedies. Record the name, dose, frequency, administration route, and adverse effects of each agent used. Also ask about drug allergies.

Find out if the patient currently takes or has previously taken medications to control pain and whether these were effective. If they currently receive analgesics, have them describe exactly how they take them. If they haven't been taking them according to instructions, they may need additional teaching on proper administration. If a particular analgesic agent or regimen didn't work for them in the past, you may be able to teach them how to use it effectively by tailoring the dosage or regimen to their needs.

Satisfaction survey

Ask the patient if they are satisfied with the level of pain relief the current medications bring. Find out how long these drugs take to work and whether the pain returns before the next dose is due.

Question the patient about adverse effects, such as nausea, constipation, and drowsiness. If they are taking opioids for pain relief, note any worries they have about becoming drug dependent. Listen carefully for concerns they may have about any medication.

Social history

Thorough pain assessment includes a social history. Many social factors can influence the patient's perception and reports of pain and vice versa. This information also helps guide interventions.

Find out how the patient feels about himself, his place in society, and their relationships with others. Ask about marital status; occupation; support systems; financial status; hobbies; exercise and sleep patterns; responsibilities; and religious, spiritual, and cultural beliefs. Determine patterns of alcohol use, smoking, and illicit drug use.

Chronic pain can have wide-ranging effects on a person's life. If your patient has chronic pain, explore the impact it has on moods, emotions, expectations, coping efforts, and resources. Also ask how family responds to their condition.

Stoics don't say much

To provide culturally sensitive care, you must determine the meaning of pain for each patient—particularly in the context of culture and religion. Determine how cultural background and religious beliefs may affect pain experience. In some cultures, pain is openly expressed. Other cultures value stoicism and denial of pain. A patient who comes from a stoic culture may lead you to believe that they are not in pain.

Be sure not to stereotype your patient. Keep in mind that, within each culture, the response to pain may vary from person to person. Also recognize your own cultural values and biases. Otherwise, you may end up evaluating the patient's response to pain according to your own beliefs instead of theirs.

Physical examination

Start the physical examination by observing the patient. They may display a broad range of behaviors to convey pain, distress, and suffering. Some behaviors are controllable. Others, such as heavy perspiring or pupil dilation, are involuntary.

As you observe the patient before or during the physical examination, note and document behaviors. (See *Pain behavior checklist.*) Use your observations to help quantify the pain.

Overt means observable

These overt behaviors may indicate that the patient is experiencing pain:
- verbal reports of pain
- vocalizations, such as sighs and moans
- altered motor activities (frequent position changes, guarded positioning, slow movements, and rigidity)
- limping
- grimacing and other expressions
- functional limitations, including reclining for long periods
- actions to reduce pain such as taking medication.

If it's acute, think "autonomic"

Next, measure the patient's blood pressure, heart and respiratory rates, and pupil size. Acute pain may raise blood pressure, speed the heart and respiratory rates, and dilate pupils.

Remember, however, that these autonomic responses may be absent in a patient with chronic pain because the body gradually

---

Pain behavior checklist

A pain behavior is something a patient uses to communicate pain, distress, or suffering. Place a check in the box next to each behavior you observe or infer while talking to your patient.

☐ Asking such questions as, "Why did this happen to me?"
☐ Asking to be relieved from tasks or activities
☐ Avoiding physical activity
☐ Being irritable
☐ Clenching teeth
☐ Frequently shifting posture or position
☐ Grimacing
☐ Holding or supporting the painful body area
☐ Limping
☐ Lying down during the day

☐ Moaning
☐ Moving in a guarded or protective manner
☐ Moving very slowly
☐ Requesting help with walking
☐ Sighing
☐ Sitting rigidly
☐ Stopping frequently while walking
☐ Taking medication
☐ Using a cane, cervical collar, or other prosthetic device
☐ Walking with an abnormal gait

adapts to pain. Don't assume lack of autonomic responses means lack of pain.

To complete the examination, use a systematic technique to perform palpation, percussion, and auscultation. If the patient is in severe pain, you may need to shorten the examination, completing it later when his pain has decreased.

Psychological characteristics of pain

If diagnostic tests don't find a physical basis for the patient's pain, some health care providers may label the pain *psychogenic*. Psychogenic pain refers to pain associated with psychological factors. A patient with psychogenic pain may have organic pathology, or a psychological disorder may be the predominant influence on pain intensity.

Common psychogenic pain syndromes include chronic headache, muscle pain, back pain, and stomach or pelvic pain of unknown cause.

Keepin' it real

Keep in mind that psychogenic pain is *real* pain and doesn't mean the patient is malingering. Remember, too, that although pain can cause emotional distress, such distress isn't necessarily the cause of the psychogenic pain.

If objective physical findings do not substantiate the patient's complaints or if their pain severity rating seems excessive in light of physical findings, consider referring them to a psychologist or psychiatrist who specializes in evaluating chronic pain.

Shopping around

Many patients with chronic pain go from doctor to doctor and undergo exhausting procedures seeking a diagnosis and effective treatment. If their pain doesn't respond to treatment, they may feel health care providers, employers, and family are blaming—or doubting—them. In time, pain may become the central focus of their lives. They may withdraw from society, lose their jobs, and alienate family and friends.

Not surprisingly, many patients with chronic pain feel anxious, depressed, demoralized, helpless, hopeless, frustrated, angry, and isolated. They may suffer from insomnia, disruption of usual activities, drug abuse and dependence, anger, and violence. Some even attempt suicide.

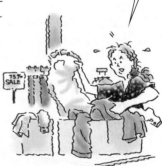

Patients with chronic pain may go from doctor to doctor trying to find someone who can give them effective treatment. Take it from me—that kind of shopping can be exhausting!

Road to success

For health care providers, assessment and management of patients with pain—especially chronic pain—can be equally frustrating. However, that doesn't mean you should lose heart or blame the patient. Through careful assessment and regular reevaluation, you can increase the odds for successful pain management—even in patients with seemingly intractable or chronic pain.

Treating pain successfully

When caring for a patient experiencing pain, you have three over-all goals:

 reduce pain intensity

improve the patient's ability to function

improve the patient's quality of life.

To accomplish these goals, you must work with the patient to agree on goals that are mutually desirable, realistic, measurable, and achievable. In addition, you'll need to focus on the nociceptive and emotional aspects of pain. A patient responds to a painful physical condition based, in part, on their subjective interpretation of illness and symptoms. The patient's beliefs about the meaning of pain and ability to function despite discomfort are important aspects of coping ability.

Harmful beliefs

Maladaptive responses to pain are more likely in a patient who believes that:
• he has a serious debilitating condition
• disability is a necessary aspect of pain
• activity is dangerous
• pain is an acceptable reason to reduce one's responsibilities.

Sometimes it pays to be a control freak

Many factors can promote or disrupt a patient's sense of control over the pain experience. They include:
• personal beliefs and expectations about pain
• coping ability
• social supports
• specific disorder that's causing the pain
• response of employers.

These factors also influence a patient's investment in treatment, acceptance of responsibility, perceptions of disability, adherence to treatment, and support from significant others. To start the patient on the road to successful pain management, consider physical, psychosocial, and behavioral factors—and the changes that occur in these relationships over time.

Interdisciplinary pain management team

An interdisciplinary team approach promotes effective pain management. Team members typically include a doctor, a nurse, a pharmacist, a social worker, a spiritual advisor, a psychologist, physical and occupational therapists, an anesthesiologist or a certified registered nurse anesthetist, a pain management specialist and, of course, the patient and his family.

Treating types of pain

In addition to the three overall goals of treating pain, consider ways to treat specific types of pain.

Treating acute pain

The cause of acute pain can be diagnosed and treated, and the pain resolves when the cause is treated or analgesics are given. Drug regimens and invasive procedures that aren't reasonable for extended periods can be used more freely in acute pain. With acute pain, it is important to stay ahead of the pain. Many physicians will order pain medication around the clock to be given to the patient.

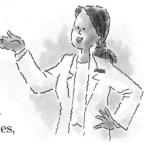

There's nothing cute about acute pain. Drug regimens and invasive procedures that aren't reasonable for extended periods can be used more freely in acute pain.

Treating chronic nonmalignant pain

Medical treatment for chronic nonmalignant pain must be based on the patient's long-term benefit, not just the current complaint of pain. Drug therapy and surgery, which typically provide only partial and temporary relief, should be individualized.

Drug treatment alone almost never effectively relieves chronic nonmalignant pain. The patient must receive a combination of treatments. These may include drugs, nondrug therapies, temporary or permanent invasive therapies (such as nerve blocks or surgery), cognitive-behavioral therapy, alternative and complementary therapies, and self-management techniques.

It pains me to say this

Even with medical management, however, chronic nonmalignant pain can be lifelong. Therefore, treatments that carry significant risks or aren't likely to prove effective over the long-term may be inappropriate.

Rehab rewards

In many cases, treatment of chronic nonmalignant pain must focus on rehabilitation rather than a cure. Rehabilitation aims to:
• maximize physical and psychological functional abilities
• minimize pain experienced during rehabilitation and for the rest of the patient's life
• teach the patient how to manage residual pain and handle pain exacerbation caused by increased activity or unexplained reasons.

Treating cancer pain

Whether pain results from cancer or its treatment, it may cause the patient to lose hope—especially if they think the pain means illness is progressing. They are then likely to suffer additional feelings of helplessness, anxiety, and depression.

However, most types of cancer pain can be managed effectively, diminishing physical and mental suffering.

Unwise to undertreat

Unfortunately, cancer pain commonly goes undertreated because of:
• inadequate knowledge of—or attention to—pain control by health care professionals
• failure of health care professionals to properly assess pain
• reluctance of patients to report their pain
• reluctance of patients and doctors to use morphine and other opioids due to fear of addiction.

Undertreated cancer pain diminishes the patient's activity level, appetite, and sleep. It may prevent the patient from working productively, enjoying leisure activities, or participating in family or social situations.

Go for the goal

The success of a pain management plan hinges on having the patient choose an appropriate goal—a pain intensity rating that will reduce his discomfort to a tolerable level and let him engage comfortably in self-care activities. Team members should work together to choose a rating scale for measuring the patient's pain intensity and to develop appropriate pain management goals.

Thorough documentation and pain assessment tools communicate vital patient information to all team members. If the patient has chronic pain, periodic team meetings also may be crucial.

Pharmacologic pain management

Pain management can be pharmacologic or nonpharmacologic. Pharmacologic pain management includes nonopioid analgesics, opioids, and adjuvant analgesics. In addition, nonpharmacologic pain management can include alternative and complementary therapies.

Nonopioid analgesics

Nonopioid (nonnarcotic) analgesics are used to treat pain that's *nociceptive* (caused by stimulation of injury-sensing receptors) or *neuropathic* (arising from nerves). These drugs are particularly effective against the somatic component of nociceptive pain such as joint and muscle pain. In addition to controlling pain, nonopioid analgesics reduce inflammation and fever.

Drug types in this category include:
- acetaminophen (Tylenol)
- nonsteroidal anti-inflammatory drugs (NSAIDs) (Advil)
- salicylates such as aspirin.

Solo or combo

When used alone, acetaminophen and NSAIDs provide relief from mild pain. NSAIDs can also relieve moderate pain; in high doses, they may help relieve severe pain. Given in combination with opioids, nonopioid analgesics provide additional analgesia, allowing a lower opioid dose and, thus, a lower risk of adverse effects.

Opioids

Opioids (narcotics) include derivatives of the opium (poppy) plant and synthetic drugs that imitate natural opioids. Unlike NSAIDs, which act peripherally, opioids produce their primary effects in the CNS. Opioids include opioid agonists, opioid antagonists, and mixed agonist-antagonists.

Opioid agonists

Opioid agonists are used to treat moderate to severe pain without causing loss of consciousness. Opioid agonists include:
- codeine
- fentanyl (Duragesic)
- hydromorphone (Dilaudid)
- methadone (Dolophine)
- morphine (Avinza) (including sustained-release tablets and intensified oral solution)
- oxycodone (Percolone).

Opioid antagonists

Opioid antagonists aren't pain medications but block the effects of opioid agonists. They're used to reverse adverse drug reactions, such as respiratory and CNS depression produced by opioid agonists. Unfortunately, by reversing analgesic effects, they may cause the patient's pain to recur.

Attached but not stimulating

Opioid antagonists attach to opiate receptors but don't stimulate them. As a result, they prevent other opioids, enkephalins, and endorphins from producing their effects. Opioid antagonists include naloxone (Narcan) and naltrexone (Depade).

Mixed opioid agonist-antagonists

As their name implies, mixed opioid agonist-antagonists have agonist and antagonist properties. The *agonist component* relieves pain while the *antagonist component* reduces the risk of toxicity and drug dependence. These agents also decrease the risk of respiratory depression and drug abuse. These agents include:
- buprenorphine (Buprenex)
- butorphanol (Stadol)
- nalbuphine (Nubain)
- pentazocine hydrochloride (Talwin) (combined with pentazocine lactate, naloxone, aspirin, or acetaminophen).

Potent potential

Originally, mixed agonist-antagonists seemed to have less addiction potential than pure opioid agonists as well as a lower risk of drug dependence. However, butorphanol and pentazocine reportedly have caused dependence.

Adjuvant analgesics

Adjuvant analgesics are drugs that have other primary indications but are used as analgesics in some circumstances. Adjuvants may be given in combination with opioids or used alone to treat chronic pain. Patients receiving adjuvant analgesics should be reevaluated periodically to monitor their pain level and check for adverse reactions.

A real potpourri

Drugs used as adjuvant analgesics include certain anticonvulsants, local and topical anesthetics, muscle relaxants, tricyclic antidepressants, serotonin 5-hydroxytryptamine agonists, selective serotonin reuptake inhibitors, ergotamine alkaloids, benzodiazepines, psych stimulants, cholinergic blockers, and corticosteroids.

Nonpharmacologic pain management

Managing pain doesn't necessarily involve capsules, syringes, I.V. lines, or medication pumps. Many nonpharmacologic therapies are available, too—and they're gaining popularity among the general public and health care professionals alike.

What accounts for this trend? For one thing, many people are concerned about the overuse of drugs for conventional pain management. For another, some people simply prefer to self-manage their health problems.

> Nonpharmacologic approaches offer something for nearly everyone—from whirlpools to massage. Ahhh, I'm feeling better already!

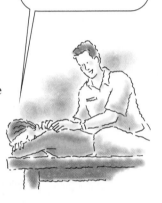

Something for everyone

Collectively speaking, nonpharmacologic approaches offer something for nearly everyone. They range from the relatively conventional (whirlpools, hot packs) to the electrifying (vibration, electrical nerve stimulation), sensual (aromatherapy, massage), serene (meditation, yoga), and high-tech (biofeedback).

These therapies fall into three main categories:

- physical therapies
- alternative and complementary therapies
- cognitive and behavioral therapies.

Many of these therapies can be used alone or combined with drug therapy. A combination approach may improve pain relief by enhancing drug effects and allowing lower dosages.

Plenty of perks

Nonpharmacologic approaches have other benefits in addition to pain management. For example, they help reduce stress, improve mood, promote sleep, and give the patient a sense of control over pain.

Opt for more options

By understanding how these techniques work and how best to use them, you can provide additional options for patients who experience pain. Although the techniques discussed in this chapter can be effective for a wide range of patients, they're best administered, prescribed, or taught by licensed practitioners or experienced, credentialed lay people. A few require a doctor's order.

Physical therapies

Physical therapies use physical agents and methods to aid rehabilitation and restore normal functioning after an illness or injury. These therapies are relatively cheap and easy to use. With appropriate teaching, patients and their families can use them on their own, which helps them participate in pain management.

Physical therapies include:
- hydrotherapy
- thermotherapy
- cryotherapy
- vibration
- transcutaneous electrical nerve stimulation (TENS).

Therapeutic goals

In addition to easing pain, physical therapies reduce inflammation, ease muscle spasms, and promote relaxation. The goals of physical therapies are to:
- promote health
- prevent physical disability
- rehabilitate patients disabled by pain, disease, or injury.

Hydrotherapy

Hydrotherapy uses water to treat pain and disease. Sometimes called the *ultimate natural pain reliever*, water comforts and soothes while providing support and buoyancy. Depending on the patient's problem, the water can be hot or cold, and liquid, solid (ice), or steam. It can be applied externally or internally.

Most commonly prescribed for burns, hydrotherapy relaxes muscles, raises or lowers tissue temperature (depending on water temperature), and eases joint stiffness (as in rheumatoid arthritis or osteoarthritis). In pain management, hydrotherapy is most commonly used to treat acute pain—for instance, from muscle sprains or strains.

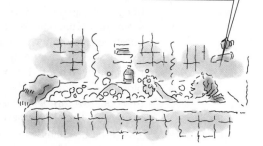

I don't need a medical book to tell me that baths are therapeutic. It's a no-brainer!

Jet set

Whirlpool baths—bathtubs with jets that force water to circulate—aid in rehabilitating injured muscles and joints. Depending on the desired effect, the water can be hot or cold. The water jets act to massage soothing muscles. (See *Pools that ease pain*, page 530.)

Pools that ease pain

Hydrotherapy commonly takes the form of a whirlpool bath, which uses water jets to help ease pain.

Pool tips

• When administering whirlpool therapy, keep water temperature between 52° and 109° F (11.1° and 42.8° C), depending on the body surface area being treated and the patient's physical condition.

• Use a hydraulic chair to help the patient get into and out of the whirlpool tub.

This illustration shows a patient whose leg injury is being treated in a whirlpool.

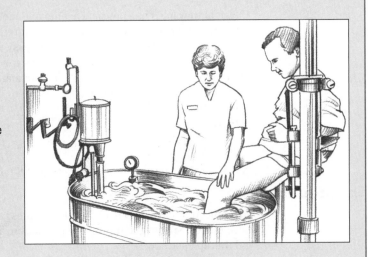

Whirlpools and certain other hydrotherapy treatments can be done at home. However, the more intensive forms are best done in a supervised clinical setting where the treatment and the patient's response can be monitored.

And that isn't all

Other forms of hydrotherapy include a neutral bath and a sitz bath. In a *neutral bath*, the patient is immersed fully (up to the neck) in water that's near body temperature. This soothing bath calms the nervous system. In a *sitz bath*, the pelvic area is immersed in a tub of water to relieve perianal pain, swelling, or discomfort; boost circulation; and reduce inflammation.

Secrets revealed

Hydrotherapy's pain-relieving properties are related to the physics and mechanics of water and its effect on the human body. When a body is immersed in water, the resulting weightlessness reduces stress on joints, muscles, and other connective tissues. This buoyancy may relieve some types of pain instantly.

Hot water hydrotherapy eases pain through a sequence of events triggered by increased skin temperature. As skin temperature rises, blood vessels widen and skin circulation increases. As resistance to blood flow through veins and capillaries drops, blood pressure decreases. The heart rate then rises to maintain blood pressure. The result is a significant drop in pain and greater comfort.

Some restrictions apply

As with any treatment, be aware of these potential hazards of hydrotherapy:
• Hydrotherapy may cause burns, falls, or light-headedness.
• Stop the treatment session if the patient feels light-headed, dizzy, or faint.
• Don't keep the patient in a heated whirlpool for more than 20 minutes.
• Instruct the patient to wipe their face frequently with a cool washcloth so they won't get overheated.
• Know that hydrotherapy isn't recommended for pregnant women; children; elderly patients; or patients with diabetes, hypertension, hypotension, or multiple sclerosis.

Thermotherapy

Thermotherapy refers to application of dry or moist heat to decrease pain, relieve stiff joints, ease muscle aches and spasms, improve circulation, and increase the pain threshold. Dry heat can be applied with a K-pad or an electric heating pad. Moist heat can be applied with a hot pack, a warm compress, or a special heating pad. Dry and moist heat involves conductive heating—heat transfer that occurs when the skin directly contacts a warm object.

What's the use?

Thermotherapy is used to treat pain caused by:
• headache
• muscle aches and spasms
• earache
• menstrual cramps
• temporomandibular joint disease
• fibromyalgia (syndrome of chronic pain in the muscles and soft tissues surrounding joints).

Five for the price of one

Thermotherapy enhances blood flow, increases tissue metabolism, and decreases vasomotor tone. It produces analgesia by suppressing free nerve endings. It also may reduce the perception of pain in the cerebral cortex.

Regional heating—heat therapy of selected body areas—can bring immediate temporary pain relief. This method may have a systemic effect, too, resulting from autonomic reflex responses to localized heat application. The reflex-mediated responses may raise body temperature, enhance blood flow, and cause other physiologic changes in areas distant from the heat application site. (See *Thermo thoughts* for considerations when using heat therapy.)

Thermo thoughts

Before administering thermotherapy, take these considerations into account:
• Determine the patient's awareness level and ability to communicate their response to the treatment.
• If the patient has a cognitive impairment, measure the temperature of the heating agent before applying it. It should be 104° to 113° F (40° to 45° C) when it contacts the skin.
• Be aware that some patients may prefer a slightly lower (or higher) temperature. Keep the heating agent at a temperature that's comfortable for the patient.
• Wrap the heating agent so it doesn't directly contact the patient's skin.

• Regularly assess skin at the heat application site for irritation and redness.
• Frequently evaluate the patient's response to treatment and his pain level.
• Stop the treatment if the patient's pain increases.
• Don't apply heat to an area that's infected, bleeding, or receiving radiation therapy or where oil or menthol has been applied.
• Know that thermotherapy is contraindicated in patients with vascular insufficiency, neuropathy, skin desensitization, or neoplasms.

Cryotherapy

Cryotherapy involves applying cold to a specific body area. In addition to reducing fever, this technique can provide immediate pain relief and help reduce or prevent edema and swelling.

Cryotherapy methods include cold packs and ice bags for pain relief measures. These measures should only be left on a patient for 20 minutes. Ice is used in acute injury along with rest, compression, and elevation.

Quite a contrast

In another cryotherapy technique, known as *contrast therapy*, cold and heat application are applied alternately during the same session. Contrast therapy may benefit patients with rheumatoid arthritis and certain other conditions.

Typically, the session begins by immersing the patient's feet and hands in warm water for 10 minutes. Next come four cycles of cold soaks (each lasting 1 to 4 minutes) alternating with warm soaks (each lasting 4 to 6 minutes).

Freezing out pain

Cryotherapy is commonly used for acute pain—especially when caused by a sports injury (such as a muscle sprain). It may also be indicated for pain resulting from:
• acute trauma
• joint disorders such as rheumatoid arthritis

- headache such as migraine
- muscle aches and spasms
- incisions
- surgery.

Constrict and reduce

Cryotherapy constricts blood vessels at the injury site, reducing blood flow to the site. This, in turn, thickens the blood, resulting in decreased bleeding and increased blood clotting.

Cold application also slows edema development, prevents further tissue damage, and minimizes bruising.

Cryotherapy also decreases sensitivity to pain by cooling nerve endings. It eases muscle spasms by cooling muscle spindles—the part of the muscle tissue responsible for the stretch reflex. (See *Applying cold to a muscle sprain*, page 534.) Contrast therapy is thought to stimulate endocrine function, reduce inflammation, decrease congestion, and improve organ function.

> ### RICE Therapy
> R – Rest
> I – Ice
> C – Compression
> E – Elevation

Remember this

When administering cryotherapy, remember these points:
- As appropriate, encourage your patient to try cold application. Many patients aren't aware that cold relieves pain.
- Before applying cold, assess the pain or injury site and the patient's pain level. Evaluate him for impaired circulation (such as from Raynaud's disease), inability to sense temperature (as from neuropathy), extreme skin sensitivity, and inability to report the response to treatment (for instance, a young child or a confused elderly patient).
- If the patient has a cognitive impairment, measure the temperature of the cooling agent. It should be no colder than 59° F (15° C).
- When administering moist cold, keep in mind that moisture intensifies cold.
- Wrap cold packs so they don't directly contact the patient's skin. Keep them at a comfortable temperature.
- Stop the treatment if the patient's skin becomes numb.
- Use caution when applying ice to the elbow, wrist, or outer part of the knee. These sites are more susceptible to cold-induced nerve injury.
- Be aware that refreezable gel packs and chemical packs may be colder than ice. Also, they may leak.
- Regularly assess the patient for adverse effects such as skin irritation, joint stiffness, numbness, frostbite, and nerve injury.
- Don't apply cold to areas that have poor circulation or have received radiation.

> Explaining the benefits of cryotherapy to a patient may be a bit more of a challenge. I can understand why! Brrrrr . . .

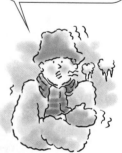

Applying cold to a muscle sprain

Cryotherapy helps reduce pain and edema when used during the first 24 to 72 hours after an injury. For best results, follow these guidelines.

Method and materials
• Apply cold to the painful area four times daily for 20 to 30 minutes each time.
• Use enough crushed ice to cover the area.
• Place the ice in a plastic bag, and place the bag inside a pillowcase or a large piece of cloth, as shown here. Then apply the bag over the

painful area for the specified treatment time.

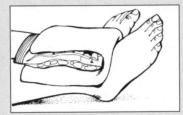

The old switcheroo
• After 24 to 72 hours, when swelling has subsided or when cold can no longer help, switch to thermotherapy.

Wise words
• Inform the patient that ice eases pain in a joint that has begun to stiffen—but caution him not to let the analgesic effect lull him into overusing the joint.

Vibration

Vibration therapy eases pain by inducing numbness in the treated area. This technique, which works like an electric massage, may be effective in such disorders as:
• muscle aches
• headache
• chronic nonmalignant pain
• cancer pain
• fractures
• neuropathic pain.

Hospitalized patients need a doctor's order to use a vibrating device. Outpatients may choose from various devices available without a prescription.

Good vibrations

A vibrating device can be stationary or handheld. Stationary devices range from vibrating cushions to full beds and recliners. The patient lies or sits on the device and receives the treatment passively.

With a handheld vibrator, the patient or a caregiver moves the device over the painful area. Some handheld vibrators are battery-operated; others plug into a wall outlet.

Handheld vibrators come in many shapes and sizes. Some are relatively heavy and may be hard for frail or arthritic patients to use.

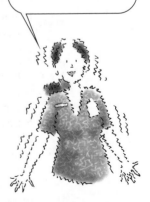

For more effective pain relief, use the highest vibration speed the patient can tolerate. Whoa! I think this speed is a little too fast for me!

Don't forget

Remember these points when administering vibration therapy:
• Before using vibration therapy, teach your patient about this method, including how it works and when it should and shouldn't be used.
• Tell the patient they may feel a warm sensation initially.
• Apply the vibrator to an area above or below the pain site.
• For more effective pain relief, use the highest vibration speed the patient can tolerate.
• Apply the vibrating device for 1 to 15 minutes at a time, two to four times daily, or as ordered.
• Determine the length of treatment needed to achieve adequate pain relief. Continue to assess the patient's response to treatment.
• Stop the treatment if the patient experiences discomfort, pain, or excessive skin redness or irritation.
• Don't use vibration therapy if the patient has thrombophlebitis or bruises easily.
• Don't apply the vibrator over burns, cuts, or incision sites.
• If the patient will self-administer this therapy, provide appropriate teaching. Advise them to assess their pain level before the session, immediately afterward, and at a later time to assess how long pain relief lasts. Doing so helps determine the optimal length of treatment. (Usually, the longer the session, the longer the duration of pain relief.)

TENS

In TENS therapy, a portable, battery-powered device transmits painless alternating electric current to peripheral nerves or directly to a painful area. Used postoperatively and for patients with chronic pain, TENS reduces the need for analgesic drugs and helps the patient resume normal activities. TENS therapy must be prescribed by a doctor.

Belt it on

The patient usually wears the TENS unit on a belt. Units have several channels and lead placements. The settings allow adjustment of wave frequency, duration, and intensity. (See *Positioning TENS electrodes*, page 536.)

Typically, a course of TENS therapy lasts 3 to 5 days. Some conditions (such as phantom limb pain) may require continuous simulation. Others, such as a painful arthritic joint, call for shorter treatment periods—perhaps 3 to 4 hours.

Top TENS list

TENS can provide temporary relief of acute pain (such as postoperative pain) and ongoing relief of chronic pain (such as in

Positioning TENS electrodes

In transcutaneous electrical nerve stimulation (TENS), electrodes placed around peripheral nerves or incision sites transmit mild electrical impulses, which presumably block pain messages.

Perfect placement

Electrode placement usually varies, even for patients with similar complaints. Electrodes can be placed in several ways:
• to cover or surround the painful area, as for muscle tenderness or spasm or painful joints
• to capture the painful area between electrodes, as for incisional pain.

These illustrations show combinations of electrode placement (dark squares) and areas of nerve stimulation (shaded strips) for low back and leg pain.

Placement tips

• If the patient has peripheral nerve injury, place electrodes proximal to the injury (between the brain and the injury site) to avoid increasing his pain.
• If a site lacks sensation, place electrodes on adjacent dermatomes (areas of skin innervated by sensory fibers from a single spinal nerve).

• Don't place electrodes in a hypersensitive area. Doing so can increase pain.

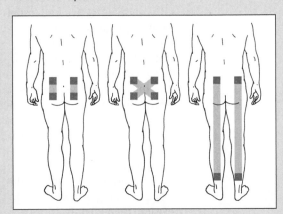

sciatica). Specific pain problems that have responded to TENS include:
• chronic nonmalignant pain
• cancer pain
• bone fracture pain
• low back pain
• sports injuries
• myofascial pain
• neurogenic pain (as in neuralgia and neuropathy)
• phantom limb pain
• arthritis
• menstrual pain.

Still a mystery

Although TENS has existed for about 30 years, experts still aren't sure exactly how it relieves pain. Some believe that it works according to the gate-control theory, which proposes that painful impulses pass through a "gate" in the brain. According to this theory, TENS alters the patient's perception of pain by closing the gate to painful stimuli.

TENS to-do list

Consider these points when administering TENS therapy:
• To ensure that your patient is a willing and active participant in TENS therapy, provide complete instructions on using and caring for the TENS unit as well as expected results of treatment.
• Before TENS therapy begins, assess the patient's pain level and evaluate for skin irritation at the sites where electrodes will be placed.
• Be aware that the safety of TENS during pregnancy hasn't been established.

TENS taboos

• Don't use TENS if the patient has undiagnosed pain, uses a pacemaker, or has a history of heart arrhythmias.
• Don't apply a TENS unit over the carotid sinus, an open wound, or anesthetized skin.
• Don't place the unit on the head or neck of a patient who has a vascular disorder or seizure disorder.

Alternative and complementary therapies

Alternative and complementary therapies greatly expand the range of therapeutic choices for patients suffering pain. Today, patients are increasingly seeking these therapies—not just to treat pain but also to address many other common health conditions. Various theories have been offered to explain the increased interest in alternative and complementary therapies. (See *Understanding the alternative trend*, page 538.)

Wholly holistic

Regardless of the problem for which they're used, alternative and complementary therapies address the whole person—body, mind, and spirit—rather than just signs and symptoms.

Defining the terms

Although alternative and complementary therapies are usually discussed together, they aren't exactly the same:
• *Alternative* therapies are those used *instead* of conventional or mainstream therapies—for example, the use of acupuncture rather than analgesics to relieve pain.
• *Complementary* therapies are those used *in conjunction with* conventional therapies—such as meditation used as an adjunct to analgesic drugs.

Alternative and complementary therapies address the whole person rather than just symptoms . . . and who doesn't want to be treated like a person?!

Understanding the alternative trend

Why are more people turning to alternative and complementary therapies to treat health problems? One reason is that most therapies are noninvasive and cause few adverse reactions.

People with certain chronic conditions may be drawn to these therapies because conventional medicine has few, if any, effective treatments for them. Also, people are encouraged by reports that document their effectiveness.

Hoopla about holism

Conventional medicine tends to treat only signs and symptoms, whereas alternative and complementary therapies focus on the whole person, thus holism.

Time—and more time

Many people also value the extra time alternative practitioners spend with the patient and the attention they pay to the patient's temperament, behavioral patterns, and perceived needs. In an increasingly stressful world, people are searching for someone who will take the time to listen to them and treat them as people, not just bodies displaying signs and symptoms.

Spiritual hunger

Some people view modern society as spiritually malnourished and hungry for meaning. Alternative practitioners seem to be more responsive to this need.

Cultural connections

Lastly, in a culturally diverse country such as the United States, a wide variety of traditional healing practices and beliefs exist. Some are based on the same principles that underlie alternative and complementary therapies.

East meets West

Some of the alternative and complementary therapies practiced today have been used since ancient times and come from the traditional healing practices of many cultures—particularly in the Eastern part of the world.

Many mainstream Western doctors have become more open-minded about these therapies. In fact, some medical doctors even administer them. However, others still object to them on the grounds that they aren't based solely on empirical science.

Pain relief prospects

Nonetheless, alternative and complementary therapies commonly relieve some types of pain that don't respond to Western techniques. They may prove especially valuable when a precise cause evades Western medicine, as typically occurs in chronic low back pain.

Cognitive and behavioral approaches

Cognitive approaches to pain management focus on influencing the patient's interpretation of the pain experience. *Behavioral* approaches help the patient develop skills for managing pain and changing his reaction to it.

Cognitive and behavioral approaches to managing pain include meditation, biofeedback, and hypnosis. These techniques improve the patient's sense of control over pain and allow him to participate actively in pain management.

Meditation

Meditation is thought to relieve stress and reduce pain through an effect called the *relaxation response*—a natural protective mechanism against overstress. Learning to activate the relaxation response through meditation may offset some of the negative physiologic effects of stress.

Biofeedback

Biofeedback uses electronic monitors to teach patients how to exert conscious control over autonomic functions. By watching the fluctuations of various body functions on a monitor, patients learn how to change a particular body function by adjusting thoughts, breathing pattern, posture, or muscle tension.

As they modify vital functions, patients may develop the ability to control pain without using conventional treatments.

Hypnosis

Hypnosis harnesses the power of suggestion and altered levels of consciousness to produce positive behavior changes and treat various conditions. Under hypnosis, a patient typically relaxes and experiences changes in respiration, which may lead to a positive shift in behavior and a greater sense of well-being.

References

Egan, M., & Cornally, N. (2013). Identifying barriers to pain management in long-term care. *Nursing Older People, 25*(7), 25–31.

Fielding, F., Sanford, T. M., & Davis, M. P. (2013). Achieving effective control in cancer pain: A review of current guidelines. *International Journal of Palliative Nursing, 19*(12), 584–591.

Quick quiz

1. Which medication is used to reverse the effects of narcotic overdose?
    A.   Meperidine
    B.   Naloxone
    C.   Acetaminophen
    D.   Fentanyl

Answer: B. Naloxone is an opioid antagonist and is used to reverse or counter an opioid overdose (e.g., morphine or heroin).

2. Thermotherapy causes which effect?
    A.   Vasodilation
    B.   Paresthesia
    C.   Vasoconstriction
    D.   Vasocompression

Answer: A. Thermotherapy causes vasodilation, which enhances blood flow to the affected area.

3. Massage promotes increased circulation and softening of connective tissues. It also has which effect?
    A.   Narrows blood vessels
    B.   Eases muscle spasms
    C.   Causes hyperventilation
    D.   Widens blood vessels

Answer: B. Massage decreases muscle tension, thereby easing muscle spasms.

Scoring

☆☆☆ If you answered all three questions correctly, wow! You must be feelin' great!

☆☆ If you answered two questions correctly, good job! You sure don't have any opioids clouding your brain.

☆ If you answered fewer than two questions correctly, feel no pain! Review the chapter and try again.

18

Nutrition

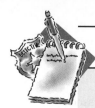

Just the facts

In this chapter, you'll learn:

♦ role nutrients play in health promotion

♦ ways to differentiate between good nutrition and poor nutrition

♦ current nutrient standards for health promotion

♦ purpose of digestion and absorption

♦ structures of the GI tract wall, digestive organs, and accessory organs as well as their functions in digestion and absorption

♦ ways to promote proper diet.

A look at nutrition

Nutrition refers to the processes by which a living organism ingests, digests, absorbs, transports, uses, and excretes *nutrients* (food and other nourishing material). Nutrition as a clinical area is primarily concerned with the properties of food that build sound bodies and promote health.

More than just a pretty process

Because good nutrition is essential to good health and disease prevention, any person involved in health care needs a thorough knowledge of nutrition and the body's nutritional requirements throughout the life span. What's more, the study of nutrition must focus on health promotion.

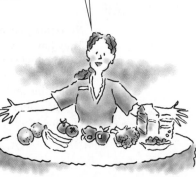

Understanding and practicing good nutrition can make you and your patients healthier throughout your life spans!

Nutrients

There are two types of nutrients:

Nonessential nutrients are nutrients that aren't needed in the diet because they're manufactured by the body.

Essential nutrients are nutrients that must be acquired through food because the body can't produce them on its own in adequate quantities.

Certain and essential

For nutrition to be adequate, a person must receive certain essential nutrients—carbohydrates, fats, proteins, vitamins, minerals, and water. These nutrients must be present for proper growth and functioning. In addition, the digestive system must function properly to make use of these nutrients.

No lone nutrients

Each nutrient has several specific metabolic functions, but no nutrient works alone. Close metabolic relationships exist among all of the basic nutrients as well as among their metabolic products.

Nutrient breakdown dance

Nutrients can be used by the body for its immediate needs, or they can be stored for later use. The body breaks down nutrients into simpler compounds for absorption in the stomach and intestines in two ways:

mechanical breakdown, which begins in the gastrointestinal (GI) tract with chewing

chemical breakdown, which starts with salivary enzymes in the mouth and continues with acid and enzyme action through the rest of the GI tract.

Role of a lifeline

Nutrients play a vital role in maintaining health and wellness. They have several important functions:
• providing energy, which can be stored in the body or transformed for vital activities
• building and maintaining body tissue
• controlling metabolic processes, such as growth, cell activity, enzyme production, and temperature regulation.

Metabolism

Regulated mostly by hormones, metabolism is a combination of several processes by which energy is extracted from certain nutrients (carbohydrates, proteins, and fats) and then used by the body. Vitamins and minerals don't directly provide us with energy, but they're an important part of the metabolic process. Metabolism can be broken down into two parts:

Catabolism is the breakdown of complex substances into simpler ones, resulting in the release of energy.

Anabolism is the synthesis of simple substances into more complex substances. This process provides the energy necessary for tissue growth, maintenance, and repair.

> Metabolism, regulated mostly by hormones like us, is a combination of several processes by which energy is extracted from certain nutrients and then used by the body.

Energy

Energy, in the form of adenosine triphosphate, is produced as a by-product of carbohydrate, fat, and protein metabolism. The amount of energy in food products is measured in kilocalories (kcal), which are commonly referred to as *calories*.

Through the processes of digestion and absorption, energy is released from food into the body. Small amounts of energy are stored within cells for immediate use. Larger amounts of energy are stored in glycogen and fat tissue to fuel long-duration activities.

Balancing act

In a healthy adult, the rate of anabolism equals the rate of catabolism, and energy balance is obtained. In other words, energy balance occurs when the caloric intake from food equals the number of calories expended. These calories may be used for voluntary activities (such as physical activity) or involuntary activities (such as basal metabolism).

Nutrition and health promotion

Many patients may consider themselves healthy because they don't feel sick. However, you must be concerned about a more holistic meaning of the term *health*—one that incorporates aspects of the patient's internal and external environments—in order to best care for your patients.

For you, health promotion must consider all of a patient's needs, including physical, emotional, mental, and social needs. Only when these needs are met can it be said that a person is healthy or well. Furthermore, wellness implies a state of balance between a person's activities and goals. Maintaining this balance allows the patient to maintain his vitality and ability to function productively in society. A nutritious diet provides the basis for health promotion and disease prevention, making it an important part of caring for any patient.

Approaches to health promotion

There are two main approaches to health promotion:

☝ The *traditional approach* is reactive; it focuses on treating symptoms after they appear.

✌ The *preventive approach* involves identifying and eliminating risk factors to stop health problems from developing.

The current wellness and fitness movement in the United States is grounded in the preventive approach, with individuals educating themselves about maintaining health and preventing illness and disease. Most Americans, however, still don't get the recommended amount of physical activity, which can put them at greater risk for such disorders as heart disease, diabetes, and hypertension.

2020 vision

The U.S. national health goals, which were originally published in the Department of Health and Human Services' report *Healthy People 2000* and have been updated for *Healthy People 2020*, also reflect this preventive wellness philosophy. Prominent themes in the latest report include:
• choosing a healthy diet
• maintaining weight control through physical exercise and diet
• monitoring for and reducing high-risk factors for disease.

Not one, not two, but three!

Promoting health, establishing wellness, and preventing disease is a three-part process. (See *Three parts to prevention.*)

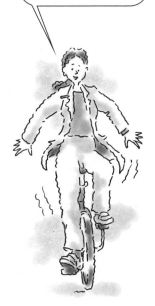

> Wellness implies a state of balance between a person's activities and goals. Maintaining this balance allows the patient to maintain his vitality and ability to function productively in society.

Three parts to prevention

Health promotion and disease prevention efforts can be categorized into three groups.

Primary prevention

Examples of primary prevention measures, which focus on health promotion, include:
• conducting nutrition classes to promote healthy eating patterns
• modifying menus in restaurants and offering low-fat alternatives
• offering fresh fruit and vegetables in workplace cafeterias.

Secondary prevention

Secondary prevention, which focuses on risk reduction, may include such measures as:
• screening for potential diseases (hypercholesterolemia, osteoporosis)
• nutritional counseling for people at risk for cardiovascular diseases and diabetes
• immunizations.

Tertiary prevention

Examples of tertiary prevention measures, which focus on disease treatment and rehabilitation, include:
• physical rehabilitation for the stroke patient
• cardiac rehabilitation for the cardiac patient
• diabetes education classes for the patient with newly diagnosed type 1 or type 2 diabetes.

Nutrition and a balanced diet

You're part of a health care team that's responsible for making sure the patient maintains optimal nutritional health, even though he may be battling illness or recovering from surgery. It's also your job to stress to the patient the importance of good nutrition in maintaining health and recovering from illness, so that he can continue sound nutritional practices when he's no longer in your care.

Optimal nutrition requires a varied diet of carbs, proteins, fats, vitamins, minerals, water, and fiber in sufficient amounts.

Nutritional status

You must use your knowledge of nutrition to promote health through education and counseling of sick and healthy patients. This counseling includes encouraging patients to consume appropriate types and amounts of food. It also means considering poor food habits as a contributing factor in a patient with chronic illness. Therefore, assessing nutritional status and identifying nutritional needs to meet the requirements of a balanced diet are primary activities in planning patient care.

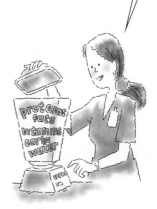

Assessing nutritional status

A patient's nutritional status can influence the body's response to illness and treatment. Regardless of your patient's overall condition, an evaluation of his nutritional health is an essential part of your assessment. Assessment of the patient's nutritional status includes determining nutritional risk factors as well as individual needs.

Good nutrition

Good nutrition, or *optimal nutrition*, is essential in promoting health, preventing illness, and restoring health after an injury or illness. To achieve optimal nutrition, a person must eat a varied diet containing carbohydrates, proteins, fats, vitamins, minerals, water, and fiber in sufficient amounts. Although excesses of certain nutrients can be detrimental to a patient's health, intake of essential nutrients should be greater than minimum requirements to allow for variations in health and disease and to provide stores for later use.

Poor nutrition

Poor nutrition, or *malnutrition*, is a state of inadequate or excess nutritional intake. It's most common among people living in poverty—especially those with greater nutritional requirements, such as elderly people, pregnant women, children, and infants. It also occurs in hospitals and long-term care facilities because the patients in these situations have illnesses that place added stress on their bodies, raising nutritional requirements.

Don't underestimate undernutrition

Undernutrition occurs when a patient consumes fewer daily nutrients than his body requires, resulting in a nutritional deficit. Typically, an undernourished patient is at greater risk for physical illnesses. He may also suffer from limitations in cognitive and physical status.

Undernutrition can result from:
- inability to metabolize nutrients
- inability to obtain the appropriate nutrients from food
- accelerated excretion of nutrients from the body
- illness or disease that increases the body's need for nutrients.

Don't overdo it

In contrast, overnutrition occurs when a patient consumes an excessive amount of nutrients. For example, overnutrition may occur in patients who self-prescribe megadoses of vitamins and mineral supplements and in those who overeat. These practices can result in damage to body tissue or obesity.

Nutrient standards

To maintain healthy populations, most developed countries have established nutrition standards for major nutrients. These standards serve as guidelines for nutrient intake based on the nutritional needs of most healthy population groups.

U.S. standards

The U.S. nutrient standards, called *recommended dietary allowances (RDAs)*, were first published during World War II as a guide for planning and acquiring food supplies and promoting good nutrition. To keep up with increasing scientific information and social concerns about nutrition and health, these standards are revised and expanded approximately every 5 years.

DRIs versus RDAs

Dietary reference intakes (DRIs) are the most recent version of the U.S. nutrient standards. Because DRIs consider an individual's sex and age-group and aren't limited to preventing deficiency diseases, these standards are more comprehensive than RDAs in measuring a patient's nutritional status and long-term health. (See *Dietary reference intakes.*)

Dietary reference intakes

Dietary reference intakes (DRIs) consist of a still-evolving set of four nutrient-based reference values being developed by the Food and Nutrition Board (FNB) of the National Academy of Sciences. These values, intended to replace and expand on the familiar recommended dietary allowances (RDAs), can be used for planning and assessing diets. They include updated values for RDAs as well as values for estimated average requirement (EAR), adequate intake (AI), and tolerable upper intake level (UL).

The new DRI system will be fully implemented over the next 3 to 4 years. Until then, reference standards will be a mix of old and new.

Recommended dietary allowance
The RDA of a nutrient is the average daily dietary intake needed to meet the requirements of virtually all healthy people in a given life stage or gender group. Critics have argued that RDAs merely prevent nutritional deficiencies rather than promote optimal health.

Estimated average requirement
The EAR of a nutrient is the average daily dietary intake needed to meet the requirements of one half of all healthy people in a given life stage or gender group. Determination of this value isn't based solely on preventing nutritional deficiencies but also includes concepts related to risk reduction and bioavailability of a given nutrient.

Adequate intake
An AI value is assigned to a nutrient if the FNB lacks sufficient information to establish an RDA and an EAR. The AI value is a recommended daily intake level based on estimates of nutrient intake by a group of healthy people.

Tolerable upper intake level
The UL is the highest level of nutrient intake that doesn't pose an adverse health effect to almost all individuals in the general population.

Other standards

The published standards of other countries, such as Canada and Britain, are similar to U.S. standards. In impoverished countries, where quality of food and nutrition are lacking, standards are set by the Food and Agriculture Organization and the World Health Organization. No matter who sets forth the standards, the goal is the same: to promote good health and prevent disease through sound nutrition.

Dietary guidelines

Dietary guidelines have been developed by governmental agencies, nutritionists, and special groups to provide recommendations that promote healthy eating habits. The U.S. dietary guidelines recommend that people age 2 and older eat a healthy assortment of foods from the basic food groups. They also emphasize the importance of:
• choosing foods that are low in added sugars, refined grains, sodium (salt), cholesterol, and saturated and trans fats
• eating more foods such as fruits, vegetables, whole grains, fat-free and low-fat dairy products
• eating reasonable portions and balance calories with physical activity to manage weight
• getting at least 30 minutes of moderate physical exercise on most days for adults. (The guidelines for children recommend at least 60 minutes of physical activity on most days of the week.)

Dietary Guidelines for Americans 2010

The U.S. Department of Agriculture and the Department of Health and Human Services released the first Dietary Guidelines and Food Guide Pyramid in 1980 to enable an individual to prepare a well-balanced diet through variety, balance, and moderation of choices. These guidelines have been revised several times, with the most recent Dietary Guidelines released in January 2011.

All mine

Dietary Guidelines for Americans 2010 introduces an updated food pyramid—called *MyPlate*—that replaces the previous *MyPyramid*. These new guidelines promote an interactive and individualized approach to improving diet and lifestyle. MyPlate helps people transfer the principles of the *Dietary Guidelines* into healthy eating and lifestyle choices. (See *Anatomy of* MyPlate.)

New features

MyPlate uses wedges of different widths and colors on a plate to represent the recommended amount of food a person should choose from a food group.

Anatomy of *MyPlate*

The U.S. Department of Agriculture's new food guidance system—called "MyPlate"—symbolizes a personalized approach to healthy eating. Designed to be simple, the symbol has been developed to remind consumers to make healthy food choices and to be active every day. The five food groups are illustrated on a familiar family place setting that emphasizes the five food groups. These five food groups consist of fruits, vegetables, grains, proteins, and dairy.

Key Behaviors:

Balancing Calories
• Enjoy your food, but eat less.
• Avoid oversized portions.

Foods to Increase
• Make half your plate fruits and vegetables.
• Make at least half your grains whole grains.
• Switch to fat-free or low-fat (1%) milk.

Foods to Reduce:
• Compare sodium in foods like soup, bread, and frozen meals, and choose foods with lower numbers.
• Drink water instead of sugary drinks.

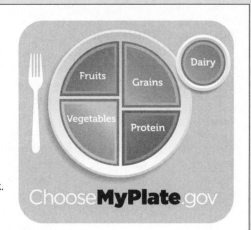

Source: U.S. Department of Agriculture. Center for Nutrition Policy and Promotion. (2010). *Getting started with MyPlate: ChooseMyPlate.gov.* Retrieved from http://www.cnpp.usda.gov/publications/myplate/gettingstartedwithmyplate.pdf

Another new feature of MyPlate is that it promotes an online, interactive approach through the website (http://www.choose myplate.gov) in which the individual can plan their meals and activity and even track it.

The new food pyramid also makes recommendations based on health needs for specific populations, such as children and adolescents, women of childbearing age, pregnant and breast-feeding women, people with hypertension, older adults, various ethnic groups, and overweight children and adults. (See *Daily Food Plans*, page 550.)

Daily Food Plans

To determine which food intake pattern to use for an individual, this chart gives an estimate of individual calorie needs. The calorie range is based on age, gender, height and weight, and physical activity level. Each Daily Food Plan is associated with a worksheet that is personally developed based on the above factors to give the individual a plan that is unique to that individual.

Age-group	Calorie range	
	Sedentary	*Active*
Children 2 to 3 years	1,000	1,400
Females		
4 to 8 years	1,200	1,800
9 to 13	1,600	2,200
14 to 18	1,800	2,400
19 to 30	2,000	2,400
31 to 50	1,800	2,200
51+	1,600	2,200
Males		
4 to 8 years	1,400	2,000
9 to 13	1,800	2,600
14 to 18	2,200	3,200
19 to 30	2,400	3,000
31 to 50	2,200	3,000
51+	2,000	2,800

Sedentary means a lifestyle that includes only the light physical activity associated with typical day-to-day life.

Active means a lifestyle that includes physical activity equivalent to walking more than 3 miles per day at 3 to 4 miles per hour, in addition to the light physical activity associated with typical day-to-day life.

Source: U.S. Department of Agriculture. (2010). *Daily food plans and worksheets*. Retrieved from http://www.choosemyplate.gov/supertracker-tools/daily-food-plans.html

Food group recommendations

Each portion on the place setting represents one of the five food groups: grains, vegetables, fruits, protein, and dairy. Each portion is designated in size with relation to the amount that is needed.

Grain group

Foods in the grain group are sources of complex carbohydrates, vitamins, minerals, and fiber. To help your patient obtain his recommended servings of foods from this food group, suggest that he:
• consume what is recommended by the Daily Food Plan based off of your age, sex, and physical activity level

- make sure that one half of all grains consumed each day (at least 3 oz) are whole grains, such as whole-grain cereals, breads, crackers, rice, or pasta
- be aware that 1 oz is approximately 1 slice of bread, 1 cup of breakfast cereal, or ½ cup of cooked rice, cereal, or pasta
- choose items made with little fat and sugar, such as bread, English muffins, rice, and pasta
- select several servings of food made from whole grains to add fiber
- avoid baked products that are high in fat and sugar, such as cakes and cookies
- use only one half of the fat suggested when preparing package mixes.

Vegetable group

Vegetables provide sources of vitamin A, vitamin C, folate, iron, magnesium, and fiber. To help your patient make healthy food choices from the vegetable group, recommend that he follow these recommendations:

- Consume at least half your plate of vegetables and fruits.
- Consume plenty of dark green vegetables, such as broccoli; spinach; and other dark, leafy greens.
- Select orange vegetables, such as carrots and sweet potatoes.
- Eat dry beans and peas, such as pinto beans, kidney beans, and lentils.
- Vary the types of vegetables consumed, being sure to choose from all vegetable subgroups (dark green, orange, legumes, starchy vegetables, and other vegetables) several times per week.

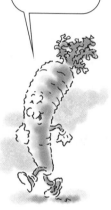

Trust me. I know what I'm talking about! Eat your veggies!

Fruit group

The fruit group provides sources of vitamin A, vitamin C, and potassium. The foods in this group are naturally low in fat and sodium. To help your patient make the right choices from the fruit group, recommend that he follow these recommendations:

- Consume at least half your plate of fruits and vegetables.
- Select a variety of fruits. Although fruits can be consumed in various forms, including fresh, frozen, canned, or dried fruits, the use of fruit juices should be limited.
- When drinking fruit juice, choose 100% fruit juice over fruit flavored juices.
- When choosing canned fruits, choose fruits that are canned in their own juice, not in syrup.

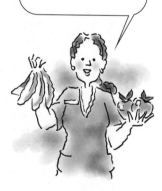

Vitamins A and C and potassium are important elements in an optimal diet. Fruit has all these, plus it's low in fat and sodium!

Dairy group

Foods in this group provide protein, vitamins, and minerals. To help your patient make healthy milk group choices, recommend that he follow these recommendations:
- Eat or drink up to 3 cups a day based on your Daily Food Plan that is specific to age and sex nutritional requirements.
- Pick low-fat or fat-free milk, yogurt, and other milk products.
- Choose lactose-free products or other calcium sources, such as fortified foods, if the patient doesn't or can't have milk.

Protein group

Foods in this group provide protein, vitamins, and minerals. To help your patient make healthy meat and bean food group choices, suggest that he follow these recommendations:
- Consume the required nutritional amount for your age and sex based on your Daily Food Plan.
- Consume low-fat or lean meats and poultry.
- Eat meats that are baked, broiled, or grilled.
- Vary selections among fish, beans, peas, nuts, and seeds.

Vegetarian diets

For various reasons, including religious, environmental, ethical, and health reasons, people may choose to follow vegetarian diets. Typically, vegetarian diets are lower in saturated fat and cholesterol and higher in fiber, carbohydrates, magnesium, boron, folate, antioxidants, carotenoids, and phytochemicals. Vegetarians have a lower risk of obesity, cancer, heart disease, hypertension, dementia, type 2 diabetes mellitus and, possibly, kidney disease, gallstones, and diverticular disease. On the other hand, vegetarians are at risk for protein, iron, and vitamin B_{12} deficiencies. If they avoid dairy products, they're also at risk for calcium and vitamin D deficiencies.

The three basic types of vegetarian diets vary according to the needs or beliefs of the person following the diet:
- Lactoovo vegetarians include dairy products and eggs in their diet.
- Lactovegetarians include only dairy products as an animal food source in their diet.
- Vegans include no animal food sources in their diet. For patients on such a diet, the use of soybeans and its by-products, along with plant foods, can help provide a balanced diet.

Well-planned vegetarian diets can be nutritionally balanced diets for any patient, including a pregnant or nursing woman. (See Tips for the vegetarian.)

Tips for the vegetarian

If your patient is a vegetarian, suggest these tips to help ensure that he's meeting his daily protein requirements:
- Eat a variety of foods from all food groups, being sure to include all nutrients.
- Consume adequate calories for your lifestyle to prevent your body from using amino acids for fuel.
- Use low-fat or nonfat products and moderately consume nuts and seeds to maintain a low-fat diet.
- Select whole grains whenever possible to increase fiber and iron content.
- Include a vitamin C source at every meal to aid iron absorption.
- Use vitamin supplements, especially vitamin B_{12} (for strict vegans).

To help a vegetarian patient meet all the nutrition recommendations of *Dietary Guidelines for Americans 2010 with the use of the MyPlate plan,* offer the following suggestions:
- Eat a variety of foods to meet caloric needs.
- Plan meals around sources of protein that are low in fat. This includes beans, lentils, and rice. Avoid using cheeses that are high in fat to replace meat.
- Increase calcium intake by using calcium-fortified, soy-based beverages, which are typically low in fat and cholesterol.
- Prepare food dishes that are usually made with meat or poultry, such as lasagna or pizza, as vegetarian dishes. Doing so increases the number of servings of vegetables while reducing saturated fat and cholesterol.
- Consider vegetarian products that look, and commonly taste, like meat dishes, such as soy-based sausages and "veggie burgers." These vegetable products are usually low in saturated fat and cholesterol-free.

A look at digestion and absorption

The basic purpose of digestion and absorption is to deliver essential nutrients to the cells in order to sustain life. To break food down into these essential nutrients, the body sends it through various mechanical and chemical processes in the GI tract or *alimentary canal.* Successful digestion and absorption depend on the coordinated function of the GI tract wall's muscles and nerves, the GI tract organs, and the accessory organs of digestion. (See *Structures of the GI system,* page 554.)

Structures of the GI system

The GI system includes the alimentary canal (pharynx, esophagus, stomach, and small and large intestines) and the accessory organs (liver, biliary duct system, and pancreas).

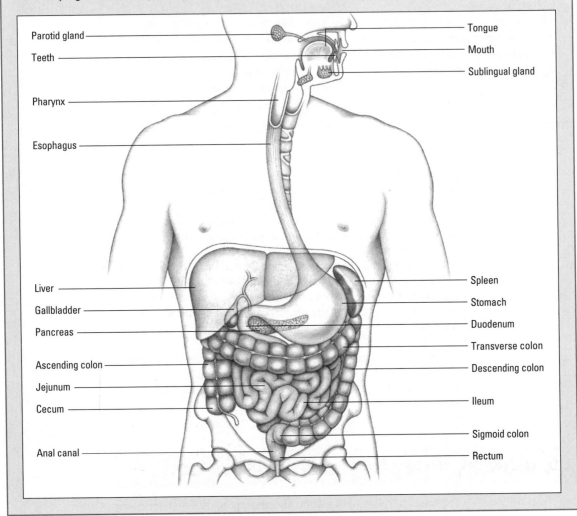

Parotid gland
Teeth
Pharynx
Esophagus

Tongue
Mouth
Sublingual gland

Liver
Gallbladder
Pancreas
Ascending colon
Jejunum
Cecum
Anal canal

Spleen
Stomach
Duodenum
Transverse colon
Descending colon
Ileum
Sigmoid colon
Rectum

GI tract wall structures

The wall of the GI tract consists of four major layers:

 visceral peritoneum

 tunica muscularis

 submucosa

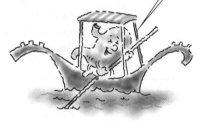 mucosa.

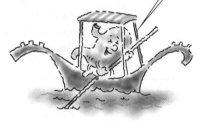

Ah, there's nothing like a trip down the alimentary canal after a good meal. Oh, sole mio!

Visceral peritoneum

The *visceral peritoneum* is the GI tract's outer covering. It covers most of the abdominal organs and lies next to an identical layer, the *parietal peritoneum*, which lines the abdominal cavity.

To serve and protect

The main job of this outer layer of the GI tract wall is to protect the blood vessels, nerves, and lymphatics. It also attaches the jejunum, ileum, and transverse colon to the posterior abdominal wall to prevent twisting.

Many names, one layer

The visceral peritoneum has many names. In the esophagus and rectum, it's called the *tunica adventitia*. Elsewhere in the GI tract, it's called the *tunica serosa*.

Tunica muscularis

The *tunica muscularis*, which lies within the visceral peritoneum, is a layer composed of skeletal muscle in the mouth, pharynx, and upper esophagus.

Elsewhere in the tract . . .

The tunica muscularis is made up of longitudinal and circular smooth muscle fibers. At points along the tract, the circular fibers thicken to form sphincters.

Pucker pouches

In the large intestine, these fibers gather into three narrow bands *(teniae coli)* down the middle of the colon and pucker the intestine into characteristic pouches *(haustra)*.

Nerve network

Between the two muscle layers lies a nerve network—the *myenteric plexus*, also known as *Auerbach's plexus*. The stomach wall contains a third muscle layer made up of oblique fibers.

Submucosa

The *submucosa*, also called the *tunica submucosa*, lies under the tunica muscularis. It's composed of loose connective tissue, blood and lymphatic vessels, and another nerve network called the *submucosal plexus* or *Meissner's plexus*.

Mucosa

The *mucosa*, the innermost layer of the GI tract wall, is also called the *tunica mucosa*. This layer consists of epithelial and surface cells and loose connective tissue. Villi from surface cells secrete gastric and protective juices and absorb nutrients.

GI tract wall functions

The nerves and muscles of the GI tract wall work jointly to ensure that food moves spontaneously through the digestive system (motility). GI tract functions include innervation and secretion.

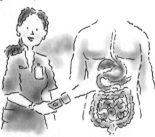

The nerves and muscles of the GI tract wall work jointly to ensure that food moves spontaneously through the digestive system (motility).

GI tract innervation

Distention of the submucosal plexus in the submucosa or myenteric plexus in the tunica muscularis stimulates transmission of nerve signals to the smooth muscle, which initiates contraction and relaxation of these muscles, called *peristalsis*. During peristalsis, longitudinal fibers of the tunica muscularis shorten the lumen length and circular fibers reduce the lumen diameter.

GI tract secretion

Five major substances secreted by the GI tract contribute to the chemical process of digestion:

Mucus protects the lining of the GI tract and aids in motility.

Enzymes are proteins that break down nutrients.

Acid and various buffer ions contribute to the level of alkalinity or acidity (pH) needed to activate digestive enzymes.

Electrolytes and water carry nutrients through the GI tract and aid in the absorption process.

Bile emulsifies fat to promote intestinal absorption of fatty acids, cholesterol, and other lipids.

How digestion and absorption work

The organs of the GI tract play the major role in mechanical and chemical digestion and absorption of food and fluid. (See *Functions of the digestive system organs*, page 558.) Aided by the GI tract wall and accessory organs, the organs of the GI tract process nutrients in three phases of digestion:

 cephalic

 gastric

 intestinal.

Cephalic phase

The cephalic phase of digestion uses the GI tract organs of the mouth, pharynx, and esophagus to begin the mechanical processes of digestion. Mechanical digestion breaks down food into smaller particles, which increases the surface area on which digestive enzymes can work.

Mouth

Digestion begins in the mouth (also called the *buccal cavity* or *oral cavity*). Ducts connect the mouth with the three major pairs of salivary glands:
• parotid
• submandibular
• sublingual.

These glands secrete the enzyme *ptyalin* (a salivary amylase) to moisten food during chewing (mastication) and begin breaking down starch into maltose. (See *Causes of dry mouth in older adults*, page 558.)

Pharynx

The *pharynx* is a cavity extending from the base of the skull to the esophagus. The pharynx aids swallowing by grasping food and propelling it toward the esophagus.

Esophagus

A muscular tube, the esophagus extends from the pharynx through the mediastinum to the stomach.

Functions of the digestive system organs

This chart lists the digestive system organs and their primary functions.

Organ	Function
Mouth	• Breaks down food into smaller particles • Releases saliva to promote chewing and swallowing • Secretes amylase (ptyalin)
Esophagus	• Propels food downward into the stomach
Stomach	• Acts as a food reservoir • Mixes food with gastric secretions (hydrochloric acid, pepsin, mucus, intrinsic factor) • Begins protein digestion • Absorbs water, alcohol, and some drugs
Liver	• Produces bile • Metabolizes carbohydrates, protein, and fat • Stores nutrients • Detoxifies drugs and waste products
Gallbladder	• Concentrates and stores bile • Releases bile into the duodenum
Pancreas	• Produces and secretes insulin and glucagon • Produces and secretes digestive enzymes: proteases, lipase, and amylase
Small intestine	• Secretes hormones to stimulate the secretion of pancreatic juices, bile, and intestinal enzymes • Secretes digestive enzymes: peptidases, disaccharidases • Absorbs iron, magnesium, and calcium (duodenum) • Absorbs water-soluble vitamins and simple sugars (jejunum) • Absorbs amino acids, peptides, fat-soluble vitamins, fats, cholesterol, bile salts, and vitamin B_{12} (ileum)
Large intestine	• Absorbs water, sodium, potassium, and vitamin K formed by colonic bacteria • Eliminates solid waste

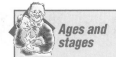

Ages and stages

Causes of dry mouth in older adults

As people age, salivation decreases, leading to dry mouth and a reduced sense of taste. Certain drugs, such as anticholinergics, antihistamines, tricyclic antidepressants, phenothiazines, clonidine (Catapres), and opioid analgesics, can also decrease salivation. Be sure to take a drug history for older adults. Other causes of dry mouth in older adults include facial nerve paralysis, salivary duct obstruction, Sjögren's syndrome, and radiation of the mouth or face.

Down the hatch

When a person swallows, the cricopharyngeal sphincter in the upper esophagus relaxes, allowing food to enter the esophagus. In the esophagus, the glossopharyngeal nerve activates peristalsis, which moves the food bolus down toward the stomach.

One slippery bolus

As food passes through the esophagus, glands in the esophageal mucosal layer secrete mucus, which lubricates the bolus and protects the mucosal membrane from damage caused by poorly chewed foods.

Stomach express

Because food is only in the mouth for a short time, digestion of starch is limited. The salivary amylase that's swallowed continues to work for another 15 to 30 minutes in the stomach before it's inactivated by gastric acids. By the time the food bolus is traveling toward the stomach, the stomach has begun secreting digestive juices (hydrochloric acid [HCl] and pepsin).

Gastric phase

When food enters the stomach, the gastric phase of digestion begins. (See *Sites and mechanisms of gastric secretion*, page 560.)

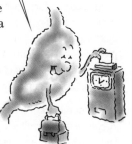

I punch the clock for chemical digestion. Yep, it all starts with me!

Stomach

Chemical digestion, which occurs as food mixes with digestive enzymes, begins in the stomach. The stomach acts, in part, as a temporary storage area for food and has four main regions:

 cardia

 fundus

 body

 antrum.

Cardia

The cardia lies near the junction of the stomach and esophagus. Relaxation of the cardiac sphincter in this region allows food to pass from the esophagus to the stomach.

Fundus

The *fundus* is an enlarged portion above and to the left of the esophageal opening into the stomach. Continued peristaltic activity in this region propels the intact food bolus toward the stomach body.

Body

The *body* is the middle portion of the stomach. In this region, distention of the stomach wall due to the food bolus stimulates secretion of gastrin.

Sites and mechanisms of gastric secretion

The body of the stomach lies between the lower esophageal, or *cardiac*, sphincter and the pyloric sphincter. Between these sphincters lie the fundus, body, antrum, and pylorus. These areas have a rich variety of mucosal cells that help the stomach carry out its tasks.

Glands and gastric secretions

Cardiac glands, pyloric glands, and gastric glands secrete 2 to 3 L of gastric juice daily through the stomach's gastric pits.

• The *cardiac gland* (near the lower esophageal sphincter [LES]) and the *pyloric gland* (near the pylorus) secrete thin mucus.

• The *gastric gland* (in the body and fundus) secretes hydrochloric acid (HCl), pepsinogen, intrinsic factor, and mucus.

Protection from self-digestion

Specialized cells line the gastric glands, gastric pits, and surface epithelium. Mucous cells in the necks of the gastric glands produce thin mucus. Mucous cells in the surface epithelium produce alkaline mucus. Both substances lubricate food and protect the stomach from self-digestion by corrosive enzymes.

Other secretions

Argentaffin cells produce gastrin, which stimulates gastric secretion and motility. *Chief cells* produce pepsinogen, which breaks proteins down into polypeptides.

Large parietal cells scattered throughout the fundus secrete HCl and intrinsic factor. HCl degrades pepsinogen, maintains an acid environment, and inhibits excess bacteria growth. Intrinsic factor promotes vitamin B_{12} absorption in the small intestine.

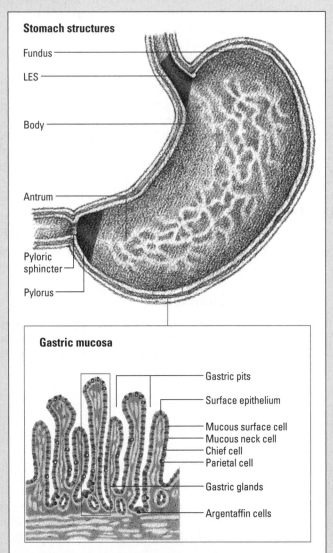

Stomach structures

- Fundus
- LES
- Body
- Antrum
- Pyloric sphincter
- Pylorus

Gastric mucosa

- Gastric pits
- Surface epithelium
- Mucous surface cell
- Mucous neck cell
- Chief cell
- Parietal cell
- Gastric glands
- Argentaffin cells

Gassing up with gastrin

Gastrin, in turn, stimulates the stomach's motor functions and release of digestive secretions by the gastric glands. Highly acidic (pH of 0.9 to 1.5), these secretions consist mainly of HCl, intrinsic factor (which helps the body absorb vitamin B_{12}), and proteolytic enzymes (which help the body use proteins). (See *GI system changes in older adults*.)

HCl helps absorb calcium and iron and activates gastric enzymes that kill most food-borne bacteria. HCl is also needed to convert the enzyme pepsinogen into pepsin.

Enzyme with pep

Pepsin becomes the major protein-splitting enzyme and, in turn, activates the secretion of the gastric mucus that protects the gastric lining. The mucus also helps move the food bolus along the path to the small intestine.

Not much at all but alcohol

Normally, except for alcohol, little food absorption occurs in the stomach. Peristaltic contractions in the stomach body churn the food into tiny particles and mix it with gastric juices, forming chyme.

Antrum

The *antrum* is the lower portion of the stomach, lying near the junction of the stomach and duodenum. Stronger peristaltic waves move the chyme from the stomach body into the antrum. Here, the chyme backs up against the pyloric sphincter before being released into the small intestine and triggering the intestinal phase of digestion. (See *Stomach emptying*.)

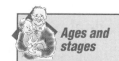

Ages and stages

GI system changes in older adults

Age-related changes in the GI system can lead to conditions that impact nutrition. Reduced gastric acid secretion in older adults can result in pernicious anemia, iron deficiency anemia, and reduced calcium absorption. Reduced production of bile acid, enlargement of the common bile duct, and increased output of cholecystokinin can lead to biliary stasis, cholelithiasis, and reduced appetite.

Stomach emptying

The rate of stomach emptying depends on several factors, including gastrin release, neural signals generated when the stomach wall distends, and the enterogastric reflex.

Enterogastric reflex

The *enterogastric reflex* is a response in which the duodenum releases secretin and gastric-inhibitory peptide, and the jejunum secretes cholecystokinin. Both reactions decrease gastric motility.

Intestinal phase

Most absorption occurs during the intestinal phase of digestion, which involves the small and large intestines.

Small intestine

The longest organ of the GI tract, the *small intestine* is a tube measuring about 20′ (6.1 m) long. It performs most of the work of digestion and absorption. (See *Digestion and absorption in the small intestine*.)

The small intestine has three major divisions:

 The *duodenum* is the longest and most superior division.

 The *jejunum*, the middle portion, is the shortest segment.

 The *ileum* is the most inferior portion.

Break it down, please

In the small intestine, intestinal wall contractions and digestive enzymes break down carbohydrates, proteins, and fats so the

---

Digestion and absorption in the small intestine

The small intestine performs most of the work of digestion and absorption. Here's a summary of the small intestine's major tasks.

Mechanical digestion
• Small muscles mix chyme.
• Peristaltic motions propel the food mass over the length of the intestine.
• Surface villi mix chyme at the intestinal wall, enhancing absorption.
• Long muscle moves the food mass in a circular motion, providing new surface sites for absorption.
• Segmentation rings from circular muscle mix the food into soft masses and then mix it with secretions.

Chemical digestion
• Lipase breaks fats into fatty acids and glycerides.
• Amylase converts starch to the disaccharides maltose and sucrose.
• Enterokinase activates trypsinogens, which become trypsin.
• Trypsin and chymotrypsin split protein molecules into small peptides and then into individual amino acids.

• Disaccharidases convert their respective disaccharides to monosaccharides.
• Bile from the liver helps to digest and absorb fat.
• Carbohydrate foods are changed into simple sugars.
• Fats are changed into fatty acids and glycerides.
• Proteins are changed into amino acids.
• Vitamins and minerals are also released.

Absorption
• Microvilli, villi, and mucus absorb essential nutrients.
• Absorption is controlled by diffusion—passive for the small materials and carrier-assisted for larger items.
• Digestive contents are mostly water soluble and can be absorbed directly into the circulation.
• Fatty contents aren't water soluble; they must pass through the villi, then into the lymph system, and finally into the bloodstream.

intestinal mucosa can facilitate absorption of these nutrients into the bloodstream (along with water and electrolytes). These nutrients are then available for use by the body.

The great intestinal wall

The intestinal wall has structural features that significantly increase its absorptive surface area. These features include:
- *plicae circulares*—circular folds of the intestinal mucosa or mucous membrane lining
- *villi*—fingerlike projections on the mucosa
- *microvilli*—tiny cytoplasmic projections on the surface of epithelial cells.

Secretion police

The small intestine also releases hormones that help control the secretion of bile, pancreatic juice, and intestinal juice.

Large intestine

The main tasks of the large intestine are absorption of body water and elimination of digestive waste. In addition, the large intestine harbors the bacteria *Escherichia coli*, *Enterobacter aerogenes*, *Clostridium perfringens*, and *Lactobacillus bifidus*. All of these bacteria help synthesize vitamin K and break down cellulose into usable carbohydrates. Bacterial action also produces *flatus*, which helps propel stools toward the rectum.

Protection from bacterial action

The mucosa of the large intestine also produces alkaline secretions from tubular glands composed of goblet cells. This alkaline mucus lubricates the intestinal walls as food pushes through, protecting the mucosa from acidic bacterial action.

From start to finish

The large intestine extends from the ileocecal valve (the valve between the ileum of the small intestine and the first segment of the large intestine) to the anus. The large intestine has five segments:

 cecum

 ascending colon

 transverse colon

 descending and sigmoid colons

 rectum.

Cecum

The *cecum*, a saclike structure, makes up the first few inches of the large intestine. The cecum is connected to the ileum of the small intestine by the ileocecal pouch.

Ascending colon

The ascending colon rises on the right posterior abdominal wall, and then turns under the liver at the hepatic flexure. By the time chyme passes through the ileocecal valve and enters the ascending colon of the large intestine, it has been reduced to mostly indigestible substances.

Transverse colon

The transverse colon is located above the small intestine, passing horizontally across the abdomen and below the liver, stomach, and spleen. It proceeds to turn downward at the left colic flexure. Through blood and lymph vessels, the large intestine has absorbed all but about 100 ml of water from the chyme by the time it leaves the transverse colon. It also absorbs large amounts of sodium and chloride at this point.

Got to have your fiber

Because dietary fiber isn't digested, it travels through the large intestine unabsorbed and contributes to the formation of feces.

Descending and sigmoid colons

The descending colon starts near the spleen and extends down the left side of the abdomen into the pelvic cavity. The sigmoid colon descends through the pelvic cavity, where it becomes the rectum. The descending and sigmoid colons are responsible for evacuation. Contents move slowly along the tract, enabling water and electrolytes to be absorbed.

Rectum

The *rectum*, the last few inches of the large intestine, terminates at the anus.

Mass movement

In the lower colon, long and relatively sluggish contractions cause propulsive waves or *mass movements*. Normally occurring several times per day, these movements propel intestinal contents into the rectum and produce the urge to defecate.

Accessory organs of digestion and absorption

Accessory organs of the digestive system—the liver, biliary duct system, and pancreas—contribute hormones, enzymes, and bile vital to digestion and absorption.

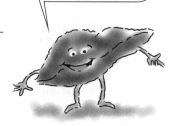

Hey, I don't mean to brag, but it says right here I'm the body's largest gland and highly vascular at that!

Liver

The body's largest gland, the highly vascular liver is enclosed in a fibrous capsule in the right upper quadrant of the abdomen. The *lesser omentum*, a fold of peritoneum, covers most of the liver and anchors it to the lesser curvature of the stomach. The *hepatic artery* and *hepatic portal vein* as well as the common bile duct and hepatic veins pass through the lesser omentum.

Functioning features

The liver's functional unit, the *lobule*, consists of a plate of hepatic cells, or *hepatocytes*, that encircle a central vein and radiate outward. Separating the hepatocyte plates from each other are *sinusoids*, the liver's capillary system. Reticuloendothelial macrophages (*Kupffer's cells*) lining the sinusoids remove bacteria and toxins that have entered the blood through the intestinal capillaries.

Go with the blood flow

The sinusoids carry oxygenated blood from the hepatic artery and nutrient-rich blood from the portal vein. Unoxygenated blood leaves through the central vein and flows through hepatic veins to the inferior vena cava.

All that and a bag of chips

The liver performs many important functions in the processes of digestion and absorption. The liver:
- aids in carbohydrate metabolism
- detoxifies various endogenous and exogenous toxins, such as drugs and alcohol
- synthesizes plasma proteins, nonessential amino acids, and vitamin A
- stores essential nutrients, such as vitamins K, D, B_{12}, and iron
- removes ammonia from body fluids, converting it to urea for excretion in urine

• converts glucose to glycogen and stores it as fuel for the muscles
• produces and secretes bile to aid in digestion
• stores fats and converts the excess sugars to fats to store in other parts of the body
• removes naturally occurring ammonia from body fluids, converting it to urea for excretion in the urine.

Biliary duct system

The biliary duct system consists of a network of ducts and includes the gallbladder.

Ducts

Think of ducts as a subway system transporting bile through the GI tract. *Bile* is a greenish liquid composed of water, cholesterol, bile salts, and phospholipids. From the liver, bile travels via the common bile duct to the small intestine, entering through the duodenum.

When bile salts are MIA

When bile salts are absent from the intestinal tract, lipids are excreted and fat-soluble vitamins are absorbed poorly.

Report on bile production

The liver recycles about 80% of bile salts into bile, combining them with bile pigments (biliverdin and bilirubin, the breakdown products of red blood cells) and cholesterol. The liver secretes this alkaline bile continuously. Bile production may increase from stimulation of the vagus nerve, release of the hormone secretin, increased blood flow in the liver, and the presence of fat in the intestine. (See *GI hormones: Production and function.*)

Gallbladder

The *gallbladder* is a pear-shaped organ joined to the ventral surface of the liver by the cystic duct. The gallbladder:
• stores and concentrates bile produced by the liver
• releases bile into the common bile duct for delivery to the duodenum in response to the contraction and relaxation of the sphincter of Oddi.

Cholecystokinin contraction

The secretion of the hormone cholecystokinin causes the gallbladder to contract. This contraction allows the release of bile into the common bile duct for delivery to the duodenum.

GI hormones: Production and function

When stimulated, GI structures secrete four hormones. Each hormone plays a different part in digestion.

Hormone and production site	Stimulating factor or agent	Function
Gastrin Produced in pyloric antrum and duodenal mucosa	• Pyloric antrum distention • Vagal stimulation • Protein digestion products • Alcohol	Stimulates gastric secretion and motility
Gastric inhibitory peptides Produced in duodenal and jejunal mucosa	• Gastric acid • Fats • Fat digestion products	Inhibits gastric secretion and motility
Secretin Produced in duodenal and jejunal mucosa	• Gastric acid • Fat digestion products • Protein digestion products	Stimulates secretion of bile and alkaline pancreatic fluid
Cholecystokinin Produced in duodenal and jejunal mucosa	• Fat digestion products • Protein digestion products	Stimulates gallbladder contraction and secretion of enzyme-rich pancreatic fluid

Pancreas

The *pancreas* is a somewhat flat organ that lies behind the stomach. Its head and neck extend into the curve of the duodenum and its tail lies against the spleen. The pancreas performs exocrine and endocrine functions.

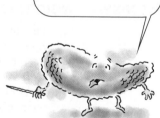

I may not be as large as the liver but I perform important exocrine and endocrine functions.

Exocrine function

The pancreas's exocrine function involves scattered cells that secrete more than 1,000 ml of digestive enzymes every day. Lobules and lobes of the clusters (*acini*) of enzyme-producing cells release their secretions into ducts that merge into the pancreatic duct. The pancreatic duct runs the length of the pancreas and joins the bile duct from the gallbladder before entering the duodenum. The vagus nerve stimulates the production and release of secretin and cholecystokinin, which are the two hormones responsible for regulating the rate and amount of pancreatic secretions.

Endocrine function

The endocrine function of the pancreas involves the islets of Langerhans. Two types of cells formulate the islets of Langerhans: alpha and beta cells.

The ABC's of alpha and beta cells

Over 1 million of these alpha and beta cells are in the islets. Alpha cells secrete *glucagon*, a hormone that stimulates glycogenolysis in the liver; beta cells secrete insulin to promote carbohydrate metabolism. Both hormones flow directly into the blood. Their release is stimulated by blood glucose levels.

Pancreatic duct

Running the length of the pancreas, the *pancreatic duct* joins the bile duct from the gallbladder before entering the duodenum. Vagal stimulation and release of the hormones secretin and chole-cystokinin control the rate and amount of pancreatic secretion.

A look at altered nutrition

Patients with nutritional problems may experience such signs and symptoms as excessive weight loss or gain, anorexia, or muscle wasting. Lifestyle habits, culture, and economic resources can also affect a person's nutritional status. Remember that clinical signs of nutritional deficiencies appear late. Also, be aware that patients hospitalized for more than 2 weeks risk developing a nutritional disorder. (See *Evaluation of nutritional findings*.)

> Remember that patients hospitalized for more than 2 weeks risk developing a nutritional disorder.

Excessive weight loss

Patients with nutritional deficiencies usually experience weight loss. Weight loss may result from decreased food intake, decreased food absorption, increased metabolic requirements, or a combination of the three. Other possible causes include endocrine, neoplastic, GI, and psychiatric disorders; chronic disease; infection; and neurologic lesions that cause paralysis and dysphagia.

Consumption conundrums

Excessive weight loss may also occur if the patient has a condition that prevents him from consuming a sufficient amount of

Evaluation of nutritional findings

This chart will help you interpret your nutritional assessment findings.

Body system or region	Sign or symptom	Implications
General	• Weakness and fatigue • Weight loss	• Anemia or electrolyte imbalance • Decreased calorie intake, increased calorie use, or inadequate nutrient intake or absorption
Skin, hair, and nails	• Dry, flaky skin • Dry skin with poor turgor • Rough, scaly skin with bumps • Petechiae or ecchymoses • Sore that won't heal • Thinning, dry hair • Spoon-shaped, brittle, or ridged nails	• Vitamin A, vitamin B complex, or linoleic acid deficiency • Dehydration • Vitamin A or essential fatty acid deficiency • Vitamin C or K deficiency • Protein, vitamin C, or zinc deficiency • Protein or zinc deficiency • Iron deficiency
Eyes	• Night blindness; corneal swelling, softening, or dryness; Bitot's spots (gray triangular patches on the conjunctiva) • Red conjunctiva	• Vitamin A deficiency • Riboflavin deficiency
Throat and mouth	• Cracks at corner of mouth • Magenta tongue • Beefy, red tongue • Soft, spongy, bleeding gums • Swollen neck (goiter)	• Riboflavin or niacin deficiency • Riboflavin deficiency • Vitamin B_{12} deficiency • Vitamin C deficiency • Iodine deficiency
Cardiovascular	• Edema • Tachycardia and hypotension	• Protein deficiency • Fluid volume deficit
GI	• Ascites	• Protein deficiency
Musculoskeletal	• Bone pain and bow leg • Muscle wasting • Pain in calves and thighs	• Vitamin D or calcium deficiency • Protein, carbohydrate, and fat deficiency • Thiamine deficiency
Neurologic	• Altered mental state • Paresthesia	• Dehydration and thiamine or vitamin B_{12} deficiency • Vitamin B_{12}, pyridoxine, or thiamine deficiency

food, such as painful oral lesions, ill-fitting dentures, or a loss of teeth. In addition, poverty, fad diets, excessive exercise, or certain drugs may contribute to excessive weight loss.

Excessive weight gain

When a person consumes more calories than his body requires for energy, his body stores excess adipose tissue, resulting in weight gain. Emotional factors (such as anxiety, guilt, and depression) as well as social factors can trigger overeating, resulting in excessive weight gain. Excessive weight gain is also a primary sign of many endocrine disorders. In addition, patients with conditions that limit activity, such as cardiovascular or respiratory disorders, may also experience excessive weight gain. (See *Overweight children*.)

Anorexia

Defined as a lack of appetite despite a physiologic need for food, *anorexia* commonly occurs with GI and endocrine disorders. It can also result from anxiety, chronic pain, poor oral hygiene, and changes in taste or smell that normally accompany aging. Short-term anorexia rarely jeopardizes health, but chronic anorexia can

Ages and stages

Overweight children

Like adults, the number of children considered overweight has dramatically increased in recent years. An estimated 15% of children and teens are overweight (as determined by their body mass index); another 15% risk becoming overweight. Most overweight children become overweight or obese adults.

More weight, more risks
Children who are overweight are more likely to have high cholesterol and high blood pressure (risk factors for heart disease) as well as type 2 diabetes. They also tend to suffer from poor self-esteem and depression because of their weight.

Counting causes
During your nutritional assessment, look for these common causes of excessive weight gain in children:

• lack of exercise
• sedentary lifestyle (involving an excessive amount of watching television, using computers, or playing video games)
• unhealthy eating habits.

Healthy habits
Help the child develop an exercise plan and suggest nutritious eating habits to prevent weight gain and promote a healthy lifestyle.

lead to life-threatening malnutrition. *Anorexia nervosa* is a psychological condition in which the patient severely restricts food intake, resulting in excessive weight loss.

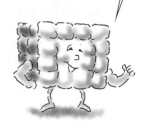

You need me to avoid atrophy, which can lead to lots of other undesirable conditions!

Muscle wasting

Usually a result of chronic protein deficiency, muscle wasting, or *atrophy*, results when muscle fibers lose bulk and length. The muscles involved shrink and lose their normal contour, appearing emaciated or even deformed. Associated signs and symptoms include chronic fatigue; apathy; anorexia; dry skin; peripheral edema; and dull, sparse, dry hair.

Lifestyle habits

Eating habits are usually set in childhood and can vary greatly from one person to another. Peer pressure and gender role stereotypes can affect a person's eating patterns. Food fads can also affect dietary patterns and may interfere with a healthy eating pattern. Nutritional supplements may not always have a scientific basis for their claims of better nutrition.

Today's fast-paced lives place families in tough situations when trying to provide well-balanced meals while maintaining busy schedules. The availability of prepackaged foods and fast food options is tempting.

Culture and beliefs

Culture plays a large role in the type of food eaten and dietary habits and patterns. Asians may eat rice with most meals, whereas Mexican Americans may have spicy, hot foods and Italians may prefer pasta.

Religious beliefs also play a large role in dietary habits. Certain religions restrict a particular food during a religious holiday, whereas others may encourage fasting. Still others restrict the kinds of foods that can be eaten in the same meal. (See *Religious practices and dietary restrictions*.)

Economic resources

A person's economic resources or lack of resources can severely alter his eating patterns and food choices. The lower a person's income, the less likely he'll be to have good nutrition. Low-income families, especially the

Religious practices and dietary restrictions

Religious beliefs can greatly impact dietary practices and, therefore, dietary nursing considerations. For example:
• Orthodox Jews who follow Kosher laws don't consume milk and other dairy products with meat or poultry.
• Many Seventh-Day Adventists are lactoovo vegetarians. Among those who do eat meat, pork is avoided.
• Hindus and Buddhists may also avoid consuming meat.

elderly, may have to sacrifice their food money to buy much needed prescriptions or to pay other bills, such as for heat and electricity. Because their income is lower, they may make poorer food choices because of their budgets. These choices may result in meals that are low in protein and high in starch.

Preventing altered nutrition

The most important role a nurse can provide to prevent altered nutrition is to teach the patient about proper diet and health promotion. To accomplish this goal, try to increase the patient's understanding of what a healthy diet includes. Knowledge doesn't always guarantee that the patient will follow the healthy diet, but the odds are greater if he has an understanding of what he should or shouldn't eat.

Promoting optimal intake

Illness greatly affects a person's eating habits and desire for food. Food should be served in an attractive, appetizing manner and be at the right temperature. The room should be pleasant and void of distractions. The patient's food preferences should be considered.

Pain medications and medications given to control nausea and pain should be timed to help the patient achieve optimal relief at mealtimes. Providing oral care before meals promotes taste and comfort. If possible and the patient's condition permits, the patient should receive meals sitting upright and out of bed in a chair. This position facilitates chewing and prevents choking and reflux of stomach contents.

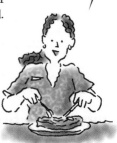

Now this looks mighty appetizing!

Assisting an adult with feeding

Confusion, arm or hand immobility, injury, weakness, or restrictions on activities or positions may prevent a patient from feeding himself. Feeding the patient then becomes a key nursing responsibility. An injured or debilitated patient may experience depression and subsequent anorexia. Meeting such a patient's nutritional needs requires determining food preferences; conducting the feeding in a friendly, unhurried manner; encouraging self-feeding to promote independence and dignity; and documenting intake and output.

What you need

Meal tray * overbed table * linen-saver pad or towels * clean linens * flexible straws * basin of water * feeding syringe * assistive feeding devices if necessary

Getting ready

- Raise the head of the bed if allowed. Fowler's or semi-Fowler's position makes swallowing easier and reduces the risk of aspiration and choking.
- Before the meal tray arrives, give the patient soap, a basin of water or a wet washcloth, and a hand towel *to clean his hands*. If necessary, you may wash his hands for him.
- Wipe the overbed table with soap and water or alcohol, especially if a urinal or bedpan was on it.
- When the meal tray arrives, compare the name on the tray with the name on the patient's wristband. Check the tray to make sure it contains foods appropriate for the patient's condition. (See *Special diets*.)

Special diets

Patients who are hospitalized may have different diets according to the reason for their hospitalization. Dietary intake is commonly changed to promote healing or to prevent complications such as a nothing-by-mouth status before surgery. Always check the doctor's orders before giving patients their meals to make sure that they're receiving the correct diet.

Nothing by mouth

The term *nothing by mouth*, or *NPO* (non per os), is actually the withholding of food or liquids. It may be indicated to:

- clear the GI tract of contents before surgery or a diagnostic procedure
- prevent aspiration in high-risk patients
- treat severe nausea and vomiting
- prevent aspiration during surgery
- rest the GI tract to promote healing
- treat medical problems such as a bowel obstruction.

Clear liquid

A clear-liquid diet includes only liquids that don't contain residue. It includes juices without pulp (such as apple or cranberry), tea, gelatin, clear broth, and soda. It's commonly used as the first diet ordered after surgery or before some diagnostic tests.

Full liquid

A full-liquid diet includes all foods and fluids that become a liquid at room temperature, such as ice cream or sherbet. This diet is commonly ordered for postoperative patients after a clear-liquid diet has been tolerated. It's

also used for patients who can't chew properly such as after a stroke.

Soft

A soft diet includes foods that are soft with reduced fiber. They may be further chopped or pureed for patients who have difficulty chewing or have no teeth. They're most commonly used for patients after surgery when a full-liquid diet has been tolerated.

Diet as tolerated

A diet classified as *as tolerated* can change as the patient's tolerance changes. For instance, a postoperative patient may start out with clear liquids but may progress to a regular diet if he hasn't had nausea or vomiting.

Restrictive diets

A restrictive diet is a diet that limits certain foods or a particular nutrient, such as sodium, potassium, and fat, or calorie content, depending on the patient's disease or metabolic status. For example, a patient who's obese may need to limit calorie intake and a cardiac patient may need to limit sodium intake.

How you do it

• *Because many adults consider being fed demeaning,* allow the patient some control over mealtime, such as letting him set the pace of the meal or decide the order in which he eats various foods.
• Encourage the patient to feed himself if he can. If he's restricted to the prone or the supine position but can use his arms and hands, encourage him to try foods he can pick up such as sandwiches. If he can assume Fowler's or semi-Fowler's position but has limited use of his arms or hands, teach him how to use assistive feeding devices. (See *Using assistive feeding devices.*)
• If necessary, tuck a napkin or towel under his chin *to protect his gown from spills.* Use a linen-saver pad or towel *to protect bed linens.*
• Position a chair next to the patient's bed so you can sit comfortably if you need to feed him yourself.
• Set up the patient's tray, remove the plate from the tray warmer, and discard all plastic wrappings. Then cut the food into bite-size pieces.

Peas at 12, corn at 3

• To help the blind or visually impaired patient feed himself, tell him that placement of various foods on his plate corresponds to the hours on a clock face. Maintain consistent placement for subsequent meals.
• Ask the patient which food he prefers to eat first *to promote his sense of control over the meal.* Some patients prefer to eat one food at a time, whereas others prefer to alternate foods.
• If the patient has difficulty swallowing, offer liquids carefully with a spoon or feeding syringe *to help prevent aspiration.* Pureed or soft foods, such as custard or flavored gelatin, may be easier to swallow than liquids. If the patient doesn't have difficulty swallowing, use a flexible straw *to reduce the risk of spills.*

We now pause for a break

• Ask the patient to indicate when he's ready for another mouthful. Pause between courses and whenever the patient wants to rest. During the meal, wipe the patient's mouth and chin as needed.
• When the patient finishes eating, remove the tray. If necessary, clean up spills and change the bed linens. Provide mouth care.

Using assistive feeding devices

Various feeding devices, available through consulting occupational therapy, can help the patient who has limited arm mobility, grasp, range of motion (ROM), or coordination. Before introducing your patient to an assistive feeding device, assess his ability to master it. Don't introduce a device he can't manage. If his condition is progressively disabling, encourage him to use the device only until his mastery of it falters.

Introduce the assistive device before mealtime, with the patient seated in a natural position. Explain its purpose, show the patient how to use it, and encourage him to practice. After meals, wash the device thoroughly and store it in the patient's bedside stand. Document the patient's progress and share it with staff and family members to help reinforce the patient's independence. Specific devices are discussed here.

Plate guard

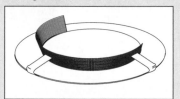

A plate guard blocks food from spilling off the plate. Attach the guard to the side of the plate opposite the hand the patient uses to feed himself. Guiding the patient's hand, show him how to push food against the guard to secure it on the utensil. Then have him try again with food of a different consistency. When the patient tires, feed him the rest of the meal. At subsequent meals, encourage the patient to feed himself for progressively longer periods until he can feed himself an entire meal.

Swivel spoon

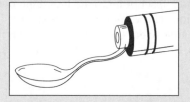

A swivel spoon helps the patient with limited ROM in his forearm and will fit in universal cuffs.

Universal cuffs

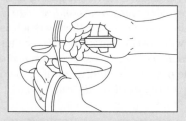

Universal cuffs are flexible bands that help the patient with flail hands or diminished grasp. Each cuff contains a slot that holds a fork or spoon. Attach the cuff to the hand the patient uses to feed himself. Then place the fork or spoon in the cuff slot. Bend the utensil to facilitate feeding.

Long-handled utensils

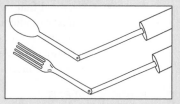

Long-handled utensils have jointed stems to help the patient with limited ROM in his elbow and shoulder.

Utensils with built-up handles

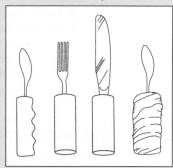

Utensils with built-up handles can help the patient with diminished grasp. They can be purchased or improvised by wrapping tape around the handles.

Practice pointers

- Don't feed the patient too quickly *because this can upset him and impair digestion.*
- If the patient is restricted to the supine position, provide foods that he can chew easily. If he's restricted to the prone position, feed him liquids carefully and only after he has swallowed his food *to reduce the risk of aspiration.*
- If the patient won't eat, try to find out why. For example, confirm his food preferences. Also, make sure the patient isn't in pain at mealtimes or that he hasn't received any treatments immediately before a meal that could upset or nauseate him. Find out if any medications cause anorexia, nausea, or sedation. Of course, clear the bedside of emesis basins, urinals, bedpans, and similar distractions at mealtimes.

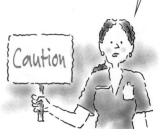

Don't feed a patient too quickly or you might upset him and impair digestion.

Caution

A plausible pattern

- Establish a pattern for feeding the patient, and share this information with the rest of the staff *so the patient doesn't need to repeatedly instruct staff members about the best way to feed him.*
- If the patient and his family are willing, suggest that family members assist with feeding. *Involving the family may make the patient feel more comfortable at mealtimes and ease discharge planning.*
- If the patient has a swallowing difficulty (such as in stroke or head injury), consult with speech therapy before feeding *to best determine the type of foods the patient requires (thickened and so forth).*
- Document the patient's feeding according to your facility's policy. (See *Recording fluid intake and output.*)

Feeding tube insertion and removal

Inserting a feeding tube into the stomach or duodenum allows patients who can't or won't eat to receive nourishment. The feeding tube also permits administration of supplemental feedings to patients who have high nutritional requirements, such as unconscious patients or those with extensive burns. The preferred feeding tube route is nasal, but the oral route may be used for patients with such conditions as a deviated septum or a head or nose injury.

Can't stomach this

The doctor may order duodenal feeding when the patient can't tolerate gastric feeding or when he expects gastric feeding to produce aspiration. Absence of bowel sounds or possible intestinal obstruction contraindicates using a feeding tube.

Recording fluid intake and output

Accurate intake and output records help evaluate a patient's fluid and electrolyte balance, suggest various diagnoses, and influence the choice of fluid therapy. These records are mandatory for patients with burns, renal failure, electrolyte imbalance, recent surgical procedures, heart failure, or severe vomiting and diarrhea, and for patients receiving diuretics or corticosteroids. Intake and output records are also significant in monitoring patients with nasogastric (NG) tubes or drainage collection devices, and those receiving I.V. therapy.

Fluid intake consists of all fluid entering the patient's body, including beverages, fluids contained in solid foods taken by mouth, and foods that are liquid at room temperature, such as flavored gelatin, custard, ice cream, and some beverages. Additional intake includes GI instillations, bladder irrigations, and I.V. fluids.

Fluid output consists of all fluid that leaves the patient's body, including urine, loose stools, vomitus, aspirated fluid loss, and drainage from surgical drains, NG tubes, and chest tubes.

When recording fluid intake and output, enlist the patient's help if possible. Record amount in cubic centimeters (cc) or milliliters (ml). Measure; don't estimate. For a small child, weigh diapers if appropriate. Monitor intake and output during each shift, and notify the doctor if amounts differ significantly over a 24-hour period. Document your findings in the appropriate location; describe any fluid restrictions and the patient's compliance.

Flexibility rules!

Feeding tubes are made of silicone, rubber, or polyurethane and have small diameters and great flexibility. To ease passage, some feeding tubes are weighted with tungsten, and some need a guide wire to keep them from curling in the back of the throat. These small-bore tubes usually have radiopaque markings and a water-activated coating, which provides a lubricated surface.

What you need

For gastric feedings

Feeding formula ✳ graduated container ✳ 120 ml of water ✳ gavage bag with tubing and flow regulator clamp ✳ towel or linen-saver pad ✳ 60-ml syringe ✳ pH test strip ✳ optional: infusion controller and tubing set (for continuous administration), adapter to connect gavage tubing to feeding tube

For nasal and oral care

Cotton-tipped applicators ✳ water-soluble lubricant ✳ lemon glycerin swabs ✳ petroleum jelly

Bulbs, catheters, and pumps

A bulb syringe or large catheter-tip syringe may be substituted for a gavage bag after the patient demonstrates tolerance for a gravity drip infusion. The doctor may order an infusion pump to ensure accurate delivery of the prescribed formula.

Getting ready

- Be sure to refrigerate formulas prepared in the dietary department or pharmacy. Refrigerate commercial formulas only after opening them.
- Check the date on all formula containers.
- Discard expired commercial formula.
- Use powdered formula within 24 hours of mixing.

Shake . . .

- Always shake the container well to mix the solution thoroughly.
- Allow the formula to warm to room temperature before administration. *Cold formula can increase the chance of diarrhea.*
- Never warm it over direct heat or in a microwave *because heat may curdle the formula or change its chemical composition. Also, hot formula may injure the patient.*

. . . and pour

- Pour 60 ml of water into the graduated container.
- After closing the flow clamp on the administration set, pour the appropriate amount of formula into the gavage bag.
- Hang no more than a 4- to 6-hour supply at one time *to prevent bacterial growth.*
- Open the flow clamp on the administration set *to remove air from the lines and prevent air from entering the patient's stomach, causing distention and discomfort.*

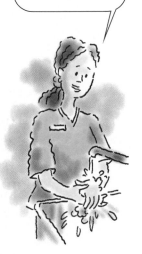

This is an important first step.

How you do it

- Provide privacy and wash your hands.
- Inform the patient that he'll receive nourishment through the tube, and explain the procedure to him. If possible, give him a schedule of subsequent feedings.
- If the patient has a nasal or oral tube, cover his chest with a towel or linen-saver pad *to protect him and the bed linens from spills.*
- Assess the patient's abdomen for bowel sounds and distention.

Delivering a gastric feeding

- Elevate the bed to semi-Fowler's or high-Fowler's position *to prevent aspiration by gastroesophageal reflux and to promote digestion.*
- Check placement of the feeding tube *to make sure it hasn't slipped out since the last feeding.*

- Never give a tube feeding until you're sure the tube is properly positioned in the patient's stomach. *Administering a feeding through a misplaced tube can cause formula to enter the patient's lungs.*
- *To check tube patency and position,* remove the cap or plug from the feeding tube, and use the syringe to aspirate gastric secretions gently.

Proper pH please!

- Examine the aspirate and place a small amount on the pH test strip. Proper placement of the gastric tube is likely if the aspirate has a typical gastric fluid appearance (grassy-green, clear and colorless with mucous shreds, or brown) and the pH is 5.0 or less.
- *To assess gastric emptying,* aspirate and measure residual gastric contents. Hold feedings if residual volume is greater than the predetermined amount specified in the doctor's order (usually 50 to 100 ml). Reinstill any aspirate obtained.
- Connect the gavage bag tubing to the feeding tube. Depending on the type of tube used, you may need to use an adapter to connect the two.
- If you're using a bulb or catheter-tip syringe, remove the bulb or plunger and attach the syringe to the pinched-off feeding tube *to prevent excess air from entering the patient's stomach, causing distention.*
- If you're using an infusion controller, thread the tube from the formula container through the controller according to the manufacturer's directions.
- Blue food dye can be added to food *to quickly identify aspiration.*
- Purge the tubing of air and attach it to the feeding tube.
- Open the regulator clamp on the gavage bag tubing and adjust the flow rate appropriately.
- When using a bulb syringe, fill the syringe with formula and release the feeding tube *to allow formula to flow through it.* The height at which you hold the syringe will determine flow rate. When the syringe is three-quarters empty, pour more formula into it.
- *To prevent air from entering the tube and the patient's stomach,* never allow the syringe to empty completely.
- If you're using an infusion controller, set the flow rate according to the manufacturer's directions.

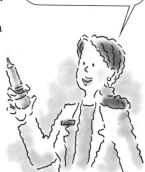

When using a bulb syringe, fill it with formula and release the feeding tube to allow formula to flow through it.

Slowly please!

- Always administer a tube feeding slowly—typically 200 to 350 ml over 15 to 30 minutes, depending on the patient's tolerance and the doctor's order—*to prevent sudden stomach distention, which can cause nausea, vomiting, cramps, or diarrhea.*

- After administering the appropriate amount of formula, flush the tubing by adding about 60 ml of water to the gavage bag or bulb syringe, or manually flush it using a barrel syringe. *Flushing maintains the tube's patency by removing excess formula, which could occlude the tube.*
- If you're administering a continuous feeding, flush the feeding tube every 4 hours *to help prevent tube occlusion.* Monitor gastric emptying every 4 hours by assessing gastric residuals.

We're all done

- To discontinue gastric feeding (depending on the equipment you're using), close the regulator clamp on the gavage bag tubing, disconnect the syringe from the feeding tube, or turn off the infusion controller.
- Cover the end of the feeding tube with its plug or cap *to prevent leakage and contamination of the tube.*
- Leave the patient in semi-Fowler's or high-Fowler's position for at least 30 minutes.
- Rinse all reusable equipment with warm water.
- Dry it and store it in a convenient place for the next feeding. Change equipment every 24 hours or according to the facility's policy.

Practice pointers

- If the feeding solution doesn't initially flow through a bulb syringe, attach the bulb and squeeze it gently *to start the flow.* Then remove the bulb. Never use the bulb to force the formula through the tube.
- If the patient becomes nauseated or vomits, stop the feeding immediately. *The patient may vomit if the stomach becomes distended from overfeeding or delayed gastric emptying.*
- *To reduce oropharyngeal discomfort from the tube,* allow the patient to brush his teeth or care for his dentures regularly, and encourage frequent gargling.
- If the patient is unconscious, administer oral care with wet sponge-tipped swabs every 4 hours. Use petroleum jelly on dry, cracked lips.

I'm parched

- Dry mucous membranes may indicate dehydration, which requires increased fluid intake.
- Clean the patient's nostrils with cotton-tipped applicators, apply lubricant along the mucosa, and assess the skin for signs of breakdown.
- During continuous feedings, assess the patient frequently for abdominal distention. Flush the tubing by adding about 50 ml

of water to the gavage bag or bulb syringe. *Flushing the tubing maintains the tube's patency by removing excess formula, which could occlude the tube.*
• If the patient develops diarrhea, administer small, frequent, less concentrated feedings, or administer bolus feedings over a longer time.
• Make sure that the formula isn't cold and that proper storage and sanitation practices have been followed. The loose stools associated with tube feedings make extra perineal and skin care necessary. Changing to a formula with more fiber may eliminate liquid stools.

More fruits and veggies

• If the patient becomes constipated, the doctor may increase the fruit, vegetable, or sugar content of the formula.
• Assess the patient's hydration status *because dehydration may produce constipation.* Increase fluid intake as necessary. If the condition persists, administer an appropriate drug or enema, as ordered.
• Drugs can be administered through the feeding tube.
• Except for enteric-coated drugs or time-released medications, crush tablets or open and dilute capsules in water before administering them. Be sure to flush the tubing afterward *to ensure full instillation of medication.* Keep in mind that some drugs may change the osmolarity of the feeding formula and cause diarrhea.

Hold the wire

• Small-bore feeding tubes may kink, making instillation impossible. If you suspect this problem, try changing the patient's position, or withdraw the tube a few inches and restart. Never use a guide wire to reposition the tube.
• Constantly monitor the flow rate of a blended or high-residue formula *to determine if the formula is clogging the tubing as it settles.* To prevent such clogging, squeeze the bag frequently *to agitate the solution.*
• Collect blood samples as ordered.
• Glycosuria, hyperglycemia, and diuresis can indicate an excessive carbohydrate level, leading to hyperosmotic dehydration, which may be fatal. Monitor blood glucose levels *to assess glucose tolerance.* (A patient with a serum glucose level of less than 200 mg/dl is considered stable.) Also monitor serum electrolytes, blood urea nitrogen, serum glucose, serum osmolality, and other pertinent findings *to determine the patient's response to therapy and assess his hydration status.*

Take note!

Documenting tube feedings

When documenting tube feedings be sure to include the details listed below:

• On the intake and output sheet, record the date, volume of formula, and volume of water.

• In your notes, include abdominal assessment (including tube exit site if appropriate); amount of residual gastric contents; verification of tube placement; amount, type, and time of feeding; and tube patency.

• Discuss the patient's tolerance of the feeding, including nausea, vomiting, cramping, diarrhea, and distention.

• Note the result of blood and urine tests, hydration status, and any drugs given through the tube.

• Include the date and time of administration set changes, oral and nasal hygiene, and results of specimen collections.

Check the flow, Flo!

• Check the flow rate hourly *to ensure correct infusion.* (With an improvised administration set, use a time tape to record the rate *because it's difficult to get precise readings from an irrigation container or enema bag.*)

• For duodenal or jejunal feeding, most patients tolerate a continuous drip better than bolus feedings. *Bolus feedings can cause such complications as hyperglycemia and diarrhea.*

• Until the patient acquires a tolerance for the formula, you may need to dilute it to one-half or three-quarters strength to start, and increase it gradually.

• Patients under stress or who are receiving steroids may experience a pseudodiabetic state. Assess them frequently *to determine the need for insulin.*

• Document the procedure and the feeding according to your facility's policy. (See *Documenting tube feedings.*)

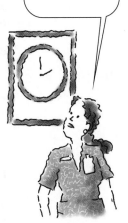

Check the flow rate hourly to ensure correct infusion.

References

U.S. Department of Agriculture. (n.d.). *MyPlate.* Retrieved from http://www.choosemyplate.gov

U.S. Department of Health and Human Services & U.S. Department of Agriculture. (2010). *Dietary Guidelines for Americans, 2010* (7th ed.). Washington, DC: U.S. Government Printing Office. Retrieved from http://www.health.gov/dietaryguidelines/dga2010/dietaryguidelines2010.pdf

Quick quiz

1. Through metabolism, energy is extracted from which nutrients?
   A.   Carbohydrates, proteins, and fats
   B.   Carbohydrates, fats, and sodium
   C.   Fats, adenosine triphosphate, and minerals
   D.   Vitamins, minerals, and electrolytes

Answer: A. Energy is produced through the metabolism of carbohydrates, proteins, and fats.

2. Essential nutrients are supplied to the body by:
   A.   vitamin or mineral supplements.
   B.   certain food combinations.
   C.   body functions.
   D.   food in many different combinations.

Answer: D. Essential nutrients are supplied by the many combinations of food consumed.

3. Which GI hormone stimulates gastric secretion and motility?
   A.   Gastric inhibitory peptides
   B.   Gastrin
   C.   Secretin
   D.   Pepsinogen

Answer: B. Gastrin is produced in the pyloric antrum and duodenal end mucosa and stimulates gastric secretion and motility.

4. In which phase of digestion does the stomach secrete the digestive juices HCl and pepsin?
   A.   Cephalic
   B.   Gastric
   C.   Intestinal
   D.   Mastication

Answer: A. By the time the food is traveling toward the stomach, the cephalic phase—during which the stomach secretes digestive juices—has begun.

Scoring

★★★   If you answered all four questions correctly, gee whiz! Your nutritional knowledge is optimal.

★★   If you answered three questions correctly, great! Your ingestion of nutrition facts is quite sufficient.

★   If you answered fewer than three questions correctly, no worries! Review the chapter, absorb some more facts, and start over.

19

Urinary elimination

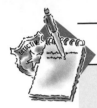

Just the facts

In this chapter, you'll learn:

♦ process of urine formation
♦ factors that affect urinary elimination
♦ common urinary abnormalities
♦ proper methods for obtaining urine specimens
♦ proper method for obtaining urine specific gravity
♦ steps for insertion, care, and removal of an indwelling urinary catheter
♦ proper method for applying a condom catheter.

A look at the urinary system

The urinary system consists of the kidneys, ureters, bladder, and urethra.

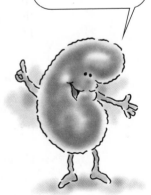

I'm essential to a well-balanced urinary system.

Kidneys

The essential functions of the urinary system—such as forming and excreting urine to maintain the proper balance of fluids and electrolytes, minerals, and organic substances for homeostasis—take place in the highly vascular kidneys. These bean-shaped organs are 4½″ to 5″ (11.4 to 12.7 cm) long and 2½″ (6.4 cm) wide.

Located retroperitoneal on either side of the lumbar vertebrae, the kidneys lie posterior to the abdominal organs and are protected by the contents of the abdomen. The right kidney extends slightly lower than the left kidney. A layer of fat surrounds each kidney, offering further protection. Each kidney consists of three regions:

 renal cortex (outer region)

 renal medulla (middle region)

 renal pelvis (inner region). (See *A close look at the kidneys.*)

A close look at the kidneys

The kidneys are located in the lumbar area, with the right kidney situated slightly lower than the left to make room for the liver, which is just above it. The position of the kidneys shifts somewhat with changes in body position. Covering the kidneys are the fibrous capsule, perirenal fat, and renal fasciae.

Blood's cleansing journey

The kidneys receive waste-filled blood from the renal artery, which branches off the abdominal aorta. After passing through a complicated network of smaller blood vessels and nephrons, the filtered blood returns to the circulation by way of the renal vein, which empties into the inferior vena cava.

Continuing the cleanup

The kidneys excrete waste products that the nephrons remove from the blood. These excretions combine with other waste fluids (such as urea, creatinine, phosphates, and sulfates) to form urine. An action called *peristalsis* (the circular contraction and relaxation of a tube-shaped structure) passes the urine through the ureters and into the urinary bladder. When the bladder has filled, nerves in the bladder wall relax the sphincter. In conjunction with a voluntary stimulus, this relaxation causes urine to pass into the urethra for elimination from the body.

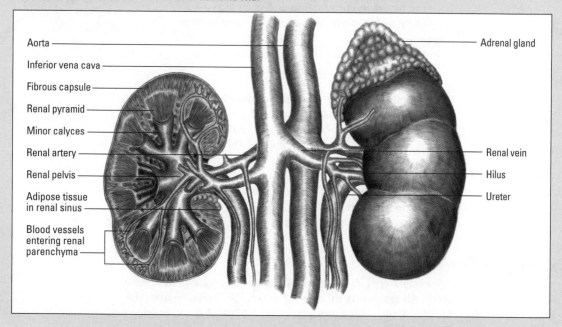

Filtering station

The outer portion of the kidney is called the *renal cortex*. It contains blood-filtering mechanisms called *nephrons* and is protected by a fibrous capsule and layers of fat.

Renal wonder

The *renal medulla* contains 8 to 12 renal pyramids—striated wedges that are composed mostly of tubular structures. The tapered portion of each pyramid empties into a cuplike calyx that channels formed urine from the pyramids into the renal pelvis. The renal pelvis receives urine through the major calyces and then urine moves into the ureters and lastly to the bladder.

All in a day's work

Kidney functions include:
• elimination of wastes and excess ions (in the form of urine)
• blood filtration (by regulating chemical composition and blood volume)
• maintenance of fluid–electrolyte and acid–base balances
• production and release of renin to promote angiotensin II activation and aldosterone production in the adrenal gland
• promotion of erythropoietin (a hormone that stimulates red blood cell production and such enzymes as renin, which governs blood pressure and kidney function)
• conversion of vitamin D to a more active form.

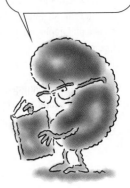

Hmm . . . It appears that I'm responsible for several important functions.

Makin' urine

The nephron is the functional unit of the kidneys. Each kidney contains roughly 1 million nephrons. Urine gathers in the collecting tubules and ducts of the nephrons and then drains into the ureters, down into the bladder, and out through the urethra.

A wealth of minerals

Formed urine consists of water, sodium, chloride, potassium, calcium, magnesium, sulfates, phosphates, bicarbonates, uric acid, ammonium ions, creatinine, and urobilinogen (a derivative of bilirubin).

Go with the flow

Approximately 250 to 400 ml of urine is expressed when someone voids. All but 5 to 10 ml of urine is typically emptied from the bladder. Daily urine output averages 720 to 2,400 ml, varying with fluid intake and climate.

Ureters

The ureters are a pair of muscular tubes that extend 10″ to 12″ (25.5 to 30.5 cm) from the urinary bladder. The left ureter is slightly longer than the right because of the left kidney's higher position. The diameter of each ureter varies from ⅛″ to ¼″ (3 to 6 mm), with the narrowest part at the ureteropelvic junction.

Where the action is

Located along the posterior abdominal wall, the ureters enter the bladder anteromedially. They carry urine from the kidneys to the bladder by peristaltic contractions that occur one to five times per minute.

Color clues

Normal urine color ranges from straw yellow to dark yellow. Certain medications and reduced or increased fluid intake can alter its color. Amitriptyline (Elavil) can turn urine blue green, and phenazopyridine (Pyridium) may produce bright orange urine. Very dilute urine is almost colorless, and concentrated urine can be dark amber or orange-brown.

Clear is cool

Freshly voided urine should appear clear with no sediment. Urine collected from an indwelling urinary catheter bag may contain mucus shreds, but urine in the tubing should still be clear.

Odor alert

The more dilute urine is, the fainter the odor. Concentrated urine will have a strong odor, and collected urine that's long-standing may develop a strong ammonia smell. Certain infections may also cause urine to have a foul or offensive odor.

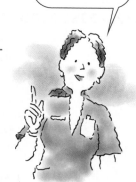

A full bladder can contain about 1 L of urine.

Bladder

Located in the pelvis, the bladder is a hollow, muscular organ that serves as a temporary storage reservoir for urine collection. When the bladder is empty, it lies behind the pelvic bone; when it's full, it becomes displaced under the peritoneal cavity. Bladder capacity ranges from 500 to 1,000 ml in healthy adults and is lower in children and the elderly.

Urethra

The urethra is a small duct that carries urine from the bladder and out of the body. A woman's urethra is only 1″ to 2″ (2.5 to 5 cm) long and is anterior to the vaginal opening. Because a man's urethra must pass through the erectile tissue of the penis, it's about 6″ (15.2 cm) longer than a woman's.

Dual role

In men, the urethra is part of the reproductive system because it also transports semen.

Factors affecting urinary elimination

Several factors can affect how urine is eliminated, including body position, decreased muscle tone, fluid intake, hypotension, infection, loss of body fluid, medications, neurologic injury, nutrition, obstruction of urinary flow, psychological problems, and surgery.

Body position

The ability to empty the bladder during each voiding is dependent on proper body positioning, which is normally standing for men and sitting for women.

Up or down

Offering a urinal to a male patient who's flat in bed will affect his ability to initiate a urine stream and empty his bladder completely. Conversely, placing a female patient on a bedpan while she's lying flat in bed will affect her ability to urinate and empty her bladder completely.

Decreased muscle tone

A voluntary contraction and relaxation of the abdominal and perineal muscles controls urination. Weakened perineal detrusor or abdominal muscles can result from trauma, surgery, obesity, multiple pregnancies, stretching during childbirth, and chronic constipation. When these muscles become weak and muscle tone is decreased, it becomes more difficult for the patient to control the urge to void, which results in incontinence.

A cystocele is a protrusion of the bladder into the vaginal canal that occurs when the vaginal wall musculature weakens as a result of muscle straining during childbirth or other straining such as heavy lifting. It can cause stress incontinence, dribbling, frequency, and an inability to empty the bladder completely.

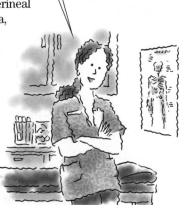

When abdominal and perineal muscles become weak and muscle tone is decreased, it becomes more difficult for the patient to control the urge to void.

Stretch and tone

A patient who has had a long-standing indwelling urinary catheter may have trouble regaining bladder control when the catheter is removed. The continuous drainage caused by the indwelling catheter doesn't allow the bladder to fill or stretch to capacity. Because the bladder wall doesn't stretch, atrophy can develop. Dribbling after the catheter is removed is usually temporary until bladder tone returns.

Fluid intake

A patient's fluid intake is directly related to urinary volume and frequency. Urine output will decrease if fluid intake decreases. Similarly, urine output will increase if fluid intake increases. If fluid intake increases significantly, frequency of urination will also increase.

Yin and yang

The correlation of intake affecting output is regulated by several hormones, such as angiotensin I and II, aldosterone, erythropoietin, and antidiuretic hormone (ADH). The most important hormone is ADH, which regulates the amount of reabsorption that occurs in the nephrons of the kidney and conserves body water by reducing urine output. ADH is released when fluid intake is decreased. The kidney then reabsorbs more water and produces more highly concentrated urine. When fluid intake increases, ADH suppression is reduced.

Hypotension

Hypotension (low arterial blood pressure) reduces blood flow to the kidneys. Adequate blood flow to the kidneys is necessary for urine production. Thus, hypotension prevents filtration from occurring. Surgery, trauma, or a severe fluid loss from vomiting or diarrhea can cause hypotension, which results in a decrease in circulating blood volume and decreased filtration and urinary excretion.

Infection

The urinary tract is sterile, except at the urinary meatus, and microorganisms there usually get washed away during urination. Urinary tract infections (UTIs) occur when microorganisms from the perineal or anal area come in contact with the urinary meatus and ascend into the urethra. This contact is usually the result of sexual intercourse, poor hygiene after bowel movements, or insertion of a urinary catheter or a diagnostic instrument. UTIs can cause urgency, frequency, and dysuria.

Infection protection

Lower UTIs are more common and occur in the urethra or bladder. Upper UTIs occur in the ureters, kidneys, pelvis, or renal tubule system. They're more serious and can lead to kidney damage and renal failure. If left untreated, however, lower UTIs can progress to the kidneys and result in renal damage and renal failure (and become upper UTIs).

Women are particularly susceptible to UTIs due to the proximity of the urinary meatus to the vagina and rectum and because their urethra is much shorter.

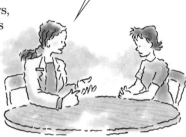

Women are particularly susceptible to UTIs.

Loss of body fluid

Loss of body fluid can result from excessive diuresis caused by fever, exercise, vomiting, diarrhea, and excessive wound drainage or blood loss from surgery or trauma. The kidneys respond to this loss by increasing water absorption to conserve water, causing a decrease in urine output.

Medications

Diuretics are used to promote the excretion of water and electrolytes by the kidneys.

To go . . .

Commonly used diuretics include furosemide (Lasix), chlorothiazide (Diuril), triamterene (Dyrenium), hydrochlorothiazide (HydroDIURIL), and spironolactone (Aldactone).

Cholinergic medications, such as bethanechol (Urecholine), may be prescribed because they stimulate contraction of the detrusor muscle, which promotes voiding.

Urinary frequency or urgency may be treated with oxybutynin (Ditropan) because of its antispasmodic effect on the detrusor muscle.

. . . or not to go

Other medications can also affect urinary output. Opioids can decrease the glomerular filtration rate and the sensation of a full bladder. Phenothiazines, belladonna alkaloids, tricyclic antidepressants, and antihistamines have anticholinergic effects and can increase urine retention.

Neurologic injury

The frontal lobe of the brain controls voluntary urination. Hemorrhage, trauma, or a tumor in this lobe can result in urinary incontinence. A spinal cord injury or a stroke also can interfere with normal urinary elimination.

Reflex control

Injury to the sacral area of the spinal cord, which controls the urination reflex, can change urinary elimination patterns. When the bladder becomes full and stretched to capacity, it contracts and urination occurs. This is called *reflex neurogenic bladder*. An *autonomous neurogenic bladder* that can occur as a result of neurologic injury results in urine retention because the bladder fills without the bladder stretch mechanism in place.

Nutrition

A diet consisting of foods high in water content, such as soups, gelatin desserts, vegetables, and fruits, will increase urine output. Salty foods can decrease urine output, especially if water intake doesn't increase. Food and drinks containing caffeine (chocolate, coffee, tea, and cola), which is a diuretic, and alcohol can increase urine output.

Obstruction of urine flow

Obstruction of urine flow can lead to decreased urinary elimination. Structural abnormalities in the urinary system can cause such obstructions as urinary tumors, renal stones, and an enlarged prostate gland. Obstruction can also result from clogs or kinks in an indwelling catheter. Unrelieved obstruction causes increased resistance to urine flow and can lead to hydronephrosis (distention of the renal pelvis).

An infection connection

Prolonged obstruction can lead to urinary stasis, a condition that provides a breeding ground for microorganisms and resulting UTIs.

Psychological factors

Urination is a voluntary function that's affected by internal and external factors.

Into the void

Stress and anxiety can cause a patient to contract his muscles involuntarily, making urination impossible or making the urge to urinate uncontrollable. In addition, asking a patient for a urine sample or to urinate "on demand" can make him unable to urinate.

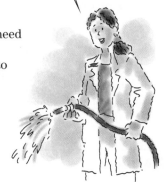

The sound or feel of running water can intensify the need to urinate.

Babbling brook

The sound or feel of running water can intensify the need to urinate. If a patient has difficulty voiding, try pouring warm water over his inner thigh or perineal area to initiate urination.

Privacy, please

Always consider a patient's need for privacy, especially when a bedpan or urinal must be used.

Surgery

Most patients should be able to urinate within 6 to 8 hours after surgery. If a patient can't urinate following surgery, limited fluid intake and fluid and blood loss during surgery with a resulting depletion in fluid volume may be the cause. The stress that accompanies surgery can cause the release of ADH, which also decreases urinary output. Urine retention is also an adverse effect of some pain medications such as opioids.

Edema dilemma

Urinary, intestinal, or reproductive surgery also predisposes a patient to postoperative urinary retention. Trauma to the tissues causes edema and can obstruct urinary flow.

How dry am I?

Medications used for spinal anesthesia or regional blocks can cause temporary urinary problems because they impair sensory and motor impulses that control urination. When the anesthetic wears off, the patient should be able to resume his normal voiding pattern.

Common urinary abnormalities

Common abnormalities in the urinary system include dysuria; hematuria; nocturia; polyuria; urinary frequency, urgency, and hesitancy; and urinary incontinence.

Dysuria

Pain during urination, or *dysuria*, commonly signals a lower UTI. The onset of the pain signifies the cause. Pain immediately before urination indicates bladder irritation or distention, whereas pain at the onset usually signals a bladder outlet obstruction. Bladder spasm can cause pain at the end of the stream. Pain throughout urination may indicate pyelonephritis, especially when accompanied by fever, chills, hematuria, and flank pain.

Hematuria

Brown or bright red urine is a sign of hematuria or blood in the urine. When the bleeding occurs during elimination, it can indicate the location of the underlying problem. For example, a urethral disorder will cause bleeding at the onset of urination. Bleeding at the end of the stream suggests a disorder of the bladder neck or prostate gland.

From the neck up

Bleeding throughout urination indicates a disorder located above the bladder neck. Hematuria can also be caused by gastrointestinal (GI), vaginal, or some coagulation disorders or cancer.

Only temporary

In addition, males may experience hematuria temporarily following urinary tract or prostate surgery or after a urethral catheterization.

Nocturia

Excessive urination at night, known as *nocturia*, is a common sign of kidney or lower urinary tract disorders. It can result from a disruption of normal urine patterns or overstimulation of the nerves and muscles that control urination. Cardiovascular, endocrine, or metabolic disorders; diuretics; and increased fluid intake can also produce nocturia.

In men, nocturia can result from benign prostatic hyperplasia (BPH), when significant urethral obstruction develops, or from prostate cancer.

Polyuria

Polyuria is the production and excretion of more than 2,500 ml of urine per day. It's a fairly common condition that's usually a result of diabetes insipidus, diabetes mellitus, or diuretic use. Other causes of polyuria include urologic disorders, such as pyelonephritis and postobstructive uropathy, and some psychological, neurologic, and renal disorders. Patients with polyuria are at risk for developing hypovolemia.

It's a classic! Urinary frequency is a classic symptom of a UTI.

Urinary frequency, urgency, and hesitancy

Urinary frequency commonly results from decreased bladder capacity and is a classic symptom of a UTI. Frequency also occurs with urethral stricture, neurologic disorders, pregnancy, and uterine tumors.

In men, urinary frequency also occurs with BPH, urethral stricture, or a prostate tumor, all of which can put pressure on the bladder.

Pain picture

The sudden urge to urinate, or *urinary urgency*, when accompanied by bladder pain is another symptom of a UTI. Even small amounts of urine in the bladder can cause pain because inflammation decreases bladder capacity. Urgency without pain may be a symptom of an upper motor neuron lesion.

Start 'er up?

Difficulty starting a urine stream, or *urinary hesitancy*, can occur with a UTI, a partial obstruction of the lower urinary tract, neuromuscular disorders, or the use of certain drugs.

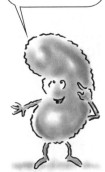

What to do, what to do! I just can't decide if I want to go or not.

Stalling

Urinary hesitancy is most common in older male patients with an enlarged prostate gland, which can cause partial obstruction of the urethra.

Urinary incontinence

Urinary incontinence is a common condition that may be transient or permanent with a minimal or significant release of urine. Possible causes include stress incontinence, tumor, bladder cancer and calculi, and such neurologic disorders as Guillain-Barré syndrome, multiple sclerosis, and spinal cord injury.

In men, urinary incontinence may also be a symptom of BPH, prostate infection, or prostate cancer.

Nursing interventions for altered urinary elimination

Nursing interventions for altered urinary elimination include bedpan and urinal use; collecting urine specimens; obtaining urine specific gravity; applying a condom catheter or male incontinence device; and insertion, care, and removal of an indwelling urinary catheter.

Bedpan and urinal use

Bedpans and urinals permit elimination by a bedridden patient and provide a way to accurately observe and measure urine and stool. A female patient can use a bedpan for urination and defecation. A male patient normally uses a urinal for urination and a bedpan for defecation. Be sure to offer these devices frequently—before meals, visiting hours, morning and evening care, and treatments or procedures. Always allow the patient privacy.

What you need

Fracture or regular bedpan or urinal with cover ✳ toilet tissue ✳ two washcloths ✳ soap ✳ gloves ✳ towel ✳ linen-saver pad ✳ bath blanket ✳ pillow ✳ optional: air freshener and talcum powder

Big and little

Bedpans are available in adult and pediatric sizes and disposable and reusable (must be sterilized) models. The fracture pan, a type of bedpan, is used when spinal injuries, body or leg casts, or other conditions prohibit or restrict turning the patient.

Getting ready

• Obtain the appropriate bedpan or urinal.
• If you're using a metal bedpan, warm it under running water to avoid startling the patient and stimulating muscle contraction, which hinders elimination.
• Dry the bedpan thoroughly and test its temperature.
• If necessary, sprinkle talcum powder on the edge of the bedpan to reduce friction during placement and removal.
• For a thin patient, place a linen-saver pad at the edge of the bedpan or use a fracture pan to minimize pressure on the coccyx.

How you do it

- Always provide privacy.
- Put on gloves *to prevent contact with body fluids and comply with standard precautions.*

Placing a bedpan

- If allowed, elevate the head of the bed slightly *to prevent hyperextension of the spine when the patient raises their buttocks.*
- Rest the bedpan on the edge of the bed. Then turn down the corner of the top linens and draw up the patient's gown. Ask the patient to raise the buttocks by flexing their knees and pushing down on their heels. While supporting the patient's lower back with one hand, center the curved, smooth edge of the bedpan beneath the buttocks.
- If the patient can't raise their buttocks, lower the head of the bed to the horizontal position and help the patient roll onto one side with the buttocks toward you. Position the bedpan properly against the buttocks, and then help the patient roll back onto the bedpan. When the patient is positioned comfortably, raise the head of the bed as indicated.

Be sure to put on gloves before performing a procedure where there's a risk of contact with body fluids.

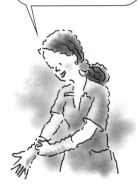

Position is everything

- After positioning the bedpan, elevate the head of the bed further, if allowed, until the patient is sitting erect. *This position aids in defecation and urination.*
- If elevation of the head of the bed is contraindicated, tuck a small pillow or folded bath blanket under the patient's back *to cushion the sacrum against the edge of the bedpan and support the lumbar region.*
- If the patient can be left alone, place the bed in a low position and raise the side rails to ensure his safety. Place toilet tissue and the call button within the patient's reach, and instruct them to push the button after elimination. If the patient is weak or disoriented, remain with them.
- Before removing the bedpan, lower the head of the bed slightly. Then ask the patient to raise the buttocks off the bed. Support the lower back with one hand, and gently remove the bedpan with the other *to avoid skin injury caused by friction.* If the patient can't raise their buttocks, ask them to roll off the pan while you assist with one hand. Hold the pan firmly with the other hand *to avoid spills.* Cover the bedpan and place it on the chair.
- Help clean the anal and perineal area, as necessary, *to prevent irritation and infection.* Turn the patient onto their side, wipe carefully with toilet tissue, clean the area with a damp washcloth and soap, and dry with a towel. Clean a female patient from front to back *to avoid introducing rectal contaminants into the vaginal or urethral openings.*

Placing a urinal

• Lift the corner of the top linens, hand the urinal to the patient, and allow them to position it.
• If the patient can't position the urinal themselves, spread the legs slightly and hold the urinal in place *to prevent spills*.
• After the patient voids, carefully withdraw the urinal.

After use of a bedpan or urinal

• Give the patient a clean, damp, warm washcloth for their hands. Check the bed linens for wetness or soiling, and straighten or change them, if needed. Make the patient comfortable. Place the bed in the low position and raise the side rails.
• Take the bedpan or urinal to the bathroom. Observe the color, odor, amount, and consistency of its contents. If ordered, measure urine output or liquid stool, or obtain a specimen for laboratory analysis.
• Empty the bedpan or urinal into the toilet or hopper. Rinse with cold water and clean it thoroughly, using a disinfectant solution. Dry and return it to the patient's bedside stand.
• Use an air freshener, if necessary, *to eliminate offensive odors and minimize embarrassment.*
• Remove and discard your gloves. Wash your hands.

Practice pointers

• Explain to the patient that drug treatment and changes in environment, diet, and activities may disrupt the usual elimination schedule. Try to anticipate elimination needs, and offer the bedpan or urinal frequently *to help reduce embarrassment and minimize incontinence.*
• Avoid placing a bedpan or urinal on top of the bedside stand or overbed table to avoid contamination of clean equipment and food trays. Similarly, avoid placing it on the floor *to prevent the spread of microorganisms from the floor to the patient's bed linens when the device is used.*
• If the patient experiences pain or discomfort on a standard bedpan, use a fracture pan. The fracture pan is slipped under the buttocks from the front rather than the side. It's also shallower than a standard bedpan, so you need to lift the patient only slightly to position it. If the patient is obese or otherwise difficult to lift, ask a coworker to help you.
• If the patient has an indwelling urinary catheter, carefully position and remove the bedpan *to avoid tension on the catheter, which could dislodge it or irritate the urethra.* After the patient defecates, wipe, clean, and dry the anal region, taking care to avoid catheter contamination. If necessary, clean the urinary meatus with povidone-iodine solution.

• Avoid leaving the urinal, fracture pan, or bedpan in place for extended periods *to prevent skin breakdown.*

Collecting a random urine specimen

A random urine specimen is collected as part of the physical examination or at various times during hospitalization. It permits laboratory screening for urinary and systemic disorders as well as drug screening.

What you need

Bedpan, fracture pan, or urinal with cover ✳ toilet tissue ✳ two washcloths ✳ soap ✳ gloves ✳ towel ✳ linen-saver pad ✳ specimen container and cover ✳ specimen label ✳ optional: air freshener and talcum powder

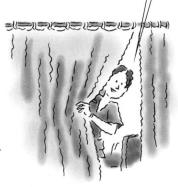

It's important to maintain a patient's dignity by providing as much privacy as the patient's condition allows.

Getting ready

• Tell the patient that a urine specimen is needed for laboratory analysis.
• Explain the procedure to the patient and their family, if necessary, to promote cooperation and prevent accidental disposal of specimens.

How you do it

• Provide privacy. Instruct the patient on bed rest to void into a clean bedpan or urinal, or ask the ambulatory patient to void into either one in the bathroom.

Pour, record, discard

• Put on gloves. Pour at least 120 ml of urine into the specimen container and cap it securely. If the patient's urine output must be measured and recorded, pour the remaining urine into the graduated container. Otherwise, discard it. If you inadvertently spill urine on the outside of the container, clean and dry it *to prevent cross-contamination.* Remove and discard gloves. Wash your hands.
• Label the specimen container with the patient's name, room number, current date, and time of collection. Attach the request form and send the specimen container immediately to the laboratory.

Clean and return

• Put on gloves. Clean the graduated container and urinal or bedpan, and return them to their proper storage area. Discard your gloves and disposable items.

• Wash your hands thoroughly after removing your gloves *to prevent cross-contamination.* Offer the patient a washcloth and soap and water to wash his hands.
• Document the urine collection according to your facility policy. (See *Documenting urine specimen collection.*)

Practice pointers

• Be sure to send the specimen to the laboratory immediately *because delayed transport of the specimen may alter test results.*
• If your patient is collecting a random urine specimen at home, instruct the patient to collect the specimen in a clean container with a tight-fitting lid and to keep it in the refrigerator (away from food items) for up to 24 hours.

Take note!

Documenting urine specimen collection

Be sure to record the times of urine specimen collection and transport to the laboratory. Specify the test as well as the appearance, odor, color, and unusual characteristics of the specimen. If necessary, record urine volume in the intake and output record.

Obtaining urine specific gravity

Urine specific gravity is determined by comparing the weight of a urine specimen with the weight of an equivalent volume of distilled water, which is 1.000. Because urine contains dissolved salts and other substances, it's heavier than 1.000. Urine specific gravity ranges from 1.003 (very dilute) to 1.035 (highly concentrated); normal values range from 1.010 to 1.025.

The light does it

Urine specific gravity is commonly measured with a refractometer, which measures the refraction of light as it passes through a urine specimen.

High and low

Elevated specific gravity reflects an increased concentration of urine solutes, which occurs in conditions that cause renal hypoperfusion, and may indicate heart failure, dehydration, hepatic disorders, or nephrosis. Low specific gravity reflects failure to reabsorb water and concentrate urine. It may indicate hypercalcemia, hypokalemia, alkalosis, acute renal failure, pyelonephritis, glomerulonephritis, or diabetes insipidus.

Controlled accuracy

Although urine specific gravity is commonly measured with a random urine specimen, a more accurate measurement is possible with a controlled specimen collected after withholding fluids for 12 to 24 hours.

What you need

Refractometer * gloves * graduated specimen container

Getting ready

• Explain the procedure to the patient, including when you'll need a urine specimen.
• Explain why you're withholding fluids and for how long *to ensure patient cooperation.*

How you do it

• Put on gloves, and collect a random or controlled urine specimen.
• Place a single drop of urine on the refractometer slide.
• Turn on the light and look through the eyepiece to see the specific gravity indicated on the scale. (Some instruments have a digital display.)
• Remove and discard your gloves and disposable equipment. Wash your hands.
• Document the procedure according to your facility policy. (See *Documenting urine specific gravity collection.*)

Practice pointers

• Follow the manufacturer's directors for calibrating the refractometer as appropriate.
• Replace the refractometer battery as needed.

Take note!

Documenting urine specific gravity collection

Be sure to record the specific gravity, volume, color, odor, and appearance of the collected urine specimen.

Applying a condom catheter

Many patients don't require an indwelling urinary catheter to manage incontinence. For male patients, a condom catheter or male incontinence device reduces the risk of a UTI associated with catheterization. It also promotes bladder retraining when possible, helps prevent skin breakdown, and maintains the patient's self-image.

A condom catheter is secured to the shaft of the penis and connected to a leg bag or drainage bag. It can cause skin irritation and edema.

What you need

Condom catheter * drainage bag * extension tubing * hypoallergenic tape or incontinence sheath holder * commercial adhesive strip or skin-bond cement * elastic adhesive or Velcro, if needed * gloves * razor, if needed * basin * soap * washcloth * towel * optional: solvent

A condom catheter or male incontinence device reduces the risk of a UTI associated with catheterization.

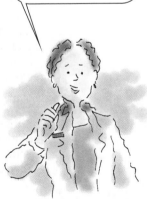

Getting ready

- Explain the procedure to the patient.
- Fill the basin with lukewarm water.
- Bring the basin and other equipment to the bedside.

How you do it

- Wash your hands thoroughly, put on gloves, and provide privacy.

Applying the device

- If the patient is circumcised, wash the penis with soap and water, rinse well, and pat dry with a towel. If the patient isn't circumcised, gently retract the foreskin, and clean beneath it. Rinse well and dry. Replace the foreskin *to avoid penile constriction.*
- If necessary, shave the base and shaft of the penis *to prevent the adhesive strip or skin-bond cement from pulling pubic hair.*

Making it stick

- If you're using a precut commercial adhesive strip, insert the glans penis through its opening, and position the strip 1″ (2.5 cm) from the scrotal area. If you're using uncut adhesive, cut a strip to fit around the shaft of the penis. Remove the protective covering from one side of the adhesive strip and press this side firmly to the penis *to enhance adhesion.* Remove the covering from the other side of the strip. If a commercial adhesive strip isn't available, apply skin-bond cement, and let it dry for a few minutes.

Positioning the catheter

- Position the rolled condom catheter at the tip of the penis, with its drainage opening at the urinary meatus. Allow 1″ to 2″ (2.5 to 5 cm) of space at the tip of the penis *to prevent erosion and to allow for expansion when the patient voids.*
- Unroll the catheter upward, past the adhesive strip on the shaft of the penis. Then gently press the sheath against the strip until it adheres. (See *How to apply a condom catheter.*)
- After the condom catheter is in place, secure it with hypoallergenic tape or an incontinence sheath holder.
- Using extension tubing, connect the condom catheter to the leg bag or drainage bag. Remove and discard your gloves. Wash your hands.

How to apply a condom catheter

Apply an adhesive strip to the shaft of the penis about 1″ (2.5 cm) from the scrotal area.

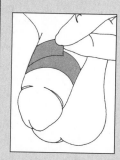

Then roll the condom catheter on to the penis past the adhesive strip, leaving about ½″ (1.3 cm) clearance at the end. Press the sheath gently against the strip until it adheres.

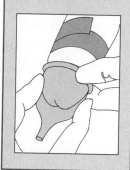

- Change the condom catheter at least every other day to protect the patient's skin and prevent UTIs.

Removing the device
- Put on gloves. Simultaneously roll the condom catheter and adhesive strip off the penis and discard them. If you've used skin-bond cement rather than an adhesive strip, remove it with solvent. Also remove and discard the hypoallergenic tape or incontinence sheath holder.
- Clean the penis with lukewarm water, rinse thoroughly, and dry. Check for swelling or signs of skin breakdown.
- Remove the leg bag by closing the drain clamp, unlatching the leg straps, and disconnecting the extension tubing at the top of the bag. Discard your gloves and wash your hands.

Practice pointers
- If hypoallergenic tape or an incontinence sheath holder isn't available, secure the condom with a strip of elastic adhesive or Velcro. Apply the strip snugly; however, make sure that it isn't too tight *to avoid circulatory constriction.*
- Inspect the condom catheter for twists and the extension tubing for kinks *to prevent obstruction of urine flow, which could cause the condom to balloon and eventually dislodge.* (See *Documenting use of a male incontinence device.*)

> **Take note!**
>
> ## Documenting use of a male incontinence device
>
> Be sure to record the date and time that the incontinence device was applied and removed. Also, note skin condition and the patient's response to the device, including voiding pattern, to assist with bladder retraining.

Inserting an indwelling urinary catheter

An indwelling urinary catheter, also called a *Foley* or *retention catheter,* provides the patient with continuous urine drainage. It's inserted into the bladder and a balloon is inflated at the catheter's distal end to prevent it from slipping out. Insert the catheter with extreme care to prevent injury and infection.

What you need

Sterile indwelling catheter (latex or silicone #10 to #22 French [average adult size: #16 to #18 French]) ✳ syringe filled with 5 to 8 ml of normal saline solution ✳ washcloth ✳ towel ✳ soap and water ✳ two linen-saver pads ✳ sterile gloves ✳ gloves ✳ sterile drape ✳ sterile fenestrated drape ✳ sterile cotton-tipped applicators (or cotton balls and plastic forceps) ✳ povidone-iodine or other antiseptic cleaning agent ✳ urine receptacle ✳

> A Foley catheter has a balloon at the distal end to prevent it from slipping out. That's handy!

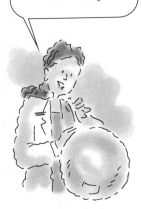

sterile water-soluble lubricant ✳ sterile drainage collection bag ✳ intake and output sheet ✳ optional: urine-specimen container and laboratory request form, leg band with Velcro closure, gooseneck lamp or flashlight, pillows or rolled blankets or towels

At your disposal

Prepackaged, commercial, sterile disposable kits containing all necessary equipment are available.

In case of contamination

Have an extra pair of sterile gloves and two appropriate-size catheters available at the bedside in case of contamination during insertion.

Getting ready

- Explain the procedure to the patient.
- Check the order on the patient's chart *to determine if a catheter size or type has been specified.*
- Verify the patient's identity using two patient identifiers (not including the patient's room number).
- Wash your hands.
- Select the appropriate equipment and assemble it at the patient's bedside.

How you do it

- Provide privacy. Check the patient's chart and ask when he voided last. Percuss and palpate the bladder *to establish baseline data.* Ask if the patient feels the urge to void. Make sure that the patient isn't allergic to iodine solution; if they *are* allergic, obtain another antiseptic cleaning agent.
- Have a coworker hold a flashlight or place a gooseneck lamp next to the patient's bed *so you can see the urinary meatus clearly.*

Assume the position

- Place the female patient in the supine position, with her knees flexed and separated and her feet flat on the bed, about 2′ (61 cm) apart. If this position is uncomfortable, have her flex one knee and keep the other leg flat on the bed. (See *Positioning the elderly female.*)
- Place the male patient in the supine position with his legs extended and flat on the bed. Ask the patient to hold this position *to give you a clear view of the urinary meatus and to prevent contamination of the sterile field.*

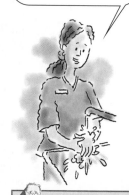

It's important to wash your hands before and after performing a procedure.

Ages and stages

Positioning the elderly female

The elderly female patient may need pillows or rolled towels or blankets for positioning support. If necessary, ask her to lie on her side with one knee drawn up to her chest during catheterization (as shown here). This position may also be helpful for a disabled patient.

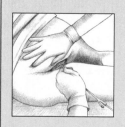

Sterile fieldwork

- Put on gloves. Clean the patient's genital area and perineum thoroughly with soap and water. Dry the area with the towel. Remove the gloves and wash your hands.
- Place the linen-saver pads on the bed between the patient's legs and under the hips. *To create the sterile field,* open the pre-packaged kit or equipment tray and place it between the female patient's legs or next to the male patient's hip. If the sterile gloves are on the top of the tray, put them on. Place the sterile drape under the patient's hips. Then drape the patient's lower abdomen with the sterile fenestrated drape so that only the genital area remains exposed. Take care not to contaminate your gloves.
- Open the rest of the kit or tray. Put on the sterile gloves if you haven't already done so.
- Tear open the packet of povidone-iodine or other antiseptic cleaning agent, and saturate the sterile cotton balls or applicators.
- Open the packet of water-soluble lubricant and apply it to the catheter tip; attach the drainage bag to the other end of the catheter. (If you're using a commercial kit, the drainage bag may be attached.) Make sure that all tubing ends remain sterile and that the clamp at the emptying port of the drainage bag is closed *to prevent urine leakage from the bag.*
- Before inserting the catheter, inflate the balloon with normal saline solution *to inspect it for leaks.* To inflate the balloon, attach the saline-filled syringe to the luer lock, and then push the plunger and check for seepage as the balloon expands. Aspirate the saline *to deflate the balloon.*

Female facts

- For the female patient, separate the labia majora and labia minora as widely as possible with the thumb, middle, and index fingers of your nondominant hand *so you have a full view of the urinary meatus.* Keep the labia well separated throughout the procedure *so they don't obscure the urinary meatus or contaminate the area when it's cleaned.*

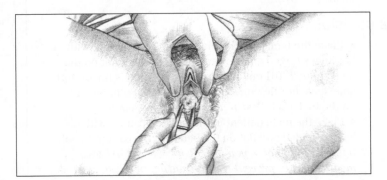

• Use your dominant hand, use a sterile, cotton-tipped applicator (or pick up a sterile cotton ball with the plastic forceps) and wipe one side of the urinary meatus with a single downward motion (as shown here). Similarly, wipe the other side with another sterile applicator or cotton ball. Then wipe directly over the meatus with still another sterile applicator or cotton ball. Take care not to contaminate your sterile gloves.

Male matters

• For the male patient, hold the penis with your nondominant hand. If he's uncircumcised, retract the foreskin. Then gently lift and stretch the penis to a 60- to 90-degree angle. Grasp the penis firmly and hold the penis this way throughout the procedure *to straighten the urethra and maintain a sterile field.*
• Use your dominant hand to clean the glans with a sterile cotton-tipped applicator or a sterile cotton ball held in the forceps. Clean in a circular motion, starting at the urinary meatus and working outward.
• Repeat the procedure, using another sterile applicator or cotton ball and taking care not to contaminate your sterile glove.
• Pick up the catheter with your dominant hand and prepare to insert the lubricated tip into the urinary meatus. *To facilitate insertion by relaxing the sphincter*, ask the patient to cough as you insert the catheter. Tell him to breathe deeply and slowly *to further relax the sphincter and spasms*. Hold the catheter close to its tip *to ease insertion and control its direction*. (See *Preventing indwelling catheter problems*.)

Preventing indwelling catheter problems

These precautions can help prevent problems with an indwelling urinary catheter:
• Never force the catheter during insertion. Instead, maneuver it gently as the patient bears down or coughs. If you still meet resistance, stop and notify the doctor. Sphincter spasms, strictures, misplacement in the vagina (in females), or an enlarged prostate (in males) may cause resistance.
• Establish urine flow, and then inflate the balloon to ensure that the catheter is in the bladder.

More helpful hints
Observe the patient carefully for hypovolemic shock and other adverse reactions caused by removing excessive volumes of residual urine. Check your facility's policy in advance to determine the maximum amount of urine that may be drained at one time; some facilities limit the amount to 700 to 1,000 ml. (Be aware, however, that controversy exists over the wisdom of limiting the amount of urine drainage.) Clamp the catheter at the first sign of an adverse reaction, and notify the doctor.

Advanced class

• For the female patient, advance the catheter 2″ to 3″ (5.1 to 7.5 cm)—while continuing to hold the labia apart—until urine begins to flow (as shown in this illustration). If the catheter is inadvertently inserted into the vagina, leave it there as a landmark. Then begin the procedure again using new supplies.

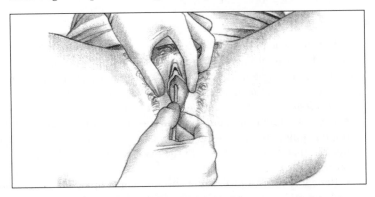

• For the male patient, advance the catheter to the bifurcation and check for urine flow (as shown below). If the foreskin was retracted, replace it *to prevent compromised circulation and painful swelling.*

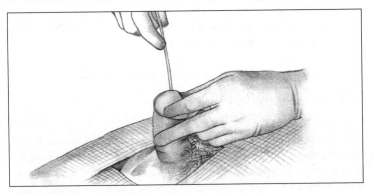

Inflate, hang, and secure

• When urine stops flowing, attach the saline-filled syringe to the luer lock.
• Push the plunger and inflate the balloon to keep the catheter in place in the bladder.
• Hang the collection bag below bladder level *to prevent urine reflux into the bladder, which can cause infection, and to promote gravity drainage of the bladder.* Make sure that the tubing doesn't get tangled in the bed's side rails.
• Secure the catheter to the patient's thigh per your facility's policy.
• Dispose of all used supplies properly. Wash your hands.

Practice pointers

• The balloon size determines the amount of solution needed for inflation. The exact amount is usually printed on the distal extension of the catheter used for inflating the balloon.
• For monitoring purposes, empty the collection bag at least every 8 hours. Excessive fluid volume may require more frequent emptying *to prevent traction on the catheter wall.* (See *Documenting indwelling catheter insertion.*)

Indwelling catheter care and removal

When performed, catheter care is completed after the patient's morning bath, immediately after perineal care. When the patient's condition warrants catheter removal, you must also remove the indwelling catheter.

Difference of opinion

Individual facility policy dictates whether a patient receives daily catheter care. Many health care facilities don't recommend daily catheter care because some studies suggest it increases the risk of infection and other complications rather than reducing it. However, regardless of the facility's catheter care policy, the equipment and the patient's genitalia require inspection twice daily.

What you need

For catheter care

Povidone-iodine solution (or other antiseptic cleaning agent) ✳ sterile gloves ✳ eight sterile 4″ × 4″ gauze pads ✳ basin ✳ sterile absorbent cotton balls or cotton-tipped applicators ✳ leg bag ✳ collection bag ✳ adhesive tape ✳ optional: safety pin, rubber band, adhesive remover, antibiotic ointment, specimen container

Now a word from our sponsor

Commercially prepared catheter care kits containing all necessary supplies are available.

For catheter removal

Absorbent cotton ✳ gloves ✳ alcohol pad ✳ 10-ml syringe with a luer lock ✳ bedpan ✳ linen-saver pad ✳ optional: clamp for bladder retraining

Take note!

Documenting indwelling catheter insertion

If your patient has an indwelling catheter, be sure to record:
• date and time of catheter insertion
• size and type of catheter used
• amount, color, and other characteristics of urine drainage
• patient's tolerance of the procedure (if large volumes of urine were drained)
• whether a urine specimen was sent for laboratory analysis.

Only on I & O
Be aware that your facility may require you to record fluid-balance information only on the intake and output sheet.

Getting ready

- Explain the procedure to the patient and provide privacy.
- Wash your hands and bring all equipment to the patient's bedside.

How you do it

Catheter care

- Open the gauze pads, place several in the first basin, and pour some povidone-iodine solution or other cleaning agent over them.

Avoid irritation

- Some facilities specify that, after wiping the urinary meatus with cleaning solution, you should wipe it off with wet, sterile gauze pads *to prevent possible irritation from the cleaning solution*. If this is your facility's policy, pour water into the second basin, and moisten three more gauze pads.
- Make sure that the lighting is adequate and the perineum and catheter tubing are clearly visible.
- Inspect the catheter for problems, and check the collected urine for mucus, blood clots, sediment, and turbidity. Then pinch the catheter between two fingers *to determine if the lumen contains any material*. If any of these conditions exist (or if your facility's policy requires it), obtain a urine specimen and notify the doctor.
- Inspect the outside of the catheter where it enters the urinary meatus for encrusted material and suppurative drainage. Also inspect the tissue around the meatus for irritation or swelling.

> Adequate lighting isn't just important for photography. It's also essential for proper indwelling catheter care.

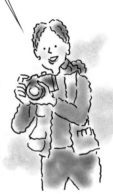

Wipe away

- Put on the sterile gloves. Use a saturated, sterile gauze pad or cotton-tipped applicator to clean the outside of the catheter and the tissue around the meatus. *To avoid contaminating the urinary tract*, always clean by wiping away from—never toward—the urinary meatus. Use a dry gauze pad to remove encrusted material. Don't pull on the catheter while you're cleaning it. *Doing so can injure the urethra and the bladder wall. What's more, it can expose a section of the catheter that was inside the urethra and, when you release the catheter, the newly contaminated section will reenter the urethra, introducing potentially infectious organisms.*
- Remove your gloves and wash your hands.
- Most drainage bags have a plastic clamp on the tubing to attach them to the sheet. If this clamp isn't available, wrap a rubber band around the drainage tubing, insert a safety pin through a loop of

the rubber band, and pin the tubing to the sheet below bladder level. Then attach the collection bag, below bladder level, to the bed frame.

Catheter removal

• Wash your hands. Assemble the equipment at the patient's bedside. Explain the procedure to the patient and tell them that they may feel slight discomfort. Tell the patient that you'll check them periodically during the first 6 to 24 hours after catheter removal *to make sure that voiding resume.*

• Put on gloves. Attach the syringe to the luer-lock mechanism on the catheter. Place a linen-saver pad under the patient's buttocks.

Deflating the balloon

• Pull back on the plunger of the syringe *to deflate the balloon by aspirating the injected fluid.* The amount of fluid injected is usually indicated on the tip of the catheter's balloon lumen and on the patient's chart.

• Before removing the catheter, offer the patient a bedpan. Then grasp the catheter with the absorbent cotton and gently pull it from the urethra. Inspect the balloon to make sure that it's intact. If it isn't intact, notify the doctor.

• Measure and record the amount of urine in the collection bag before discarding it. (See *Documenting indwelling catheter care and removal.*)

Take note!

Documenting indwelling catheter care and removal

When providing care for a patient with an indwelling catheter, be sure to record:
• care you performed
• care modifications required
• patient complaints
• condition of the perineum and urinary meatus
• characteristics of urine in the drainage bag
• whether a specimen was sent for laboratory analysis
• fluid intake and output. (Usually, an hourly record is required for critically ill patients and hemodynamically unstable patients with renal insufficiency.)

Catheter removal
When removing a catheter, be sure to record:
• date and time of catheter removal
• patient's tolerance of the procedure
• when and how much the patient voided after removal (usually for first 24 hours)
• associated problems.

Bladder retraining
For bladder retraining, be sure to record:
• date and time the catheter was clamped and released
• volume and appearance of urine.

Practice pointers

• Your facility may require the use of specific cleaning agents for catheter care, so check the policy manual before the procedure.
• A doctor's order is needed to apply antibiotic ointments to the urinary meatus after cleaning.

Stay low

• Avoid raising the drainage bag above bladder level *to prevent urine reflux, which may contain bacteria.*
• If the patient will be discharged with an indwelling catheter, teach him how to use a leg bag.
• When changing catheters after long-term use (usually 30 days), you may need a larger size catheter *because the meatus enlarges, causing urine to leak around the catheter.*

Collecting urine from an indwelling catheter

Obtain an indwelling catheter specimen by clamping the drainage tube and emptying the accumulated urine into a container or by aspirating a specimen with a syringe. Both procedures require sterile collection technique to prevent catheter contamination and a UTI. Clamping the drainage tube and emptying the urine into a container are contraindicated after genitourinary surgery.

What you need

Gloves ✳ alcohol pad ✳ 10-ml syringe ✳ 21G or 22G 1½″ needle ✳ tube clamp ✳ sterile specimen container with lid ✳ label ✳ laboratory request form

Getting ready

• About 30 minutes before collecting the specimen, clamp the drainage tube to allow urine to accumulate.

How you do it

• Put on gloves. If the drainage tube has a built-in sampling port, wipe the port with an alcohol pad. Uncap the needle on the syringe and insert the needle into the sampling port at a 90-degree angle to the tubing. Aspirate the specimen into the syringe. (See *Aspirating a urine specimen.*)

Aspirating a urine specimen

To aspirate a urine specimen when the patient has an indwelling urinary catheter in place, clamp the tube distal to the aspiration port for about 30 minutes. Wipe the port with an alcohol pad, and insert a needle and a 10- or 20-ml syringe into the port perpendicular to the tube. Aspirate the required amount of urine, and expel it into the specimen container. Remove the clamp on the drainage tube.

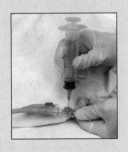

Rubber made

• If the drainage tube doesn't have a sampling port and the catheter is made of rubber, obtain the specimen from the catheter. *Other types of catheters will leak after you withdraw the needle.* To withdraw the specimen from a rubber catheter, wipe it with an alcohol pad just above where it connects to the drainage tube. Insert the needle into the rubber catheter at a 45-degree angle and withdraw the specimen. Never insert the needle into the shaft of the catheter *because doing so may puncture the lumen leading to the catheter balloon.*
• Transfer the specimen to a sterile container, label it, and send it to the laboratory immediately or place it on ice. If a urine culture is ordered, include a list of current antibiotic therapy on the laboratory request form. Remove your gloves and wash your hands.

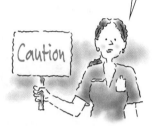

Don't forget to clamp the drainage tube before collecting urine.

Not rubber made

• If the catheter isn't made of rubber or has no sampling port, wipe the area where the catheter joins the drainage tube with an alcohol pad. Disconnect the catheter, and allow urine to drain into the sterile specimen container. Avoid touching the inside of the sterile container with the catheter, and don't touch anything with the catheter drainage tube *to avoid contamination.* When you've collected the specimen, wipe both connection sites with an alcohol pad and join them. Cap the specimen container, label it, and send it to the laboratory immediately or place it on ice. Remove your gloves and wash your hands.

Needleless ports

If the catheter has a needleless sampling port, wipe the port with an alcohol pad. Insert the needleless syringe into the port and withdraw the specimen. Transfer the specimen to a sterile container, label it, and send it to the laboratory immediately or place it on ice. If a urine culture is ordered, include a list of current antibiotic therapy on the laboratory request form. Remove your gloves and wash your hands.

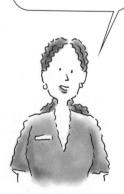

Collecting urine can be easy and safe if you follow the proper steps!

Practice pointers

• Make sure that you unclamp the drainage tube after collecting the specimen *to prevent urine backflow, which may cause bladder distention and infection.*

Reference

Gould, C. V., Umscheid, C. A., Agarwal, R. K., Kuntz, G., & Pegues, D. A. (2009). *Guideline for prevention of catheter-associated urinary tract infections 2009.* Retrieved from http://www.cdc.gov/hicpac/pdg/cauti/cautiguideline2009Final.pdf

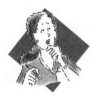

Quick quiz

1. A patient complains of lower abdominal pressure, and you note a firm mass extending above the symphysis pubis. You suspect:

    A.   distended bladder.
    B.   enlarged kidney.
    C.   UTI.
    D.   inflamed ovary.

Answer: A. The bladder is usually nonpalpable unless it's distended. The feeling of pressure is usually relieved with urination.

2. Although the male and female urinary systems function in the same way, there's a difference in the length of the:

    A.   bladder neck.
    B.   ureter.
    C.   epididymis.
    D.   urethra.

Answer: D. A man's urethra passes through the erectile tissue of the penis, it's about 6″ (15.2 cm) longer than a woman's urethra.

3. In a healthy adult, what's the normal range of bladder capacity?

    A.   50 to 100 ml
    B.   200 to 300 ml
    C.   500 to 600 ml
    D.   700 to 900 ml

Answer: C. In a healthy adult, bladder capacity ranges from 500 to 600 ml.

4. The left ureter is slightly longer than the right ureter because the:

    A.   left kidney is higher than the right.
    B.   right kidney is higher than the left.
    C.   left kidney performs more functions.
    D.   left ureter has a three-layered wall.

Answer: A. The left kidney is slightly higher than the right kidney. Therefore, the left ureter needs to be longer to reach the bladder.

Scoring

☆☆☆ If you answered all four questions correctly, sensational! You're as smooth as a perfect indwelling catheter removal.

☆☆ If you answered three questions correctly, great! You've got a great capacity for knowledge.

☆ If you answered fewer than three questions correctly, don't worry. Review the chapter, and you'll begin to filter all the important facts!

Bowel elimination

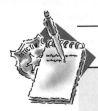

Just the facts

In this chapter, you'll learn:

♦ organs and structures that make up the GI system

♦ causes and characteristics of abnormalities in the GI system

♦ factors that affect bowel elimination

♦ abnormalities of bowel elimination

♦ methods for obtaining a stool specimen

♦ proper way to perform a test for occult blood

♦ proper way to administer an enema

♦ proper colostomy and ileostomy care.

A look at the GI system

The gastrointestinal (GI) system consists of two major divisions: the GI tract and the accessory organs.

GI tract

The GI tract, also called the *alimentary canal*, is a hollow tube that begins at the mouth and ends at the anus. It consists of smooth muscle alternating with blood vessels and nerve tissue. About 25′ (7.5 m) long, the GI tract includes the pharynx, esophagus, stomach, small intestine, and large intestine.

Open wide

Digestion begins in the mouth with chewing, salivating, and swallowing. Three pairs of glands—

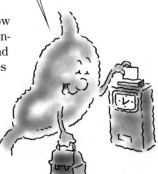

I couldn't do my job without my coworkers—the pharynx, the esophagus, and the small and large intestines.

the parotid, submandibular, and sublingual—produce saliva. The tongue provides the sense of taste.

Proceed to the pharynx

The pharynx, or throat, allows the passage of food from the mouth to the esophagus. It assists in swallowing and secretes mucus that aids in digestion. The epiglottis—a thin, leaf-shaped structure made of fibrocartilage—is directly behind the root of the tongue. When food is swallowed, the epiglottis closes over the larynx and the soft palate lifts to block the nasal cavity, preventing food and fluid from aspirating into the airway.

Down the esophagus

The esophagus is a muscular, hollow tube about 10″ (25.5 cm) long that moves food from the pharynx to the stomach. When food is swallowed, the upper esophageal sphincter relaxes and the food moves into the esophagus. Specialized circular and longitudinal fibers contract, causing peristalsis, which propels food through the GI tract toward the stomach. The gastroesophageal sphincter at the lower end of the esophagus remains closed to prevent the reflux of gastric contents.

Sitting in the stomach

The stomach is a dilated, saclike structure that serves as a reservoir for food. It lies obliquely in the left upper quadrant below the esophagus and diaphragm, to the right of the spleen, and partially under the liver. The stomach contains two important sphincters: the cardiac sphincter, which protects the entrance to the stomach, and the pyloric sphincter, which guards the exit.

The stomach has three major functions:

stores food

mixes food with gastric juices (hydrochloric acid [HCl])

passes chyme—a watery mixture of partly digested food and digestive juices—into the small intestine for further digestion and absorption.

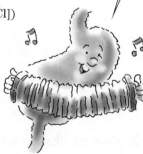

Large amounts of food are like music to my rugae!

Expands to size

Accordion-like folds in the stomach lining, called *rugae*, allow the stomach to expand when large amounts of food and fluid are ingested.

Slipping through the small intestine

The small intestine is about 20′ (6.1 m) long. Named for its diameter, not its length, it consists of the duodenum, the jejunum, and the ileum. As chyme passes into the small intestine, the end products of digestion are absorbed through its thin mucous membrane lining into the bloodstream.

Leaping through the large intestine

The large intestine, or colon, is about 5′ (1.5 m) long. Its main functions are:
- absorbing excess water and electrolytes
- storing food residue
- eliminating waste products in the form of feces.

The large intestine includes the cecum; the ascending, transverse, descending, and sigmoid colons; the rectum; and the anus—in that order. The appendix, a fingerlike projection, is attached to the cecum. Bacteria in the colon produce gas or flatus.

Accessory organs

Accessory GI organs include the liver, pancreas, gallbladder, and bile ducts. The abdominal aorta and the gastric and splenic veins also aid the GI system.

Spotting the liver

The liver is located in the right upper quadrant under the diaphragm and is the heaviest organ in the body, weighing about 3 lb (1.4 kg) in a healthy adult. It's divided into two major lobes by the falciform ligament.

The liver's functions include:
- metabolizing carbohydrates, fats, and proteins
- detoxifying blood
- converting ammonia to urea for excretion
- synthesizing plasma proteins, nonessential amino acids, vitamin A, and essential nutrients, such as iron and vitamins D, K, and B_{12}.

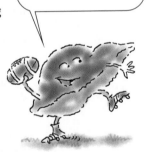

I'm a key player when it comes to digesting fats and absorbing fatty acids.

Believe in bile

The liver also secretes bile, a greenish fluid that helps digest fats and absorb fatty acids, cholesterol, and other lipids.

Gaping at the gallbladder

The gallbladder is a small, pear-shaped organ about 4″ (10 cm) long that lies halfway under the right lobe of the liver. Its main function is to store bile. The small intestine initiates chemical impulses that cause the gallbladder to contract and empty bile into the duodenum.

Probing the pancreas

The pancreas, which measures 6″ to 8″ (15 to 20.5 cm) in length, lies horizontally in the abdomen, behind the stomach. It consists of a head, tail, and body. The body of the pancreas is located in the right upper quadrant and the tail is in the left upper quadrant, attached to the duodenum.

The pancreas releases insulin and glycogen into the bloodstream and produces pancreatic enzymes that are released into the duodenum for digestion.

Beholding the bile ducts

The bile ducts provide passageways for bile to travel from the liver to the intestines. Two hepatic ducts drain the liver and the cystic duct drains the gallbladder. These ducts converge into the common bile duct, which then empties into the duodenum.

Visualizing the vascular structures

The abdominal aorta supplies blood to the GI tract. It enters the abdomen, separates into the common iliac arteries, and branches into many arteries that extend the length of the GI tract.

The gastric and splenic veins drain absorbed nutrients into the portal vein of the liver. After entering the liver, the venous blood circulates and exits the liver through the hepatic vein, emptying into the inferior vena cava.

Digestion and elimination

Digestion starts in the oral cavity, where chewing (mastication), salivation (the beginning of starch digestion), and swallowing (deglutition) all take place. When a patient swallows, the hypopharyngeal sphincter in the upper esophagus relaxes, allowing food to enter the esophagus.

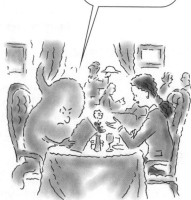

Fill and empty. Fill and empty. Do I ever get a break?

Long day's journey into the stomach

In the esophagus, the glossopharyngeal nerve activates peristalsis, which moves food down toward the stomach. As food passes through the esophagus, glands in the esophageal mucosa layer secrete mucus, which lubricates the bolus and protects the mucosal membrane from damage caused by poorly chewed food.

Stomach emptying

Food can remain in the stomach for 3 to 4 hours. The rate of stomach emptying depends on gastrin release, neural signals generated when the stomach wall distends, and the enterogastric reflex. This reflex causes the duodenum to release secretin and gastric-inhibiting peptide and the jejunum to secrete cholecystokinin—both of which decrease gastric motility.

Small intestine

Nearly all digestion and absorption takes place in the small intestine. (See *Small intestine: How form affects absorption.*)

Small but mighty

In the small intestine, intestinal contractions and various digestive secretions break down carbohydrates, proteins, and fats—actions that enable the intestinal mucosa to absorb these nutrients into the bloodstream (along with water and electrolytes) for use by the body. Pancreatic enzymes, bile, and hormones from glands of the small intestine mix with chyme and aid in digestion.

By the time the chyme passes through the small intestine and enters the ascending colon of the large intestine, it's reduced to mostly indigestible substances.

Large intestine

The food bolus begins its journey through the large intestine where the ileum and the cecum join with the ileocecal pouch. The bolus moves up the ascending colon and past the right abdominal cavity to the liver's lower border. It crosses horizontally below the liver and stomach, by way of the transverse colon, and descends the left abdominal cavity to the iliac fossa through the descending colon.

The journey continues

From there, the bolus travels through the sigmoid colon to the lower midline of the abdominal cavity, then to the rectum, and finally to the anal canal. The anus opens to the exterior through two sphincters. The internal sphincter contains thick, circular smooth muscle under autonomic control; the external sphincter contains skeletal muscle under voluntary control.

Super absorption

The large intestine doesn't produce hormones or enzymes. It continues the absorption process through blood and lymph vessels in its submucosa. The proximal half of the large intestine absorbs all but about 100 ml of the remaining water in the colon. It also absorbs large amounts of sodium and chloride.

Bacteria in action

The large intestine harbors the bacteria *Escherichia coli, Enterobacter aerogenes, Clostridium perfringens,* and *Lactobacillus*

Small intestine: How form affects absorption

Nearly all digestion and absorption take place in the 20′ (6.1 m) of small intestine. The structure of the small intestine, as shown here, is key to digestion and absorption.

Specialized mucosa

Multiple projections of the intestinal mucosa increase the surface area for absorption several hundredfold, as shown in the enlarged views.

Circular projections (Kerckring's folds) are covered by villi. Each villus contains a lymphatic vessel (lacteal), a venule, capillaries, an arteriole, nerve fibers, and smooth muscle.

Each villus is densely fringed with about 2,000 microvilli, making it resemble a fine brush. The villi are lined with columnar epithelial cells, which dip into the lamina propria between the villi to form intestinal glands (crypts of Lieberkühn).

Types of epithelial cells

The type of epithelial cell dictates its function:
• Mucus-secreting *goblet cells* are found on and between the villi on the crypt mucosa.
• Specialized *Brunner's glands* in the proximal duodenum also secrete large amounts of mucus to lubricate and protect the duodenum from potentially corrosive acidic chyme and gastric juices.
• Duodenal *argentaffin cells* produce the hormones secretin and cholecystokinin.
• *Undifferentiated cells* deep within the intestinal glands replace the epithelium.
• *Absorptive cells* consist of large numbers of tightly packed microvilli over a plasma membrane that contains transport mechanisms for absorption and produces enzymes for the final step in digestion.

Intestinal glands

The intestinal glands primarily secrete a watery fluid that bathes the villi with chyme particles. Fluid production results from local irritation of nerve cells and, possibly, from hormonal stimulation by secretin and cholecystokinin. The microvillous brush border secretes various hormones and digestive enzymes that catalyze final nutrient breakdown.

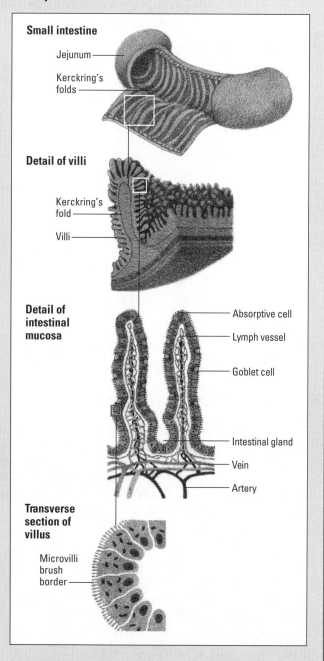

Small intestine

Jejunum

Kerckring's folds

Detail of villi

Kerckring's fold

Villi

Detail of intestinal mucosa

Absorptive cell

Lymph vessel

Goblet cell

Intestinal gland

Vein

Artery

Transverse section of villus

Microvilli brush border

bifidus. These bacteria help synthesize vitamin K and break down cellulose into usable carbohydrates. Bacterial action also produces flatus, which helps propel stool toward the rectum.

Mucosa on a mission

In addition, the mucosa of the large intestine produces alkaline secretions from tubular glands composed of goblet cells. This alkaline mucus lubricates the intestinal walls as food pushes through, protecting the mucosa from acidic bacterial action.

Mass movement

In the lower colon, long and relatively sluggish contractions cause propulsive waves or mass movements. These movements occur several times per day and propel intestinal contents into the rectum, producing the urge to defecate.

Defecation normally results from the defecation reflex, a sensory and parasympathetic nerve-mediated response, along with voluntary relaxation of the external anal sphincter. (See *GI changes with aging.*)

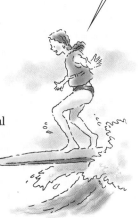

In the lower colon, long and relatively sluggish contractions cause propulsive waves or mass movements.

Ages and stages

GI changes with aging

The physiologic changes that accompany aging usually prove less debilitating in the GI system than in most other body systems. Normal changes include diminished mucosal elasticity and reduced GI secretions that, in turn, modify some processes—for example, digestion and absorption. GI tract motility, bowel wall and anal sphincter tone, and abdominal muscle strength may also decrease with age. Any of these changes may cause complaints in an older patient, ranging from loss of appetite to constipation.

Changes in the oral cavity also occur. Tooth enamel wears away, leaving the teeth prone to cavities. Periodontal disease increases and the number of taste buds decline. The sense of smell diminishes and salivary gland secretion decreases, leading to appetite loss.

Liver changes
Normal physiologic changes in the liver include decreased liver weight, reduced regenera-tive capacity, and decreased blood flow to the liver. Because liver enzymes involved in oxidation and reduction markedly decline with age, the liver metabolizes drugs and detoxifies substances less efficiently.

Characteristics of normal stool

Stool is 25% solids and 75% water. The solids consist of bacteria, undigested fiber, fat, inorganic matter, and some protein.

Bili Brown

The chemical conversion of bilirubin produces the brown color of stool. Certain foods and medications can alter stool's color. Beets will turn stool to a reddish color, and medications, such as bismuth subsalicylate (Pepto-Bismol), can turn stool black. Stool color can also be indicative of certain medical conditions. White or clay-colored stools, for example, can signal a malabsorption disorder or a blockage in the liver or biliary system.

Pardon my odor!

Bacterial decomposition of protein in the solids produces stool's characteristic, unpleasant odor.

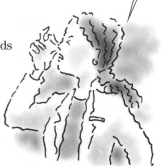

Bacterial decomposition of protein in the solids produces stool's characteristic, unpleasant odor.

Let's get in shape

Stool normally has a soft consistency and a cylindrical form that mimics the shape of the rectum. Thin and ribbon like stools may be a result of internal hemorrhoids or are a warning sign of colorectal cancer.

Different strokes for different folks

Each patient's elimination pattern differs. The frequency of bowel movements can range from one or two bowel movements per day to one bowel movement every 2 or 3 days. If dietary fiber intake is reduced, fewer stools will be produced.

Factors affecting bowel elimination

Many factors affect bowel elimination including body position, exercise and activity, fecal diversion, fluid intake, ignoring the urge to defecate, lifestyle, medications, nutrition, and surgery.

Body position

Semisquatting or sitting is the most conducive position for having a bowel movement because it allows gravity to aid in stool movement. It also promotes contraction of the abdominal and pelvic muscles that are used during bowel elimination. A patient who uses a bedpan while he's flat in bed may have difficulty having a bowel movement.

Exercise and activity

Good muscle tone and regular exercise facilitates peristalsis and aids in bowel elimination. Abdominal and pelvic muscles create the intra-abdominal pressure needed to have a bowel movement. Lack of or reduced physical activity can increase the chances of developing constipation. Also, loss of neurologic control due to illness or trauma will impair muscle tone.

Fecal diversion

Fecal diversion is the creation of an alternate route for bowel elimination. This procedure removes all or part of the colon, rectum, and anus. An alternative exit site, called a *stoma*, is created that redirects a portion of the remaining bowel through the abdominal wall to a spot on the abdomen. Fecal diversions may be temporary or permanent and are sometimes performed in a patient with bowel cancer or a bowel obstruction or to rest the bowel in disorders such as Crohn's disease.

All those ostomies

When a part of the small intestine is redirected through the abdominal wall, it's called an *ileostomy*. *Colostomy* refers to a fecal diversion that brings a portion of the large intestine or colon through the abdominal wall. (See *Reviewing types of ostomies.*)

Reviewing types of ostomies

The appropriate type of ostomy for a patient depends on the patient's condition. Temporary ostomies, such as a double-barrel or loop colostomy, help treat perforated sigmoid diverticulitis and other conditions in which intestinal healing is expected. Permanent colostomy or ileostomy accompanies extensive abdominal surgery such as the removal of a malignant tumor.

Double-barrel colostomy

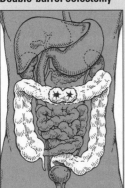

Loop colostomy

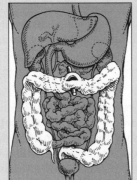

Permanent colostomy

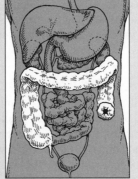

Ileostomy

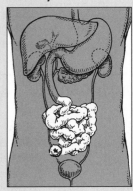

Fluid intake

Stool is 75% water. If the body doesn't take in enough fluid, the bowel will conserve more water by absorbing it from the stool. Stools then become hard and difficult to pass.

A storage problem

The longer stool remains in the colon, the greater the amount of water absorbed, resulting in hard, dry stool. Conversely, stool that doesn't remain in the colon long enough for water to be absorbed will be watery, resulting in fluid loss.

Ignoring the urge to defecate

If the initial reflex urge to defecate is ignored, it subsides in a few minutes. Stool remains in the rectum until another mass movement propels more stool into the rectum, creating another urge. A patient with a chronic condition, such as hemorrhoids, may ignore the urge because of painful bowel movements. Lack of privacy may also cause a patient to ignore the urge to defecate. Ignoring the urge to have a bowel movement can lead to constipation.

Lifestyle

Bowel elimination patterns are commonly part of patients' daily routines and are convenient for their lifestyle. Some patients may be used to waiting until they have the urge to defecate. An early riser may consistently have a bowel movement in the morning, whereas a patient who works the night shift may have their daily bowel movements in the late afternoon.

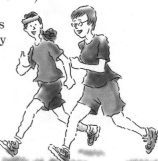

A person's bowel elimination pattern is commonly part of her daily routine and is convenient for her lifestyle.

Here we go—or not

Vacation, changing jobs, and such strong emotions as anxiety, anger, fear, depression, or excitement can alter bowel habits. Hospitalization or a disruption in personal relationships can also be stressful enough to alter bowel habits.

Medications

Medications, such as opioids and iron preparations, can cause constipation. Antibiotics can cause diarrhea. Antacids can cause constipation or diarrhea.

To go or not to go

Stool softeners and laxatives are normally prescribed to increase stool consistency or bowel elimination. Other medications, such as antidiarrheals, are given to decrease stool frequency.

Nutrition

A high fiber diet (20 to 30 g of dietary fiber per day) should produce enough bulk to assist in bowel elimination. Foods high in fiber include fruits, vegetables, and cereal grains.

Hard to tolerate

Certain patients may not be able to tolerate lactose (a sugar contained in milk products) or gluten (a protein found in barley, rye, buckwheat, and wheat) and should avoid foods containing these substances. If a lactose-intolerant patient eats or drinks milk products, it may cause abdominal distention, gas formation, abdominal cramping, and diarrhea. If a gluten-intolerant patient ingests foods containing gluten, bulky greasy stools, abdominal distention, and bloating will likely result.

Surgery

Surgery can significantly impact bowel elimination patterns. A patient who's scheduled for operative procedures is commonly required to restrict food and water intake preoperatively and postoperatively.

A surgical pause

Anesthesia slows GI motility for 1 to 2 days following surgery. GI or abdominal surgery may hinder a return of full bowel function for 3 to 4 days. Decreased bowel motility may also result from the bowel's exposure to air and handling during the surgical procedure.

A painless pause

Opioids used to manage pain postoperatively can reduce bowel motility. Fear of pain upon defecation, especially if the patient has an abdominal incision, can also inhibit normal bowel function.

Altered bowel function

Alterations in bowel function include constipation, diarrhea, distention, fecal impaction, fecal incontinence, and flatulence.

Constipation

Constipation is most common in older patients. It can be caused by immobility, a sedentary lifestyle, and certain medications. A patient who's constipated may complain of a dull abdominal ache and a full feeling. Hyperactive bowel sounds, which may signal irritable bowel syndrome, are sometimes present. A patient with complete intestinal obstruction won't pass flatus or stool, with an absence of bowel sounds below the obstruction.

Diarrhea

Toxins, medications, or a GI condition, such as Crohn's disease, can result in diarrhea. Typical symptoms include cramping, abdominal tenderness, anorexia, and hyperactive bowel sounds. Diarrhea accompanied by a fever suggests a toxin as the causative agent.

Distention

Distention may result from gas, a tumor, or a colon filled with stool. It can also suggest an incisional hernia, which may protrude when the patient lifts his head and shoulders.

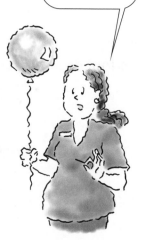

Do you sometimes feel like a balloon ready to pop?

Fecal impaction

Fecal impaction is a large, hard, dry mass of stool in the folds of the rectum or in the sigmoid colon. It's the result of prolonged retention and stool accumulation. Poor bowel habits, inactivity, dehydration, improper diet (especially inadequate fluid intake), the use of constipation-inducing drugs, and incomplete bowel cleaning after a barium enema or barium swallow are all possible causes.

Fecal incontinence

Fecal incontinence is the involuntary elimination of feces from the bowel and may result from watery or loose stool. In an elderly patient, fecal incontinence commonly follows loss or impairment of anal sphincter control.

Flatulence

Flatus is the accumulation of gas in the GI tract resulting from swallowing air, diffusion in the blood, and bacterial action in the large intestine. Certain foods, such as cabbage and onions, large amounts of carbonated beverages, smoking, and anxiety (which can cause excessive swallowing) can also produce flatus.

Nursing interventions for bowel elimination

Nursing interventions for bowel elimination include stool specimen collection, testing the stool for occult blood, administering enemas, colostomy or ileostomy care, and irrigating a colostomy.

Stool specimen collection

Stool is collected to determine if blood, ova and parasites, bile, fat, pathogens, or ingested drugs are present. Stool characteristics—such as color, consistency, and odor—can reveal such conditions as GI bleeding and steatorrhea.

Random or specific

Stool specimens are collected randomly or for specified periods such as for 72 hours. Proper collection requires careful instructions to the patient to ensure an uncontaminated specimen.

What you need

Specimen container with lid ✳ gloves ✳ tongue blade ✳ paper towel or paper bag ✳ bedpan or portable commode ✳ three patient-care reminders (for timed specimens) ✳ laboratory request form

Getting ready

• Verify the patient's identity using two patient identifiers (not including the patient's room number).
• Inform the patient that a stool specimen is needed for laboratory analysis.
• Explain the procedure to the patient and his family, if possible, to ensure cooperation and prevent the disposal of timed stool specimens.

How you do it

Collecting a random specimen

- Ask the patient to notify you when he has the urge to defecate. Have him defecate into a clean, dry bedpan or portable commode. Instruct him not to contaminate the specimen with urine or toilet tissue *because urine inhibits fecal bacterial growth and toilet tissue contains bismuth, which interferes with test results.*
- Put on gloves.

Stands out from the crowd

- Using a tongue blade, transfer the most representative stool specimen from the bedpan to the specimen container, and cap the container. If the patient passes blood, mucus, or pus with the stool, include this with the specimen.
- Wrap the tongue blade in a paper towel or place it in a paper bag and discard it. Remove and discard your gloves, and wash your hands thoroughly *to prevent cross-contamination.*

Collecting a timed specimen

- Place a patient-care reminder stating SAVE ALL STOOL over the patient's bed, in his bathroom, and in the utility room.
- After putting on gloves, collect the first specimen and include it in the total specimen.

Complete transfer

- Obtain the timed specimen as you would a random specimen. Remember to transfer all stool to the specimen container.
- If stool must be obtained with an enema, use only tap water or normal saline solution.
- Send each specimen to the laboratory immediately with a laboratory request form or, if permitted, refrigerate the specimens and send them all when collection is complete. Remove and discard gloves. Wash your hands.
- Make sure that the patient is comfortable after the procedure and has the opportunity to thoroughly clean his hands and perianal area. Offer assistance if help with perineal care is indicated.

Practice pointers

- Never place a stool specimen in a refrigerator that contains food or medication *to prevent contamination.* (See *Collecting a stool specimen.*)
- Notify the doctor if the stool specimen looks unusual. (See *Documenting stool collection*, page 628.)

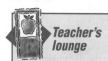

Teacher's lounge

Collecting a stool specimen

If the patient is to collect a stool specimen at home, instruct him to collect it in a clean container with a tight-fitting lid, to wrap the container in a brown paper bag, and to keep it in the refrigerator (separate from food items) until it can be transported.

Assessing stool for occult blood

Take note!

Fecal occult blood tests are valuable for detecting occult blood (hidden GI bleeding), which may signal colorectal cancer, and can distinguish between true melena and melena-like stools. Certain medications, such as iron supplements and bismuth compounds, can darken stools to resemble *melena*, which is black, tarry stool containing blood.

Look for blue

The Hematest (an orthotolidine reagent tablet) and the Hemoccult slide (filter paper impregnated with guaiac) are two common occult blood screening tests. Both tests produce a blue reaction in a fecal smear if occult blood loss exceeds 5 ml in 24 hours. A newer test, ColoCARE, requires no fecal smear. (See *Home tests for fecal occult blood*.)

Repeat three times

To confirm a positive result, the test must be repeated at least three times while the patient follows a meatless, high-residue diet. A positive result doesn't necessarily

Documenting stool collection

In your notes, be sure to record:
• time of specimen collection and transport to the laboratory
• color, odor, and consistency of the stool
• unusual characteristics
• whether the patient had difficulty passing the stool.

Teacher's lounge

Home tests for fecal occult blood

Most fecal occult blood tests require the patient to collect a specimen of his stool and smear some of it on a slide. In contrast, some new tests don't require the patient to handle stool, making the procedure safer and simpler. One example is a test called *ColoCARE*. If your patient will be performing the ColoCARE test at home, include these instructions in your patient teaching:
• Tell him to avoid red meat and vitamin C supplements for 2 days before the test.
• Advise him to check with his doctor about the need for discontinuing medications before the test. Drugs that can interfere with test results include aspirin, indomethacin, corticosteroids, phenylbutazone, reserpine, dietary supplements, anticancer drugs, and anticoagulants.

• Tell him to flush the toilet twice just before performing the test to remove any toilet-cleaning chemicals from the tank.
• Instruct him to defecate into the toilet—but to throw no toilet paper into the bowl—and, within 5 minutes, to remove the test pad from its pouch and float it printed-side-up on the surface of the water.
• Tell him to watch the pad for 15 to 30 seconds for evidence of blue or green color changes, and have him record the result on the reply card.
• Emphasize that he should perform this test with three consecutive bowel movements and then send the completed card to his doctor. However, he should call his doctor immediately if he notes a positive color change in the first test.

confirm colorectal cancer, but it does indicate the need for further diagnostic studies. GI bleeding can result from conditions other than cancer, such as ulcers and diverticula.

These tests are easily performed on collected specimens or smears from a digital rectal examination.

What you need

Test kit ✳ gloves ✳ glass or porcelain plate ✳ tongue blade or other wooden applicator

Getting ready

- Explain the procedure to the patient and his family, if possible, *to ensure cooperation and prevent disposal of timed stool specimens.*
- Provide privacy.
- Wash your hands and bring all equipment to the patient's bedside.
- Verify the patient's identity using two patient identifiers (not including the patient's room number).

How you do it

- Put on gloves, and collect a stool specimen.

Hematest reagent tablet test

- Use a tongue blade or other wooden applicator to smear a bit of the stool specimen on the filter paper supplied with the test kit. Alternatively, after performing a digital rectal examination, wipe the finger you used for the examination on a square of the filter paper.
- Place the filter paper with the stool smear on a glass plate.
- Remove a reagent tablet from the bottle, and immediately replace the cap tightly. Then place the tablet in the center of the stool smear on the filter paper.
- Add one drop of water to the tablet, and allow it to soak in for 5 to 10 seconds. Add a second drop, letting it run from the tablet onto the specimen and filter paper. If necessary, tap the plate gently to dislodge water from the top of the tablet.

If a test is timed, be sure to read the results exactly when specified to ensure you're documenting the correct result.

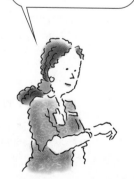

2-minute read

- If the test is positive, the filter paper will turn blue after 2 minutes. Don't read the color on the tablet or the color that develops on the filter paper after the 2-minute period.
- Note the results and discard the filter paper.
- Remove and discard your gloves, and wash your hands thoroughly.

Hemoccult slide test

• Open the flap on the slide packet, and use a tongue blade or other wooden applicator to apply a thin smear of the stool specimen to the guaiac-impregnated filter paper exposed in box A. Alternatively, after performing a digital rectal examination, wipe the finger you used for the examination on a square of the filter paper.

• Apply a second smear from another part of the specimen to the filter paper exposed in box B *because some parts of the specimen may not contain blood.*

• Allow the specimens to dry for 3 to 5 minutes.

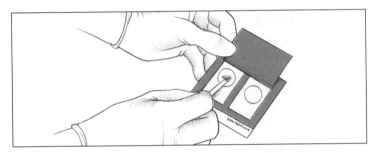

Positive result

• Open the flap on the reverse side of the slide package, and place 2 drops of Hemoccult-developing solution on the paper over each smear, as shown.

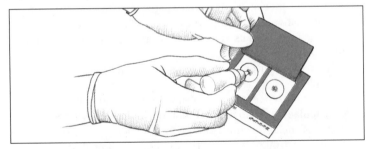

• If the test result is positive, a blue reaction will appear in 30 to 60 seconds.

• Record the results, and discard the slide package.

• Remove and discard your gloves, and wash your hands thoroughly.

Practice pointers

• Make sure that stool specimens aren't contaminated with urine, soap solution, or toilet tissue, and test them as soon as possible after collection.

• Test samples from several portions of the same specimen because occult blood from the upper GI tract isn't always evenly dispersed throughout the formed stool. Blood from colorectal bleeding occurs mostly on the outer stool surface.

• Protect Hematest tablets from moisture, heat, and light. Discard outdated tablets.

Repeat if positive

• If repeat testing is necessary after a positive result, explain the test to the patient. Instruct him to maintain a high-fiber diet and refrain from eating red meat, poultry, fish, turnips, and horseradish for 48 to 72 hours before the test and throughout the collection period *because these substances may alter test results.*

• As ordered, have the patient discontinue the use of iron preparations, bromides, iodides, rauwolfia derivatives, indomethacin (Indocin), colchicine, salicylates, potassium, bismuth compounds, steroids, and ascorbic acid for 48 to 72 hours before the test and during it *to ensure accurate test results and avoid possible bleeding.* (See *Documenting a fecal occult blood test.*)

Take note!

Documenting a fecal occult blood test

Be sure to record the time and date of the test, the result, and unusual characteristics of the stool tested. Report positive results to the doctor.

Enema administration

Enema administration involves instilling a solution into the rectum and colon. In a retention enema, the patient holds the solution for 30 minutes to 1 hour. In an irrigating enema, the patient expels the solution almost completely within 15 minutes. Both enemas stimulate peristalsis by mechanically distending the colon and stimulating rectal wall nerves.

Enem-ies

Enemas are contraindicated after a recent colon or rectal surgery or a myocardial infarction and in a patient with an acute abdominal condition of unknown origin such as suspected appendicitis. They also should be administered cautiously to a patient with an arrhythmia.

> Enemas are contraindicated after some surgeries or MIs.

What you need

Prescribed solution ✴ bath (utility) thermometer ✴ enema administration bag with attached rectal tube and clamp ✴ I.V. pole ✴ gloves ✴ linen-saver pads ✴ bath blanket ✴ two bedpans with covers or bedside commode ✴ water-soluble lubricant ✴ toilet tissue ✴ bulb syringe or funnel ✴ plastic bag for equipment ✴ water ✴ gown ✴ washcloth ✴ soap

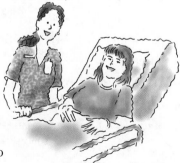

and water ✳ if observing enteric precautions: plastic trash bags, labels ✳ optional (for patients who can't retain the solution): plastic rectal tube guard, indwelling urinary catheter or Verden rectal catheter with 30-ml balloon and syringe

Prep package

Prepackaged disposable enema sets are available, as are small volume enema solutions in irrigating and retention types and pediatric sizes.

Getting ready

- Verify the patient's identity using two patient identifiers (not including the patient's room number).
- Explain the procedure to the patient and his family, if possible, *to ensure cooperation.*
- Provide privacy.
- Wash your hands and bring all equipment to the patient's bedside.
- Prepare the prescribed type and amount of solution, as indicated. (See *Understanding types of enemas.*) The standard volume of an irrigating enema for an adult is 750 to 1,000 ml.

Understanding types of enemas

Enemas are used primarily for three purposes: cleaning, lubricating (or emollient), and carminative (to promote expulsion of flatus). This chart outlines the preparation steps and purposes of common irrigating and retention enemas.

Solution	Preparation	Purpose
Irrigating enemas		
Harris flush	Instill 1,000 ml of tap water.	Cleaning
Magnesium sulfate	Add 2 tbsp of magnesium sulfate to 3 tbsp of salt in 1,000 ml of tap water.	Carminative
Saline solution	If a commercially prepared solution isn't available, add 2 tsp of salt to 1,000 ml of tap water.	Cleaning
Soap and water	Add 1 packet of mild soap to 1,000 ml of tap water, and remove all bubbles before administering solution.	Cleaning
Retention enemas		
Oil	Instill 150 ml of mineral, olive, or cottonseed oil.	Cleaning and lubricating
1-2-3	Add 30 ml of 50% magnesium sulfate to 60 ml of glycerin. Add mixture to 90 ml of warm tap water.	Cleaning

Ages and stages

Giving an enema to a child

Unless contraindicated, help the child into left lateral Sims' position. After lubricating the end of the tube, separate the child's buttocks and push the tube gently into the anus, aiming it toward the umbilicus. Insert the tube 2" to 3" (5.1 to 7.6 cm); for an infant, insert it 1" to 1½" (2.5 to 3.8 cm).

Try this solution

Avoid forcing the tube to prevent rectal wall trauma. If it doesn't advance easily, let a little solution flow in to relax the inner sphincter enough to allow passage.

Standard irrigating enema volumes for pediatric patients are 500 to 1,000 ml for a school-age child, 250 to 500 ml for a toddler or preschooler, and 250 ml or less for an infant.

A matter of degree (and inches)

To avoid burning rectal tissues, don't administer an enema solution that's warmer than 100° F (37.8° C). Be sure not to raise the solution container higher than 12" (30.5 cm) above bed level for a child or 6" to 8" (15.2 to 20.3 cm) for an infant. Excessive pressure can force colonic bacteria into the small intestine or cause the colon to rupture.

• Warm the solution (if for use with an adult) to 100° to 105° F (37.8° to 40.6° C) *to reduce patient discomfort.*

Working toward the right solution

• Clamp the tubing and fill the solution bag with the prescribed solution. Unclamp the tubing, flush the solution through the tubing, and then reclamp it. *Flushing detects leaks and removes air that could cause discomfort if introduced into the colon.*
• Hang the solution container on the I.V. pole and take supplies to the patient's room. If you're using an indwelling urinary catheter or Verden catheter, fill the syringe with 30 ml of water.

How you do it

• Check the doctor's order and assess the patient's condition.
• Provide privacy. If you're administering an enema to a child, familiarize them with the equipment and allow a parent or another relative to remain with them during the procedure. (See *Giving an enema to a child.*)
• Instruct the patient to breathe through their mouth *to relax the anal sphincter, which will ease catheter insertion.*

If you're administering an enema to a child, familiarize them with the equipment and allow a parent or another relative to remain with them during the procedure.

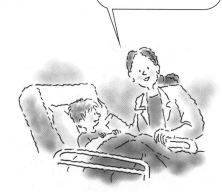

- Wash your hands and put on gloves. If there's a chance you could become soiled, put on a gown.
- Assist the patient into left lateral Sims' position *to facilitate the solution's flow into the descending colon*. If contraindicated or if the patient reports discomfort, reposition them on their back or right side.

Prep procedures

- Place linen-saver pads under the patient's buttocks *to prevent soiling the linens*. Replace the top bed linens with a bath blanket.
- Have a bedpan or commode nearby and toilet tissue within the patient's reach. If the patient can use the bathroom, make sure that it's easily accessible.
- Lubricate the distal tip of the rectal catheter with water-soluble lubricant *to facilitate rectal insertion and reduce irritation*.

Contraction reaction

- Separate the patient's buttocks and touch the anal sphincter with the rectal tube *to stimulate contraction*. Then, as the sphincter relaxes, tell the patient to breathe deeply through their mouth as you gently advance the tube.
- If the patient feels pain or if the tube meets continued resistance, notify the doctor. *This may signal an unknown stricture or abscess.*
- An indwelling urinary catheter or a Verden catheter can also be used as a rectal tube if your facility's policy permits. Insert the lubricated catheter as you would a rectal tube. Then gently inflate the catheter's balloon with 20 to 30 ml of water. Gently pull the catheter back against the patient's internal anal sphincter *to seal off the rectum*. If leakage still occurs with the balloon in place, add more water to the balloon in small amounts. When using either catheter, avoid inflating the balloon above 45 ml *because overinflation can compromise blood flow to the rectal tissues and may cause necrosis from pressure on the rectal mucosa*.
- If you're using a rectal tube, hold it in place throughout the procedure. *Bowel contractions and the pressure of the tube against the anal sphincter can cause tube displacement.*

Go with the flow

- Hold the solution container slightly above bed level, and release the tubing clamp. Raise the container gradually to start the flow— usually at a rate of 75 to 100 ml/minute for an irrigating enema. Use the slowest possible rate for a retention enema *to avoid stimulating peristalsis and promote retention*. Adjust the flow rate of an irrigating enema by raising or lowering the solution container according to the patient's retention ability and comfort. However, be sure not to raise it higher than 18″ (46 cm) above bed level for an adult.

- Assess the patient's tolerance frequently during instillation. If they complain of discomfort, cramps, or the need to defecate, stop the flow by pinching or clamping the tubing. Instruct the patient to breathe slowly and deeply through the mouth *to help relax the abdominal muscles and promote retention.* Resume administration at a slower flow rate after a few minutes when discomfort passes. Interrupt the flow any time the patient complains of discomfort.

Sudden slowdown

- If the flow slows or stops, the catheter tip may be clogged with feces or pressed against the rectal wall. Gently turn the catheter slightly *to free it without stimulating defecation.* If the catheter tip remains clogged, withdraw the catheter, flush it with solution, and reinsert it.

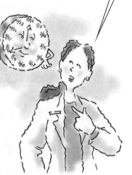

Use the slowest possible rate for a retention enema to avoid stimulating peristalsis and promote retention.

- After administering most of the prescribed amount of solution, clamp the tubing. Stop the flow before the container empties completely *to avoid introducing air into the bowel.*
- To administer a commercially prepared, small-volume enema, first remove the cap from the rectal tube. Insert the rectal tube into the rectum and squeeze the bottle to deposit the contents in the rectum. Remove the rectal tube, replace the used enema unit in its original container, and discard.
- For a flush enema, stop the flow by lowering the solution container below bed level and allowing gravity to siphon the enema from the colon. Continue to raise and lower the container until gas bubbles cease or the patient feels more comfortable and abdominal distention subsides. Don't allow the solution container to empty completely before lowering it *because this may introduce air into the bowel.*

Time frame

- For an irrigating enema, instruct the patient to retain the solution for 15 minutes, if possible.
- For a retention enema, instruct the patient to avoid defecation for the prescribed time or 30 minutes or longer for oil retention and 15 to 30 minutes for anthelmintic and emollient enemas. If you're using an indwelling catheter, leave the catheter in place *to promote retention.*
- Position the patient on the bedpan with the call button within reach. If they will be using the bathroom or the commode, instruct to call for help before attempting to get out of bed *because the procedure may make the patient—particularly an elderly patient—feel weak or faint.* Also instruct to call if they feel weak or in pain at any time.

- When the solution has remained in the colon for the recommended time or for as long as the patient can tolerate it, assist the patient onto a bedpan or to the commode or bathroom.
- If an indwelling catheter is in place, deflate the balloon and remove the catheter, if applicable.

Wrapping it up

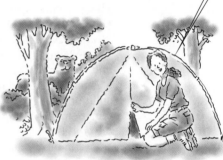

I like to have a little privacy when I'm camping in the middle of nowhere. So, imagine how much privacy your patient desires when they have an indwelling catheter!

- Provide privacy. Instruct the patient not to flush the toilet.
- Assist the patient with cleaning, if necessary, and help them into bed. Place clean linen-saver pad under them *to absorb rectal drainage.*
- Observe the contents of the toilet or bedpan. Carefully note fecal color, consistency, amount, and foreign matter, such as blood, rectal tissue, worms, pus, mucus, or other unusual matter.
- Send specimens to the laboratory, if ordered.
- Rinse and wash the bedpan or commode.
- Properly dispose of the enema equipment. Store clean, reusable equipment. Discard your gloves and gown, and wash your hands.

Practice pointers

- Schedule a retention enema before meals. A full stomach may stimulate peristalsis and make retention difficult. Follow an oil retention enema with a soap and water enema 1 hour later to help expel the softened feces completely.
- If the patient has hemorrhoids, instruct them to bear down gently during tube insertion *because bearing down causes the anus to open and facilitates insertion.*

A failed solution

- If the patient fails to expel the enema solution within 1 hour, it may need to be removed. You may need a doctor's order, so review your facility's policy and inform the doctor. To siphon the enema solution from the patient's rectum, assist the patient to a side-lying position on the bed. Place a bedpan on a bedside chair so that it rests below mattress level. Disconnect the tubing from the solution container, place the distal end in the bedpan, and reinsert the rectal end into the patient's anus. If gravity fails to drain the solution into the bedpan, instill 30 to 50 ml of warm water (105° F [40.6° C]) for an adult. Then quickly direct the distal end of the tube into the bedpan. In both cases, measure the return *to ensure all of the solution has drained.*

• If the doctor orders enemas until returns are clear, give no more than three in succession *to avoid excessive irritation of the rectal mucosa*. Notify the doctor if the returned fluid isn't clear after three administrations. (See *Documenting enema administration*.)

Colostomy and ileostomy care

A patient with a colostomy or an ileostomy must wear an external pouch to collect emerging fecal matter. The pouch also helps control odor and protect the stoma and peristomal skin. Most disposable pouching systems can be used for 2 to 7 days, although some models exceed 7 days.

Half-full

An external pouch must be emptied when it's one-third to one-half full. A patient with an ileostomy may need to empty the pouch more frequently, four or five times daily. A pouch should be changed immediately if a leak develops.

After meals

The best time to change a pouching system is when the bowel is least active, usually 2 to 4 hours after meals. After a few months, most patients can determine which time is best for them.

A protective seal

The type of pouch selected depends on the stoma's location and structure, availability of supplies, wear time, consistency of effluent, personal preference, and finances. The best adhesive seal and skin protection for the individual patient should also be considered.

What you need

Pouching system ✳ stoma measuring guide ✳ stoma paste (if drainage is watery to pasty or stoma secretes excess mucus) ✳ plastic bag ✳ water ✳ washcloth and towel ✳ closure clamp ✳ toilet or bedpan ✳ water or pouch cleaning solution ✳ gloves ✳ facial tissues ✳ optional: ostomy belt, paper tape, mild nonmoisturizing soap, skin shaving equipment, liquid skin sealant, pouch deodorant

Choices, choices, choices

Pouching systems may be drainable or closed-bottomed, disposable or reusable, adhesive-backed, and one-piece or two-piece. (See *Comparing ostomy pouching systems*, page 638.)

Take note!

Documenting enema administration

If you have administered an enema, be sure to record:
• date and time of administration
• type and amount of solution administered
• special equipment used
• retention time
• approximate amount returned
• color, consistency, and amount of the return
• abnormalities within the return
• complications.

Comparing ostomy pouching systems

Available in many shapes and sizes, ostomy pouches are fashioned for comfort, safety, and easy application. A disposable closed-end pouch may meet the needs of a patient who irrigates, wants added security, or wants to discard the pouch after each bowel movement. Another patient may prefer a reusable, drainable pouch. Some commonly available pouches are described here.

One-piece disposable pouch

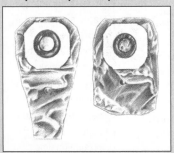

The patient who must empty the pouch often (because of diarrhea or a new colostomy or ileostomy) may prefer a one-piece, drainable, disposable pouch with a closure clamp attached to a skin barrier (see above).

This odor-proof, plastic pouch comes with an attached adhesive or karaya seal. The bottom opening allows for easy draining. This pouch may be used permanently or temporarily, until stoma size stabilizes.

A one-piece closed-end pouch (above right) is also disposable and made of odor-proof plastic. It may come in a kit with an adhesive seal, belt tabs, a skin barrier, or a carbon filter for gas release. A patient with a regular bowel elimination pattern may choose this style.

Two-piece disposable pouch

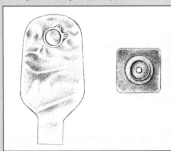

A two-piece disposable drainable pouch with a separate skin barrier (above) permits frequent changes and minimizes skin breakdown. Also made of odor-proof plastic, this style comes with belt tabs and usually snaps to the skin barrier with a flange mechanism.

Reusable pouch

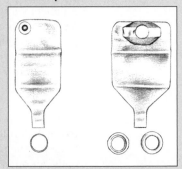

Typically made of sturdy, hypoallergenic plastic, the reusable pouch (above) comes with a separate custom-made faceplate and o-ring. Some reusable pouches have pressure valves for releasing gas. The device has a 1- to 2-month life span, depending on how frequently the patient empties the pouch.

Reusable equipment may benefit a patient who needs a firm faceplate or who wishes to minimize cost. However, many reusable ostomy pouches aren't odor-proof.

Getting ready

- Explain the procedure to the patient and family, if possible.
- Wash your hands and bring all equipment to the patient's bedside.

How you do it

- Provide privacy and emotional support.

Fitting the pouch and skin barrier

• For a pouch with an attached skin barrier, measure the stoma with the stoma measuring guide. Select the opening size that matches the stoma.

• For an adhesive-backed pouch with a separate skin barrier, measure the stoma with the measuring guide and select the opening that matches the stoma. Trace the selected size opening onto the paper back of the skin barrier's adhesive side. Cut out the opening. (If the pouch has precut openings, which can be handy for a round stoma, select an opening that's ⅛″ (0.3 cm) larger than the stoma. If the pouch comes without an opening, cut the hole ⅛″ wider than the measured tracing.) The cut-to-fit system works best for an irregularly shaped stoma.

• For a two-piece pouching system with flanges, see *Applying a skin barrier and pouch*.

Applying a skin barrier and pouch

Fitting a skin barrier and ostomy pouch properly can be done in a few steps. Shown here is a commonly used two-piece pouching system with flanges.

Measure the stoma using a measuring guide.

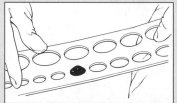

Trace the appropriate circle carefully on the back of the skin barrier.

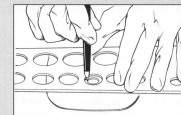

Cut the circular opening in the skin barrier. Bevel the edges to keep them from irritating the patient.

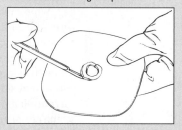

Remove the backing from the skin barrier and moisten it or apply barrier paste, as needed, along the edge of the circular opening.

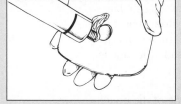

Center the skin barrier over the stoma, adhesive side down, and gently press it to the skin.

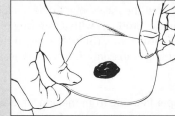

Gently press the pouch opening onto the ring until it snaps into place.

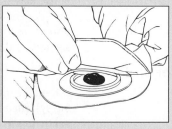

Can't feel a thing

• Avoid fitting the pouch too tightly because the stoma has no pain receptors. A constrictive opening could injure the stoma or skin tissue without the patient feeling warning discomfort. Also avoid cutting the opening too big *because this may expose the skin to fecal matter and moisture.*

• If the patient has a descending or sigmoid colostomy, has formed stools, and has an ostomy that doesn't secrete much mucus, he may choose to wear only a pouch. In this case, make sure the pouch opening closely matches the stoma size.

• Between 6 weeks and 1 year after surgery, the stoma will shrink to its permanent size. At that point, pattern-making preparations will be unnecessary unless the patient gains weight, has additional surgery, or injures the stoma.

Applying or changing the pouch

• Collect all equipment.

• Wash your hands and provide privacy.

• Explain the procedure to the patient because the patient will eventually perform the procedure themselves.

• Put on gloves.

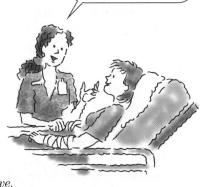

I'm going to explain each step so that you can understand the procedure and, eventually, learn to do it yourself.

Out with the old

• Remove and discard the old pouch in a plastic bag. Wipe the stoma and peristomal skin gently with a facial tissue.

• Carefully wash the peristomal skin with mild soap and water and dry it by patting gently. Allow the skin to dry thoroughly. Inspect the peristomal skin and stoma. If necessary, shave surrounding hair (in a direction away from the stoma) *to promote a better seal and avoid skin irritation from hair pulling against the adhesive.*

• If applying a separate skin barrier, peel off the paper backing of the prepared skin barrier, center the barrier over the stoma, and press gently *to ensure adhesion.*

• You may want to outline the stoma on the back of the skin barrier (depending on the product) with a thin ring of stoma paste *to provide extra skin protection.* (Skip this step if the patient has a sigmoid or descending colostomy, formed stools, and little mucus.)

Peel and press

• Remove the paper backing from the adhesive side of the pouching system and center the pouch opening over the stoma. Press gently *to secure.*

• For a pouching system with flanges, align the lip of the pouch flange with the bottom edge of the skin barrier flange. Gently press around the circumference of the pouch flange, beginning at the bottom, until the pouch securely adheres to the barrier flange. (The pouch will click into its secured position.) Holding the barrier against the skin, gently pull on the pouch *to confirm the seal between flanges.*

Warm to the task

• Encourage the patient to stay quietly in position for about 5 minutes to improve adherence. The patient's body warmth also helps to improve adherence and soften a rigid skin barrier.
• Attach an ostomy belt to further secure the pouch, if desired. (Some pouches have belt loops, and others have plastic adapters for belts.)
• Leave a bit of air in the pouch *to allow drainage to fall to the bottom.*
• Apply the closure clamp, if necessary.
• If desired, apply paper tape in a picture frame fashion to the pouch edges for additional security.

Emptying the pouch

• Put on gloves. Tilt the bottom of the pouch upward and remove the closure clamp.
• Turn up a cuff on the lower end of the pouch and allow it to drain into the toilet or bedpan.
• Wipe the bottom of the pouch and reapply the closure clamp.
• If desired, the bottom portion of the pouch can be rinsed with cool tap water. Don't aim water up near the top of the pouch *because this may loosen the seal on the skin.*
• A two-piece flanged system can also be emptied by unsnapping the pouch. Let the drainage flow into the toilet.

Gas release

• Release flatus through the gas release valve if the pouch has one. Otherwise, release flatus by tilting the pouch bottom upward, releasing the clamp, and expelling the flatus. To release flatus from a flanged system, loosen the seal between the flanges.
• Never make a pinhole in a pouch to release gas *because doing so destroys the odor-proof seal.*

Practice pointers

• After performing and explaining the procedure to the patient, encourage self-care.
• Use adhesive solvents and removers only after patch-testing the patient's skin. Some products may irritate the skin or produce

hypersensitivity reactions. Consider using a liquid skin sealant, if available, *to give skin tissue additional protection from drainage and adhesive irritants.*

• Remove the pouching system if the patient reports burning or itching beneath it or if there's purulent drainage around the stoma. Notify the doctor or therapist of skin irritation, skin breakdown, a rash, or an unusual appearance of the stoma or peristomal area.

• Use commercial pouch deodorants, if desired. Most pouches are odor-free, and odor should only be evident when emptying the pouch or if it leaks. Instruct the patient to avoid odor-causing foods such as fish, eggs, onions, and garlic.

• If the patient wears a reusable pouching system, suggest that they have two or more systems *so one can be worn while one is being cleaned.* Clean the pouching system with soap and water or a commercially prepared cleaning solution.

• Document the procedure according to facility policy. (See *Documenting colostomy and ileostomy care.*)

Colostomy irrigation

Irrigation of a colostomy serves two purposes. It allows a patient with a descending or sigmoid colostomy to regulate bowel function, and it cleans the large bowel before and after tests, surgery, or other procedures.

Colostomy irrigation may begin as soon as bowel function resumes after surgery. However, most clinicians recommend waiting until bowel movements are more predictable, which may take 4 to 6 weeks. Initially, the nurse or the patient irrigates the colostomy at the same time daily, recording the output and any spillage between irrigations.

What you need

Colostomy irrigation set (contains an irrigation drain or sleeve, an ostomy belt [if needed] to secure the drain or sleeve, water-soluble lubricant, a drainage pouch clamp, an irrigation bag with clamp, tubing, and a cone tip) ✳ 1,000 ml (1 quart) of tap water ✳ irrigant warmed to about 100° F (37.8° C) ✳ normal saline solution (for cleaning enemas) ✳ I.V. pole or wall hook ✳ washcloth and towel ✳ water ✳ ostomy pouching system ✳ linen-saver pad ✳ bedpan or chair ✳ mild nonmoisturizing soap ✳ rubber band or clip ✳ small dressing or bandage ✳ stoma cap ✳ optional: gloves

Take note!

Documenting colostomy and ileostomy care

In your notes, be sure to record:
• date and time of the pouching system change
• characteristics of drainage, including color, amount, type, and consistency
• appearance of the stoma and peristomal skin
• patient teaching
• patient's response to self-care and evaluation of his learning progress.

Getting ready

- Explain each step of the procedure to the patient *to promote self-care.*
- Provide privacy and wash your hands.
- If the patient is in bed, place a linen-saver pad under them *to protect the sheets from soiling.*
- Put on gloves.
- Remove the ostomy pouch if the patient uses one.

How you do it

- Depending on the patient's condition, colostomy irrigation may be performed in bed using a bedpan or in the bathroom using the chair and the toilet.
- Set up the irrigation bag with the tubing and cone tip. If the patient remains in bed, place the bedpan beside the bed and elevate the head of the bed between 45 and 90 degrees, if allowed. If irrigation occurs in the bathroom, have the patient sit on the toilet or on a chair facing the toilet, which-ever offers more comfort.

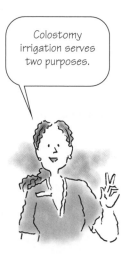

> *Colostomy irrigation serves two purposes.*

Shoulder level

- Fill the irrigation bag with warmed tap water (or normal saline solution, if the irrigation is for bowel cleaning). Hang the bag on the I.V. pole or wall hook. The bottom of the bag should be at the patient's shoulder level to prevent the fluid from entering the bowel too quickly. Most irrigation sets also have a clamp that regulates the flow rate.
- Prime the tubing with irrigant *to prevent air from entering the colon and possibly causing cramps and gas pains.*

Belt, please

- Place the irrigation sleeve over the stoma. If the sleeve doesn't have an adhesive backing, secure the sleeve with an ostomy belt. If the patient has a two-piece pouching system with flanges, snap off the pouch and save it. Snap on the irrigation sleeve.
- Place the open-ended bottom of the irrigation sleeve in the bed-pan or toilet *to promote drainage by gravity.* If necessary, cut the sleeve so that it meets the water level inside the bedpan or toilet. *Effluent may splash from a short sleeve or may not drain from a long sleeve.*
- Lubricate your gloved small finger with water-soluble lubricant and insert the finger into the stoma. If you're teaching the patient, have them do this *to determine the bowel angle at which to insert the cone safely.* Expect the stoma to tighten when the finger enters the bowel and then to relax in a few seconds.

- Lubricate the cone with water-soluble lubricant *to prevent it from irritating the mucosa.*
- Insert the cone into the top opening of the irrigation sleeve and then into the stoma. Angle the cone to match the bowel angle. Insert it gently but snugly; never force it in place.

A slow flow

- Unclamp the irrigation tubing and allow the water to flow slowly. If you don't have a clamp to control the irrigant's flow rate, pinch the tubing *to control it.* The water should enter the colon over 10 to 15 minutes. (If the patient reports cramping, slow or stop the flow, keep the cone in place, and tell the patient take a few deep breaths until the cramping stops.) *Cramping during irrigation may result from a bowel that's ready to empty, water that's too cold, a rapid flow rate, or air in the tubing.*

It's so draining

- Have the patient remain stationary for 15 or 20 minutes *so that the initial effluent can drain.*
- If the patient is ambulatory, they can stay in the bathroom until all effluent empties, or they can clamp the bottom of the drainage sleeve with a rubber band or clip and return to bed. Explain that ambulation and activity stimulate elimination. Suggest that the nonambulatory patient lean forward or massage their abdomen *to stimulate elimination.*
- Wait about 45 minutes for the bowel to finish eliminating the irrigant and effluent. Then remove the irrigation sleeve.

A clean machine

- If the irrigation was intended to clean the bowel, repeat the procedure with warmed normal saline solution until the return solution appears clear.
- Using a washcloth, mild soap, and water, gently clean the area around the stoma. Rinse and dry the area thoroughly with a clean towel.
- Inspect the skin and stoma for changes in appearance. Usually dark pink to red, stoma color may change with the patient's status. Notify the doctor of marked stoma color changes *because a pale hue may result from anemia, and substantial darkening suggests a change in blood flow to the stoma.*
- Apply a clean pouch. If the patient has a regular bowel elimination pattern, they may prefer a small dressing, bandage, or commercial stoma cap.
- Discard a disposable irrigation sleeve. Rinse a reusable irrigation sleeve and hang it to dry along with the irrigation bag, tubing, and cone.

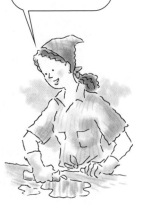

Cleaning is the name of the game in kitchens and with stomas!

Practice pointers

• Irrigating a colostomy to establish a regular bowel elimination pattern doesn't work for all patients. If the bowel continues to move between irrigations, try decreasing the volume of irrigant. Increasing the irrigant won't help because it serves only to stimulate peristalsis. Keep a record of results. Also consider irrigating every other day.

Regulation station

• Irrigation may help to regulate bowel function in a patient with a descending or sigmoid colostomy. A patient with an ascending or transverse colostomy won't benefit from irrigation, and a patient with descending or sigmoid colostomy who's missing part of the ascending or transverse colon may not be able to irrigate successfully.

Diet and exercise

• If diarrhea develops, discontinue irrigations until stools regain form. Irrigation alone won't achieve regularity. The patient must also observe a nutritionally adequate diet and exercise regimen.
• If the patient has a stricture stoma that prohibits cone insertion, remove the cone from the irrigation tubing and replace it with a soft silicone catheter. Angle the catheter gently 2″ to 4″ (5.1 to 10.2 cm) into the bowel to instill the irrigant. Don't force the catheter into the stoma, and don't insert it further than the recommended length *because it may perforate the bowel.*
• Document the procedure according to your facility policy. (See *Documenting colostomy irrigation.*)

Take note!

Documenting colostomy irrigation

• Record the date and time of irrigation and the type and amount of irrigant.
• Note the stoma's color and characteristics of drainage, including color, consistency, and amount.
• Record patient teaching.
• Describe teaching content and patient response to self-care instruction.
• Evaluate the patient's learning progress.

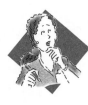

Quick quiz

1. What role does the epiglottis play in swallowing?
  A.   Opens to allow air to enter
  B.   Closes to prevent aspiration
  C.   Opens or closes depending on the food type
  D.   Rotates to aid in swallowing

Answer: B. The epiglottis, a thin flap of tissue over the larynx, closes during swallowing to prevent aspiration.

2. An adhesive-backed ostomy opening should be how much larger than the stoma?

     A.   ¼″

     B.   ½″

     C.   ⅓″

     D.   ⅛″

Answer: D. In general, the opening should be ⅛″ larger than the stoma itself. An opening that fits too tightly can injure the stoma. If the opening is too large, skin surrounding the stoma may come in contact with feces, causing skin breakdown.

3. Which GI hormone stimulates gastric secretion and motility?

     A.   Gastrin

     B.   Gastric-inhibitory peptides

     C.   Secretin

     D.   Cholecystokinin

Answer: A. Gastrin is produced in the pyloric antrum and duodenal end mucosa and stimulates gastric secretion and motility.

Scoring

☆☆☆   If you answered all three questions correctly, super! You've really digested this chapter.

  ☆☆   If you answered two questions correctly, great! Your functions (brain, that is) are all in line.

    ☆   If you answered fewer than two questions correctly, don't worry. Reread the chapter and you'll soon swallow all the facts you need!

Appendices and Index

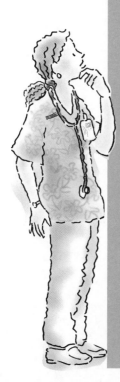

Glossary

abduct: to move away from the midline of the body; the opposite of *adduct*

activities of daily living: activities performed every day, such as bathing, eating, and toileting

adduct: to move toward the midline of the body; the opposite of *abduct*

advance directive: written legal document that identifies a patient's wishes in advance about the types of health care he desires should the patient be unable to decide for himself

aerobic: oxygen necessary for growth

affective: pertaining to emotions or feelings

agent: factor that by its presence or absence can lead to disease

agonist: drug that binds to a receptor to elicit a physiologic response

alveolus: in the lung, a small saclike dilation of the terminal bronchioles

American Nurses Association: professional organization for nurses made up of individual state nursing organizations with specialized units representing all nursing practice specialty areas

anaerobic: oxygen not required for growth

anion: ion with a negative electrical charge

anorexia: loss of appetite

antagonist: drug that binds to a receptor but doesn't produce a response or blocks the response at the receptor

antigen: foreign substance that causes antibody formation when introduced into the body

antiseptic: agent applied to living tissue to stop or slow the growth of microorganisms

apnea: cessation of breathing

asepsis: condition in which disease-producing microorganisms aren't present

assessment: first step in the nursing process; involves data collection

atrophy: wasting away

auscultation: listening to body sounds using a stethoscope

autonomy: degree of independence of action

basal metabolic rate: amount of energy used by the body at absolute rest when in an awake state

base: substance with the ability to combine with hydrogen ions; alkali

binder: large bandage used to support a body part or keep a dressing in place

blood pressure: force exerted by the blood on the walls of the vessels; expressed in millimeters of mercury (mm Hg)

body image: feelings about one's body

body mechanics: use of body positioning or movement to prevent or correct problems related to activity or immobility

bone: dense, hard, connective tissue that composes the skeleton

bone marrow: soft tissue in the cancellous bone of the epiphyses; crucial for blood cell formation and maturation

bradycardia: abnormally slow heart rate; usually fewer than 60 beats/minute

bradypnea: abnormally slow respiratory rate; usually fewer than 10 breaths/minute

bronchiole: small branch of the bronchus

buccal: pertaining to the cheek

buffer: substance that helps to control pH through neutralization

bursa: fluid-filled sac lined with synovial membrane

calorie: unit of heat

capillary: microscopic blood vessel that links arterioles with venules

carpal: pertaining to the wrist

cartilage: connective supporting tissue occurring mainly in the joints, thorax, larynx, trachea, nose, and ear

case management: means of providing care that involves coordination of patient services

cation: positively charged ion

central nervous system: one of the two main divisions of the nervous system; consists of the brain and spinal cord

cilia: small, hairlike projections on the outer surfaces of some cells

colloid: fluid containing starches or proteins

communication: exchange of information

conceptual framework: formal explanation of how concepts are linked, with an emphasis on the relationship among them

confidentiality: maintenance of patient information as private

consciousness: state involving full awareness and ability to respond to stimuli

continuity of care: provision of services uninterrupted as the patient moves within the health care system

coping mechanism: method used to manage stress

coronary: pertaining to the heart or its arteries

cortex: outer part of an internal organ; the opposite of *medulla*

costal: pertaining to the ribs

crystalloid: solution that's clear

critical thinking: process that's purposeful and disciplined and requires the use of reason and reflection to achieve insight and determine conclusions

cultural diversity: wide ranging ideas and opinions of persons for behavior that add to the fabric of society

culture: behavior and beliefs of a specific group that's passed from one generation to the next

cutaneous: pertaining to the skin

cyanosis: bluish discoloration of the skin and mucous membranes

debridement: removal of dead tissue or foreign material from a wound

dehiscence: separation of a wound's edges

deltoid: shaped like a triangle (as in the deltoid muscle)

dermis: skin layer beneath the epidermis

diaphragm: membrane that separates one part from another; the muscular partition separating the thorax and abdomen

diarrhea: frequent elimination of watery stool

diffusion: movement of particles from an area of higher concentration to one of lower concentration

discharge planning: coordination and arrangement of the patient's transition from one health care setting to another

disinfectant: solution used to kill microorganisms on inanimate objects

distal: far from the point of origin or attachment; the opposite of *proximal*

diuresis: formation and excretion of large amounts of urine

documentation: process of writing a record of patient information and care

dorsal: pertaining to the back or posterior; the opposite of *ventral* or *anterior*

duct: passage or canal

dyspnea: difficulty or labored breathing

edema: accumulation of fluid in the interstitial space

empathy: process of putting one's self into the feelings of another

endocrine: pertaining to secretion into the blood or lymph rather than into a duct; the opposite of *exocrine*

epidermis: outermost layer of the skin; lacking vessels

ethics: professional standards of behavior that indicate right and wrong

evaluation: last step of the nursing process; determines the effectiveness of nursing care

evidence-based care: approach that emphasizes decision making based on the best pertinent research-based evidence

evisceration: internal organ protrusion through an opening in a wound

exocrine: pertaining to secretion into a duct; the opposite of *endocrine*

extracellular fluid space: space outside of cells that contains fluid

febrile: state of temperature elevation

fistula: abnormal opening between organs or between an organ and body surface

flatus: gas or air in the GI tract

focused health assessment: data collection directly related to the patient's problems

fossa: hollow or cavity

functional health assessment: data collection focusing on the ability of the patient to perform activities of daily living

fundus: base of a hollow organ; the part farthest from the organ's outlet

gait: characteristics associated with a patient's walking

gastric lavage: instillation and removal of solution into the stomach

gland: organ or structure body that secretes or excretes substances

goal: intended purpose; that which is to be achieved with the delivery of care

health: optimal state of well-being

hematuria: blood in the urine

hemoglobin: protein found in red blood cells that contains iron

homeostasis: balance in the body

hormone: substance secreted by an endocrine gland that triggers or regulates the activity of an organ or cell group

host: person or thing that harbors a microorganism and allows it to grow

hypertension: elevated blood pressure

hypertonic: having a greater concentration than body fluid

hypotension: low blood pressure

hypotonic: having a lesser concentration than body fluid

hypoxemia: state in which the blood contains a lower than normal amount of oxygen

hypoxia: state in which the tissues have a decreased amount of oxygen

implementation: fourth step of the nursing process in which the care plan is carried out

infarction: death of tissue due to ischemia

infiltration: seepage or leakage of fluid into the tissues

informed consent: legal document that a patient or legal guardian signs giving permission for a procedure after the patient or guardian has demonstrated an understanding of the procedure

inferior: lower; the opposite of *superior*

inspection: assessment technique that involves systematic observation

interstitial fluid: fluid contained between the cells

intracellular fluid compartment: fluid contained within the cells

intravascular fluid: fluid contained within the blood vessels and lymphatics

ion: charged particle that forms when an electrolyte separates in solution

ipsilateral: on the same side; the opposite of *contralateral*

ischemia: insufficient blood supply to a part

isotonic: having the same concentration as body fluid

joint: fibrous, cartilaginous, or synovial connection between bones

justice: treatment of all patients fairly and equally

Korotkoff sounds: sounds heard when auscultating blood pressure denoting systolic and diastolic pressures

laceration: wound caused by tearing of the tissues

laws: standards for human conduct and enforced by the government

lacrimal: pertaining to tears

lateral: pertaining to the side; the opposite of *medial*

leukocyte: white blood cell

ligament: band of white fibrous tissue that connects bones

living will: advance directive that states the medical care that a person would want or would refuse should the person be unable to give consent or refusal

lumbar: pertaining to the area of the back between the thorax and the pelvis

lymph: watery fluid in lymphatic vessels

maceration: tissue softening resulting from excessive moisture

malpractice: professional negligence

mammary: pertaining to the breast

meatus: opening or passageway

medial: pertaining to the middle; the opposite of *lateral*

medical asepsis: clean technique involving measures to reduce and control the number of microorganisms

membrane: thin layer or sheet

muscle: fibrous structure whose contraction initiates movement

National League for Nursing: organization responsible for accrediting nursing educational programs

nerve: cordlike structure consisting of fibers that convey impulses from the central nervous system to the body

networking: process of interacting with colleagues who share common interests

neutropenia: decreased number of neutrophils

neutrophil: white blood cell that removes and destroys bacteria, cellular debris, and solid particles

noncompliance: inability to adhere to a prescribed regimen

normal flora: organisms that inhabit the body but usually cause no harm

nurse practice acts: state-established guidelines that govern the practice of nursing

nursing diagnosis: statement of potential or actual health problems for which the nurse can intervene

nursing process: systematic method for delivering nursing care

objective data: information that's observable and measurable and that can be verified and validated

oliguria: urine output of less than 500 ml in 24 hours

ophthalmic: pertaining to the eye

osmosis: movement of water through a semipermeable membrane from an area of higher water concentration (lower solute concentration) to a lower one (higher solute concentration)

outcome: end product of nursing care, that which is hoped to be achieved

palpation: use of touch to determine size, shape, and consistency of underlying structures

parenteral nutrition: administration of nutrients by I.V. route

pathogen: organism capable of causing disease

percussion: use of tapping on a body surface with fingers to determine density of underlying structure or area

peristalsis: wavelike movement to progress contents through the intestines

phrenic: pertaining to the diaphragm

plantar: pertaining to the sole of the foot

plasma: colorless, watery fluid portion of lymph and blood

platelet: small, disk-shaped blood cell necessary for coagulation

pleura: thin serous membrane that encloses the lung

plexus: network of nerves, lymphatic vessels, or veins

popliteal: pertaining to the back of the knee

posterior: back or dorsal; the opposite of *anterior* or *ventral*

primary source: patient

pronate: to turn the palm downward; the opposite of *supinate*

proximal: situated nearest the center of the body; the opposite of *distal*

pruritus: itching

pulse deficit: difference between the apical and radial pulse rates

pulse pressure: difference between the systolic blood pressure and diastolic blood pressure readings

purulent: pus producing or pus containing

range of motion: extent to which a person can move his joints or muscles

reflex: involuntary action

renal: pertaining to the kidney

respiration: exchange of carbon dioxide and oxygen in tissue and the lungs

restraint: device used to prevent a patient from moving or gaining access

role: expected function and behavior of a person

sanguineous: referring to or containing blood

secondary source: anyone other than the patient who supplies information

self-concept: mental image that a person has of one's self

serosanguineous: containing blood and serum

serous: serumlike, watery, and thin

spasticity: sudden, involuntary increase in muscle tone or contractions

standard precautions: set of guidelines developed by the Centers for Disease Control and Prevention to protect against infection transmission

sternum: long, flat bone that forms the middle portion of the thorax

striated: marked with parallel lines such as striated (skeletal) muscle

subcutaneous: related to the tissue layer under the dermis

sublingual: under the tongue

superior: higher; the opposite of *inferior*

supinate: to turn the palm of the hand upward; the opposite of *pronate*

surgical asepsis: sterile technique involving measures to keep an object free from all microorganisms

symphysis: growing together; a type of cartilaginous joint in which fibrocartilage firmly connects opposing surfaces

synapse: point of contact between adjacent neurons

tachycardia: rapid heart rate; usually greater than 100 beats/minute

tachypnea: rapid respiratory rate; usually greater than 20 breaths/minute

temporal artery thermometer: measures the core arterial temperature 0.4 degrees higher than an oral temperature

tendon: band of fibrous connective tissue that attaches a muscle to a bone

therapeutic communication: use of special techniques to interact, enabling a person to express feelings and work out problems

thrombus: blood clot

total parenteral nutrition: administration of highly concentrated nutrient solutions via a central intravenous site

transfusion: administration of whole blood or blood products directly into a person's circulation

urinal: metal or plastic device used by male patients for urinary elimination

valve: structure that permits fluid to flow in only one direction

venipuncture: insertion of a needle or catheter into a vein

ventilation: movement of air in and out of the lungs

ventral: pertaining to the front or anterior; the opposite of *dorsal* or *posterior*

ventricle: small cavity, such as one of several in the brain or one of the two lower chambers of the heart

viscera: internal organs

Z-track: technique of I.M. medication administration that prevents medication from seeping into the tissue

Index

Note: i refers to an illustration; t refers to a table.

Note: i refers to an illustration; t refers to a table.

Note: i refers to an illustration; t refers to a table.

Note: i refers to an illustration; t refers to a table.

Note: i refers to an illustration; t refers to a table.

Note: i refers to an illustration; t refers to a table.

Note: i refers to an illustration; t refers to a table.

Note: i refers to an illustration; t refers to a table.

Note: i refers to an illustration; t refers to a table.

Note: i refers to an illustration; t refers to a table.

Note: i refers to an illustration; t refers to a table.